I0044562

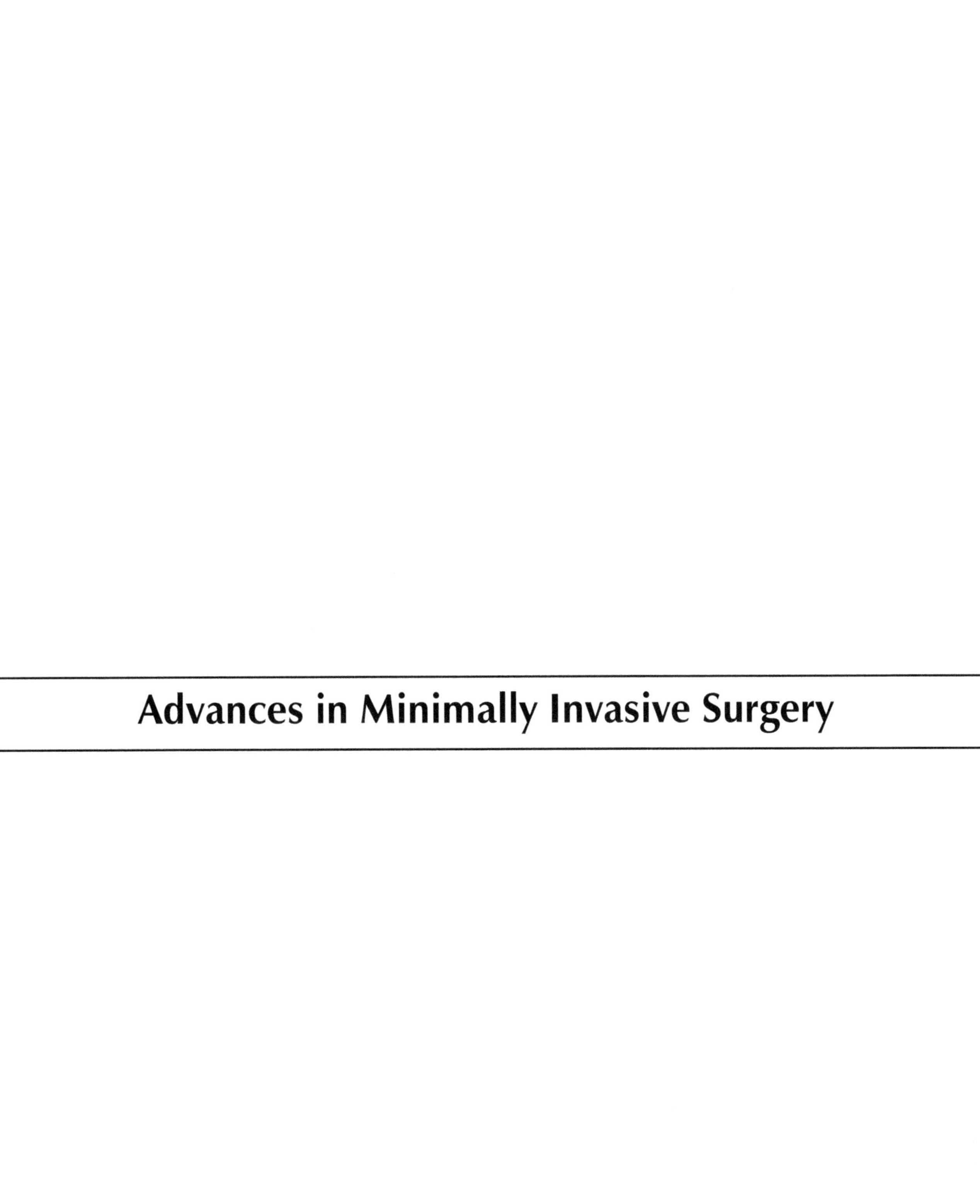

Advances in Minimally Invasive Surgery

Advances in Minimally Invasive Surgery

Editor: Philip Rudolf

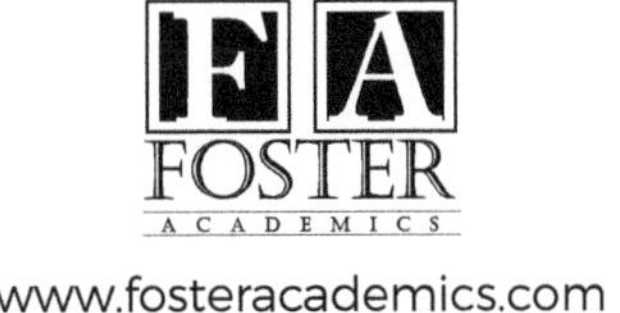

www.fosteracademics.com

www.fosteracademics.com

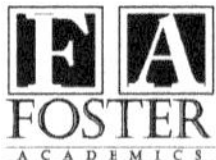

Cataloging-in-Publication Data

Advances in minimally invasive surgery / edited by Philip Rudolf.
p. cm.
Includes bibliographical references and index.
ISBN 978-1-63242-809-7
1. Endoscopic surgery. 2. Laparoscopic surgery. 3. Surgery, Operative.
4. Endoscopy. 5. Laparoscopy. 6. Microsurgery. I. Rudolf, Philip.
RD33.53 .A37 2019
617.05--dc23

Foster Academics,
118-35 Queens Blvd., Suite 400,
Forest Hills, NY 11375, USA

ISBN 978-1-63242-809-7 (Hardback)

Contents

Preface

Minimally invasive surgery is a surgical technique, characterized by smaller incisions, quicker healing, lower pain and reduced risk of infection. Such procedures have been made possible due to advancement in medical technologies. These procedures are guided by laparoscopic or arthroscopic devices, large scale display panel and remote-control manipulation of instruments. Refractive eye surgery, cryosurgery, keyhole surgery, stereotactic surgery, the Nuss procedure, etc. are some examples of minimally invasive surgical procedures. Laparoscopic surgery is performed within the abdominal or pelvic cavities, and thoracoscopic surgery is done on the chest or thoracic cavity. Minimally invasive spine surgeries such as laminotomy, artificial disc replacement, anterior cervical discectomy, laminectomy, etc. are performed to treat degenerative disc disease, disc fractures, herniation, tumors, infections, etc. This book is compiled in such a manner, that it will provide in-depth knowledge about the theories and practices of minimally invasive surgeries. It aims to present researches that have transformed this discipline and aided its advancement. Coherent flow of topics, student-friendly language and extensive use of examples make this book an invaluable source of knowledge.

The researches compiled throughout the book are authentic and of high quality, combining several disciplines and from very diverse regions from around the world. Drawing on the contributions of many researchers from diverse countries, the book's objective is to provide the readers with the latest achievements in the area of research. This book will surely be a source of knowledge to all interested and researching the field.

In the end, I would like to express my deep sense of gratitude to all the authors for meeting the set deadlines in completing and submitting their research chapters. I would also like to thank the publisher for the support offered to us throughout the course of the book. Finally, I extend my sincere thanks to my family for being a constant source of inspiration and encouragement.

Editor

1

Hybrid Coronary Revascularization as a Safe, Feasible, and Viable Alternative to Conventional Coronary Artery Bypass Grafting: What Is the Current Evidence?

Arjan J. F. P. Verhaegh, Ryan E. Accord, Leen van Garsse, and Jos G. Maessen

Department of Cardiothoracic Surgery, Maastricht University Medical Center, P. Debyelaan 25, P.O. Box 5800, 6202 AZ Maastricht, The Netherlands

Correspondence should be addressed to Ryan E. Accord; ryan.accord@gmail.com

Academic Editor: Casey M. Calkins

The "hybrid" approach to multivessel coronary artery disease combines surgical left internal thoracic artery (LITA) to left anterior descending coronary artery (LAD) bypass grafting and percutaneous coronary intervention of the remaining lesions. Ideally, the LITA to LAD bypass graft is performed in a minimally invasive fashion. This review aims to clarify the place of hybrid coronary revascularization (HCR) in the current therapeutic armamentarium against multivessel coronary artery disease. Eighteen studies including 970 patients were included for analysis. The postoperative LITA patency varied between 93.0% and 100.0%. The mean overall survival rate in hybrid treated patients was 98.1%. Hybrid treated patients showed statistically significant shorter hospital length of stay (LOS), intensive care unit (ICU) LOS, and intubation time, less packed red blood cell (PRBC) transfusion requirements, and lower in-hospital major adverse cardiac and cerebrovascular event (MACCE) rates compared with patients treated by on-pump and off-pump coronary artery bypass grafting (CABG). This resulted in a significant reduction in costs for hybrid treated patients in the postoperative period. In studies completed to date, HCR appears to be a promising and cost-effective alternative for CABG in the treatment of multivessel coronary artery disease in a selected patient population.

1. Introduction

Coronary artery bypass grafting (CABG) is considered to be the "gold standard" in patients with multivessel disease and remains the treatment of choice for patients with severe coronary artery disease, including three-vessel or left main coronary artery disease [1]. The use of CABG, as compared with both percutaneous coronary intervention (PCI) and medical therapy, is superior with regard to long-term symptom relief, major adverse cardiac or cerebrovascular events and survival benefit [1–4]. However, because of the use of cardiopulmonary bypass and median sternotomy, CABG is associated with significant surgical trauma leading to a long rehabilitation period and delayed postoperative improvement of quality of life [5]. An alternative "hybrid" approach to multivessel coronary artery disease combines surgical left internal thoracic artery (LITA) to left anterior descending coronary artery (LAD) bypass grafting and percutaneous coronary intervention of the remaining lesions [3, 6–8]. Ideally, the LITA to LAD bypass graft is performed in a minimally invasive fashion through minimally invasive direct coronary artery bypass grafting (MIDCAB) [9]. This hybrid approach takes advantage of the survival benefit of the LITA to LAD bypass, while minimizing invasiveness and lowering morbidity by avoiding median sternotomy, rib retraction, aortic manipulation, and cardiopulmonary bypass [3, 8, 10–14]. The purpose of the hybrid approach is to achieve complete coronary revascularization with outcomes equivalent to conventional coronary artery bypass grafting, while ensuring faster patient recovery, shorter hospital stays, and earlier return to work due to lower morbidity and mortality rates.

Angelini and colleagues reported the first hybrid coronary revascularization (HCR) procedure in 1996, and several patient series using hybrid coronary revascularization have been published since then [3]. These series support the above-mentioned presumptions and indicate that the hybrid

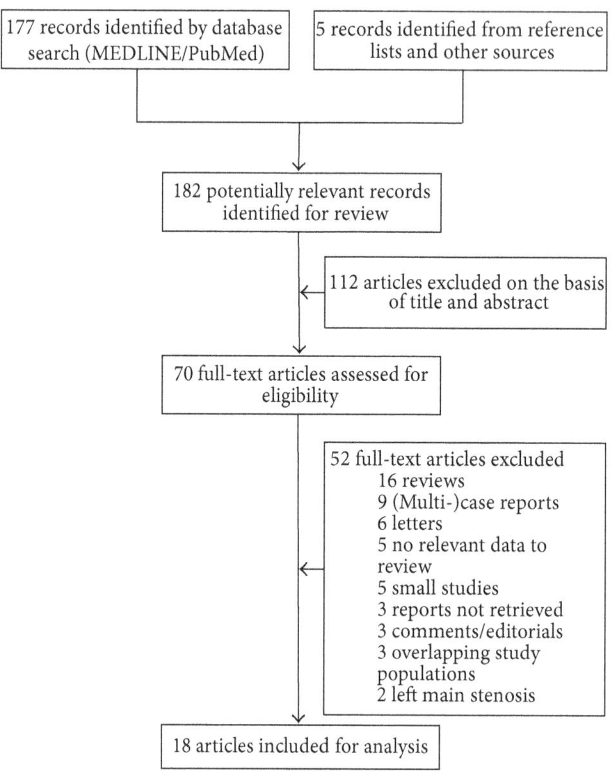

FIGURE 1: Study selection.

approach is a feasible option for the treatment of selected patients with multivessel coronary artery disease involving the left main. Moreover, the introduction of drug-eluting stents (DESs) with lower rates of restenosis and better clinical outcomes may make hybrid coronary revascularization a more sustainable and feasible option than previously reported [9, 15].

Nevertheless, this hybrid approach has not been widely adopted because practical and logistical concerns have been expressed. These concerns implicate the need for close cooperation between surgeon and interventional cardiologist, logistical issues regarding sequencing and timing of the procedures, and the use of aggressive anticoagulant therapy for percutaneous coronary intervention that may worsen bleeding in the surgical patient [7, 14, 16].

This review aims to clarify the place of hybrid coronary revascularization in the current therapeutic armamentarium against multivessel coronary artery disease. First, the patient selection for the HCR procedure is clarified. Second, the results of previous patient series using the hybrid approach are summarized and interpreted. Finally, the cost effectiveness of the HCR procedure is analysed.

2. Materials and Methods

2.1. Search Strategy. The MEDLINE/PubMed database was searched in January 2012 using the medical subject headings (MESH) for "coronary artery disease" and "angioplasty, balloon, coronary" combined with the following free-text keywords: "multivessel coronary artery disease," "minimally invasive coronary artery bypass," "percutaneous coronary intervention," and "hybrid coronary revascularization". One hundred seventy-seven articles matching these search criteria were found, and the search for additional papers was continued by analysing the reference lists of relevant articles.

2.2. Selection Criteria. Randomized controlled trials, nonrandomized prospective and retrospective (comparative) studies were selected for inclusion. Publications in languages other than English were excluded beforehand. Letters, editorials, (multi)case reports, reviews, and small studies ($n < 15$) were also excluded. Studies examining the HCR procedure for multivessel coronary disease were included, while studies investigating the HCR procedure for left main coronary stenosis were excluded. Authors and medical centres with two or more published studies were carefully evaluated and were represented by their most recent publication to avoid multiple reporting of the same patients. A total of eighteen included studies remained eligible for analysis after applying these in- and exclusion criteria (Figure 1).

2.3. Review Strategy. The primary outcome measures were in-hospital major adverse cardiac and cerebrovascular events (MACCEs), packed red blood cells (PRBCs) transfusion rate, LITA patency, hospital length of stay (LOS), 30-day mortality, survival, and target vessel revascularization (TVR). Secondary outcome measures were intensive care unit (ICU) LOS and intubation time, as only a limited number of studies reported these outcome measures. In addition, the period

Table 1: Overview of 18 series describing hybrid coronary revascularization.

Author	Date	N	Age (years)	Followup (months)	Strategy	Surgical procedure	PCI
Zenati et al. [17]	1999	31	69 (46–86)	10.8 ± 3.8	Staged	Open MIDCAB	PTCA/BMS
Lloyd et al. [18]	1999	18	63.2 (35–87)	6 (5–8)	Simultaneous (4) and staged (14)	Open MIDCAB	PTCA/BMS
Wittwer et al. [19]	2000	35	56.7 ± 17	11.4 ± 7.7	Staged	Open MIDCAB	PTCA/BMS
de Cannière et al. [12]	2001	20	62 ± 9	24.0	Staged	Open MIDCAB	PTCA/BMS
Riess et al. [20]	2002	57	65.7 ± 7.9	23.2 ± 8.7	Staged	Inversed L-shaped ministernotomy	PTCA/BMS
Stahl et al. [21]	2002	54	62.4 (36–86)	11.6 (1–23)	Staged	Robotic endo-ACAB	PTCA/BMS
Cisowski et al. [22]	2002	50	54.8 ± 20.1	3–32	Staged	Thoracoscopic endo-ACAB	PTCA/BMS
Davidavicius et al. [11]	2005	20	65 ± 9	19 ± 10	Staged	Robotic endo-ACAB	BMS/DES
Katz et al. [13]	2006	27	59.8 ± 8.9	3.0	Simultaneous (4) and staged (23)	Arrested-heart TECAB	BMS/DES
Us et al. [23]	2006	17	63.1 ± 20.9	21.3 ± 6.5	Staged	Reversed J-shaped inferior ministernotomy	PTCA/BMS
Gilard et al. [6]	2007	70	68.5 ± 10	33 (2–70)	Staged	On-pump (64) or off-pump (6) CABG	Stent to RCA
Kon et al. [7]	2008	15	61 ± 10	12.0	Simultaneous	Open MIDCAB	DES
Kiaii et al. [14]	2008	58	59.9 ± 11.7	20.2 (1.1–40.8)	Simultaneous	Robotic endo-ACAB	BMS/DES
Holzhey et al. [24]	2008	117	64.6 ± 12.0	21.3	Simultaneous (5) and staged (112)	Open MIDCAB (107); beating-heart TECAB (8); arrested-heart TECAB (8)	DES/BMS
Zhao et al. [25]	2009	112	63 (32–85) (median)	NR	Simultaneous	On-pump (90) or off-pump (22) CABG	DES/BMS
Delhaye et al. [26]	2010	18	62 (55–77) (median)	12.0	Staged	On-pump (13) or off-pump (5) CABG	DES
Halkos et al. [27]	2011	147	64.3 ± 12.8	38.4 (median)	Mainly staged	Thoracoscopic endo-ACAB and robotic endo-ACAB	DES
Hu et al. [28]	2011	104	61.8 ± 10.2	18 ± 7.9	Simultaneous	Reversed J-shaped inferior ministernotomy	PTCA/BMS/DES

Unless otherwise indicated, data are expressed as mean ± standard deviation. N: number; PCI: percutaneous coronary intervention; MIDCAB: minimally invasive direct coronary artery bypass; PTCA: percutaneous transluminal coronary angioplasty; BMS: bare metal stent; endo-ACAB: endoscopic atraumatic coronary artery bypass; DES: drug-eluting stent; TECAB: totally endoscopic coronary artery bypass; NR: not reported; CABG: coronary artery bypass grafting; RCA: right coronary artery.

of time between PCI and LITA to LAD bypass grafting and the cost effectiveness of HCR were examined. The long-term LITA patency was not included as an outcome measure, since only a limited number of studies report this outcome measure in a clear and concise manner.

In-hospital major adverse cardiac and cerebrovascular events were defined as postoperative stroke, myocardial infarction (MI), or death during hospital stay. Only the Fitzgibbon patency class A (widely patent) was considered as a patent LITA to LAD bypass graft, while the Fitzgibbon patency class B (flow limiting) and C (occluded) were defined as a nonpatent LITA to LAD bypass graft. Hospital LOS was defined as the number of days spent in hospital from operation to discharge. If the need for repeated revascularization involved a coronary artery initially treated with either bypass grafting or PCI, this repeated revascularization was considered to be target vessel revascularization.

One observer extracted all available outcome measures of each article and a second observer checked and supervised the first observer thoroughly. When an article did not disclose one or more of these outcome measures or reported medians and ranges as central tendency instead of means and standard deviations, the study was excluded from the analysis of that particular variable.

2.4. Statistical Analysis. The results were analysed using IBM SPSS Statistics 19 software (IBM Inc., Armonk, NY, USA). Continuous data were presented as mean and standard deviation (SD), while categorical data were expressed as numbers and percentages.

3. Outline and Interpretation of the Results of HCR

Nine hundred seventy patients undergoing HCR procedures were included for analysis (Tables 1 and 2) [6, 7, 11–14, 17–28]. The most important findings are reported below.

TABLE 2: Outcomes of 18 series describing hybrid coronary revascularization.

Author	MACCE (%)	PRBC (%)	LITA patency (%)	Hospital LOS (days)	TVR (%)	30-day mortality (%)	Survival (%)
Zenati et al. [17]	0 (0.0)	2 (6.5)	100.0	2.7 ± 1.0	9.6	0.0	100.0
Lloyd et al. [18]	0 (0.0)	1 (5.6)	100.0	5 ± 1.5	0.0	0.0	100.0
Wittwer et al. [19]	0 (0.0)	1 (2.9)	100.0	7.5 ± 4	NR	0.0	100.0
de Cannière et al. [12]	0 (0.0)	0 (0.0)	100.0	6.7 ± 0.7	15.0	0.0	100.0
Riess et al. [20]	0 (0.0)	2 (3.5)	97.2	5.7 ± 1.8	15.8	0.0	98.2
Stahl et al. [21]	0 (0.0)	16 (29.6)	100.0	3.54 (2–12)	1.9	0.0	100.0
Cisowski et al. [22]	0 (0.0)	2 (4.0)	98.0	4.4 ± 1.7	12.7	0.0	100.0
Davidavicius et al. [11]	0 (0.0)	5 (25.0)	100.0	8.1 ± 1.6	0.0	0.0	100.0
Katz et al. [13]	1 (3.7)	NR	NR	NR	29.6	0.0	100.0
Us et al. [23]	0 (0.0)	1 (5.9)	NR	5.3 ± 1.4	17.6	0.0	100.0
Gilard et al. [6]	1 (1.4)	12 (17.1)	NR	NR	4.3	1.4	98.6
Kon et al. [7]	0 (0.0)	NR	100.0	3.7 ± 1.4	6.7	0.0	100.0
Kiaii et al. [14]	2 (3.4)	9 (15.5)	93.0	4.3 ± 1.42	5.2	0.0	100.0
Holzhey et al. [24]	3 (2.6)	NR	NR	NR	4.3	1.7	84.8 at 5 years
Zhao et al. [25]	5 (4.5)	NR	NR	6 (1–97) (median)	NR	2.6	NR
Delhaye et al. [26]	1 (5.6)	2 (11.1)	NR	10.0 (10.0–11.2) (median)	5.6	0.0	100.0
Halkos et al. [27]	3 (2.0)	52 (35.4)	NR	6.6 ± 6.7	8.8	0.7	86.8 at 5 years
Hu et al. [28]	0 (0.0)	30 (28.8)	NR	8.2 ± 2.6	1.0	0.0	100.0

Unless otherwise indicated, data are expressed as mean ± standard deviation or number (%). MACCE: major adverse cardiac and cerebrovascular events; PRBC: packed red blood cells; LITA: left internal thoracic artery; LOS: length of stay; TVR: target vessel revascularization; NR: not reported.

3.1. Patient Selection. The classical indication for an HCR procedure is multivessel coronary artery disease involving LAD lesion judged suitable for minimally invasive LITA to LAD bypass grafting but unsuitable for PCI (type C), and (a) non-LAD lesion(s) (most of the time right coronary artery (RCA) and/or circumflex coronary artery (Cx) lesions) amenable to PCI (type A or B) [7, 11, 12, 14, 17, 18, 20, 22, 23, 26–28]. High-risk patients especially with severe concomitant diseases (e.g., diabetes mellitus, malignancies, significant carotid disease, severely impaired LV function, and neurological diseases), who are more prone to develop complications after cardiopulmonary bypass and sternotomy, might benefit from the circumvention of CPB and sternotomy [11, 18, 20, 22–24].

Exclusion criteria for HCR consist of contraindications to minimally invasive LITA to LAD bypass grafting or PCI. LITA to LAD bypass grafting in a minimally invasive fashion requires single-lung ventilation and chest cavity insufflation. Therefore, HCR procedures are contraindicated in patients with a compromised pulmonary function (i.e., forced expiratory volume in one second less than 50% of predicted) and a small intrathoracic cavity space [14, 27, 28]. Moreover, patients with a nongraftable or a buried intramyocardial LAD, history of left subclavian artery and/or LITA stenosis, morbid obesity (BMI > 40 kg/m^2), and previous left chest surgery are not well suited for minimally invasive LITA tot LAD bypass grafting [14, 20, 22, 27, 28]. Conditions rendering PCI unsuitable include peripheral vascular disease precluding vascular access, coronary vessel diameter smaller than 1.5 mm, tortuous calcified coronary vessels, fresh thrombotic lesions, chronic totally occluded coronary arteries, extensive coronary involvement, chronic renal insufficiency (serum creatinine ≥ 200 μmol/L), and allergy to radiographic contrast [7, 14, 18, 20, 22, 27, 28]. Finally, haemodynamic instability, need for a concomitant operation (e.g., valve repair or replacement), and decompensated congestive heart failure are regarded as exclusion criteria [7, 17, 20, 22, 27, 28].

3.2. Timing of the HCR Procedure. The best timing of the interventions remains a matter of debate. Three HCR strategies can be distinguished: (I) performing PCI first, followed by LITA to LAD bypass grafting or (II) vice versa; (III) combining LITA to LAD bypass grafting and PCI in the same setting in a hybrid operative suite. In the included studies, staged HCR procedures (I and II) were applied much more frequently than simultaneous procedures (III).

In a "staged" procedure, in which PCI and LITA to LAD bypass grafting are carried out at separate locations and/or different days, both interventions can be performed under ideal circumstances (in a modern catheterization laboratory and modern operating room, resp.) [11, 18, 29]. However, patients have to undergo 2 procedures, while they remain incompletely revascularized and at risk for cardiovascular events for an extended period of time [14, 29].

When PCI is performed first, a staged procedure takes place with an unprotected anterior wall, which could pose serious health risks in case the LAD lesion is considered the culprit lesion [13]. In addition, LITA to LAD bypass grafting is performed after aggressive platelet inhibition for prevention of acute (stent) thrombosis, which might lead to unnecessary postponement of following operation or may cause a higher than expected rate of bleeding [12, 13, 21, 29]. Moreover, stent thrombosis is risked after reversal of surgical anticoagulation and is related to the inflammatory reaction after cardiac surgery [13]. Furthermore, the opportunity for quality control of the LITA to LAD bypass graft and anastomosis by a coronary angiogram is lost and, therefore, this strategy requires a reangiography [12, 13]. These repeat control angiograms increase overall healthcare costs unnecessarily and decrease cost effectiveness [12].

Nevertheless, the potential advantages of this strategy are threefold. First, revascularization of non-LAD vessels provides an optimized overall coronary flow reserve, thereby minimizing the potential risk of ischemia and myocardial infarction during the LAD occlusion for LITA to LAD bypass grafting [6, 12]. Second, it is possible for the interventional cardiologist to fall back on conventional CABG in case of a suboptimal PCI result or major PCI complications. However, failure of PCI leading to emergency conventional CABG has become extremely rare with decreasing incidence since the introduction of coronary artery stenting [12, 20, 29–32]. Furthermore, this strategy allows HCR in patients with the immediate need for PCI in a non-LAD target and no immediate possibility for emergency bypass surgery [11, 24]. Critical stenosis in the right coronary artery (RCA) or the left circumflex coronary artery (LCx) or difficult PCI targets are considered as clear indications for a "PCI first" approach because these patients can undergo conventional CABG in case of PCI failure [11].

When the LITA to LAD bypass graft is performed first, antiplatelet therapy is routinely started after surgery to prevent antiplatelet-related bleeding complications during surgery and is present at time of PCI [6, 13, 27]. These antiplatelet agents can be administered long term, which is mandatory for preventing stent thrombosis. Moreover, the quality control of the LITA to LAD bypass graft and anastomosis can be performed simultaneously without a further angiogram [6, 12, 13, 18, 20, 23, 25, 26, 29]. In addition, PCI is performed in a "protective" environment with a revascularized anteroseptal wall, which probably reduces the procedural risks and gives the interventional cardiologist the ability to approach lesions that would be quite challenging without a revascularized LAD [13, 20, 25, 26, 29]. However, patients undergoing this strategy could require a second, much higher-risk, surgical intervention due to complications of the PCI [13, 23, 25]. Finally, the cardiac surgeon has to be aware of possible intraoperative ischemia during this HCR strategy because the collateral, non-LAD vessels are unprotected.

Nevertheless, combining the two procedures in one stage under general anaesthesia in a specific hybrid-operating room, which combines the potential of catheterization and cardiac surgery, has advantages compared with staged HCR procedures [7, 14, 25, 28]. This simultaneous approach represents a single procedure that achieves complete revascularization, while minimizing patient discomfort and reducing the need for anaesthetics [12, 14, 18, 20, 28]. This approach eliminates logistic concerns about timing and sequence of two separate procedures and maximizes patient satisfaction [7, 14, 25, 28]. Moreover, the quality of the LITA to LAD bypass graft and anastomosis can be confirmed immediately by an intraoperative angiogram, which enables direct revision of the LITA to LAD bypass graft [18, 25]. Complications and difficulties during PCI or MIDCAB can be dealt with immediately in the same setting by conversion to conventional, open-chest CABG [25].

This procedure also has its own drawbacks. Perioperative haemorrhage can become a problem because full antiplatelet therapy and incomplete heparin reversal are necessary instantly after MIDCAB to prevent a transient "rebound" increase in thrombin formation associated with stent thrombosis and ensure an optimal intraoperative DES placement [7, 14, 18]. Besides, off-pump surgery may give rise to hypercoagulability and increased platelet activation during the early postoperative period, which is associated with an increased risk of stent thrombosis [33]. This makes antiplatelet management an important safety issue in HCR. Therefore, a modified antiplatelet protocol and careful patient selection seem appropriate, especially in one-stop HCR, in order to minimize the risk of stent thrombosis without increasing perioperative bleeding risk. A tried and tested protocol of dual antiplatelet therapy (DAPT) includes continuous use of aspirin (100 mg/day) until the operation day and intraoperative administration of a loading dose clopidogrel (300 mg) via a nasogastric tube after confirming LITA graft patency, followed by a maintenance dose of 75 mg/day for 12 months [34]. However, caution is required when using DAPT, since reversal agents for clopidogrel and aspirin are not available. Moreover, newer more potent antiplatelet agents, like prasugrel and ticagrelor, should be reserved exclusively for selected cases (high risk of stent thrombosis) and managed with even more care, since the clinical experience with these newer antiplatelet agents is limited in cardiac surgery and the bleeding risk may be increased. Furthermore, intraoperative collaboration and communication among cardiac surgeons, interventional cardiologists, and anaesthesiologists should be outstanding and ongoing to optimize continuity of care [11, 14]. Currently, this simultaneous procedure is used in only a few centres, and some authors state that this might be caused by the need to possess catheterization laboratories outfitted to accommodate cardiac surgery or hybrid operating rooms equipped with a mobile coronary angiography C-arm or permanent fluoroscopic equipment [7, 13].

The latter is reflected in the small number of patients undergoing a simultaneous procedure in our sample of included studies [7, 13, 14, 18, 24, 25, 28]. Expansion of other percutaneous and hybrid procedures like "hybrid AF ablation" may help to make these hybrid, multipurpose operating rooms more common in the future. However, staged HCR procedures could offer a more realistic alternative for many institutions without a so-called hybrid operating room, and this is supported by the fact that staged HCR procedures are applied much more frequently than simultaneous procedures in the included studies [6, 11–13, 17–24, 26, 27].

Tables 3 and 4 present the period of time between both procedures in a staged HCR strategy, and this period of time varied notably from 0 to 180 days. Therefore, some patients remained incompletely revascularized and were in theory at risk for cardiovascular events for a considerable length of time, while complete myocardial revascularization should be the main goal of treatment in patients with multivessel coronary artery disease. Moreover, Delhaye et al. found that PCI with clopidogrel preloading can be performed within

Table 3: Two-stage HCR procedure, LITA to LAD bypass grafting followed by PCI ($n = 322$).

Author	Number	Delay (mean ± SD or median)	Range
Zenati et al. [17]	29	NR	From 0–4 days
Lloyd et al. [18]	14	NR	From 1–3 days
Wittwer et al. [19]	35	7 days (median)	From 1–54 days
de Cannière et al. [12]	11	NR	From 2-3 days
Riess et al. [20]	53	4.7 ± 0.8 days (mean ± SD)	From 2–7 days
Stahl et al. [21]	35	16 days (mean)	From 18 hours to 3 months
Cisowski et al. [22]	50	6.5 ± 4.6 days (mean ± SD)	NR
Davidavicius et al. [11]	6	NR	From 2–180 days
Katz et al. [13]	12	16 days (mean)	From 2–60 days
Holzhey et al. [24]	59	NR	From 2–45 days
Delhaye et al. [26]	18	41 hours (median)	From 37–44 hours

SD: standard deviation; NR: not reported.

Table 4: Two-stage HCR procedure, PCI followed by LITA to LAD bypass grafting ($n = 200$).

Author	Number	Delay (mean ± SD)	Range
Zenati et al. [17]	2	NR	From 1-2 days
de Cannière et al. [12]	9	NR	From 1-2 days
Riess et al. [20]	4	22 days (mean)	From 1–63 days
Stahl et al. [21]	19	15 days (mean)	NR
Davidavicius et al. [11]	14	NR	From 2–83 days
Katz et al. [13]	12	38 days (mean)	From 2–137 days
Us et al. [23]	17	NR	Within 3 hours
Gilard et al. [6]	70	16 ± 2 hours (mean)	NR
Holzhey et al. [24]	53	NR	From 4–6 weeks

SD: standard deviation; NR: not reported.

48 hours of LITA to LAD bypass grafting without increasing the bleeding risk [26]. In addition, Zenati et al. performed PCI zero to four days after LITA to LAD bypass grafting without increasing the PRBC transfusion requirements, while lowering the hospital length of stay (2.7 ± 1.0 days) [17]. The mean hospital length of stay was 5.5 ± 1.8 days (range: from 2.7 to 8.2 days), and hospital length of stay seems not to be influenced by the HCR strategy used (Table 2).

3.3. Surgical Techniques in Relation to Outcome Measures. As shown in Table 1, the surgical techniques for LITA to LAD bypass grafting have evolved continuously since the introduction of the HCR procedure in 1996 by Angelini et al. Most of the initial patient series performed the LITA to LAD bypass graft in a minimally invasive fashion carrying out a mini-thoracotomy on the anterolateral chest wall in imitation of Angelini et al. [3, 7, 12, 17–19]. In this so-called minimally invasive direct coronary artery bypass (MIDCAB) approach, the LITA is harvested under direct vision using specially designed LITA retractors. The anastomosis to the LAD is performed with 8-0 or 4-0 Prolene sutures on the beating heart (without CPB) with the help of mechanical stabilizers. In more recent patient series, the LITA was identified and harvested thoracoscopically or robotically, which decreased rib retraction, chest wall deformity, and trauma [11, 14, 21, 22, 27]. This approach significantly minimizes the typical thoracotomy-type incisional pain and wound complications of conventional MIDCAB, while optimizing graft length and retaining the reliability of manually sewn LITA to LAD anastomosis [21, 22]. Some teams prefer to place the LITA bypass graft to the LAD through a ministernotomy (inversed L-shaped or reversed J-shaped), which makes it possible to switch to full sternotomy in case complications may occur during the original operation [20, 23, 28]. Nevertheless, this surgical technique increases surgical trauma and, therefore, may raise morbidity and mortality. In addition, some centres even decided to perform the LITA to LAD bypass graft through a full sternotomy on the beating heart (off-pump CABG), thereby further increasing invasiveness [6, 25, 26]. If the LITA bypass graft is placed on the LAD through a sternotomy on the arrested heart (on-pump CABG), circumvention of CPB is lost too [6, 25, 26]. Thus, both on-pump and off-pump CABG can be seen as suboptimal procedures to carry out the LITA to LAD bypass graft. This might explain the higher MACCE rates found by Zhao et al. and Delhaye et al. and the high 30-day mortality discovered by Zhao et al. and Gilard et al., who decided to place the LITA to LAD bypass graft on the arrested heart through full sternotomy in the majority of the patients [6, 25, 26]. Lastly, some authors prefer to perform the LITA to LAD bypass graft in a totally endoscopic, port-only fashion using totally endoscopic coronary artery bypass grafting (TECAB) [13, 24]. This most challenging form of LITA to LAD bypass grafting using robotic telemanipulation techniques was initially performed on the arrested heart with the use of peripherally introduced cardiopulmonary bypass with intraaortic balloon occlusion and cardioplegic arrest [13, 24]. A major disadvantage of this approach is the use of the heart lung machine, which increases the risk of stroke, bleeding, and an inflammatory response to surgery. The latter can be solved by using beating heart TECAB (BH-TECAB), in which CPB and its considerable drawbacks are avoided [24]. Total endoscopic completion of the LITA to LAD bypass graft on the beating heart requires an additional port subxiphoidally to place a specially designed endoscopic stabilizer, which stabilizes the heart to optimize the quality of the anastomosis [24]. This so-called beating heart totally endoscopic coronary artery bypass (BH TECAB) procedure might be the least invasive approach for coronary bypass surgery without making concessions to graft patency [24, 35–38]. However, the TECAB procedure is an extremely challenging and a potentially expensive procedure with an extensive learning curve, which may raise concerns about widespread adoption and application [11].

The postoperative LITA patency seemed to be independent of the surgical technique of LITA to LAD bypass grafting, since LITA patency has shown to be approximately equal for all surgical techniques (Table 2). The postoperative LITA patency varied between 93.0% and 100.0% (mean: 98.8% ± 2.3%). The mean in-hospital MACCE rate was 1.3% ± 1.9% (range: from 0,0% to 5.6%) with relatively high MACCE rates shown by Katz et al. (3.7%), Kiaii et al. (3.4%), Zhao et al. (4.5%) and Delhaye et al. (5.6%) [13, 14, 25, 26]. Strikingly, three of these authors (Katz et al., Zhao et al., and Delhaye et al.) performed LITA to LAD placement on the arrested heart [13, 25, 26]. The percentage of patients requiring PRBC transfusion varied considerably between 0.0% and 35.4% (mean: 13.6% ± 11.7%). The surgical technique or HCR strategy (staged versus simultaneous) used did not appear to affect the percentage of patients requiring PRBC transfusion. Overall, the 30-day mortality rate was 0.4% ± 0.8% (range: from 0.0% to 2.6%). Interestingly, higher than expected 30-day mortality rates were found in studies (Gilard et al. and Zhao et al.) using on-pump CABG to perform the LITA to LAD bypass graft in the majority of patients [6, 25]. Finally, the mean overall survival rate in hybrid treated patients was 98.1% ± 4.7% (range: from 84.8% to 100.0%).

3.4. PCI Techniques and Target Vessel Revascularization. Besides the technical improvements of LITA to LAD bypass grafting, innovations occurred in the field of PCI. This development was supported by the increased rate of DES implantation in later patient series compared to earlier patient series, which used percutaneous transluminal coronary angioplasty (PTCA) only or PTCA in combination with BMS implantation. Application of drug-eluting stents should lower the restenosis rate, but their potentially beneficial effect on the target vessel revascularization (TVR) is not supported by data from the included studies (Table 2). The TVR ranged between 0.0% and 29.6% (mean: 8.6% ± 7.9%). However, the (early and late) patency rate of new generation drug-eluting stents in non-LAD lesions, provided that proper DAPT is applied, may already be superior to that of saphenous vein grafts. Hard evidence is however lacking, since a head-to-head comparison of (early and late) patency rates between DES (in non-LAD lesions) and saphenous vein grafts is not available [9]. Finally, the introduction of bioresorbable scaffold (BRS) technology may improve sustainability, safety and feasibility of future HCR interventions. The application of BRS technology can make long-term DAPT redundant reducing bleeding complications without increasing the risk of stent thrombosis and may allow future reinterventions or reoperations on the same vessel if necessary due to its bioresorbable features [39].

3.5. HCR Procedure versus On- or Off-Pump CABG. A relatively small number of studies in our sample (Table 5) compared the HCR procedure using minimally invasive LITA to LAD bypass grafting with conventional CABG or off-pump coronary artery bypass (OPCAB) [7, 12, 27, 28]. All four of these studies selected matched controls who had undergone elective CABG or OPCAB with LITA and saphenous vein grafts through median sternotomy during the same period using propensity score matching [7, 12, 27, 28]. Kon et al. and Hu et al. found that patients in the hybrid group had a statistically significant shorter hospital length of stay, ICU length of stay, and intubation time compared with OPCAB, while de Cannière et al. reported that hospital and ICU length of stay was statistically shorter in hybrid treated patients compared with patients treated with CABG [7, 12, 28]. Halkos et al. showed that intubation time, ICU, and hospital length of stay were similar between the hybrid and OPCAB group [27]. Moreover, these studies revealed that PRBC transfusion requirements were reduced by the hybrid approach [12, 27, 28]. Lastly, the in-hospital MACCE rates were considerably lower in the hybrid groups compared with both the CABG and the OPCAB groups.

3.6. Cost Effectiveness. Currently, only a few studies have explicitly explored the costs associated with hybrid coronary revascularization. De Cannière and colleagues were the first to quantify costs associated with HCR and to compare these costs with costs involved in conventional double CABG [12]. Costs were calculated using six major expenditure categories: costs of hospital admission (including intensive care unit and postsurgical cardiac ward cost as well as costs associated with delayed repeat procedures), pharmaceutical costs, surgical costs, PCI-related costs, costs of blood products, and other miscellaneous fees (including physiotherapy and consultants). The extra cost associated with PCI (including stents) in the hybrid group in comparison with the CABG group (€2.517 ± 288 versus €0 ± 0), which uses autologous grafts to treat non-LAD lesions, counterbalanced the cost savings on all other expenditure categories, which resulted in a nonsignificant cost difference at 2 years between both groups (€10.622 ± 1329 versus €9699 ± 2500; not statistically significant). It is worth mentioning that the reduced ICU and hospital length of stay due to faster recovery were largely responsible for the cost reduction in the hybrid group compared with the CABG group (€3.033 ± 499 versus €4.156 ± 1.413).

Kon et al. showed that shorter intubation times, shorter ICU and hospital length of stay, and less PRBC transfusions resulted in a significant reduction in costs for hybrid treated patients in the postoperative period [7]. Conversely, intraoperative costs were statistically significant higher in patients undergoing HCR compared with OPCAB, largely because of longer operative times and the use of coated stents (DES) rather than autologous grafts ($14.691 ± 2.967 versus $9.819 ± 2.229; $P < 0.001$). In conclusion, the difference in intraoperative costs was almost completely outweighed by the lower postoperative costs in the hybrid group. This resulted in slightly, but not significantly, higher overall costs in the hybrid group.

The nonhealthcare costs after HCR will presumably be lower than after CABG or OPCAB because both Kon et al. and de Cannière et al. showed that return to work was

Table 5: Comparison of hospital outcomes.

Outcome	de Cannière et al. [12]		Kon et al. [7]		Halkos et al. [27]		Hu et al. [28]	
	Hybrid ($n = 20$) Mean ± SD or no. (%)	CABG ($n = 20$) Mean ± SD or no. (%)	Hybrid ($n = 15$) Mean ± SD or no. (%)	OPCAB ($n = 30$) Mean ± SD or no. (%)	Hybrid ($n = 147$) Mean ± SD or no. (%)	OPCAB ($n = 588$) Mean ± SD or no. (%)	Hybrid ($n = 104$) Mean ± SD or no. (%)	OPCAB ($n = 104$) Mean ± SD or no. (%)
Hospital LOS (days)	6.7 ± 0.7*	9.0 ± 1.2*	3.7 ± 1.4**	6.4 ± 2.2**	6.6 ± 6.7	6.1 ± 4.7	8.2 ± 2.6*	9.5 ± 4.5*
ICU LOS (hours)	20.2 ± 1.8*	26.6 ± 11.2*	23.5 ± 10.1**	58.1 ± 37.7**	57.4 ± 145.0	52.7 ± 87.8	34.5 ± 35.6**	55.3 ± 46.4**
Intubation time (hours)	NR	NR	1.3 ± 3.4**	20.6 ± 25.7**	17.0 ± 30.8	22.7 ± 89.5	11.6 ± 6.3*	13.8 ± 6.8*
PRBC transfusion	0 (0.0)	4 (20.0)	NR	NR	52 (34.4)**	329 (56.0)**	30 (28.8)**	54 (51.9)**
In-hospital MACCE	0 (0.0)	2 (10.0)	0 (0.0)*	7 (23.3)*	3 (2.0)	12 (2.0)	0 (0.0)	0 (0.0)
Death	0 (0.0)	0 (0.0)	0 (0.0)	0 (0.0)	1 (0.7)	5 (0.9)	0 (0.0)	0 (0.0)
Stroke	0 (0.0)	0 (0.0)	0 (0.0)	1 (3.3)	1 (0.7)	4 (0.7)	0 (0.0)	0 (0.0)
MI	0 (0.0)	2 (10.0)	0 (0.0)	6 (20.0)	1 (0.7)	3 (0.5)	0 (0.0)	0 (0.0)
Conclusion	Favours hybrid		Favours hybrid		Favours hybrid		Favours hybrid	

*P value <0.05.
**P value <0.005.
CABG: coronary artery bypass grafting; OPCAB: off-pump coronary artery bypass; SD: standard deviation; LOS: length of stay; ICU: intensive care unit; NR: not reported; PRBC: packed red blood cells; MACCE: major adverse cardiac and cerebrovascular events; MI: myocardial infarction.

significantly faster in the hybrid group, leading to a marked reduction in absenteeism from work in hybrid treated patients [7, 12]. This difference in nonhealthcare costs should be able to compensate the opposite difference in healthcare costs, resulting in a negligible difference in total societal costs. Moreover, the emergency of simultaneous hybrid procedures in especially designed multipurpose operating rooms combining the potential of catheter-based procedures and cardiac surgery will reduce the unnecessary costs incurred by staged HCR procedures [12, 25]. Lastly, more experience with minimally invasive cardiac surgery will shorten operative times, which might help reduce total healthcare costs [7].

4. Discussion

4.1. Key Results. This review is the largest and most comprehensive report to date comparing the clinical outcomes of patients who underwent either hybrid coronary revascularization or conventional on- or off-pump CABG for multivessel coronary artery disease. Three principal findings were revealed as follows: (1) hybrid treated patients showed a significantly faster recovery with lower PRBC transfusion requirements and less in-hospital major adverse cardiac and cerebrovascular events than patients treated by on- or off-pump CABG; (2) staged procedures were associated with considerable period of times between both procedures, leaving patients incompletely revascularized and in theory at risk for cardiovascular events for a considerable length of time; and (3) the invasiveness of surgical LITA to LAD bypass grafting appeared to influence the clinical outcome, with higher MACCE and 30-day mortality rates in patients treated by more invasive surgical techniques using CPB and/or median sternotomy.

4.2. Limitations. As with any review, this report shares the limitations of the original studies. First, the initial reports especially included a relatively small number of patients, which may have resulted in biased results due to outliers. Furthermore, almost all studies were performed retrospectively with inherent patient selection bias, since the decision to perform the HCR procedure was taken on an individual and highly selective basis according to cardiac surgeon and interventional cardiologist discretion. Likewise, the inclusion and exclusion criteria used to select high-risk patients for the HCR procedure differed notably between the included studies, yielding a very heterogenic population. In addition, the used surgical techniques to perform the LITA to LAD bypass graft varied considerably, with learning curve issues and different levels of expertise and equipment. All these factors potentially contribute to heterogeneity, which may reduce the certainty of the evidence presented in this review. Moreover, the mean length of followup was generally short, almost never exceeding two years, which made it difficult to assess long-term clinical outcomes of hybrid treated patients. Therefore, this review relies mainly on in-hospital and short-term outcomes to assess the safety and feasibility of the HCR procedure. Another limitation was the lack of long-term systematic and routine angiographic followup of graft and stent patency in the majority of studies included in the present review, which precluded any conclusions about the graft and stent longevity of the HCR procedure. Furthermore, the comparative studies lacked randomization and nonblinded assessment of outcome, which might have led to selection bias and might have influenced outcome measures by preconceived notions about the superiority of the HCR procedure. Finally, postoperative pain, which might be higher in patients treated with conventional MIDCAB, was not included as outcome measure in the present review, because only a limited number of studies assessed this outcome measure. Notwithstanding these weaknesses and limitations, this review selected the best evidence currently available to give a broad and comprehensive overview of the preliminary results of the HCR procedure.

4.3. Recommendations for Future Research. Larger, multicenter, prospective, randomized trials with long-term clinical and angiographic followup and cost analysis comparing HCR with both conventional on-pump and off-pump CABG or multivessel PCI will be necessary to further evaluate whether this hybrid approach is associated with similar promising long-term results. In the meantime, the first prospective, randomized pilot trial to compare HCR with conventional CABG in patients with multivessel coronary artery disease has been started [40]. These data are also needed to identify patient populations that would benefit most from this hybrid approach. Furthermore, more insights in the different surgical techniques for LITA to LAD bypass grafting and their clinical outcomes are necessary. Therefore, the different surgical techniques for LITA to LAD bypass grafting in the HCR procedure should be integrated in these large, multicenter HCR studies in order to determine the best way of LITA to LAD bypass grafting in HCR. Moreover, different HCR strategies (staged versus simultaneous) should be compared to decide which strategy will serve which patients best. Finally, the advantages and disadvantages of a hybrid operative suite need to be explored further.

5. Conclusions

The large variability in HCR techniques makes it difficult to draw firm conclusions from the currently available evidence, but HCR appears to be a promising and cost-effective alternative for CABG in the treatment of multivessel coronary artery disease in a selected patient population. The HCR procedure was associated with short hospital stays (including ICU stay and intubation time), low MACCE and 30-day mortality rates, low PRBC transfusion requirements and TVR, high postoperative LITA patency rates, and high survival rates. These promising early outcomes warrant further research with larger sample size, multicenter RCTs to determine the definite place of HCR in the current therapeutic armamentarium against coronary artery disease. Until then, this review justifies the continued use of the hybrid approach, but careful patient selection and close cooperation between cardiac surgeons and interventional cardiologists will determine the clinical outcomes to a significant extent.

References

[1] P. W. Serruvs, M. C. Morice, A. P. Kappetein et al., "Percutaneous coronary intervention versus coronary-artery bypass grafting for severe coronary artery disease," *New England Journal of Medicine*, vol. 360, no. 10, pp. 961–972, 2009.

[2] R. L. Frye, E. L. Alderman, K. Andrews et al., "Comparison of coronary bypass surgery with angioplasty in patients with multivessel disease: the Bypass Angioplasty Revascularization Investigation (BARI) investigators," *New England Journal of Medicine*, vol. 335, no. 4, pp. 217–225, 1996.

[3] G. D. Angelini, P. Wilde, T. A. Salemo, G. Bosco, and A. M. Caiafiore, "Integrated left small thoracotomy and angioplasty for multivessel coronary artery revascularisation," *The Lancet*, vol. 347, no. 9003, pp. 757–758, 1996.

[4] R. A. Guyton, "Coronary artery bypass is superior to drug-eluting stents in multivessel coronary artery disease," *Annals of Thoracic Surgery*, vol. 81, no. 6, pp. 1949–1957, 2006.

[5] N. Bonaros, T. Schachner, D. Wiedemann et al., "Quality of life improvement after robotically assisted coronary artery bypass grafting," *Cardiology*, vol. 114, no. 1, pp. 59–66, 2009.

[6] M. Gilard, E. Bezon, J. C. Cornily et al., "Same-day combined percutaneous coronary intervention and coronary artery surgery," *Cardiology*, vol. 108, no. 4, pp. 363–367, 2007.

[7] Z. N. Kon, E. N. Brown, R. Tran et al., "Simultaneous hybrid coronary revascularization reduces postoperative morbidity compared with results from conventional off-pump coronary artery bypass," *Journal of Thoracic and Cardiovascular Surgery*, vol. 135, no. 2, pp. 367–375, 2008.

[8] D. Zimrin, P. A. Reyes, B. Reicher, and R. S. Poston, "A hybrid alternative for high risk left main disease," *Catheterization and Cardiovascular Interventions*, vol. 69, no. 1, pp. 123–127, 2007.

[9] T. A. Vassiliades Jr., J. S. Douglas, D. C. Morris et al., "Integrated coronary revascularization with drug-eluting stents: immediate and seven-month outcome," *Journal of Thoracic and Cardiovascular Surgery*, vol. 131, no. 5, pp. 956–962, 2006.

[10] M. J. Boylan, B. W. Lytle, F. D. Loop et al., "Surgical treatment of isolated left anterior descending coronary stenosis: comparison of left internal mammary artery and venous autograft at 18 to 20 years of follow-up," *Journal of Thoracic and Cardiovascular Surgery*, vol. 107, no. 3, pp. 657–662, 1994.

[11] G. Davidavicius, F. van Praet, S. Mansour et al., "Hybrid revascularization strategy: a pilot study on the association of robotically enhanced minimally invasive direct coronary artery bypass surgery and fractional flow reserve-guided percutaneous coronary intervention," *Circulation*, vol. 112, no. 9, pp. I317–I322, 2005.

[12] D. de Cannière, J. L. Jansens, P. Goldschmidt-Clermont, L. Barvais, P. Decroly, and E. Stoupel, "Combination of minimally invasive coronary bypass and percutaneous transluminal coronary angioplasty in the treatment of double-vessel coronary disease: two-year follow-up of a new hybrid procedure compared with "on-pump" double bypass grafting," *American Heart Journal*, vol. 142, no. 4, pp. 563–570, 2001.

[13] M. R. Katz, F. van Praet, D. de Canniere et al., "Integrated coronary revascularization: percutaneous coronary intervention plus robotic totally endoscopic coronary artery bypass," *Circulation*, vol. 114, no. 1, pp. I473–I476, 2006.

[14] B. Kiaii, R. S. McClure, P. Stewart et al. et al., "Simultaneous integrated coronary artery revascularization with long-term angiographic follow-up," *The Journal of Thoracic and Cardiovascular Surgery*, vol. 136, no. 3, pp. 702–708, 2008.

[15] C. Indolfi, M. Pavia, and I. F. Angelillo, "Drug-eluting stents versus bare metal stents in percutaneous coronary interventions (a meta-analysis)," *American Journal of Cardiology*, vol. 95, no. 10, pp. 1146–1152, 2005.

[16] B. Reicher, R. S. Poston, M. R. Mehra et al., "Simultaneous "hybrid" percutaneous coronary intervention and minimally invasive surgical bypass grafting: feasibility, safety, and clinical outcomes," *American Heart Journal*, vol. 155, no. 4, pp. 661–667, 2008.

[17] M. Zenati, H. A. Cohen, and B. P. Griffith, "Alternative approach to multivessel coronary disease with integrated coronary revascularization," *Journal of Thoracic and Cardiovascular Surgery*, vol. 117, no. 3, pp. 439–446, 1999.

[18] C. T. Lloyd, A. M. Calafiore, P. Wilde et al., "Integrated left anterior small thoracotomy and angioplasty for coronary artery revascularization," *Annals of Thoracic Surgery*, vol. 68, no. 3, pp. 908–912, 1999.

[19] T. Wittwer, A. Haverich, J. Cremer, P. Boonstra, U. Franke, and T. Wahlers, "Follow-up experience with coronary hybrid-revascularisation," *Thoracic and Cardiovascular Surgeon*, vol. 48, no. 6, pp. 356–359, 2000.

[20] F. C. Riess, R. Bader, P. Kremer et al., "Coronary hybrid revascularization from January 1997 to January 2001: a clinical follow-up," *Annals of Thoracic Surgery*, vol. 73, no. 6, pp. 1849–1855, 2002.

[21] K. D. Stahl, W. D. Boyd, T. A. Vassiliades, and H. L. Karamanoukian, "Hybrid robotic coronary artery surgery and angioplasty in multivessel coronary artery disease," *Annals of Thoracic Surgery*, vol. 74, no. 4, pp. S1358–S1362, 2002.

[22] M. Cisowski, W. Morawski, J. Drzewiecki et al., "Integrated minimally invasive direct coronary artery bypass grafting and angioplasty for coronary artery revascularization," *European Journal of Cardio-Thoracic Surgery*, vol. 22, no. 2, pp. 261–265, 2002.

[23] M. H. Us, M. Basaran, M. Yilmaz et al., "Hybrid coronary revascularization in high-risk patients," *Texas Heart Institute Journal*, vol. 33, no. 4, pp. 458–462, 2006.

[24] D. M. Holzhey, S. Jacobs, M. Mochalski et al., "Minimally invasive hybrid coronary artery revascularization," *Annals of Thoracic Surgery*, vol. 86, no. 6, pp. 1856–1860, 2008.

[25] D. X. Zhao, M. Leacche, J. M. Balaguer et al., "Routine intraoperative completion angiography after coronary artery bypass grafting and 1-stop hybrid revascularization results from a fully integrated hybrid catheterization laboratory/operating room," *Journal of the American College of Cardiology*, vol. 53, no. 3, pp. 232–241, 2009.

[26] C. Delhaye, A. Sudre, G. Lemesle et al., "Hybrid revascularization, comprising coronary artery bypass graft with exclusive arterial conduits followed by early drug-eluting stent implantation, in multivessel coronary artery disease," *Archives of Cardiovascular Diseases*, vol. 103, no. 10, pp. 502–511, 2010.

[27] M. E. Halkos, T. A. Vassiliades, J. S. Douglas et al., "Hybrid coronary revascularization versus off-pump coronary artery bypass grafting for the treatment of multivessel coronary artery disease," *The Annals of Thoracic Surgery*, vol. 92, no. 5, pp. 1695–1701, 2011.

[28] S. Hu, Q. Li, P. Gao et al., "Simultaneous hybrid revascularization versus off-pump coronary artery bypass for multivessel coronary artery disease," *Annals of Thoracic Surgery*, vol. 91, no. 2, pp. 432–438, 2011.

[29] T. Wittwer, J. Cremer, P. Boonstra et al., "Myocardial "hybrid" revascularisation with minimally invasive direct coronary artery bypass grafting: combined with coronary angioplasty: preliminary results of a multicentre study," *Heart*, vol. 83, no. 1, pp. 58–63, 2000.

[30] C. Loubeyre, M. C. Morice, B. Berzin et al. et al., "Emergency coronary artery bypass surgery following coronary angioplasty and stenting: results of a French multicenter registry," *Catheterization and Cardiovascular Interventions*, vol. 47, no. 4, pp. 441–448, 1999.

[31] J. A. Carey, S. W. Davies, R. Balcon et al., "Emergency surgical revascularisation for coronary angioplasty complications," *British Heart Journal*, vol. 72, no. 5, pp. 428–435, 1994.

[32] M. A. Greene, L. A. Gray Jr., A. D. Slater, B. L. Ganzel, and C. Mavroudis, "Emergency aortocoronary bypass after failed angioplasty," *Annals of Thoracic Surgery*, vol. 51, no. 2, pp. 194–199, 1991.

[33] F. Bednar, P. Osmancik, T. Vanek et al., "Platelet activity and aspirin efficacy after off-pump compared with on-pump coronary artery bypass surgery: results from the prospective randomized trial PRAGUE 11-Coronary Artery Bypass and REactivity of Thrombocytes (CABARET)," *Journal of Thoracic and Cardiovascular Surgery*, vol. 136, no. 4, pp. 1054–1060, 2008.

[34] P. Gao, H. Xiong, Z. Zheng, L. Li, R. Gao, and S. S. Hu, "Evaluation of antiplatelet effects of a modified protocol by platelet aggregation in patients undergoing "one-stop" hybrid coronary revascularization," *Platelets*, vol. 21, no. 3, pp. 183–190, 2010.

[35] J. Bonatti, T. Schachner, N. Bonaros et al., "Simultaneous hybrid coronary revascularization using totally endoscopic left internal mammary artery bypass grafting and placement of rapamycin eluting stents in the same interventional session. The COMBINATION pilot study," *Cardiology*, vol. 110, no. 2, pp. 92–95, 2008.

[36] J. Bonatti, T. Schachner, N. Bonaros et al., "Robotic totally endoscopic coronary artery bypass and catheter based coronary intervention in one operative session," *Annals of Thoracic Surgery*, vol. 79, no. 6, pp. 2138–2141, 2005.

[37] C. Gao, M. Yang, Y. Wu et al., "Hybrid coronary revascularization by endoscopic robotic coronary artery bypass grafting on beating heart and stent placement," *Annals of Thoracic Surgery*, vol. 87, no. 3, pp. 737–741, 2009.

[38] S. Srivastava, S. Gadasalli, M. Agusala et al., "Beating heart totally endoscopic coronary artery bypass," *Annals of Thoracic Surgery*, vol. 89, no. 6, pp. 1873–1880, 2010.

[39] Y. Onuma and P. W. Serruys, "Bioresorbable scaffold: the advent of a new era in percutaneous coronary and peripheral revascularization?" *Circulation*, vol. 123, no. 7, pp. 779–797, 2011.

[40] M. Zembala, M. Tajstra, M. Zembala et al., "Prospective randomised pilOt study evaLuating the safety and efficacy of hybrid revascularisation in MultI-vessel coronary artery DisEaSe (POLMIDES)—study design," *Kardiologia Polska*, vol. 69, no. 5, pp. 460–466, 2011.

2

Clinical Effectiveness of Modified Laparoscopic Fimbrioplasty for the Treatment of Minimal Endometriosis and Unexplained Infertility

Sarah E. Franjoine,[1] Mohamed A. Bedaiwy,[1,2,3] Faten F. AbdelHafez,[3] Cuiyu Geng,[4] and James H. Liu[1]

[1] *Division of Reproductive Endocrinology and Infertility, Department of Obstetrics and Gynecology, University Hospitals Case Medical Center, MacDonald Women's Hospital, Cleveland, OH 44106, USA*
[2] *Division of Reproductive Endocrinology and Infertility, Department of Obstetrics and Gynaecology, The University of British Columbia, D415A, 4500 Oak Street, Vancouver, BC, Canada V6H 3N1*
[3] *Women's Health University Center, Department of Obstetrics and Gynecology, Faculty of Medicine, Assiut University, Assiut 71515, Egypt*
[4] *Department of Biostatistics and Epidemiology, Case Western Reserve University School of Medicine, Cleveland, OH 44106, USA*

Correspondence should be addressed to James H. Liu; james.liu@uhhospitals.org

Academic Editor: Peng Hui Wang

Objective. To study the reproductive outcomes of modified laparoscopic fimbrioplasty (MLF), a surgical technique designed to increase the working surface area of the fimbriated end of the fallopian tube. We postulated that an improvement in fimbrial function through MLF will improve reproductive outcomes. *Design*. Retrospective cohort study. *Setting*. Academic tertiary-care medical center. *Patients*. Women with minimal endometriosis or unexplained infertility, who underwent MLF during diagnostic laparoscopy ($n = 50$) or diagnostic laparoscopy alone ($n = 87$). *Intervention*. MLF involved gentle, circumferential dilatation of the fimbria and lysis of fimbrial adhesions bridging the fimbrial folds. *Main Outcome Measures*. The primary outcome was pregnancy rate and the secondary outcome was time to pregnancy. *Results*. The pregnancy rate for the MLF group was 40.0%, compared to 28.7% for the control group. The average time to pregnancy for the MLF group was 13 weeks, compared to 18 weeks for the control group. The pregnancy rate in the MLF group was significantly higher for patients ≤35 ys (51.5% versus 28.8%), but not for those >35 ys (17.6% versus 28.6%). *Conclusion*. MLF was associated with a significant increase in pregnancy rate for patients ≤35 ys.

1. Introduction

Ovum pickup occurs at midcycle when the dominant follicle, ovary, and fimbrial end of the tube interact behind the uterus near the cul de sac [1]. The factors that contribute to ovum pickup, besides tubal and fimbrial structure, have not been well characterized in humans but may include chemotactic factors, elastic mucoid projections from the fimbria, and peristaltic or pressure changes of the oviduct or surrounding ligaments [2, 3]. Our group designed a procedure designated as modified laparoscopic fimbrioplasty (MLF), to improve ovum pickup by the fimbria, to target and correct subclinical fimbrial lesions, and to increase the working fimbrial surface area.

For normal fallopian tubal function, the tube must be patent, in close proximity to the ovary, and freely mobile. Additionally, the fimbria must have sufficient surface area for ovum pickup. The fimbria needs to be closely apposed to the ovarian surface in order to capture ova from all sides; this can be visualized in the endoscopic video of ovulation [4].

Abnormal tubal function can be a factor in more than 20% of couples presenting with primary infertility [5]. An assessment of tubal architecture can be made with diagnostic laparoscopy, which can detect the presence of pelvic adhesions or endometriosis. However, laparoscopy is now less frequently a part of the standard initial evaluation for infertility. Falloposcopy, a technique that cannulates and visualizes the entirety of the fallopian tube via fiber optic imaging through the uterine cavity, is able to detect and target lesions, debris, and adhesions not visible or detectable with either HSG or diagnostic laparoscopy. Even though today this technique is less popular and is infrequently utilized, the findings from falloposcopy indicate that there is often more pathology present than is recognized by HSG or laparoscopy [3].

Currently, the empiric treatment for unexplained infertility often includes three cycles of ovarian stimulation with clomiphene citrate or gonadotropins with intrauterine insemination (IUI). If this approach is unsuccessful, couples can then proceed onto in vitro fertilization (IVF) or diagnostic laparoscopy [6].

The objective of this project was to examine the effectiveness of MLF, a novel, simple surgical technique that is performed during diagnostic laparoscopy in patients with minimal endometriosis or unexplained infertility. This study analyzed retrospectively the pregnancy rate and time to pregnancy after MLF. We hypothesized that fimbrial function is enhanced by MLF.

2. Materials and Methods

2.1. Study Design. This was a retrospective cohort study that compared the reproductive outcomes of women who underwent MLF during diagnostic laparoscopy to women who underwent diagnostic laparoscopy alone. The study was approved by the Institutional Review Board of University Hospitals Case Medical Center. The reproductive history, operative information, and reproductive outcomes of all subjects were collected from preexisting records. The primary outcome for this study was pregnancy rate, and the secondary outcome was time to pregnancy.

2.2. Subject Selection. Patients were identified from a database of 511 patients who had a laparoscopic procedure performed by the reproductive endocrine division between 2006 and 2012. The MLF group was comprised of women who underwent MLF during diagnostic laparoscopy performed by James H. Liu (JHL). The control group was comprised of women who underwent diagnostic laparoscopy without MLF by other members of our reproductive endocrine division. Other inclusion criteria were age less than 42 ys, diagnosis of either minimal endometriosis or unexplained infertility, and adequate follow-up while attempting to conceive.

Minimal, or Stage I, endometriosis was defined according to the American Society for Reproductive Medicine (ASRM) classification as superficial lesions less than 3 cm [7]. A diagnosis of unexplained infertility was given when a patient was infertile with normal ovulatory and tubal functions along with a normal sperm count for her partner. These were determined by the regularity of menstrual cycles, HSG, and semen analysis, respectively. When endometriosis lesions were minimal, they could be missed laparoscopically, resulting in patients being characterized as "unexplained infertility." Thus, in many studies, minimal endometriosis and unexplained infertility were combined in the analysis.

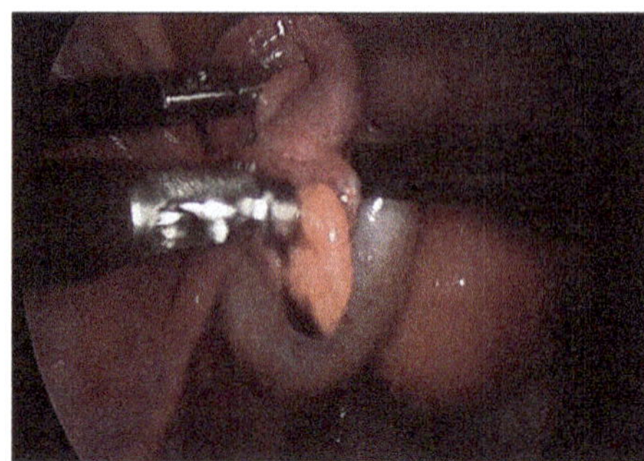

Figure 1: Endoscopic picture of MLF procedure; right angle cystic duct clamp inserted halfway into fimbria.

Preoperatively, the two groups of patients were treated as patients of the entire reproductive endocrine division with similar preoperative treatment course. The cycles of Clomid and IUI were managed in the same fashion by the same group of nurses. The decision to proceed to laparoscopy was similar between the three group clinicians, typically after three unsuccessful cycles of Clomid and IUI. The only difference in their treatment was that JHL chose to perform the MLF and the other group clinicians did not.

Patients were excluded when other procedures were performed during the laparoscopy such as removal of an ectopic pregnancy, bilateral salpingectomy or salpingostomy, ovarian drilling, or myomectomy, as these might confound the effects of MLF on fertility by altering the woman's ability to conceive. Also, 10 subjects from each group were lost to follow-up. The final sample size was 50 MLF patients and 87 control patients. The study was powered for a minimum of 50 MLF patients and 57 control patients, to support a twofold increase in pregnancy rate from a baseline of 20% [8].

2.3. Surgical Procedure. The MLF procedure was performed during diagnostic laparoscopy. For the patients of JHL, MLF was performed as an additional procedure during the laparoscopy, regardless of the presence or absence of a visible pathology.

After a pelvic survey, two 5-mm accessory ports were placed, one in the right lower quadrant and the other in the left lower quadrant. If any evidence of endometriosis was noted, a small confirmatory biopsy was taken, and any minimal adhesions in the pelvis were lysed. The fimbriated end of each tube was then elevated with a nongrasping instrument, and dye was injected in order to more readily identify the tubal lumen. At the point of dye extrusion, a small right angle cystic duct clamp was inserted into the fimbrial lumen and gently opened 5–7 times with simultaneous rotation of the clamp to achieve circumferential dilatation in an attempt to expand the working surface area of the fimbria (Figure 1). This was then repeated with the opposite tube.

Before the procedure, intraluminal adhesions beyond the fimbriated end were not visualized; however, in some cases, intraluminal adhesions were noted once the clamp began dilating the fimbriated end. The adhesions that were noted at this time were not grossly blocking the tubal lumen but rather often bridged between the fimbrial folds. These intraluminal adhesions were not consistently documented and did not result in a change in the surgical or postoperative management.

2.4. Statistical Methods. Each patient's chart was reviewed for up to 70 weeks after her procedure or until she became pregnant. Each patient attempted to conceive after her procedure either naturally or with supplemental ovarian stimulation with various treatment protocols. These included clomiphene, gonadotropins, or combination clomiphene-gonadotropins, with or without intrauterine insemination. The choice of postsurgical treatment was a joint decision made by the patient and her physician. For women attempting to conceive with ovulatory stimulation, each cycle was tracked and recorded in a paper chart, including length and dose of treatment and ultrasound monitoring of endometrial thickness and number of codominant follicles, with a dominant follicle defined by a diameter of at least 15 mm averaged from all dimensions. Pregnancies were tracked through both paper and electronic charts by serum βhCG and ultrasound, with a positive serum βhCG result defined as greater than 10 IU/L. Eight MLF and 13 control patients chose to proceed to IVF after attempting to conceive with the above methods for an average of six months. The data from treatment cycles were included until IVF began.

The demographics of the two groups were analyzed by summary statistics and by univariate analysis. Survival analysis using Kaplan-Meier plots was used to display cumulative pregnancy rates for both groups and to determine the mean time to pregnancy. Number needed to treat (NNT) was calculated by the number of treatment cycles needed to achieve one pregnancy. For each outcome, a p value less than 0.05 (two-tailed) was used to determine significance. The subjects were further dichotomized into age groups, either ≤35 or >35; then the demographics and outcomes were compared for these age groups.

3. Results

3.1. Baseline Characteristics. The demographic features of the MLF and control cohorts are shown in Table 1. The two groups were similar in terms of age, BMI, smoking history, partner's smoking history, and length of relationship. There was a statistically significant difference in the ethnic distribution between the two groups, with a higher percentage of the MLF group reporting ethnicity as white (80.8% versus 60.2%, MLF versus control) and a lower percentage as black (6.4% versus 27.9%, $p < 0.01$). No differences in these characteristics were observed for women aged ≤35 ys when comparing the MLF group to the control group; however there was a significant difference in BMI, with a lower mean BMI in the younger MLF group when compared to the younger control group (24.9 versus 28.5, $p < 0.01$).

The baseline reproductive characteristics of the patients in both groups are also shown in Table 1. The two groups were

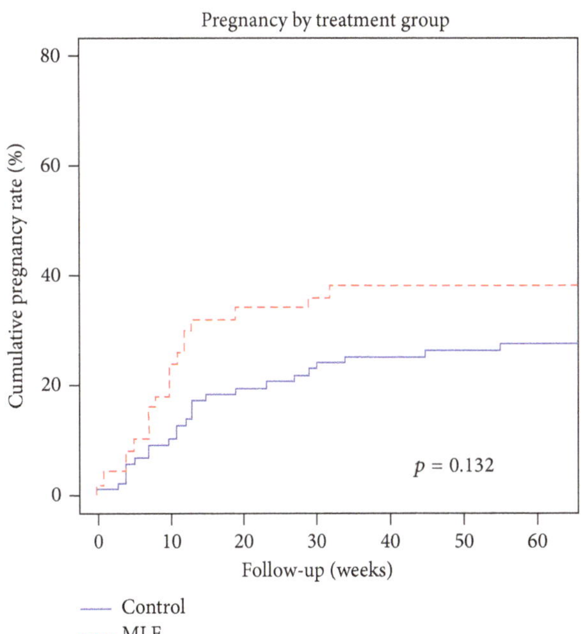

FIGURE 2: Pregnancy rate for MLF versus control over time (p = 0.13).

comparable, with no significant differences in gravidity, day 3 FSH level, day 3 estradiol level, prior use of oral contraceptive pills, intraoperative chromopertubation findings, and semen analysis results.

For individual cycles that led to pregnancy and those that did not, the endometrial thickness (9.7 ± 2.6 mm versus 8.8 ± 2.6 mm, $p = 0.07$) and the number of dominant follicles (1.6± 1.2 versus 1.6 ± 1.0, $p = 0.95$) were comparable.

Univariate analysis examined the effect of each of the variables on the reproductive outcomes, namely, age, BMI, race, smoking history, FSH level, estradiol level, HSG findings, intraoperative chromopertubation findings, and semen analysis. None of these variables were found to have a significant impact on the outcome (data not shown).

Operative times were similar for the two groups (60.1 ± 17.7 minutes versus 62.6±36.2 minutes, $p = 0.59$, MLF versus control). Minimal surgical complications were noted for each group (0% versus 3.5%, $p = 0.29$, MLF versus control).

3.2. Reproductive Outcomes. The Kaplan-Meier analysis of the cumulative pregnancy rate is shown in Figure 2. Overall, the pregnancy rate for the MLF group was 40.0%, compared to 28.7% for that of the control group ($p = 0.13$). The average time to pregnancy for the MLF group was 13.4 weeks compared to 18.4 weeks for the control group ($p = 0.27$) (Table 2).

Figure 3 shows the cumulative pregnancy rate with women dichotomized into two age groups with a cutoff of age 35 ys. This demonstrates that, for the younger cohort, a significantly higher percentage of the MLF group (n = 33) became pregnant compared to the control group (n = 66) (51.5% versus 28.8%, $p = 0.02$). However, there were no differences for women older than 35 years (17.6% versus 28.6%, $p = 0.45$). The average time to pregnancy for the MLF

Table 1: Demographic features of all subjects.

	All subjects			Age ≤ 35		
	MLF (n = 50)	Control (n = 87)	p value	MLF (n = 33)	Control (n = 66)	p value
Age	33.3 ± 6.5	32.2 ± 5.1	0.28	31.0 ± 2.9	30.1 ± 3.8	0.23
BMI	25.8 ± 5.5	28.2 ± 7.8	**0.04**	24.9 ± 4.6	28.5 ± 7.3	**<0.01**
Ethnicity						
White	38 (80.8%)	49 (62.0%)		23 (76.7%)	37 (61.7%)	
Black	3 (6.4%)	22 (27.9%)	**<0.01**	3 (10.0%)	18 (30.0%)	0.09
Others	6 (12.8%)	8 (10.1%)		4 (13.3%)	5 (8.3%)	
Smoking history						
Ever smoker	13 (26.0%)	26 (29.9%)	0.63	11 (33.3%)	21 (31.8%)	0.88
Never smoker	37 (74.0%)	61 (70.1%)		22 (66.7%)	45 (68.2%)	
Partner's smoking						
Ever smoker	15 (31.9%)	23 (27.7%)	0.61	10 (32.3%)	20 (31.8%)	0.96
Never smoker	32 (68.1%)	60 (72.3%)		21 (67.7%)	43 (68.2%)	
Length of relationship (years)	7.9 ± 5.1	6.8 ± 4.1	0.20	7.5 ± 5.8	6.3 ± 5.4	0.18
Gravidity						
0	24 (48.0%)	46 (52.9%)	0.59	36 (54.5%)	16 (48.5%)	0.57
≥1	26 (52.0%)	41 (47.1%)		30 (45.5%)	17 (51.6%)	
Day 3 FSH	57 ± 3.3	6.3 ± 3.2	0.39	6.0 ± 3.9	5.7 ± 2.3	0.78
Day 3 estradiol	45.1 ± 38.4	36.5 ± 27.1	0.22	50.7 ± 45.2	36.7 ± 26.6	0.11
Prior OCP use						
Yes	30 (78.9%)	64 (83.1%)	0.59	19 (73.1%)	47 (82.5%)	0.33
No	8 (21.1%)	13 (16.9%)		7 (26.9%)	10 (17.5%)	
Chromopertubation						
Patent	47 (97.9%)	80 (96.4%)	1.00	31 (96.9%)	61 (98.4%)	1.00
≥1 blocked	1 (2.1%)	3 (3.6%)		1 (3.1%)	1 (1.6%)	
Semen analysis						
Normal	15 (31.3%)	18 (26.1%)	0.54	12 (37.5%)	11 (22.0%)	0.13
Abnormal	33 (68.7%)	51 (73.9%)		20 (62.5%)	39 (78.0%)	

Note: MLF = women treated with modified laparoscopic fimbrioplasty. OCP = oral contraceptive pills. Data are expressed as mean ± SD for age, BMI, length of relationship, day 3 FSH level, and day 3 estradiol level. Data are expressed as numerator and percentage for all other factors (ethnicity, smoking history, gravidity, prior OCP use, chromopertubation findings, and semen analysis). p values were obtained by either Fisher's exact test or two-tailed t-test.

Table 2: Reproductive outcomes.

	All subjects			Subjects ≤ 35		
	MLF (n = 50)	Control (n = 87)	p value	MLF (n = 33)	Control (n = 66)	p value
Percent pregnant	20 (40%)	25 (28.7%)	0.13	17 (51.5%)	19 (28.8%)	**0.02**
Average time to pregnancy (weeks)	13.4	18.4	0.27	10.8	15.7	0.27

Note: MLF = women treated with modified laparoscopic fimbrioplasty. Data are expressed as numerator and percentage for the number and percent of women who conceived. Data are expressed as mean time to pregnancy for those women who became pregnant. p values were obtained by either Fisher's exact test or two-tailed t-test.

group in the younger cohort was 10.8 weeks compared to 15.7 weeks for the control group (p = 0.27).

The impact of ovulatory stimulation and IUI in postsurgical management was also evaluated. Couples in both groups often attempted to conceive multiple times with different methods. Analysis of treatment cycles indicates that the two groups, MLF versus control, attempted to conceive in comparable proportions without additional medication (16% versus 27%, p = 0.12), with clomiphene (48% versus 59.8, p = 0.18), and with gonadotropins (32% versus 26.4%, p = 0.49); however, a greater proportion of women in the MLF group attempted to conceive using combination clomiphene-gonadotropin therapy (36% versus 8.1%, $p < 0.01$).

For all conception cycles, MLF patients became pregnant without ovulatory stimulation 35% of the time compared to 28% of the time for the control group (p = 0.36). Both groups

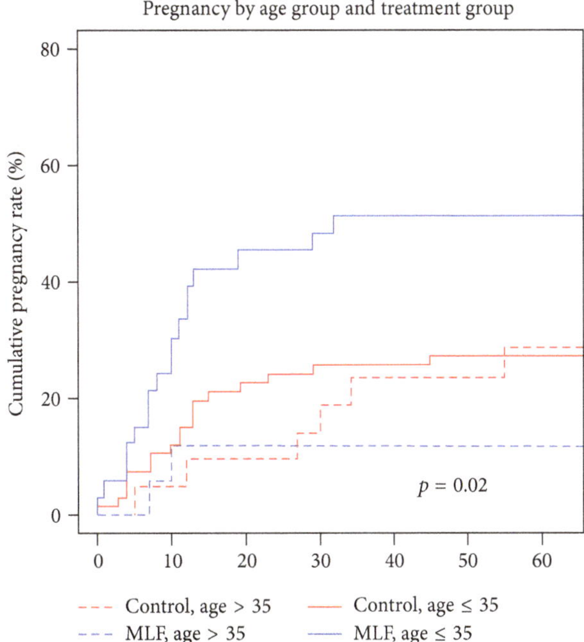

FIGURE 3: Pregnancy rate by treatment (MLF versus control) and age (women ≤35 ys, women >35 ys) over time. Significant difference for women ≤35 ys ($p = 0.02$), no significant difference for women >35 ys ($p = 0.45$).

achieved pregnancy with timed intercourse 40% of the time and with IUI 60% of the time ($p = 0.40$).

For subjects aged ≤35 ys, the overall per cycle pregnancy rate was 22.7% for MLF compared to 13.3% for control ($p = 0.06$).

The NNT was calculated as the number of postsurgical cycles needed to achieve one pregnancy. The NNT for all women was 6 for the MLF group compared to 8 for the control group. For women aged ≤35 ys, the NNT for the MLF group was 4 compared to 8 for the control group.

4. Discussion

The present cohort study showed that MLF performed during routine diagnostic laparoscopy led to a significantly greater pregnancy rate of 51.5% for women ≤35 ys and a trend towards a higher pregnancy rate of 40.0% in the overall MLF cohort when compared to diagnostic laparoscopy alone. The MLF also showed a trend towards a shorter time to pregnancy: an average of 10 weeks for women ≤35 ys and 13 weeks for all women.

The per cycle pregnancy rate for MLF was 22% for women ≤35 ys and 16% for all women; this can be compared to the per cycle pregnancy rate of 32.4% with IVF for women of all ages with tubal infertility [9]. The NNT for the MLF group was 4 for women ≤35 ys and 6 for all women, which can be compared to the NNT of 3 for IVF for women of all ages and for women ≤35 ys with infertility of all causes, based on historical data [10].

The control and MLF groups were comparable for most demographic features, except for ethnic distribution for subjects of all ages and a lower BMI for the younger cohort. These observations can be expected given that the groups were not randomized. However univariate analysis determined that neither of these factors significantly impacted the outcome.

With regards to current treatment trends, the surgical role in the treatment of unexplained infertility has been largely supplanted by IVF. However, a variety of surgical options for optimizing tubal function are available, including neosalpingostomy, traditional fimbrioplasty, and our MLF. These surgical options can be an alternative or predecessor to IVF and are potential options for younger women.

A recent committee opinion article from the ASRM supports the role of tubal surgery as an alternative to IVF. The committee describes the benefits of tubal surgery for infertility, including that it is a one-time procedure, often minimally invasive, that one procedure allows multiple attempts at conception without additional treatment, and that it can result in multiple conceptions over time. The committee recommended proximal tubal cannulation and laparoscopic fimbrioplasty or neosalpingostomy to treat mild hydrosalpinges in young women without other pathology [9].

The MLF procedure differs significantly from the traditional procedure that is termed "fimbrioplasty." The later, often associated with neosalpingostomy, is a similar, but distinct, technique, where visible periadnexal lesions are lysed, the tube is dilated with forceps, and fimbrial bridges are freed [11]. This procedure is indicated for patients with hydrosalpinx or known distal tubal obstruction secondary to pelvic infection or surgery. Modified fimbrioplasty (MLF) is used on patent tubes in patients with minimal endometriosis or unexplained infertility. Traditional fimbrioplasty targets visible lesions, while the MLF aims to correct subclinical lesions.

However one limitation of the current study is the nonrandomization of the initial surgery and the postsurgical treatments. Another limitation is the moderate loss to follow-up after the procedure as well as the modest size for the cohort groups. The conclusions would be stronger with a larger cohort size. Meanwhile, the comparability of the MLF and control groups, the comparability of the postsurgical treatment regimens, and the long follow-up period strengthen the study.

Given our promising preliminary results, the authors propose that the present described approach, MLF, would be an adjunctive procedure for women already undergoing diagnostic laparoscopy. It would be performed as an additional step during a routine diagnostic laparoscopy, similar to fulguration or excision of endometriosis or chromopertubation. At this point, the authors do not recommend undertaking diagnostic laparoscopy solely for the purpose of performing an MLF but rather only if there is already a plan to perform a laparoscopy.

5. Conclusion

MLF is a minimally invasive surgical technique that can be safely incorporated into diagnostic laparoscopy and may be an effective alternative to IVF for women with minimal endometriosis or unexplained infertility. The present findings need further validation by a larger, prospective, and randomized study to assess whether this procedure is still effective in a larger population and to assess whether the benefit extends to women over the age of 35 ys.

Capsule

Improved pregnancy rate was observed in women ≤35 ys after modified laparoscopic fimbrioplasty.

Disclosure

Abstract was presented in part at ASRM/IFFS Conjoint Meeting, Boston, MA, on October 15, 2013.

References

[1] R. J. Blandau, "Comparative aspects of tubal anatomy and physiology as they relate to reconstructive procedures," *Journal of Reproductive Medicine*, vol. 21, no. 1, pp. 7-15, 1978.

[2] C. A. Eddy and C. J. Pauerstein, "Anatomy and physiology of the fallopian tube," *Clinical Obstetrics and Gynecology*, vol. 23, no. 4, pp. 1177–1193, 1980.

[3] J. F. Kerin, D. B. Williams, G. A. San Roman, A. C. Pearlstone, W. S. Grundfest, and E. S. Surrey, "Falloposcopic classification and treatment of fallopian tube lumen disease," *Fertility and Sterility*, vol. 57, no. 4, pp. 731–741, 1992.

[4] S. Gordts, *Human Ovulation Captured on Film*, Leuven Institute for Fertility and Embryology, Leuven, Belgium, 2008, http://www.youtube.com/watch?v=2-VKgdhfNpY.

[5] The Practice Committee of the American Society for Reproductive Medicine, "Diagnostic evaluation of the infertile female: a committee opinion," *Fertility and Sterility*, vol. 98, no. 2, pp. 302–307, 2012.

[6] H. Hatasaka, "New perspectives for unexplained infertility," *Clinical Obstetrics and Gynecology*, vol. 54, no. 4, pp. 727–733, 2011.

[7] American Society for Reproductive Medicine, "Revised American Society for reproductive medicine classification of endometriosis: 1996," *Fertility and Sterility*, vol. 67, no. 5, pp. 817–821, 1997.

[8] The Practice Committee of the American Society for Reproductive Medicine, "Endometriosis and infertility: a committee opinion," *Fertility and Sterility*, vol. 98, no. 3, pp. 591–598, 2012.

[9] The Practice Committee of the American Society for Reproductive Medicine, "Committee opinion: role of tubal surgery in the era of assisted reproductive technology," *Fertility and Sterility*, vol. 97, no. 3, pp. 539–545, 2012.

[10] Society for Assisted Reproductive Technology, *Clinical Summary Report*, 2013, https://www.sartcorsonline.com/rptCSR_PublicMultYear.aspx?ClinicPKID=0.

[11] M. Yusoff Dawood, "Laparoscopic surgery of the fallopian tubes ana ovaries," *Seminars in Laparoscopic Surgery*, vol. 6, no. 2, pp. 58–67, 1999.

3

SILC for SILC: Single Institution Learning Curve for Single-Incision Laparoscopic Cholecystectomy

Chee Wei Tay,[1] Liang Shen,[2] Mikael Hartman,[1,3,4] Shridhar Ganpathi Iyer,[1] Krishnakumar Madhavan,[1] and Stephen Kin Yong Chang[1]

[1] *Department of Surgery, Division of Hepatobiliary and Pancreatic Surgery, National University Health System, Singapore 119228*
[2] *Division of Biostatistics, Yong Loo Lin School of Medicine, National University of Singapore, Singapore 119228*
[3] *Department of Medical Epidemiology and Biostatistics, Karolinska Institute, 17177 Stockholm, Sweden*
[4] *Saw Swee Hock School of Public Health, National University of Singapore, Singapore 117597*

Correspondence should be addressed to Stephen Kin Yong Chang; cfscky@nus.edu.sg

Academic Editor: Peng Hui Wang

Objectives. We report the single-incision laparoscopic cholecystectomy (SILC) learning experience of 2 hepatobiliary surgeons and the factors that could influence the learning curve of SILC. *Methods.* Patients who underwent SILC by Surgeons A and B were studied retrospectively. Operating time, conversion rate, reason for conversion, identity of first assistants, and their experience with previous laparoscopic cholecystectomy (LC) were analysed. CUSUM analysis is used to identify learning curve. *Results.* Hundred and nineteen SILC cases were performed by Surgeons A and B, respectively. Eight cases required additional port. In CUSUM analysis, most conversion occurred during the first 19 cases. Operating time was significantly lower (62.5 versus 90.6 min, $P = 0.04$) after the learning curve has been overcome. Operating time decreases as the experience increases, especially Surgeon B. Most conversions are due to adhesion at Calot's triangle. Acute cholecystitis, patients' BMI, and previous surgery do not seem to influence conversion rate. Mean operating times of cases assisted by first assistant with and without LC experience were 48 and 74 minutes, respectively ($P = 0.004$). *Conclusion.* Nineteen cases are needed to overcome the learning curve of SILC. Team work, assistant with CLC experience, and appropriate equipment and technique are the important factors in performing SILC.

1. Introduction

Single-incision laparoscopic cholecystectomy (SILC) has been increasingly performed for benign gallbladder disease over the last few years with comparable operative results with conventional 4-port laparoscopic cholecystectomy (CLC). With results from randomized controlled trials (RCTs) [1–5] and series of publications [6–9] showing that SILC is equally safe, with no obvious additional scar and potentially have less postoperative pain and earlier return to daily activity [5], more surgeons are embarking on learning the technique.

As SILC is a new approach to gallbladder disease, many aspects of this new technique have not been studied in detail. Most surgeons embarking on this technique are concerned with its learning curve, conversions, and potential longer operating time. To date, very limited work has been done to look into this important issue and few publications have looked into learning curve of SILC from conversion point of view.

To perform SILC safely and successfully, there may be changes in surgical technique, need of new equipment, and modifications in the role of assistant.

In this study, we report an SILC learning experience of a tertiary university hospital with advanced laparoscopic facility. Operating time, potential problems, and ways to overcome them as well as surgical technique were included in this report. Our paper aims at facilitating and smoothening the learning curve of surgeons especially those who are starting to perform SILC or those facing difficulty in performing SILC.

2. Methods

All patients who underwent SILC from April 2009 to August 2011 (28 months) by two HPB attending surgeons (Surgeons

A and B) who both have been attending grade for more than 7 years and routinely performed laparoscopic cholecystectomy for all benign gallbladder disease in a tertiary university hospital were studied retrospectively. The unit performs about 400 laparoscopic cholecystectomies per year.

Operating time, conversion rate, and reason for conversion of individual surgeons were recorded. Conversion is defined as adding additional port(s) at other parts of the abdomen or minilaparotomy. Identity of first assistants was collected and analysed. Risk factors of conversion such as patient's BMI, presence of acute cholecystitis, and previous abdominal surgery were recorded and compared.

Cumulative summative (CUSUM) analysis is used to identify learning curve of SILC of Surgeon A, and standard conversion rate is defined as 5%. t-test is used to compare continuous variable, and $P < 0.05$ is defined as statistical significance. SPSS Statistics version 17.0 is used to analyse the data.

Operating time of all CLC done by Surgeon A at the same period of time was collected to establish the baseline operating time for comparison with SILC operating time of Surgeons A and B.

2.1. SILC Surgical Methods. All procedures were performed under general anaesthesia. The patients were placed at supine or split-leg (French) position depends on availability of different operating tables. Marcaine 0.25% is infiltrated around the umbilicus then a 1.5 cm vertical incision is made in the umbilicus, and SILS port (Covidien, Dublin, Ireland) is then inserted. A 5 mm 30° Endo-EYE surgical videoscope (Olympus, Tokyo, Japan) is used for visualization of the entire operation. Prolene suture with straight needle is introduced percutaneously at the right hypochondrium and is made to pierce the gallbladder at the seromuscular plane before exiting the peritoneal cavity at the right hypochondrium (Figure 1); care is taken not to pierce through the mucosa to prevent bile spillage. This serves as a retraction suture to facilitate the exposure of the Calot's triangle and subsequent dissection.

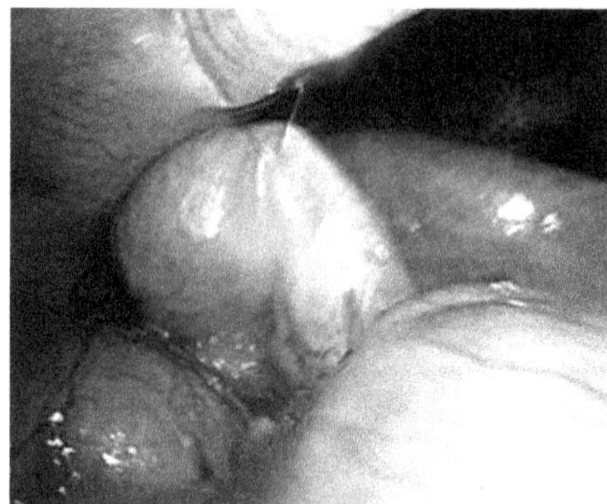

FIGURE 1: Hanging suture place at gallbladder fundus.

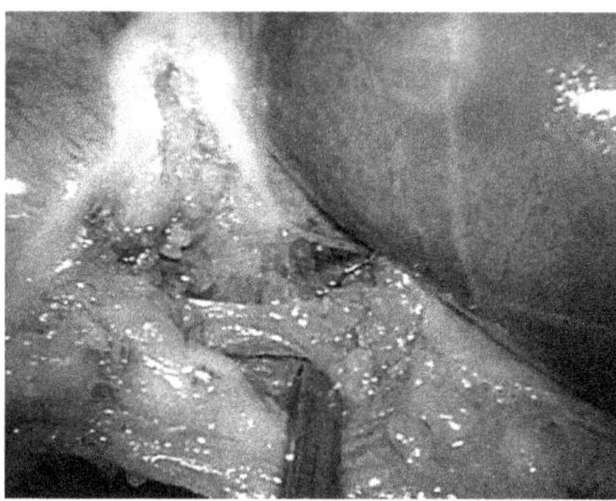

FIGURE 2: Articulating forcep used to retract Hartmann's pouch to expose Calot's triangle and critical view of safety is visualized.

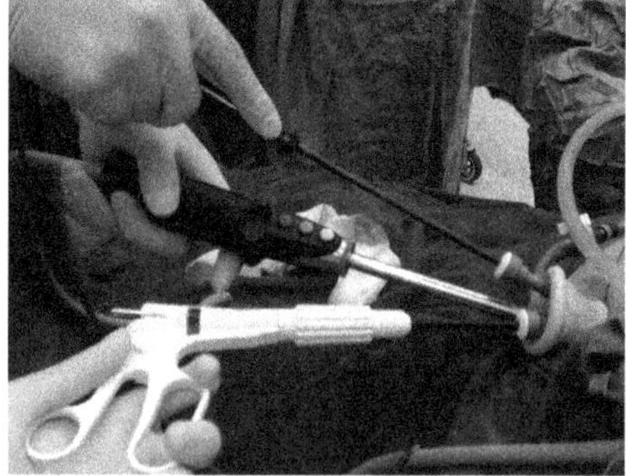

FIGURE 3: "Snooker cue guide" position.

An articulating endoforcep, Roticulator (Covidien, Dublin, Ireland), is introduced to provide lateral retraction of the gallbladder, and careful dissection to achieve critical view of safety is then completed (Figure 2).

Both the surgeon and the assistant will be on the patient's left if the patient is on supine position, whereas the operating surgeon will be standing between patient's legs and the assistant will be on the patient's left side if the patient is on split-leg position. The assistant would sit in front of the surgeon. In most parts of the surgery, he will be providing gentle lateral traction of the gallbladder by manipulating the Roticulator while the primary surgeon holds the EndoEYE and the dissecting instruments in the "snooker cue guide" position (Figure 3). This position allows the camera and the dissecting instrument to move in a coordinated fashion to ensure optimal visualization of the dissecting process which is critical in safely exposing the Calot's triangle to identify the cystic artery and duct. Five mm Hem-o-lock (Teleflex Medical, USA) clips are used to ligate both cystic artery and duct before they are divided between clips. Gallbladder is then placed into a self-constructed bag intracorporeally and removed from the abdominal cavity; fascia is closed with nonabsorbable suture in figure-of-eight fashion, and skin is closed subcuticularly.

3. Results

One hundred and nineteen patients who underwent SILC for their gallbladder diseases between April 2009 and August 2011 by 2 HPB consultants (Surgeons A and B) were retrospectively studied. One hundred and nineteen cases were performed by Surgeons A and B, respectively. 7 (5.8%) cases

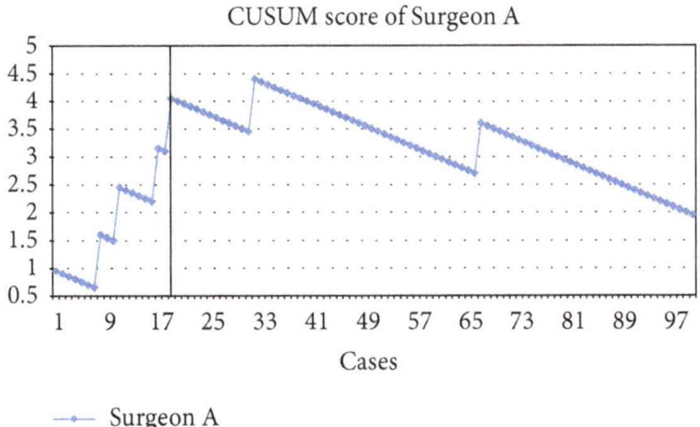

FIGURE 4: CUSUM analysis of learning curve of Surgeon A.

TABLE 1: Operative and patient profile of the first 19 cases of Surgeons A and B.

	Surgeon A	Surgeon B
Cases, *n*	19	19
Mean operative time, minutes (range, SD)	90.6 (43–135, 25.8)	124.3 (61–182, 34.1)
Conversion rate, *n* (%)	4 (21%)	2 (11%)
Acute cholecystitis, *n* (%)	3 (16%)	1 (5%)
Previous abdominal surgery, *n* (%)	3 (16%)	1 (5%)
Mean BMI (range, SD)	25.4 (19.2–36.0, 4.8)	22.4 (16.0–30.5, 4.0)

were acute cholecystitis and 75 cases (94.1%) were chronic cholecystitis. Diagnosis of gallbladder disease was achieved by clinical information and pre-op radiological investigations (ultrasound scan or CT scan). There were 8 cases (6.7%) that needed extra working port(s) to complete the procedure; no open conversion was needed in our experience.

3.1. Learning Curve of SILC. We defined acceptable conversion rate of SILC as 5% after learning curve is overcome as this is considered traditionally an acceptable conversion rate in CLC. Surgeons A and B had 6 (6%) and 2 (10.9%) conversions respectively. Figure 4 shows the CUSUM analysis of learning curve of Surgeon A; vertical line at the 19th case indicates the predicted minimal number of cases required to overcome the SILC learning curve. Surgeon B is excluded from CUSUM analysis in this study due to limited number of cases performed.

Most conversions of Surgeon A happened before the first 19 cases, and subsequently his learning curve reached a plateau except two conversions in the 32nd and 67th case. Surgeon B had two conversions in his 1st and 4th case. Most conversions were due to dense adhesion at the Calot's triangle and vital anatomical structures cannot be visualized clearly. One (5%) patient with previous abdominal surgery required conversion and one (5%) patient with active acute cholecystitis required conversion. Table 1 shows the operative and patient profile of the first 19 cases of Surgeons A and B. Table 2 shows the profile of cases that required conversion in the first 19 cases. When comparing cases which required conversion and cases which did not require conversion, there is no significant difference between patients (1) with previous, without previous, or on-going acute cholecystitis, (2) previous abdominal surgery, and (3) mean BMI. Table 3 demonstrates the comparison of potential risk factors between cases with and without conversion.

3.2. Operating Time. Surgeon A's mean operating time is significantly lower (62.5 minutes versus 90.6 minutes, $P = 0.04$) after he has overcome the learning curve. Conversion rates were lower as well (2.5% versus 21%, $P = 0.36$). Mean operating times, conversion rate, and patients' profile of Surgeons A before and after the first 19 cases is shown in Table 4.

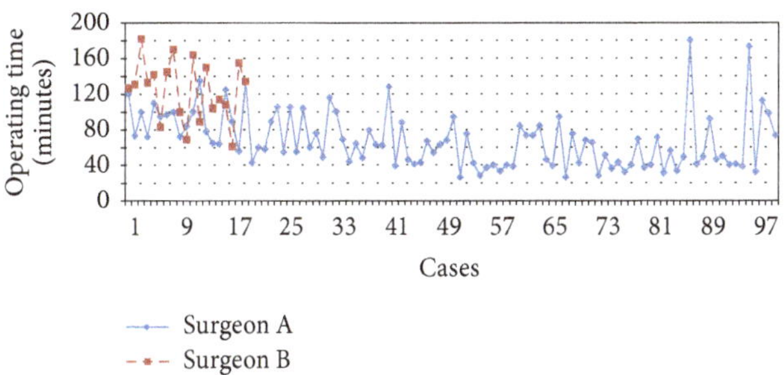

FIGURE 5: Operating times of Surgeons A and B.

Figure 5 demonstrates the operating times of Surgeons A and B as their experience increased. Figure 6 demonstrates the trend line of operating time of Surgeon A (dashed line) and B (dotted line). We found that the trend line of operating time of Surgeon B is steeper than Surgeon A, hence suggests that guidance from another surgeon who is experienced in SILC can facilitate the learning curve rapidly. Surgeon A SILC operating time trend line crosses his CLC operating time trend line (straight line) at the 82th case, which is suggestive of that SILC operating time may be faster than CLC eventually as the experience increases further.

We compared the 2 HPB fellows who have assisted in most of the SILC cases of Surgeon A in our institution, one who had previous CLC experience and the other without. We found that the mean operating time of cases assisted by the assistant with CLC experience is significantly shorter in comparison with cases assisted by the assistant without previous CLC experience (48 versus 74 minutes, $P = 0.004$). Mean operating time of cases assisted by the 2 assistants and the trend are demonstrated in Table 5 and Figure 7 respectively.

4. Discussion

4.1. Operating Time and Conversion. Our studies demonstrated that the operating time of SILC was more than 90 minutes at the beginning of both surgeons. Surgeon A was able to achieve mean operating time of below 60 minute after about 50 cases of SILC and his mean operating

TABLE 2: Profile of cases that required conversion in the first 19 cases.

Patient	Surgeon A/B	Reason	Types of conversion	Previous or on-going acute cholecystitis	Previous abdominal surgery	BMI (kg/m^2)	Operating time (minutes)
1	A	Bile leak from cystic duct	1 × additional 5 mm port	No	Yes	22.6	100
2	A	Dense adhesion at Calot's triangle	1 × additional 5 mm port	No	No	28.3	100
3	A	Acute cholecystitis with dense adhesion at Calot's triangle and gallbladder bed bleeding	2 × additional 5 mm ports	Yes	No	27.0	89
4	A	Gallbladder densely adherent to liver	2 × additional 5 mm ports	No	No	25.0	134
5	B	Dense adhesion at Calot's triangle	3 × additional 5 mm ports	No	No	29.8	127
6	B	Dense adhesion at Calot's triangle	2 × additional 5 mm ports	No	No	21.8	145

TABLE 3: Comparison of potential risk factors in cases with and without conversion.

	Cases required conversion	Cases did not require conversion	P
n	8	111	—
On-going or previous acute cholecystitis, n (%)	1 (13%)	9 (8%)	0.63
Previous abdominal surgery, n (%)	0 (0%)	6 (5%)	0.06
Mean BMI (range, SD)	25.8 (21.8–29.8, 3.2)	24.1 (17.5–36, 4.6)	0.13

TABLE 4: Mean operating times, conversion rate, and patients' profile of Surgeons A after the first 19 cases.

	Surgeon A's subsequent 81 cases	Surgeon A's first 19 cases	P
Cases, n	81	19	
Operative time, minutes (range, SD)	62.5 (26–180, 30.2)	90.6 (43–135, 25.8)	**0.04**
Conversion rate, n (%)	2 (2.5%)	4 (21%)	0.36

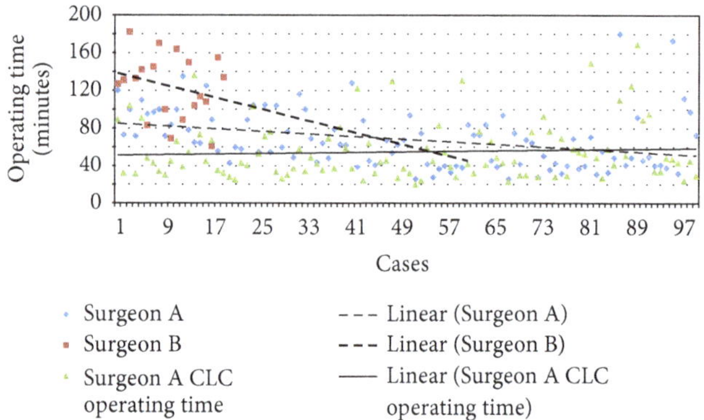

FIGURE 6: Trend lines of operating time of Surgeons A and B. Trend line of Surgeon B showed faster improvement in operating time with mentoring from Surgeon A.

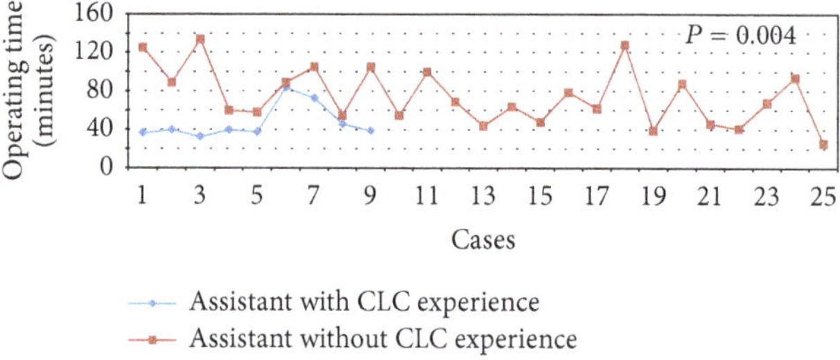

FIGURE 7: Operating time of cases assisted by assistants with and without CLC experience.

time continues to decrease to 37 minutes after 60 cases. Antoniou et al. [10] reported that the mean operative time was 70.2 minutes in a systemic review which involved 29 studies with 1166 patients. However, most of the studies included were the early experiences of surgeon performing SILC in their individual centres. In comparison, our studies showed that mean operative time continues to decrease as experiences increase after the learning curve is overcome. Other publications [11–13] that looked into SILC operative time and learning curve reported a mean operative time between 46.9 minutes and 80 minutes. Hernandez et al. [11] found that mean operative time was reduced significantly after 75 cases of SILC and was not significantly longer than mean operative time of CLC. Our institution showed similar studies data. Qiu et al. [12] reported a much shorter mean operative time of 46.9 minutes with no conversion in their highly selected 80 patients, all of whom have minimal sign of gallbladder inflammation and no surgical history of the right upper quadrant of abdomen. They were able to perform SILC with mean operative time of below 40 minutes after 40 cases. Joseph et al. [14] concluded that surgical trainees who were proficient in CLC had significant reduction in operative time along their learning curve. Recently published RCTs [1–5] reported mean operative time between 46 minutes and 88 minutes with 3 studies [1, 2, 4] which showed significant longer operative time of SILC; however, these RCTs did not

TABLE 5: Mean operating time of cases assisted by assistants with and without CLC experience.

	Mean operating time (minute)	Max (minute)	Min (minute)	SD (±)	P
Assistant with CLC experience	48	84	33	18	**0.004**
Assistant without CLC experience	74	134	26	29	

specify the surgeons' previous CLC and SILC experience and all of them did not include patients with acute cholecystitis.

There were 8 (6.7%) cases in our studies which required additional port(s) to aid dissection of the Calot's triangle due to dense adhesion at the area; no open conversion or laparotomy was needed in our studies. Four (80%) out of the 5 conversions of Surgeon A happened before his first 20 cases. Surgeon B had two conversions at his 1st and 7th case. The systemic review published by Antoniou et al. [10] reported a conversion (additional ports required) rate of 9.3% and an open conversion rate of 0.4%. Most common conversion reason that was reported was an obscured anatomy of the Calot's triangle due to adhesions, acute or chronic inflammation (71.1%). Seven out of 8 (87%) of our conversions were due to severe adhesions at the Calot's triangle as well. In conclusion, our study was found to have very similar rate and reason of conversion with Antoniou's study [10].

One of our conversions was associated with previous abdominal surgery. However, the reason for inserting an additional port was to place a clip at a leaking cystic duct. Hence, we do not think that the previous abdominal surgery has any significance on this conversion. In another conversion which was associated with an on-going acute cholecystitis, two additional ports were added to provide retraction for adequate visualization as well as to secure haemostasis from the liver bed. We performed SILC on 4 other cases of acute cholecystitis with no significant issues.

In our center, Surgeon A was the first HPB surgeon who adopted SILC into his routine treatment option for gallbladder diseases, followed by Surgeon B. From our CUSUM analysis, Surgeon B had less conversion in the early stages of his SILC learning curve in comparison to Surgeon A. Hence, we deduced that during the process of pioneering this new surgical technique in our center, Surgeon A inevitably had more conversions than other surgeons in the center before his learning curve was overcome.

Once the expertise is shared among other surgeons, we would expect less conversion and smoother learning curve in the subsequent cases. This phenomenon was demonstrated in the steeper trend line of operating time of Surgeon B, after Surgeon A has overcome his learning curve of SILC. With less skin incisions in SILC hence less closure time, we believe the operating time could be faster than CLC eventually as the experience increases, as shown in our results.

Analyzing the CUSUM, significantly less conversion was experienced after the 19th case; we therefore conclude that surgeons who routinely perform CLC for gallbladder diseases need about 19 cases to overcome SILC learning curve.

4.2. Assistant Factor. In the beginning phase of adopting new surgical technique or equipment in our center, we found that there are always benefits if the same group of surgeons and nurses can provide feedbacks among themselves to hasten the learning process.

We compared the operating times with 2 HPB fellows as assistants; one routinely performs CLC in her practice and one was new to CLC; both were new to SILC. We found that there was significant shorter mean operating time in cases that were assisted by the fellow who was familiar with CLC. SILC is a procedure that requires advanced laparoscopic skills. In addition, the surgeon and his/her assistant must be able to work closely with each other in a more limited space without colliding their instruments against each other. In addition, having CLC experience prior to assisting SILC is an invaluable advantage. Qiu et al. [12] and Solomon et al. [13] both had similar learning experience, and hence they encouraged surgeons to work with skilled assistant and obtaining preceptorship in order to overcome one's SILC learning curve.

We also encouraged other surgeons to record a video of all their SILC cases, and subsequently watch the video together with their assistant, with the aim of identifying weaknesses and mistakes and avoid them in subsequent cases.

4.3. Technique and Equipment Issues. In SILC, all surgical equipment is introduced from the umbilical port site. Manipulation of the instruments intra- and extracorporeally is thus very challenging due to the limited working space and loss of the traditional laparoscopic triangulation. We started our SILC practice with SILS port as intraperitoneal access, it accommodates all working instruments, insufflation and camera port, and is inserted through a single fascial defect. This port does increase the cost of surgery, however in our experience, there is no significant surgical or technical problems caused by the port, and we continued to improve our operating time and conversion rate with the help of this port; therefore, it remains as the port of choice for intraperitoneal access.

In order to overcome the loss of laparoscopic triangulation, we utilized the Roticulator forceps, which is held by the first assistant, who sits at the right side of the surgeon. The forceps provide lateral retraction of the gallbladder to facilitate the dissection of Calot's triangle. We realized that with SILS surgery, especially in someone who just started performing SILS surgery, loss of conventional triangulation in manipulating the instruments and loss of working space can be frustrating to the surgeons and dangerous to the patients; we recommend surgeons who are new to SILC to use articulating or prebend instruments to facilitate the surgery in the first few cases of SILC, and with the increased experience in SILC, they can make a choice to continue in using these instrument or switch to conventional laparoscopic instruments. Again, these articulating or pre-bend instruments add extra cost to the patients; however, in view of the advantages mentioned above, we believe it has an important role in SILC, especially in those surgeons who are new to SILC.

The other equipment which we found to be of value is the Olympus Endoeye, which is a very compact and highly manipulable laparoscopic camera that provides adequate visualization for the scope of SILC surgery without occupying much space.

We routinely used extracorporeal hanging suture to enhance the visualization of SILC. In this way, 2 instruments can actively be used in performing the surgery. We manipulate the straight needle laparoscopically and pierce the thickest part of the gallbladder at the seromuscular layer, to prevent bile spillage; so far, there is no issue in all the cases we performed in this series. In addition, hanging suture has been shown to reduce complication rates in comparison with instrumental anchorage [10] (3.3% versus 13.3%, $P < 0.0001$).

Port site hernia has been a concern in SILC due to the bigger umbilical fascial defect if compared to CLC, a 52-patient retrospective study [15] published a port site hernia rate of SILC of 5.8%. Multiple up-to-date meta-analysis [16–18] has not shown significant increase in port site hernia so far; the majority of the RCTs performed up-to-date utilized commercialized umbilical access port, and these studies are limited with their short follow-up period. Goel and Lomanto [19] concluded in their review that port site hernia in single-incision laparoscopic surgery can be minimized with good suture closure of the fascial defect. We close all umbilical fascial defects with 1 or 2 figure-of-eight sutures; there is no umbilical hernia detected in this series of patients during followup.

4.4. Patient Selection. Patients with risk factors such as previous abdominal surgery, history of acute cholecystitis or on-going cholecystitis and obese patient were thought to have higher chance of conversion in SILC [10]. However in our experience, all of our patients who needed conversion to CLC, did not evidently presented with the above risk factors. In fact, the most common reason for conversion was dense adhesions and failure to identify vital structures due to poor visualization. Patients with the above risk factors are shown to increase operative time [12], therefore we suggest selecting patients sensibly at the early stage of performing SILC. Once our learning curve has been overcome, we were able to perform SILC in majority of the gallbladder condition in the general patient population with minimal conversion rate.

5. Conclusion

Single-incision laparoscopic cholecystectomy is a safe and feasible procedure. Nineteen cases were needed to overcome the learning curve in our experience. Comparable conversion rate and operating time with conventional laparoscopic cholecystectomy were observed after learning curve has been overcome. Team work, careful patient selection, assistant with conventional laparoscopic cholecystectomy experiences, and appropriate equipment and technique are important factors at the beginning stage of performing SILC.

Abbreviations

SILC: Single-incision laparoscopic cholecystectomy
CLC: Conventional laparoscopic cholecystectomy
RCT: Randomized controlled trial
HPB: Hepatopancreatobiliary
CT: Computer tomography
CUSUM: Cumulative summative
SD: Standard deviation
BMI: Body mass index.

References

[1] J. Marks, R. Tacchino, K. Roberts et al., "Prospective randomized controlled trial of traditional laparoscopic cholecystectomy versus single-incision laparoscopic cholecystectomy: report of preliminary data," *American Journal of Surgery*, vol. 201, no. 3, pp. 369–373, 2011.

[2] J. Ma, M. A. Cassera, G. O. Spaun, C. W. Hammill, P. D. Hansen, and S. Aliabadi-Wahle, "Randomized controlled trial comparing single-port laparoscopic cholecystectomy and four-port laparoscopic cholecystectomy," *Annals of Surgery*, vol. 254, no. 1, pp. 22–27, 2011.

[3] P. Bucher, F. Pugin, N. C. Buchs, S. Ostermann, and P. Morel, "Randomized clinical trial of laparoendoscopic single-site versus conventional laparoscopic cholecystectomy," *British Journal of Surgery*, vol. 98, pp. 1695–1702, 2011.

[4] M. M. Lirici, A. D. Califano, P. Angelini, and F. Corcione, "Laparo-endoscopic single site cholecystectomy versus standard laparoscopic cholecystectomy: results of a pilot randomized trial," *American Journal of Surgery*, vol. 202, no. 1, pp. 45–52, 2011.

[5] E. C. H. Lai, G. P. C. Yang, C. N. Tang, P. C. L. Yih, O. C. Y. Chan, and M. K. W. Li, "Prospective randomized comparative study of single incision laparoscopic cholecystectomy versus conventional four-port laparoscopic cholecystectomy," *The Amedican Journal of Surgery*, vol. 202, pp. 254–258, 2011.

[6] P. P. Rao, S. M. Bhagwat, A. Rane, and P. P. Rao, "The feasibility of single port laparoscopic cholecystectomy: a pilot study of 20 cases," *HPB*, vol. 10, no. 5, pp. 336–340, 2008.

[7] R. Tacchino, F. Greco, and D. Matera, "Single-incision laparoscopic cholecystectomy: surgery without a visible scar," *Surgical Endoscopy and Other Interventional Techniques*, vol. 23, no. 4, pp. 896–899, 2009.

[8] J. M. Hernandez, C. A. Morton, S. Ross, M. Albrink, and A. S. Rosemurgy, "Laparoendoscopic single site cholecystectomy: the first 100 patients," *American Surgeon*, vol. 75, no. 8, pp. 681–685, 2009.

[9] S. K. Y. Chang, C. W. Tay, R. A. Bicol, Y. Y. Lee, and K. Madhavan, "A case-control study of single-incision versus standard laparoscopic cholecystectomy," *World Journal of Surgery*, vol. 35, no. 2, pp. 289–293, 2011.

[10] S. A. Antoniou, R. Pointner, and F. A. Granderath, "Single-incision laparoscopic cholecystectomy: a systematic review," *Surgical Endoscopy and Other Interventional Techniques*, vol. 25, no. 2, pp. 367–377, 2011.

[11] J. Hernandez, S. Ross, C. Morton et al., "The learning curve of laparoendoscopic single-site (LESS) cholecystectomy: definable, short, and safe," *Journal of the American College of Surgeons*, vol. 211, no. 5, pp. 652–657, 2010.

[12] Z. Qiu, J. Sun, Y. Pu, T. Jiang, J. Cao, and W. Wu, "Learning curve of transumbilical single incision laparoscopic cholecystectomy (SILS): a preliminary study of 80 selected patients with benign gallbladder diseases," *World Journal of Surgery*, vol. 35, pp. 2092–2101, 2011.

[13] D. Solomon, R. L. Bell, A. J. Duffy, and K. E. Roberts, "Single-port cholecystectomy: small scar, short learning curve," *Surgical Endoscopy and Other Interventional Techniques*, vol. 24, no. 12, pp. 2954–2957, 2010.

[14] M. Joseph, M. Phillips, and C. C. Rupp, "Single-incision laparoscopic cholecystectomy: a combine analysis of resident and attending learning curves at a single institution," *The American Surgeons*, vol. 78, no. 1, pp. 119–124, 2012.

[15] H. Alptekin, H. Yilmaz, F. Acar, M. Kafali, and M. Sahin, "Incisional hernia rate may increase after single-port cholecystectomy," *Journal of Laparoendoscopic & Advance Surgical Techniques*, vol. 22, no. 8, pp. 731–737, 2012.

[16] S. Trastulli, R. Cirocchi, J. Desiderio et al., "Systematic review and meta-analysis of randomized clinical trials comparing single-incision versus conventional laparoscopic cholecystectomy," *British Journal of Surgery*, vol. 100, pp. 191–208, 2013.

[17] A. Pisanu, I. Reccia, G. Porceddu, and A. Uccheddu, "Meta-analysis of prospective randomized studies comparing single-incision laparoscopic cholecystectomy (SILC) and conventional multiport laparoscopic cholecystectomy (CMLC)," *Journal of Gastrointestinal Surgery*, vol. 16, pp. 1790–1801, 2012.

[18] P. Garg, J. D. Thakur, M. Garg, and G. R. Menon, "Single-incision laparoscopic cholecystectomy versus conventional laparoscopic cholecystectomy: a meta-analysis of randomized controlled trials," *Journal of Gastrointestinal Surgery*, vol. 16, pp. 1618–1628, 2012.

[19] R. Goel and D. Lomanto, "Controversies in single-port laparoscopic surgery," *Surgery in Laparoscopic, Endoscopic and Percutaneous Technology*, vol. 22, pp. 380–382, 2012.

4

Stability Outcomes following Computer-Assisted ACL Reconstruction

Melissa A. Christino,[1] Bryan G. Vopat,[2] Alexander Mayer,[3] Andrew P. Matson,[4] Steven E. Reinert,[5] and Robert M. Shalvoy[3]

[1]*Division of Sports Medicine, Boston Children's Hospital, Boston, MA 02215, USA*
[2]*Department of Orthopaedic Surgery, Massachusetts General Hospital, Boston, MA 02114, USA*
[3]*Department of Orthopaedic Surgery, Rhode Island Hospital, Brown University, Providence, RI 02903, USA*
[4]*Department of Orthopaedic Surgery, Duke University Medical Center, Durham, NC 27710, USA*
[5]*Department of Information Services, Rhode Island Hospital, Lifespan, Providence, RI 02903, USA*

Correspondence should be addressed to Melissa A. Christino; melissa.christino@childrens.harvard.edu

Academic Editor: Peng Hui Wang

Purpose. The purpose of this study was to determine whether intraoperative prereconstruction stability measurements and/or patient characteristics were associated with final knee stability after computer-assisted ACL reconstruction. *Methods.* This was a retrospective review of all patients who underwent computer-assisted single-bundle ACL reconstruction by a single surgeon. Prereconstruction intraoperative stability measurements were correlated with patient characteristics and postreconstruction stability measurements. 143 patients were included (87 male and 56 female). Average age was 29.8 years (SD ± 11.8). *Results.* Females were found to have significantly more pre- and postreconstruction internal rotation than males ($P < 0.001$ and $P = 0.001$, resp.). Patients with additional intra-articular injuries demonstrated more prereconstruction anterior instability than patients with isolated ACL tears ($P < 0.001$). After reconstruction, these patients also had higher residual anterior translation ($P = 0.01$). Among all patients with ACL reconstructions, the percent of correction of anterior translation was found to be significantly higher than the percent of correction for internal or external rotation ($P < 0.001$). *Conclusion.* Anterior translation was corrected the most using a single-bundle ACL reconstruction. Females had higher pre- and postoperative internal rotation. Patients with additional injuries had greater original anterior translation and less operative correction of anterior translation compared to patients with isolated ACL tears.

1. Introduction

Anterior cruciate ligament (ACL) reconstruction surgery is common, with approximately 125,000–175,000 procedures performed annually in the United States [1, 2]. Despite the large number of ACL reconstructions performed, the success rate of this procedure lags behind those of other common orthopedic procedures, and optimizing surgical technique to minimize failures has been the focus of the majority of ACL research.

Individual factors that have been associated with higher rates of failure after ACL reconstruction include younger age [3], higher activity level [4], female gender [5, 6], and ligamentous laxity [7, 8]. Additionally, injury factors such as mechanism of injury and concomitant lesions of the meniscus and articular cartilage have been shown to predict worse long term outcomes [9–11]. Historically, subclassification of ligamentous knee injuries has improved the accuracy of diagnoses and enabled treatments to be tailored toward specific injuries [12]. The fact that outcome has been shown to be associated with patient and injury specific factors suggests ACL injuries are not all the same and that patients may benefit from individualized treatment.

Computer navigation is increasingly being used in orthopaedic surgical procedures. In ACL reconstruction surgery, it has been shown to improve accuracy of bone tunnel placement [13–16]. It has also been shown to reliably obtain quantitative intraoperative measurements of knee stability [17, 18]. Many kinematic studies utilizing computer navigation have compared stability outcomes of single-bundle versus double-bundle techniques [19–26]. Others have described translational and rotational stability characteristics in cadaver and in vivo studies [27–29].

Few studies have specifically sought to define injury instability or have investigated the amount of translational and rotational correction that can be achieved using computer-assisted ACL reconstruction techniques. Evaluating the quantitative kinematics of the knee after injury as well as the changes that occur with reconstruction may provide valuable insight into the management of ACL injuries and could influence surgical decision making. Ohkawa et al. demonstrated that preoperative AP and rotational laxity varied among patients and suggested that postoperative stabilization may vary as well [29]. However, they did not stratify these differences by patient characteristics or additional injuries. The purpose of this study was to determine whether intraoperative prereconstruction stability measurements and/or patient characteristics were associated with final stability results after computer-assisted ACL reconstruction. It was hypothesized that preoperative rotational and translational stability would predict postoperative stability and that patient characteristics and concomitant intra-articular knee injuries would be associated with more pre- and postoperative instability.

2. Materials and Methods

This study was a retrospective review of all patients who underwent computer-assisted primary single-bundle ACL reconstruction by a single surgeon from 2007 to 2012. Exclusion criteria included revision surgeries and those patients with incomplete intraoperative data.

All patients had computer-navigated ACL reconstructions using the Aesculap 2.0 Ortho Pilot Navigation System (B. Braun Aesculap, Tuttlingen, Germany). Intraoperative pre- and post-ACL reconstruction stability measurements were collected; anterior translation, internal rotation, and external rotation were measured at 30 degrees of knee flexion (see Section 3).

Patient charts were reviewed for this intraoperative stability data as well as for relevant surgical details (graft type, fixation) as well as patient characteristics (age, gender, and associated injuries).

One hundred eighty-seven anterior cruciate ligament reconstructions were performed by a single surgeon between January 2007 and January 2012. Twenty-two were revision surgeries and were excluded from data analysis, and an additional 22 patients were excluded due to incomplete charts or documented problems with intraoperative stability measurements. Thus 143 patients with primary ACL reconstructions were included for analysis.

Preoperative rotational and translational stability was compared to postoperative stability, and stability data was compared between various patient and injury characteristics. Statistical analysis was performed using Pearson's correlation coefficients, t-tests, and ANOVAs. Significance was set at $P < 0.05$ *a priori*.

3. Surgical Technique

All surgical ACL reconstructions were performed under general anesthesia with a tourniquet applied to the proximal thigh. The tourniquet was inflated for all patellar tendon graft reconstructions but not for hamstring or allograft (soft tissue) reconstructions. A diagnostic arthroscopy was performed with a 30-degree arthroscope. If present, all meniscal pathology was addressed with meniscal repair or partial meniscectomy prior to reconstruction. A modest notchplasty was performed if the notch was stenotic, and the ligament remnants were debrided to their footprints on the tibia and the femur.

For hamstring graft reconstructions, the gracilis and semitendinosus tendons were harvested prior to diagnostic arthroscopy, prepared, and doubled to create a quadrupled tendon graft construct. For patellar tendon graft reconstructions, the tourniquet was inflated after diagnostic arthroscopy and a 10 mm central strip of tendon harvested. A 20 mm bone plug was harvested from the inferior pole of the patella in line with the tendon graft and a similar 25 mm bone plug harvested from the tibial tubercle.

For all surgeries, the 2.0 Ortho Pilot (B. Braun Aesculap, Tuttlingen, Germany) Computer Navigation System was used to calculate knee kinematics before and after reconstruction. Tibial and femoral transmitters were applied with two 2.5 smooth K-wires each (Figure 1). Intra-articular and extra-articular landmarks were registered and kinematic acquisition was achieved by ranging the knee from 0 to 90 degrees of flexion. The knee was secured manually on a semirigid bolster with the knee at 30 degrees of flexion, which is the standard position for the Lachman examination of the ACL. Stability testing was performed by the senior surgeon in all cases. Maximum manual AP stress was applied to the posterior calf for three trials (Figure 1(a)), and the resulting values of AP translation, external rotation, and internal rotation were recorded for this maneuver. Maximum manual internal rotation (IR) was then applied to the foot for three trials (Figure 1(b)), and associated values of AP translation, external, and internal rotation were recorded. Maximum manual external rotation (ER) was also applied to the foot for three trials, and corresponding AP translation, external rotation, and internal rotation were again recorded (Figure 1(c)).

Computer navigation and arthroscopic visualization were used to identify anatomic tibial and femoral tunnel placement and avoid graft impingement. Soft tissue grafts were fixed by 9-10 Intrafix devices (DePuy Mitek, Raynham, MA) on the femur and 8–10 Intrafix (Depuy Mitek, Raynham, MA) devices on the tibia. Patellar tendon grafts were fixed with Biosure HA interference screws (Smith & Nephew, Andover, MA) on the femur and tibia.

With graft fixation completed, stability testing was repeated and documented in the same manner as previously described.

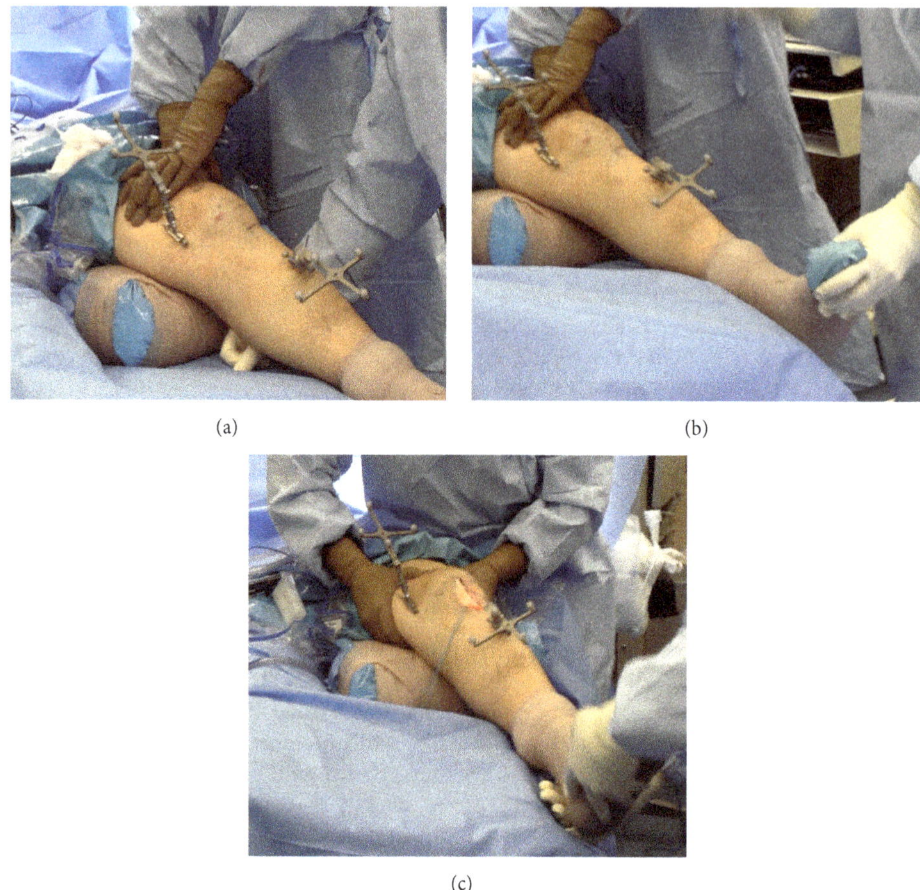

FIGURE 1: Intraoperative photographs showing positioning of the femoral and tibial navigation transmitters and demonstrating the stability testing maneuvers: anterior translation (a), internal rotation (b), and external rotation (c).

4. Results

A summary of patient demographics, injury characteristics, and type of ACL reconstructions can be seen in Table 1. The five most common mechanisms of injury were soccer (23), nonspecified sports (18), nontraumatic injuries (18) such as falls or twists while standing, skiing (14), and basketball (14).

The average pre- and postreconstruction anterior drawer, internal rotation, external rotation, and the percent of correction for each of these values can be seen in Table 2. There were no significant correlations found between prereconstruction rotation measurements and either the pre- or postreconstruction anterior drawer. When total rotation was calculated by adding maximum external and internal rotation, total rotation had a weak but significant correlation with prereconstruction anterior drawer ($r = 0.27$, $P = 0.001$).

The average percent of correction between pre- and postreconstruction anterior drawer was significantly higher than the percent of correction for pre- and postreconstruction internal rotation ($P < 0.001$) and external rotation ($P < 0.001$). The percent of correction for internal rotation was also significantly higher than the percent of external rotation correction ($P < 0.001$). Postreconstruction total rotation was found to be significantly less than prereconstruction total rotation (29.3 degrees versus 38.9 degrees, $P < 0.001$).

When examining stability data by gender, there were no statistically significant differences in prereconstruction anterior drawer or external rotation, but females had significantly more prereconstruction internal rotation than males (24.1 degrees versus 20.4 degrees, $P < 0.001$). Females were also found to have significantly higher total rotation numbers before reconstruction when compared to males (41.3 degrees versus 37.4 degrees, $P < 0.001$). Looking at postreconstruction measurements, females continued to have significantly higher internal rotation values than males (16.8 degrees versus 13.7 degrees, $P = 0.001$) as well as total rotation (30.9 degrees versus 28.2 degrees, $P = 0.002$). Table 3 summarizes these results.

Seventy-one patients (49.7%) had additional intra-articular injuries in addition to an ACL tear, and these included meniscal tears, chondral injuries, and capsular tears. Sixty-six (92.3%) of these patients had at least 1 meniscal tear, and the breakdown of injuries can be seen in Table 4. Patients with additional intra-articular injuries showed more anterior instability before reconstruction than patients with isolated ACL tears (15.7 mm versus 13.3 mm, $P < 0.001$), although there were no significant differences in rotation. After reconstruction, patients with additional injuries had statistically higher residual anterior drawer measurements than those with isolated ACL tears (5.2 mm versus 4.4 mm, $P = 0.01$).

Table 1: Patient demographics, injury characteristics, and type of ACL reconstructions.

Patient characteristics	
Total number of patients	143
Gender	
Male	87 (60.8%)
Female	56 (39.2%)
Average age in years (SD)	29.8 (±11.8)
Injury characteristics	
Knee affected:	
Right	71 (49.7%)
Left	72 (50.3%)
Isolated ACL tear	72 (50.3%)
ACL tear with additional intra-articular injuries	71 (49.7%)
Type of ACL reconstruction	
Hamstring autograft	63 (44.1%)
Patellar tendon autograft	54 (37.8%)
Allograft	24 (16.8%)
Combination of hamstring autograft with allograft augmentation	2 (1.4%)

Table 2: Pre- and postreconstruction stability measurements.

	Prereconstruction	Postreconstruction	Percent of correction
Anterior drawer mm (SD)	14.47 (±3.41)	4.80 (±2.05)	65.7% (±15.4%)
Internal rotation degrees (SD)	21.86 (±4.37)	14.99 (±4.39)	31.3% (±17.1%)
External rotation degrees (SD)	17.08 (±3.80)	14.29 (±3.52)	15.2% (±19.2%)

There were no significant differences in postreconstruction anterior translation or rotational stability measurements among the different graft types used.

5. Discussion

This is the largest series reporting intraoperative knee stability following ACL reconstruction and comparing patient and injury characteristics with computer-navigated stability data. Our study found that anterior translation was corrected more than rotation using a single-bundle reconstruction. Women were also found to have more pre- and residual postreconstruction internal rotation than men, and patients with additional intra-articular injuries had more anterior laxity both before and after reconstruction. These results suggest that subtleties exist among ACL injuries and future research needs to be done to account for individual variability related to rotation, gender, and associated injuries.

Using computer navigation for ACL reconstructions has not been shown to improve knee stability or functional outcomes in patients compared to conventional ACL reconstructions [30]. However, the value of computer navigation may lie in the ability to define and identify subtleties among injuries. Quantitatively defining injury characteristics of ACL tears and their subsequent repairs may play an important role in guiding treatment and surgical decision making. Reporting these findings may be an important first step in trying to stratify differences seen in patients and injury patterns immediately affecting pre- and postoperative stability.

Ohkawa et al. demonstrated that preoperative AP and rotational laxity varied among patients and suggested that postoperative stabilization may vary as well [29]. However, they did not stratify these differences by patient characteristics or additional injuries. Our study demonstrated that females had greater internal rotation and patients with additional intra-articular injuries had greater anterior laxity. The clinical significance of these findings has yet to be elucidated, but these patients may be considered for adjunct procedures or perhaps double-bundle reconstruction techniques, which have been proposed to control for rotation more than single-bundle reconstructions [31–33].

A recent retrospective review of 55 patients with computer-navigated ACL reconstructions found that double-bundle reconstruction had significantly greater rotational stability than single-bundle reconstructions [34]. However, female patients who had computer-navigated double-bundle ACL reconstructions had significantly worse outcome scores at 2 years than males. In this study, they also reported higher preoperative internal rotation values for females who had either single- or double-bundle reconstructions compared to males but found no difference postoperatively. This is similar to our study; however we also found increased internal rotation in women immediately postoperatively using a single-bundle reconstruction. Females have been found to have more ligamentous laxity in general when compared to males [8], and the rotational stability differences identified in this study support the idea that unique anatomic and physiologic differences may exist between sexes, and they should be taken into account with surgical decision making and management of ACL injuries.

Similarly, our study suggests that isolated ACL tears may behave differently than tears with associated additional intra-articular pathology. We showed that patients with at least one additional intra-articular injury had higher pre- as well as postreconstruction anterior translation compared to isolated ACL tears. Logically, a more severe injury would be more unstable. The menisci, capsular structures, and collateral ligaments all contribute to providing inherent stability to the knee, so it is not surprising that if these are also injured, the knee may be more unstable initially and more difficult to stabilize. Particularly if injured meniscal tissue needs to be resected with partial meniscectomy, as was the case for most of our meniscal tears, this may negatively contribute to final stability of the knee. More significant injuries may require more rigorous stabilization techniques, but the intricacies of complex injury patterns need to be further evaluated for their

Table 3: Gender differences pre- and postreconstruction.

	Prereconstruction		Postreconstruction	
	Male	Female	Male	Female
Anterior drawer mm (SD)	14.47 (±3.01)	14.4 (±3.67)	5.02 (±2.15)	4.45 (±1.86)
Internal rotation degrees (SD)	*20.45 (±4.15)	*24.05 (±3.79)	*13.86 (±4.2)	*16.75 (±4.11)
External rotation degrees (SD)	17 (±4.09)	17.21 (±3.34)	14.39 (±3.21)	14.13 (±3.97)
Total rotation degrees (SD)	*37.45 (±5.2)	*41.27 (±4.77)	*28.25 (±4.6)	*30.89 (±5.49)

*denotes significance with $P < 0.05$.

Table 4: Distribution of additional intra-articular injuries.

Additional intra-articular injuries ($n = 71$)	Number	Percentage
Isolated medial meniscus tear	27	38.0%
Isolated lateral meniscus tear	25	35.2%
Combined medial and lateral meniscal tears	8	11.3%
MCL tear (2 also with medial capsular tears)	4	5.6%
Medial meniscus tear with chondral injury	2	2.8%
Lateral meniscal tear with chondral injury	1	1.4%
Lateral meniscal tear with medial capsular tear	1	1.4%
Combined medial and lateral meniscal tears with chondral injury	1	1.4%
Combined medial and lateral meniscal tears with medial capsular injury	1	1.4%
Isolated medial capsular tear	1	1.4%

clinical significance and impact on the overall stability of the knee during ACL reconstruction.

There were limitations to this study. First, the study was retrospective in nature. Second, some patients had to be excluded due to incomplete medical records, and their data was thus not included in the analysis. Third, while surgical technique was performed by the same surgeon in a systematic standardized way, the possibility exists for error in obtaining navigation measurements as manual stress was applied in conjunction with automated measurements. Last, only intraoperative knee stability was assessed, and initial stability may not predict the final stability after healing and in the clinical setting [29]. However, our focus was to define initial injury and reconstruction characteristics using computer navigation. Follow-up evaluation of knee stability and outcome measures were beyond the scope of the current study, but they should be evaluated in the future.

6. Conclusions

Anterior translation was found to have the most correction using a single-bundle ACL reconstruction. Females were found to have higher pre- and postoperative internal rotation. Patients with additional intra-articular knee injuries had greater original anterior translation and less operative correction of anterior translation when compared to patients with isolated ACL tears.

Consent

Patients were exempt from the informed consent process due to the retrospective nature of the study.

References

[1] S. Kim, J. Bosque, J. P. Meehan, A. Jamali, and R. Marder, "Increase in outpatient knee arthroscopy in the United States: a comparison of national surveys of ambulatory surgery, 1996 and 2006," *The Journal of Bone & Joint Surgery Series A*, vol. 93, no. 11, pp. 994–1000, 2011.

[2] K. P. Spindler and R. W. Wright, "Clinical practice: anterior cruciate ligament tear," *The New England Journal of Medicine*, vol. 359, no. 20, pp. 2135–2142, 2008.

[3] A. M. Barrett, J. A. Craft, W. H. Replogle, J. M. Hydrick, and G. R. Barrett, "Anterior cruciate ligament graft failure: a comparison of graft type based on age and tegner activity level," *The American Journal of Sports Medicine*, vol. 39, no. 10, pp. 2194–2198, 2011.

[4] J. R. Borchers, A. Pedroza, and C. Kaeding, "Activity level and graft type as risk factors for anterior cruciate ligament graft failure: a case-control study," *The American Journal of Sports Medicine*, vol. 37, no. 12, pp. 2362–2367, 2009.

[5] F. K. Noojin, G. R. Barrett, C. W. Hartzog, and C. R. Nash, "Clinical comparison of intraarticular anterior cruciate ligament reconstruction using autogenous semitendinosus and gracilis tendons in men versus women," *The American Journal of Sports Medicine*, vol. 28, no. 6, pp. 783–789, 2000.

[6] L. J. Salmon, K. M. Refshauge, V. J. Russell, J. P. Roe, J. Linklater, and L. A. Pinczewski, "Gender differences in outcome after anterior cruciate ligament reconstruction with hamstring tendon autograft," *The American Journal of Sports Medicine*, vol. 34, no. 4, pp. 621–629, 2006.

[7] S.-J. Kim, T.-E. Kim, D.-H. Lee, and K.-S. Oh, "Anterior cruciate ligament reconstruction in patients who have excessive joint laxity," *The Journal of Bone & Joint Surgery—American Volume*, vol. 90, no. 4, pp. 735–741, 2008.

[8] S.-J. Kim, P. Kumar, and S.-H. Kim, "Anterior cruciate ligament reconstruction in patients with generalized joint laxity," *Clinics in Orthopedic Surgery*, vol. 2, no. 3, pp. 130–139, 2010.

[9] L. Salmon, V. Russell, T. Musgrove, L. Pinczewski, and K. Refshauge, "Incidence and risk factors for graft rupture and contralateral rupture after anterior cruciate ligament reconstruction," *Arthroscopy*, vol. 21, no. 8, pp. 948–957, 2005.

[10] K. D. Shelbourne and T. Gray, "Results of anterior cruciate ligament reconstruction based on meniscus and articular cartilage status at the time of surgery: five- to fifteen-year evaluations," *American Journal of Sports Medicine*, vol. 28, no. 4, pp. 446–452, 2000.

[11] R. P. A. Janssen, A. W. F. du Mée, J. van Valkenburg, H. A. G. M. Sala, and C. M. Tseng, "Anterior cruciate ligament reconstruction with 4-strand hamstring autograft and accelerated rehabilitation: a 10-year prospective study on clinical results, knee osteoarthritis and its predictors," *Knee Surgery, Sports Traumatology, Arthroscopy*, vol. 21, no. 9, pp. 1977–1988, 2013.

[12] J. C. Hughston, J. R. Andrews, M. J. Cross, and A. Moschi, "Classification of knee ligament instabilities. Part I. The medical compartment and cruciate ligaments," *Journal of Bone and Joint Surgery—Series A*, vol. 58, no. 2, pp. 159–172, 1976.

[13] Y. Ishibashi, E. Tsuda, A. Fukuda, H. Tsukada, and S. Toh, "Intraoperative biomechanical evaluation of anatomic anterior cruciate ligament reconstruction using a navigation system: comparison of hamstring tendon and bone-patellar tendon-bone graft," *The American Journal of Sports Medicine*, vol. 36, no. 10, pp. 1903–1912, 2008.

[14] S. Plaweski, J. Cazal, P. Rosell, and P. Merloz, "Anterior cruciate ligament reconstruction using navigation: a comparative study on 60 patients," *The American Journal of Sports Medicine*, vol. 34, no. 4, pp. 542–552, 2006.

[15] J. Eichhorn, "Three years of experience with computer navigation-assisted positioning of drilling tunnels in anterior cruciate ligament replacement (SS-67)," *Arthroscopy*, vol. 20, supplement 1, pp. e31–e32, 2004.

[16] R. Hart, J. Krejzla, P. Šváb, J. Kočiš, and V. Štipčák, "Outcomes after conventional versus computer-navigated anterior cruciate ligament reconstruction," *Arthroscopy*, vol. 24, no. 5, pp. 569–578, 2008.

[17] S. Martelli, S. Zaffagnini, S. Bignozzi, N. Lopomo, and M. Marcacci, "Description and validation of a navigation system for intra-operative evaluation of knee laxity," *Computer Aided Surgery*, vol. 12, no. 3, pp. 181–188, 2007.

[18] N. Lopomo, S. Bignozzi, S. Martelli et al., "Reliability of a navigation system for intra-operative evaluation of antero-posterior knee joint laxity," *Computers in Biology and Medicine*, vol. 39, no. 3, pp. 280–285, 2009.

[19] V. Musahl, J. E. Voos, P. F. O'Loughlin et al., "Comparing stability of different single- and double-bundle anterior cruciate ligament reconstruction techniques: a cadaveric study using navigation," *Arthroscopy*, vol. 26, no. 9, supplement, pp. S41–S48, 2010.

[20] M. Hofbauer, P. Valentin, R. Kdolsky et al., "Rotational and translational laxity after computer-navigated single- and double-bundle anterior cruciate ligament reconstruction," *Knee Surgery, Sports Traumatology, Arthroscopy*, vol. 18, no. 9, pp. 1201–1207, 2010.

[21] S. Plaweski, M. Grimaldi, A. Courvoisier, and S. Wimsey, "Intra-operative comparisons of knee kinematics of double-bundle versus single-bundle anterior cruciate ligament reconstruction," *Knee Surgery, Sports Traumatology, Arthroscopy*, vol. 19, no. 8, pp. 1277–1286, 2011.

[22] K. Miura, Y. Ishibashi, E. Tsuda, A. Fukuda, H. Tsukada, and S. Toh, "Intraoperative comparison of knee laxity between anterior cruciate ligament-reconstructed knee and contralateral stable knee using navigation system," *Arthroscopy*, vol. 26, no. 9, pp. 1203–1211, 2010.

[23] M. Komzák, R. Hart, F. Okál, and A. Safi, "Does the posterolateral bundle influence rotational movement more than the anteromedial bundle in anterior cruciate ligament reconstruction? A clinical study," *The Journal of Bone & Joint Surgery—British Volume*, vol. 94, no. 10, pp. 1372–1376, 2012.

[24] Y. Ishibashi, E. Tsuda, A. Fukuda, H. Tsukada, and S. Toh, "Stability evaluation of single-bundle and double-bundle reconstruction during navigated ACL reconstruction," *Sports Medicine and Arthroscopy Review*, vol. 16, no. 2, pp. 77–83, 2008.

[25] A. Kanaya, M. Ochi, M. Deie, N. Adachi, M. Nishimori, and A. Nakamae, "Intraoperative evaluation of anteroposterior and rotational stabilities in anterior cruciate ligament reconstruction: lower femoral tunnel placed single-bundle versus double-bundle reconstruction," *Knee Surgery, Sports Traumatology, Arthroscopy*, vol. 17, no. 8, pp. 907–913, 2009.

[26] A. Ferretti, E. Monaco, L. Labianca, F. Conteduca, and A. De Carli, "Double-bundle anterior cruciate ligament reconstruction: a computer-assisted orthopaedic surgery study," *The American Journal of Sports Medicine*, vol. 36, no. 4, pp. 760–766, 2008.

[27] P. Colombet, J. Robinson, P. Christel, J.-P. Franceschi, and P. Djian, "Using navigation to measure rotation kinematics during ACL reconstruction," *Clinical Orthopaedics and Related Research*, no. 454, pp. 59–65, 2007.

[28] E. K. Song, J. K. Seon, S. J. Park, C. I. Hur, and D. S. Lee, "In vivo laxity of stable versus anterior cruciate liagment-injured knees using a navigation system: a comparative study," *Knee Surgery, Sports Traumatology, Arthroscopy*, vol. 17, no. 8, pp. 941–945, 2009.

[29] S. Ohkawa, N. Adachi, M. Deie, A. Nakamae, T. Nakasa, and M. Ochi, "The relationship of anterior and rotatory laxity between surgical navigation and clinical outcome after ACL reconstruction," *Knee Surgery, Sports Traumatology, Arthroscopy*, vol. 20, no. 4, pp. 778–784, 2012.

[30] T. Cheng, G.-Y. Zhang, and X.-L. Zhang, "Does computer navigation system really improve early clinical outcomes after anterior cruciate ligament reconstruction? A meta-analysis and systematic review of randomized controlled trials," *Knee*, vol. 19, no. 2, pp. 73–77, 2012.

[31] J. Kongtharvonskul, J. Attia, S. Thamakaison, C. Kijkunasathian, P. Woratanarat, and A. Thakkinstian, "Clinical outcomes of double- vs single-bundle anterior cruciate ligament reconstruction: a systematic review of randomized control trials," *Scandinavian Journal of Medicine and Science in Sports*, vol. 23, no. 1, pp. 1–14, 2013.

[32] S. Lee, H. Kim, J. Jang, S. C. Seong, and M. C. Lee, "Comparison of anterior and rotatory laxity using navigation between single-

and double-bundle ACL reconstruction: prospective randomized trial," *Knee Surgery, Sports Traumatology, Arthroscopy*, vol. 20, no. 4, pp. 752–761, 2012.

[33] T. Izawa, K. Okazaki, Y. Tashiro et al., "Comparison of rotatory stability after anterior cruciate ligament reconstruction between single-bundle and double-bundle techniques," *The American Journal of Sports Medicine*, vol. 39, no. 7, pp. 1470–1477, 2011.

[34] S. Aldrian, P. Valentin, B. Wondrasch et al., "Gender differences following computer-navigated single- and double-bundle anterior cruciate ligament reconstruction," *Knee Surgery, Sports Traumatology, Arthroscopy*, vol. 22, no. 9, pp. 2145–2152, 2014.

5

Antimullerian Hormone Changes after Laparoscopic Ovarian Cystectomy for Endometrioma Compared with the Nonovarian Conditions

Chamnan Tanprasertkul,[1,2] Sakol Manusook,[1] Charintip Somprasit,[1] Sophapun Ekarattanawong,[3] Opas Sreshthaputra,[4] and Teraporn Vutyavanich[4]

[1] *Department of Obstetrics and Gynaecology, Faculty of Medicine, Thammasat University, Pathum Thani 12120, Thailand*
[2] *Center of Excellence in Applied Epidemiology, Thammasat University, Pathum Thani 12120, Thailand*
[3] *Division of Physiology, Department of Preclinical Science, Faculty of Medicine, Thammasat University, Pathum Thani 12120, Thailand*
[4] *Department of Obstetrics and Gynecology, Faculty of Medicine, Chiang Mai University, Chiang Mai 50000, Thailand*

Correspondence should be addressed to Chamnan Tanprasertkul; chamnandoctor@gmail.com

Academic Editor: Chin-Jung Wang

Laparoscopic ovarian cystectomy is recommended for surgical procedure of endometrioma. The negative impact on ovarian reserve following removal had been documented. Little evidence had been reported for nonovarian originated effects. *Objective.* To evaluate the impact of laparoscopic ovarian cystectomy for endometrioma on ovarian reserve, measured by serum antimullerian hormone (AMH), compared to nonovarian pelvic surgery. *Materials and Methods.* A prospective study was conducted. Women who underwent laparoscopic ovarian cystectomy (LOC) and laparoscopic nonovarian pelvic surgery (NOS) were recruited and followed up through 6 months. Clinical baseline data and AMH were evaluated. *Results.* 39 and 38 participants were enrolled in LOC and NOS groups, respectively. Baseline characteristics (age, weight, BMI, and height) and preoperative AMH level between 2 groups were not statistically different. After surgery, AMH of both groups decreased since the first week, at 1 month and at 3 months. However, as compared to the LOC group at 6 months after operation, the mean AMH of the NOS group had regained its value with a highly significant difference. *Conclusion.* This study demonstrated the negative impact of nonovarian or indirect effects of laparoscopic surgery to ovarian reserve. The possible mechanisms are necessary for more investigations.

1. Introduction

Endometriosis, the presence of endometrial tissue outside the lining of the uterine cavity, is one of the most common pelvic diseases in women. It is generally acknowledged that an estimated 6–10% of all women during their reproductive years are affected by this condition. In group of infertility women, 38 percent (20–50%) of them have endometriosis. If the patients have a history of chronic pelvic pain, the prevalence could be as high as 71–87 percent [1–4].

The ovarian endometriosis was recognized by the common term, namely, endometriotic cyst or endometrioma. The surgical intervention, laparoscopy, is the most useful option for further evaluation, treatment, and pathological removal [5]. Moreover, laparoscopic surgery is currently accepted as the procedure of choice for both diagnostic and therapeutic modalities. The systematic reviews showed that the excisional surgery or laparoscopic ovarian cystectomy for endometrioma provided more favorable outcomes than drainage and ablation surgery with regard to the recurrence of the endometrioma, recurrence of pain symptoms [6]. However, there were some reports that showed the negative impact on ovarian reserve, measured by serum antimullerian hormone (AMH) levels following ovarian cystectomy [7–11]. AMH levels represent the ovarian follicular pool and could be a useful marker of ovarian reserve. The clinical application of AMH measurement had been proposed in the prediction of quantitative and qualitative aspects in assisted reproductive technologies (ART). AMH seemed to be a better marker in predicting ovarian response to control ovarian stimulation

TABLE 1: Characteristics of the participants between the laparoscopic ovarian cystectomy (LOC) and nonovarian surgery (NOS) group.

	LOC ($n = 39$)	NOS ($n = 38$)*	P value
Age (yrs)	32.74 ± 6.98	34.74 ± 5.2	0.16
Weight (kg)	52.51 ± 9.42	53.79 ± 6.93	0.49
Height (cm)	159.28 ± 4.63	156.86 ± 6.11	0.05
Duration of surgery (min)	67.05 ± 29.73	92.26 ± 34.20	0.001
Blood loss (mL)	61.15 ± 42.36	105.79 ± 57.50	0.002
Size of ovarian cyst (cm)	5.46 ± 1.70		
Bilateral	6 (15.38%)		
Stage of disease/rASRM score			
III	24 (61.54%)		
IV	15 (38.46%)		

rASRM: the revised American Society for Reproductive Medicine score.
*Laparoscopic NOS: 19 hysterectomies (without adnexectomy), 16 myomectomies, and 3 adenomyomectomies.

than the patient's age, FSH (follicular stimulating hormone), estradiol, and inhibin B [12].

This negative effect had been explained by injury of adjacent ovarian follicles during the cyst wall excision. Also, the comparative study group of the most previous trials was benign, nonendometrioma ovarian cyst. To the best of our knowledge, there were a very few data which explored the possible effects of laparoscopic surgery and anesthesia on AMH in the nonovarian disease. The aim of current study was to evaluate the impact of laparoscopic ovarian cystectomy for endometrioma on ovarian reserve as measured by serum AMH, compared to nonovarian pelvic surgery.

2. Materials and Methods

This was a prospective cohort study which was conducted at Department of Obstetrics and Gynaecology in Thammasat University Hospital, Thailand. After approval from Ethical Institute Committee, the patients were enrolled with the following criteria; having 18–45 years; having regular menstrual cycles (21–35 days) at the time of operation; having no evidence of any other endocrine disorders such as diabetes mellitus, thyroid dysfunction, hyperprolactinemia, congenital adrenal hyperplasia, Cushing's syndrome, or adrenal insufficiency; undergoing laparoscopic ovarian cystectomy or laparoscopic nonovarian pelvic surgery for benign pelvic disease; having no previous history of adnexal surgery; having no suspicious findings of malignant ovarian diseases, never taking any medication such as oral pill and hormonal drugs within 3 months before the enrollment, pathological diagnosis of excised ovarian tissue confirmed it to be an endometriotic cyst in the study group and to consist of other benign pelvic diseases in control group. The participants were excluded if they had one of the following: polycystic ovarian syndrome according to the Rotterdam criteria [13] or operation conversion to exploratory laparotomy or pathological report as the malignant diseases.

All patients underwent the standard surgical procedures under general anesthesia. Each patient was appointed to visit the hospital on the seventh day and 1st, 3rd, and sixth months after laparoscopic ovarian cystectomy or nonovarian pelvic surgery. On each visit and preoperative day, blood samples would be obtained from the patients by venipuncture to measure the levels of AMH. The patient's sera were obtained from blood samples by centrifuge at 1400 ×g for 10 minutes to separate cellular contents and debris. The serum was transferred to sterile polypropylene tubes and stored at −70°C until assayed. Serum AMH levels were measured by enzyme-linked immunosorbent assay (ELISA, Diagnostic Systems Laboratories, Webster, TX, USA).

The sample size was calculated based on the determination of difference in means including confidence interval approach. The difference in means of serum AMH from previous studies was used for sample size calculation. From the study of Ercan et al. [11], mean preoperative AMH levels of the study and the control cases were 1.62 ± 1.09 and 2.06 ± 0.51 ng/mL, respectively. According to these values, the sample size was calculated by STATA program. The estimated number of women in each group was 40. In data and statistical analysis, descriptive statistics was used to describe study subjects' characteristics. Concentrations of serum AMH were interpreted between each sampling point (preoperative, postoperative first week, for 1st, 3rd and 6th months). The P value of less than 0.05 was considered as statistically significant.

3. Results

In this study, 90 women were enrolled. There were thirty-nine and 38 women in laparoscopic ovarian cystectomy (LOC) and laparoscopic nonovarian pelvic surgery (NOS), respectively, who had adequate complete data to analyze (Table 1). The mean age, weight, and height were not different between both groups. Duration of surgery and blood loss in LOC group were statistically significant in their differences from those of the NOS group. The mean diameter of endometrioma was 5.46 cm and ranged from 3 cm to 10 cm. Most of cases were unilateral but more so on the left side(58.97%). Bilateral disease was found to be only 15.38 percent. NOS group is composed of 19, 16, and 3 cases of laparoscopic hysterectomy (without adnexectomy), myomectomy, and adenomyomectomy, respectively.

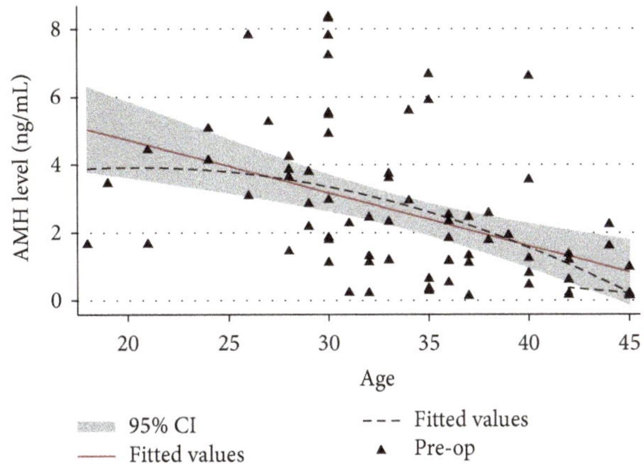

FIGURE 1: The correlation of serum AMH and age in participants. (AMH: antimullerian hormone).

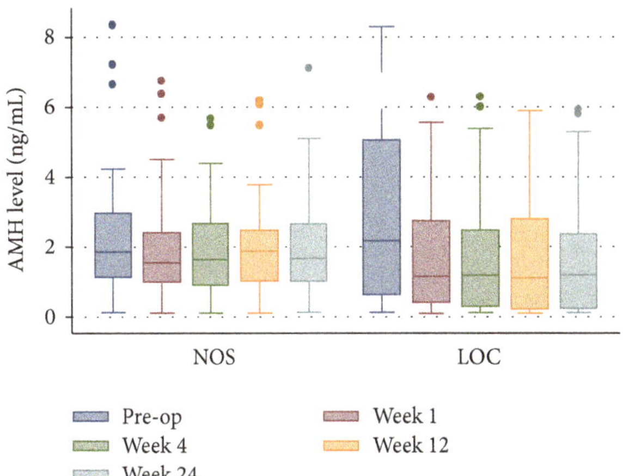

FIGURE 2: The changes in the serum AMH level at preoperative, post-op over periods of first week, 1, 3 and 6 months in the LOC and NOS groups. (AMH: antimullerian hormone, LOC: laparoscopic ovarian cystectomy, and NOS: nonovarian laparoscopic pelvic surgery).

As shown in Figure 1, the distribution of serum AMH levels was inversely correlated to the patients' age. After age of 40, the rate of declination was accelerated.

When comparing the serum AMH of LOC to NOS group, there was no statistically significant difference between groups at preoperative level, first visit on 7th day, second visit on first month, and third visit on 3rd month. However, there was statistically significant difference between groups at 6th month of operation. This negative change also occurred in the unilateral LOC group but there was no statistical difference.

4. Discussion

As shown in Figure 1, the AMH level was decreased with the advance of women age. This result demonstrated that ovarian reserve was declined throughout reproductive age. However, the cut-off value for serum AMH level for approving diminished ovarian reserve is still not determined. Previous research suggested that AMH was a promising marker [9]. But availability was limited because it was of high cost.

This study found that laparoscopic ovarian cystectomy in cases of endometrioma had negative effect on the ovarian capacity. Similar to previous studies which had been shown, the ovarian cystectomy can be harmful to ovarian reserve [7–10]. The present study showed that this adverse effect occurred immediately after operation and affected the patient for medium term, at least 6 months. In 9–12 months, we also investigated some patients; this diminished ovarian reserve effects still persist in most of them (data not available).

The results demonstrated that there is a strong negative impact of ovarian cystectomy on ovarian reserve; the guideline for management of ovarian cyst or endometrioma might be adjusted and reconsidered. Busacca et al. [14] reported that patients who underwent surgical operation for bilateral endometrioma had a prevalence of 2.4% ovarian failure immediately after surgery. This was consistent with Somigliana et al. [15] that in vitro fertilization (IVF) outcome and ovarian reserve were severely impaired in women who underwent operation for bilateral ovarian endometriomas. Similar to these findings, bilaterality is the major risk factor. Therefore, before ovarian surgery, not only morphological assessment but also careful ovarian function evaluation was needed. In case of low ovarian reserve, the surgical technique might be tailored and adjusted. The other alternative treatment may be a better option.

Most previous studies compared women who had ovarian cystectomy to the patients who had no history of surgery, for example, infertile women. Moreover, the study was cross-sectional design which did not have ability to demonstrate the causal relationship. The flaws of these were the uncertain causes of decline in ovarian reserve. Not only loss of follicles during stripping the endometriotic cyst but also blood loss in operative field could be another explainable reason. Atabekoğlu et al. [16] had reported the additional effect of total abdominal hysterectomy on serum AMH, 30% more loss of ovarian reserve. The surgery, hysterectomy, could reduce ovarian blood supply and resulted in temporary decline in ovarian reserve. In this study, we compared LOC to the NOS group in which laparoscopic surgery does not directly involve the ovaries, for example, hysterectomy and myomectomy. The postulated mechanism of decline in AMH especially in first 3 months might be due to the effect of blood loss and anaesthesia. This could be rescued by revascularisation of the ovaries.

As shown in Table 2 and Figure 2, AMH level of both groups had declined immediately after laparoscopic surgery. In LOC group the serum AMH level had declined until six months at least. However, this effect lasts only for short term, three months in NOS group. This might demonstrate that the effect of blood volume depletion includes the aesthetic impact during surgery. But it was only short term and temporary adverse effect.

There were some limitations of the study. Firstly, the ovarian reserve was measured by only single marker. Antral follicle count (AFC) is another useful marker for ovarian

TABLE 2: Comparison of serum AMH level (ng/mL) between LOC and NOS group.

Serum AMH	LOC			NOS	Diff.	P value		
	Uni* ($n = 33$)	Bi* ($n = 6$)	All* ($n = 39$)	($n = 38$)	All/NOS	All/NOS	Uni/NOS	Bi/NOS
Preoperative	2.94 ± 2.47	2.01 ± 1.02	2.84 ± 2.47	2.33 ± 1.91	0.51	0.31	0.22	0.69
Postoperative								
7 days	1.71 ± 1.41	1.48 ± 1.07	1.76 ± 1.52	1.97 ± 1.64	−0.21	0.57	0.48	0.48
1 month	1.79 ± 1.74	1.41 ± 0.77	1.80 ± 1.70	2.24 ± 1.40	−0.44	0.22	0.23	0.16
3 months	1.86 ± 1.60	0.98 ± 0.42	1.72 ± 1.55	2.28 ± 1.46	−0.56	0.11	0.25	0.03
6 months	2.03 ± 1.74	0.94 ± 0.46	1.69 ± 1.63	2.44 ± 1.59	−0.75	0.04$	0.30	0.02$

Uni: unilateral, Bi: bilateral, and *mean ± standard deviation.
$Statistically significant, Diff.: mean difference, and NOS: nonovarian laparoscopic pelvic surgery.
AMH: antimullerian hormone and LOC: laparoscopic ovarian cystectomy.

reserve. Sugita et al. [17] postulated the balancing effect of a healthy ovary which may compensate for a reduced ovarian reserve in the contralateral, affected ovary. Therefore, AFC may be a more accurate marker than AMH. However, this study did not have enough AFC data for analysis. Also, the measurement of AFC is subjective and evaluator-dependent. Secondly, the operations in the NOS group varied and were non-unique. Moreover, laparoscopic surgeons use a variety of techniques to operate on a case by case basis. Thirdly, there were some dropout participants, caused by loss follow-up and becoming pregnant.

5. Conclusion

Laparoscopic ovarian cystectomy in case of endometrioma had negative impact on the ovarian reserve, measured by serum AMH. This effect was sustained at least 6 months after operation. The negative impact occurred in patients who had nonovarian pelvic surgery but this adverse effect was only mild and temporary. This study showed the negative impact of nonovarian or indirect effects of laparoscopic surgery on ovarian reserve; however, the exact mechanisms were still unknown and needed to be explored more.

References

[1] L. C. Giudice, "Clinical practice. Endometriosis," *The New England Journal of Medicine*, vol. 362, pp. 2389–2398, 2010.

[2] N. Leyland, R. Casper, P. Laberge, and S. S. Singh, "Endometriosis: diagnosis and management," *Journal of Obstetrics and Gynaecology Canada*, vol. 32, no. 7, pp. S1–S32, 2010.

[3] S. Kennedy, A. Bergqvist, C. Chapron et al., "ESHRE guideline for the diagnosis and treatment of endometriosis," *Human Reproduction*, vol. 20, no. 10, pp. 2698–2704, 2005.

[4] "Practice bulletin no. 114: management of endometriosis," *Obstetrics & Gynecology*, vol. 116, pp. 223–236, 2010.

[5] P. P. Yeung Jr., J. Shwayder, and R. P. Pasic, "Laparoscopic management of endometriosis: comprehensive review of best evidence," *Journal of Minimally Invasive Gynecology*, vol. 16, no. 3, pp. 269–281, 2009.

[6] R. J. Hart, M. Hickey, P. Maouris, and W. Buckett, "Excisional surgery versus ablative surgery for ovarian endometriomata," *Cochrane Database of Systematic Reviews*, no. 2, Article ID :CD004992, 2008.

[7] Y.-M. Hwu, F. S. Wu, S.-H. Li, F.-J. Sun, M.-H. Lin, and R. K. Lee, "The impact of endometrioma and laparoscopic cystectomy on serum anti-Müllerian hormone levels," *Reproductive Biology and Endocrinology*, vol. 9, article 80, 2011.

[8] H. J. Chang, S. H. Han, J. R. Lee et al., "Impact of laparoscopic cystectomy on ovarian reserve: serial changes of serum anti-Müllerian hormone levels," *Fertility and Sterility*, vol. 94, no. 1, pp. 343–349, 2010.

[9] A. Iwase, W. Hirokawa, M. Goto et al., "Serum anti-Müllerian hormone level is a useful marker for evaluating the impact of laparoscopic cystectomy on ovarian reserve," *Fertility and Sterility*, vol. 94, no. 7, pp. 2846–2849, 2010.

[10] D.-Y. Lee, N. Y. Kim, M. J. Kim, B.-K. Yoon, and D. Choi, "Effects of laparoscopic surgery on serum anti-mllerian hormone levels in reproductive-aged women with endometrioma," *Gynecological Endocrinology*, vol. 27, no. 10, pp. 733–736, 2011.

[11] C. M. Ercan, M. Sakinci, N. K. Duru, B. Alanbay, K. E. Karasahin, and I. Baser, "Antimullerian hormone levels after laparoscopic endometrioma stripping surgery," *Gynecological Endocrinology*, vol. 26, no. 6, pp. 468–472, 2010.

[12] A. La Marca, G. Sighinolfi, D. Radi et al., "Anti-Müllerian hormone (AMH) as a predictive marker in assisted reproductive technology (ART)," *Human Reproduction Update*, vol. 16, no. 2, pp. 113–130, 2009.

[13] F. J. Broekmans, E. A. H. Knauff, O. Valkenburg, J. S. Laven, M. J. Eijkemans, and B. C. J. M. Fauser, "PCOS according to the Rotterdam consensus criteria: change in prevalence among WHO-II anovulation and association with metabolic factors," *BJOG*, vol. 113, no. 10, pp. 1210–1217, 2006.

[14] M. Busacca, J. Riparini, E. Somigliana et al., "Postsurgical ovarian failure after laparoscopic excision of bilateral endometriomas," *American Journal of Obstetrics and Gynecology*, vol. 195, no. 2, pp. 421–425, 2006.

[15] E. Somigliana, M. Arnoldi, L. Benaglia, R. Iemmello, A. E. Nicolosi, and G. Ragni, "IVF-ICSI outcome in women operated on for bilateral endometriomas," *Human Reproduction*, vol. 23, no. 7, pp. 1526–1530, 2008.

[16] C. Atabekoğlu, S. Taşkin, K. Kahraman et al., "The effect of total abdominal hysterectomy on serum anti-Müllerian hormone levels: a pilot study," *Climacteric*, vol. 15, no. 4, pp. 393–397, 2012.

[17] A. Sugita, A. Iwase, M. Goto et al., "One-year follow-up of serum antimüllerian hormone levels in patients with cystectomy: are different sequential changes due to different mechanisms causing damage to the ovarian reserve?" *Fertility and Sterility*, vol. 100, no. 2, pp. 516.e3–522.e3, 2013.

6

The Supraorbital Keyhole Craniotomy through an Eyebrow Incision: Its Origins and Evolution

D. Ryan Ormond and Costas G. Hadjipanayis

Department of Neurosurgery, Emory University School of Medicine, Atlanta, GA 30322, USA

Correspondence should be addressed to Costas G. Hadjipanayis; chadjip@emory.edu

Academic Editor: Joachim Oertel

In the modern era of neurosurgery, the use of the operative microscope, rigid rod-lens endoscope, and neuronavigation has helped to overcome some of the previous limitations of surgery due to poor lighting and anatomic localization available to the surgeon. Over the last thirty years, the supraorbital craniotomy and subfrontal approach through an eyebrow incision have been developed and refined to play a legitimate role in the armamentarium of the modern skull base neurosurgeon. With careful patient selection, the supraorbital "keyhole" approach offers a less invasive but still efficacious approach to a number of lesions along the subfrontal corridor. Well over 1000 cases have been reported in the literature utilizing this approach establishing its safety and efficacy. This paper discusses the nuances of this approach, including the benefits and limitations of its use described through our technique, review of the literature, and case illustration.

1. Introduction

Numerous neurosurgical approaches have been developed to operate on lesions of the frontotemporal skull base. These approaches include frontal, bifrontal, frontotemporal, pterional, orbitozygomatic, and other variations [1]. The evolution of these approaches from Dandy's frontotemporal "macrosurgical approach," to Yasargil's microsurgical pterional approach, and finally to the supraorbital keyhole approach through an eyebrow incision all have served to give the neurosurgeon the exposure they needed to safely address various pathologies [2]. The goal of "keyhole" surgery was not to perform a small incision and craniotomy for the sake of a small opening. The goal of this approach was to permit adequate access to skull base lesions while limiting trauma to surrounding structures such as the skin, bone, dura, and, most importantly, the brain [3–5].

The supraorbital craniotomy and subfrontal approach have been used to access a number of pathologies including tumors (meningiomas, craniopharyngiomas, etc.) and vascular abnormalities (e.g., aneurysms, arteriovenous malformations, and cavernous hemangiomas) [1, 2, 5–35]. Surface lesions typically require craniotomies as large as the lesion. Deep-seated lesions, however, can be accessed through a much smaller craniotomy since the intracranial field widens with increasing distance from the skull [2, 3, 5, 36–38]. Utilizing this principle, surgeons can access lesions in the subfrontal, suprasellar, Sylvian fissure, and posterior fossa regions of the brain [2–6, 21].

When considering any approach to a pathological entity, it is important to understand the advantages and disadvantages of a given procedure. Surgery through an eyebrow incision may not be appropriate for all lesions of the anterior skull base. There is a narrow viewing angle through this approach that may require frequent adjustment of the operating room table and microscope for adequate visualization of a given lesion. The microscope light is often another problem, as there may be some difficulty getting adequate light through such a small opening onto a deep-seated lesion. Microinstruments require almost coaxial control through such narrow anatomic windows [2, 5]. In the setting of vascular lesions, a smaller opening in a blood-filled field can also make it difficult to obtain adequate vascular control without damage to surrounding structures.

Use of a rigid rod-lens endoscope in combination with the operative microscope can provide a great benefit with the supraorbital craniotomy and subfrontal approach. The endoscope can provide a much greater light source at the depths of the exposure, with greater focus and better visualization. Ensuring a large enough size to the craniotomy (no smaller than 1.5–2 cm) is important as well to ensure adequate maneuverability of instruments for a bimanual approach to surgery [2, 5]. Through thoughtful consideration of appropriate lesions and adequate experience with this technique, we believe that safe surgery can be performed on numerous pathologies without brain retraction and with a superb cosmetic result.

2. Surgical Description

After general anesthesia, endotracheal intubation, and placement of a Foley catheter, the patient is fixed in a Mayfield three-pin head holder with two pins on the ipsilateral posterior cranium and the one pin site on the contralateral frontal bone. The torso is slightly elevated at ten degrees, and the head is positioned in a slightly extended position of around 15–20 degrees to allow gravity retraction of the frontal lobes away from the surgical field. No retractors are used. The head is turned approximately 15–45 degrees contralaterally to the side of surgery to allow appropriate visualization of midline lesions. The bed can be further rotated as necessary for further adjustments during surgery. Midline lesions, such as olfactory groove lesions, require more rotation, whereas laterally placed lesions require less rotation for appropriate visualization and access. The most important information in decision making regarding the side of the approach is the structure of the lesion itself and its relationship to surrounding anatomic structures. Certainly, when either side can adequately access the lesion, we typically choose a nondominant approach in order to reduce the risk of damage to the dominant frontal lobe.

The skin incision is made along the eyebrow without cutting the hair of the eyebrow (Figure 4). Previous studies have shown no increased risk of infection, and leaving the eyebrow intact allows for a better cosmetic result [2, 3, 5, 7, 46]. It is important that the skin incision be placed laterally to the supraorbital notch to avoid forehead numbness from injury to the supraorbital nerve during surgery [2, 5, 21, 22]. The incision is made through the skin and dermis, with dissection continuing superiorly just superficial to the orbicularis oculi, pericranium, and temporalis fascia. Care is taken to ensure that orbicularis oculi fibers are not damaged. This layer is important for closure purposes as well as for an optimal cosmetic result. Dissection continues in this manner approximately 1.5–2 cm superior to the supraorbital ridge. A small retractor can be used to keep the incision open at this point. The pericranium is incised medially beginning lateral to the supraorbital nerve. Pericranial dissection continues in a "C"-shaped fashion extending approximately 1.5–2 cm superior to the supraorbital ridge and laterally to the superior temporal line. This muscle and pericranial flap are reflected inferiorly and retracted out of the way with a suture.

The craniotomy is made by bluntly dissecting a small portion of temporalis muscle and fascia at the superior temporal line and drilling a 5 mm burr hole on the lateral aspect of the exposure below the temporalis for a better cosmetic result. Care is taken to avoid the use of cautery around the temporalis at this location, as this may cause damage to the frontalis branch of the facial nerve. A craniotome is then used to make two cuts. The first is from the burr hole along the floor of the anterior cranial fossa extending to a position lateral to the supraorbital notch. The second again starts from the lateral burr hole but makes an arch superiorly to then return to meet the medial edge of the first cut. The craniotomy takes the form of a "D," with the back wall of the "D" along the floor of the anterior cranial fossa. It is important to ensure a craniotomy at least 1.5–2 cm in width, or manipulation of microinstruments is very difficult. It is also important to recognize a breach of the frontal sinus, as this can be a source of CSF leak postprocedure if not adequately addressed. In fact, a very lateral extension of frontal sinus may preclude the use of this approach in a given patient because of the difficulty repairing a large opening in the frontal sinus via this approach. We have used bone wax to seal off any small breach of the frontal sinus and betadine-soaked gel foam to seal off larger defects.

The dura is now dissected off the orbital roof. At this point, the inner table of the inferior edge of the craniotomy is drilled flush with the orbital roof. Any ridges of the orbital roof can also be leveled with the high-speed drill. This not only improves visualization but also allows greater access of instruments during the procedure. A malleable brain retractor may be placed against the dura to protect against unintentional durotomy. The outer table is left intact to maintain cosmesis. Bone dust is washed out with antibiotic irrigation prior to dural opening. The dura is opened in a "C"-shaped fashion and reflected inferiorly with a stitch. The microscope is brought into the field, the frontal lobe is lightly retracted with a cottonoid, and the CSF cisterns are opened to allow CSF egress to facilitate brain relaxation. Following brain relaxation, the primary procedure may be performed safely with no fixed retractors on the brain and with use of the operative microscope, a rigid rod-lens endoscope, or both.

Wound closure is straightforward. The dural leaflets are reapproximated with a 4-0 Nurolon suture sewn in a running fashion. The craniotomy bone flap is replaced with a titanium burr hole cover and two titanium square plates to improve the cosmetic result by restoring the supraorbital ridge. The pericranium and muscle flap are then closed primarily. Buried, interrupted, and absorbable sutures are used in the dermis, and a 5-0 prolene subcuticular stitch is placed without any knots to ensure removal in the office in 7–10 days. A head wrap can be applied until the first postoperative day to lessen subgaleal edema formation.

3. Case Illustrations

A number of case series utilizing this approach have been published in the literature (Table 1). The reported morbidity and mortality in these series are similar to that reported in surgeries on similar pathologies by other approaches. It is important to understand the benefits and shortcomings of this approach so that case selection can be performed appropriately. We have provided a few case examples from our own

Table 1: Case series of keyhole supraorbital subfrontal approaches through an eyebrow incision.

Publication	Year	Patients	Tumors	Aneurysms	Other	Supraorbital hypesthesia	Frontalis palsy	Hyposmia	Wound infection	CSF leak	Hematoma	Perioperative mortality	Diabetes insipidus	Other
Jho [10]	1997	11	11	0	0	11	0	NR	0	0	NR	0	2	Vision worsened ($n = 2$)
Paladino et al. [14]	1998	37	0	40	0	4 (all recovered)	NR	NR	1	NR	NR	0	NR	Aneurysm rupture ($n = 1$)
Van Lindert et al. [21]	1998	139	0	197	0	0	0	0	0	0	0	NR	NR	Aneurysm rupture ($n = 4$)
Sánchez-Vázquez et al. [19]	1999	41	34	6	1	41 (all recovered)	41 (all recovered)	21 (2 permanent)	0	0	0	0	NR	
Czirják and Szeifert [6]	2001	155	52	102	1	2	1	2	2	NR	NR	5	NR	Aneurysm rupture ($n = 2$), PE ($n = 1$)
Dare et al. [7]	2001	10	0	10	0	10 (all recovered)	10 (all recovered)	NR	1	0	0	0	0	Wound edema
Ko et al. [11]	2001	7	3	4	0	4	NR	NR	NR	NR	NR	NR	NR	Periorbital edema ($n = 7$)
Shanno et al. [15]	2001	72	61	0	11	NR	NR	NR	5	5	1	0	NR	Tension pneumocephalus, asp pna, infarct, ICA injury, and corneal abrasion. Lateral rectus palsy (all $n = 1$)
Steiger et al. [16]	2001	33	0	33	0	NR	2	NR	1	NR	NR	0	NR	Diplopia ($n = 1$) resolved
Czirják et al. [29]	2002	36	0	74	0	0	0	0	0	0	0	1	NR	2 intraoperative ruptures
Fernandes et al. [35]	2002	16	10	2	4	NR	NR	1	1	1	0	0	NR	
Ramos-Zúñiga et al. [17]	2002	20	0	20	0	NR	20 (all recovered)	NR	NR	NR	1	0	NR	Blindness ($n = 1$), infarct ($n = 1$)
Wiedemayer et al. [23]	2004	9	7	0	2	1	1	NR	0	0	0	0	NR	
Zhang et al. [39]	2004	54	52	0	2	NR	NR	NR	NR	1	NR	0	NR	
Jallo et al. [9]	2005	28	24	0	4	NR	NR	NR	1	0	0	0	NR	Decreased vision ($n = 1$)
Melamed et al. [12]	2005	25	15	0	10	NR	NR	NR	1	1	0	0	1	Blindness ($n = 1$)
Mitchell et al. [13]	2005	47	0	47	0	1	NR	NR	0	NR	4	1	NR	Aneurysm rupture ($n = 2$), infarct ($n = 2$)
Reisch and Perneczky [2]	2005	450	199	229	22	34	25	27	6	12	4	1	NR	
Lupret et al. [25]	2006	30	0	30	0	10	NR	NR	1	NR	NR	2	NR	Aneurysm rupture ($n = 4$), mucocele ($n = 2$)
Zheng et al. [22]	2007	35	35	0	0	0	0	0	0	NR	0	0	11	

Table 1: Continued.

Publication	Year	Patients	Tumors	Aneurysms	Other	Supraorbital hypesthesia	Frontalis palsy	Hyposmia	Wound infection	CSF leak	Hematoma	Perioperative mortality	Diabetes insipidus	Other
Brydon et al. [28]	2008	50	0	50	0	NR	NR	NR	1	1	1	3	NR	New neurological deficit ($n = 12$)
Fatemi et al. [8]	2009	13	13	0	0	0	2 (both recovered)	NR	0	0	0	0	0	Vision worse ($n = 1$)
Romani et al. [34]	2009	66	66	0	0	0	0	6	4	6	1	0	NR	4 cotton granulomas
Chen and Tzaan [1]	2010	21	5	13	3	NR	NR	NR	NR	NR	NR	2	NR	Hydrocephalus ($n = 2$), infarct ($n = 1$)
Telera et al. [20]	2012	20	20	0	0	NR	NR	6	0	1	1	1	1	4 with worse vision
Abdel Aziz et al. [26]	2011	40	8	31	1	NR	NR	NR	2	1	1	0	NR	Transpalpebral approach, 1 ischemic infarct
Fischer et al. [27]	2011	793	0	989	0	0	0	0	9	9	14	NR independent of other approaches	NR	26 reoperations for inadequate clipping (19 clipping, 7 coiling), 61 intraoperative ruptures
McLaughlin et al. [31]	2011	11	11	0	0	NR	NR	NR	0	1	0	0	0	1 carotid artery injury, 1 bilateral caudate infarcts
Park et al. [40]	2011	13	0	13	0	NR	0	NR	0	0	0	0	NR	All unruptured PCoA aneurysms with CN III palsy, all resolved
Romani, et al. [32]	2011	73	73	0	0	NR	NR	1	1	3	2	3	2	New postop. neurological deficits ($n = 19$)
Chalouhi et al. [41]	2013	47	0	47	0	NR	NR	NR	1	0	1	0	NR	5 intraoperative ruptures, 4 ischemic infarcts
Romani et al. [33]	2012	52	52	0	0	NR	NR	0	0	3	0	0	4	New postop. neurological deficits ($n = 16$)
Ivan and Lawton [42]	2013	2	0	0	2	0	0	0	0	0	0	0	0	Both cavernous malformations
Kang et al. [43]	2013	4	0	4	0	NR	NR	NR	NR	NR	NR	NR	NR	
Ditzel Filho et al. [44]	2013	10	9	0	1	NR	NR	NR	0	0	0	2	NR	Deaths: 1 pulmonary embolus, 1 systemic disease
Park et al. [45]	2013	52	0	52	0	NR	26 (all recovered)	NR	NR	NR	NR	NR	NR	
Totals		2522	760	1993	64	63	57	43	38	45	31	21	21	
Percent of reported (number)		100%	30.5%	79.0%	2.6%	2.8% (53/1881)	3.0% (57/1878)	2.3% (43/1878)	1.6% (38/2364)	2.2% (45/2081)	1.5% (31/2118)	1.4% (21/1527)	8.3% (21/252)	

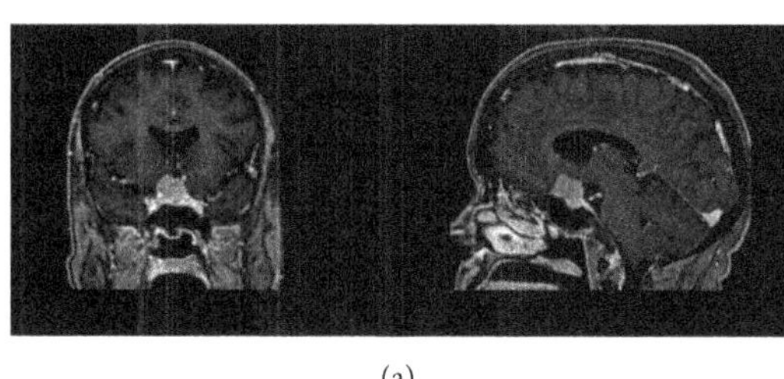

(a)

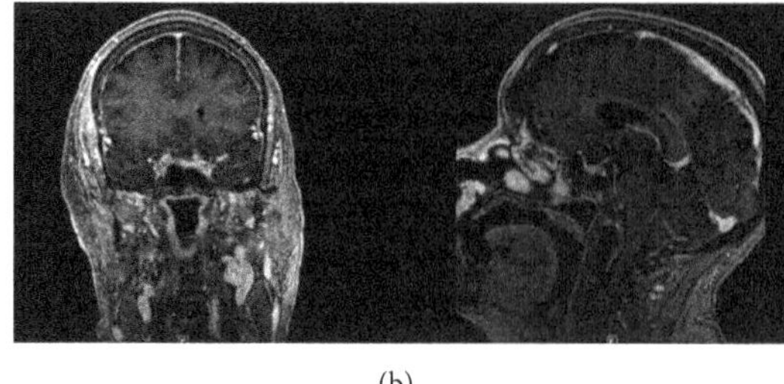

(b)

Figure 1: (a) Preoperative and (b) postoperative MR images of a homogeneously enhancing mass involving the tuberculum sellae and planum sphenoidale. Pathology was meningioma. Gross total resection was achieved.

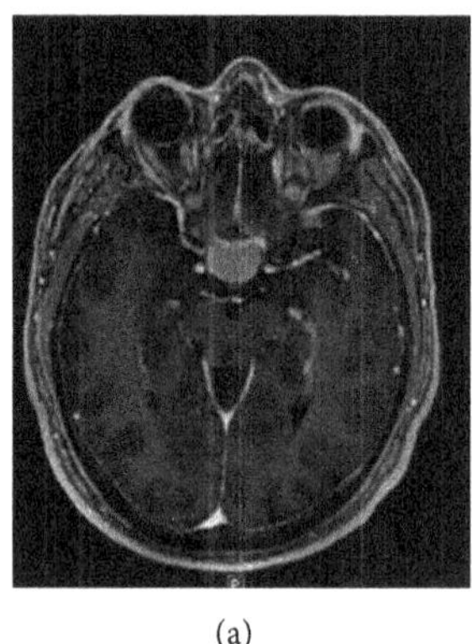

(a)

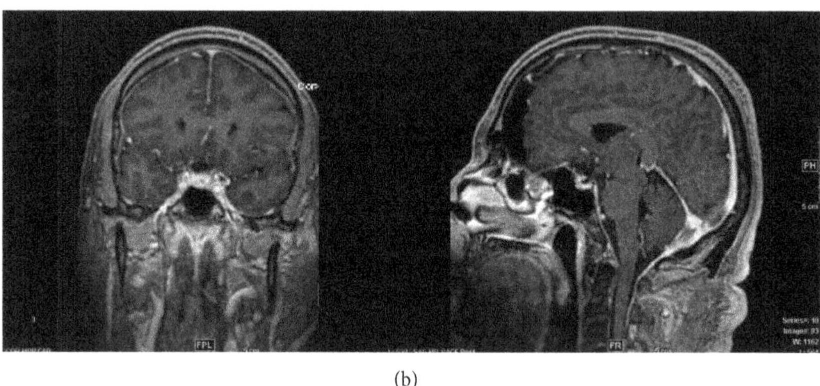

(b)

Figure 2: (a) Preoperative and (b) postoperative MR images of a homogenously enhancing mass involving the planum sphenoidale. Pathology was meningioma. Gross total resection was achieved.

series to highlight some of the benefits of this approach, as well as ways to make the approach safer and more efficacious using modern techniques, technology, and adaptation.

3.1. Case 1. A 71-year-old RH woman presents with a history of progressive headaches who underwent an MRI of the brain with gadolinium contrast administration. The MRI demonstrated a homogeneously enhancing sellar/suprasellar lesion that extended to the planum sphenoidale causing optic chiasmal compression as well as compression of the right optic nerve. The right A2 branch of the anterior cerebral artery coursed through the superior aspect of the tumor. Its imaging characteristics were most consistent with a tuberculum sellae meningioma. This increased in size on subsequent imaging, and the patient underwent elective resection of her tumor by a right supraorbital keyhole craniotomy through the right eyebrow. Preoperative and postoperative imaging are shown (Figure 1). She had a gross total resection of a WHO grade I meningioma and had no visual deficits postoperatively.

3.2. Case 2. A 46-year-old right-handed male presented with visual loss and headache. He could only finger count in the right eye and had an additional bitemporal hemianopsia on visual field testing. Imaging demonstrated a homogeneously enhancing mass involving the tuberculum sellae and planum sphenoidale causing compression of the right optic nerve and chiasm. Imaging characteristics were most consistent with a meningioma. He underwent a right supraorbital craniotomy via an eyebrow incision obtaining a Simpson grade II resection (Figure 2). Postoperatively, his vision improved substantially to where he could read with his right eye and had some improvement in his bitemporal field cut.

3.3. Case 3. A 51-year-old right-handed woman presented with vision loss and headache. Imaging demonstrated a sellar and suprasellar heterogeneously enhancing cystic mass causing optic chiasmal compression (Figure 3). She underwent a right supraorbital craniotomy via an eyebrow incision and had a gross total resection of her craniopharyngioma and preservation of her pituitary stalk (Figure 3). Postoperatively, her vision improved, but she did develop transient diabetes insipidus.

4. Discussion

When the supraorbital craniotomy and subfrontal approach through an eyebrow incision were first described, there was significant controversy over the use of this approach in neurosurgery [2, 5]. Many felt that a keyhole approach would limit exposure and not allow adequate visualization to perform safe and successful surgery. Early reports discussed difficulties with cosmesis both from the bony repair and the incision. Postoperative functional loss of the supraorbital nerve or frontalis branch of the facial nerve was common in early case series as well. In the setting of a breach of the frontal sinus, meningitis or CSF leak has also been reported.

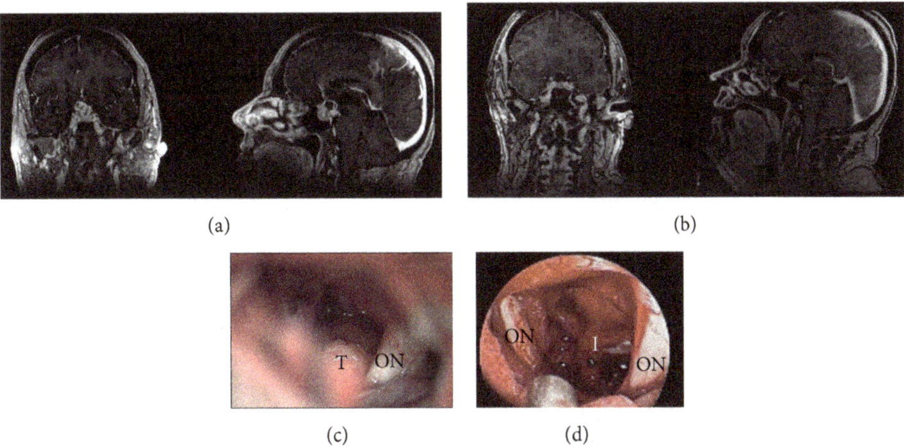

FIGURE 3: (a) Preoperative and (b) postoperative MR images of a heterogeneously enhancing cystic mass involving the sella and suprasellar region. Pathology was consistent with craniopharyngioma. Near-total resection was achieved. (c) Microscopic images from surgery demonstrate optic nerve (ON) and its relationship to tumor (T). (d) Comparison image from endoscopic view in the same patient now demonstrating both optic nerves (ON) and infundibulum (I) following tumor resection. Note the wider field of view, greater visibility, and contrast at depth. There is also significantly less blur from anatomy obscuring view superficial to focal point as clearly noted in microscopic image (c).

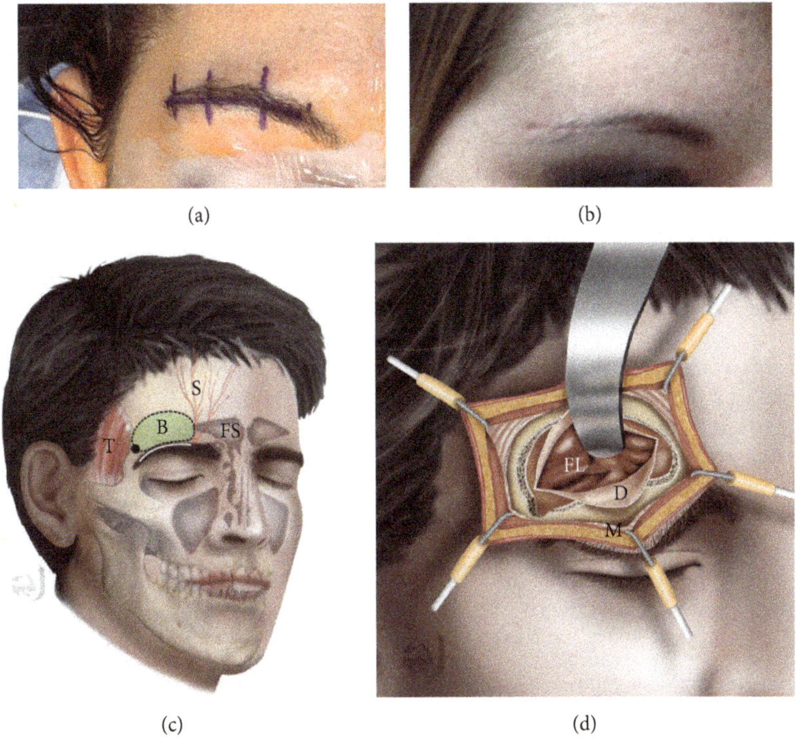

FIGURE 4: (a) Preoperative image of planned right eyebrow incision and (b) six-week postoperative image in the same patient. (c) Illustration of supraorbital craniotomy through an eyebrow incision. The incision is within the eyebrow (white), lateral to the supraorbital nerve (S) and frontal sinus (FS). The temporalis (T) is separated just posterior to the zygomatic process for the burr hole. Bone flap is approximately 1.5 × 2 cm (B). (d) Illustration after opening demonstrating dural opening (D), retracted frontal lobe (FL). The orbicularis oculi muscle (M) is reflected inferiorly with the pericranium.

Experience has helped to demonstrate the limitations of the approach, and many of these early limitations have been overcome. A number of case series reported in the literature demonstrate the efficacy of this approach (see Table 1). Gross total resection was achieved in a similar extent as much larger craniotomies, being reported as 89.2% gross total resection of skull base meningiomas in the largest series [2–5]. Morbidity also does not appear to be higher than in other procedures for similar pathologies including a low cerebrospinal fluid (CSF) leak rate (see Table 1).

4.1. Limitations of Supraorbital Craniotomy through the Eyebrow Incision. Entering through the eyebrow historically led to postoperative loss of supraorbital sensation or to a palsy of the frontalis branch of the facial nerve (see Table 1). Placement of the incision lateral to the supraorbital notch is important in preserving function of the supraorbital nerve. Avoiding the use of cautery laterally over the temporalis fascia and muscle can also avoid injury to the frontalis nerve. The use of neuronavigation can help prevent a breach of the frontal sinus during the craniotomy. Avoidance of the frontal sinus will lower the risk of CSF leak or postoperative wound infection. A lateral frontal sinus may even be considered a contraindication for this approach.

In the setting of vascular pathologies, there may be some difficulty with using two suction tubes in managing prematurely ruptured aneurysms or to obtain proximal control [13, 22, 46, 47]. Some have even recommended against this approach for vascular lesions for this reason [47]. A prominent orbital rim may impede the surgical degree of freedom, and some authors have advocated the addition of an orbital osteotomy to improve surgical freedom and access for vascular pathologies [16, 48]. A similar concept led to similar adaptations to traditional approaches to frontal base and parasellar lesions in the past [46, 49–52]. A number of authors have described different vascular pathologies safely treated through this approach, but we feel it should be limited to those with significant experience with the approach, and it may not be the best approach for some lesions (such as in subarachnoid hemorrhage, giant aneurysms, or vascular lesions in the posterior circulation) in comparison to more traditional approaches (see Table 1) [13, 22, 46, 47].

Numerous shortcomings have been overcome since the introduction of this approach in the 1980s. Probably the biggest limitation was the problem of lighting with the operating microscope down such a narrow corridor. Endoscopes have dramatically improved visualization of this region through this approach and allow for safer dissection with better visualization through this smaller incision than can often be achieved with the microscope alone. Endoscopic-assisted surgery is a common adjunct to the modern skull-based surgeon wishing to employ this keyhole approach in his armamentarium, and is discussed in more detail in what follows.

4.2. Head Positioning with the Keyhole Supraorbital Craniotomy and Subfrontal Approach. Proper positioning of the head for the keyhole supraorbital craniotomy can play an important role in surgical access of skull base lesions. Extension of the neck permits frontal lobe relaxation in combination with mannitol. Contralateral rotation of the head is also performed [2–5, 9, 13, 48]. The degree of head rotation is related to the anatomic location of the pathology in the subfrontal corridor. One author has recommended 10–15 degrees of rotation for suprasellar lesions and the temporomesial surface, 30 degrees for lesions of the planum sphenoidale, and 45 degrees for lesions involving the cribriform plate [48]. Adjustments in the viewing angle can also be made by rotating the operating room table or by adjusting the microscope or endoscope for appropriate visualization during the procedure. Lumbar drainage is rarely used in any of the case series reported [1, 2, 5–35].

4.3. Avoidance of the Supraorbital and Frontalis Nerves. Multiple cadaveric studies have been performed in an attempt to increase the safety of the supraorbital keyhole approach. One study looked at the location and course of the supraorbital nerve and the frontalis branch of facial nerve. This study of ten specimens noted a supraorbital notch in 12/20 sides (right or left) and a supraorbital foramen in the remaining 8 [53]. The lateral branch of the supraorbital nerve has no branches within 10 mm after exiting the supraorbital foramen and notch and courses on the pericranium with an angle with the supraorbital margin of $74 \pm 3^{\circ}$ (68–80°) [53]. The authors suggest that a more medial craniotomy can be performed without damage to the supraorbital nerve by dissecting below calvarium and elevating pericranium with the supraorbital nerve to expose calvarium for craniotomy without damage to the nerve [53]. Certainly, staying at least 5 mm lateral to the supraorbital notch or foramen with the craniotomy has significantly reduced the risk of supraorbital palsy as well [13, 22, 46]. Incision into the orbicularis oculi should be made along the margin of the muscle superiorly with the muscle dissected with pericranium inferiorly to spare the fibers. The frontalis branch of facial nerve can be injured if the incision extends greater than 13 mm lateral to the zygomatic process of the frontal bone [53]. Therefore, limiting the lateral extension of the incision as well as the use of cautery in the temporalis muscle below the zygomatic process also reduces the risk of frontalis palsy [3, 4, 13, 53]. Finally, another author also recommends sparing the insertion of the temporalis muscle for a better cosmetic result [53]. Using these techniques, among others, has likely played a role in the reduction in supraorbital and frontalis nerve problems in more recent series (Table 1).

4.4. Keyhole Approach and Optical Field. An additional cadaveric study sought to quantitatively verify the accuracy of the claims of Perneczky's group that the optical field widened with increasing distance from the keyhole and that contralateral parasellar structures could be visualized well [2–5, 46]. In this study, the supraorbital keyhole approach was compared to the pterional and larger more traditional supraorbital craniotomies. Their findings demonstrate that the difference in area of exposure between approaches was less than 1 cm, and there was no difference in the total or contralateral side area of exposure in the parasellar region between the three approaches [46]. The authors conclude that the limitations in this approach have more to do with "surgical freedom" of microinstruments than in the field of view at depth [46]. Similar results were found in another cadaveric study noting that, for approaching anterior communicating artery aneurysms, the supraorbital keyhole and transorbital keyhole approaches both afforded more area of exposure than the standard pterional approach [54].

4.5. Supraorbital Keyhole Approach with Endoscopic Assistance. Endoscopes have aided in overcoming one of the main disadvantages to the keyhole approach: illumination. Use of the microscope in keyhole surgery requires frequent changing of the visual angle to allow illumination of the area of interest deep in the surgical field. Endoscopes produce illumination at depth rather than from a distance and therefore can illuminate the area of interest without casting shadows on the field. Endoscopes can be held either by an assistant or with a retractor arm, allowing the surgeon to continue to work bimanually with microinstruments running in a parallel axis with the endoscope [21]. Angled lenses also allow visualization around corners without requiring retraction of important neurovascular structures. This aids in minimizing trauma to the collateral tissue field. A "second look" with the endoscope can also improve the gross total resection of tumors despite the smaller craniotomy with better visualization [21, 22]. The use of angled endoscopes has allowed the supraorbital window to be extended to regions as distant as the interpeduncular cisterns and contralateral cerebellopontine angle by some authors [21]. A secondary advantage to improved illumination with the endoscope is improved ability to achieve hemostasis, which is more difficult through a keyhole approach and listed often as a disadvantage [22].

4.6. Supraorbital Keyhole Approach for Resection of Tuberculum Sellae Meningiomas in Comparison to Endoscopic Endonasal Extended Approaches. A few case series have been reported regarding both supraorbital keyhole approach or endoscopic endonasal extended approaches for resection of tuberculum sellae meningiomas. One author performed a meta-analysis comparing the endoscopic endonasal extended approach for tuberculum sellae meningioma resection with an open craniotomy approach [55]. In this meta-analysis, abstracts that did not differentiate tumor type and location with outcome were excluded. There were 38 retrospective references, 33 were for open cases and 8 for endoscopic endonasal approaches (3 had both approaches). Results demonstrated a similar rate of gross total resection between approaches (85% versus 84% of open versus endoscopic cases, resp.). However, there was a much higher rate of cerebrospinal fluid (CSF) in the endoscopic cases (26.8% versus 3.5% open cases). This rate differed greatly between endoscopic series, with series utilizing a rigid reconstruction and/or a vascularized nasoseptal flap having a 16% leak rate versus 64% for series with other closure methods. Vision loss was significantly higher for open approaches (9.2% versus 1.3% for open versus endoscopic, resp.), but the open series included much larger tumors, potentially accounting for this difference [55]. Rates of pituitary dysfunction were similarly low across series. Unfortunately, this comparison included multiple types of open approaches and lumped them all together. We were interested in the subset of open series performed through a supraorbital keyhole approach through an eyebrow incision. We performed a MEDLINE search for tuberculum sellae meningiomas similar to Bohman et al. and extracted data on case series that performed surgery through a keyhole approach through an eyebrow incision where outcomes data specific to the location were reported. We found 78 cases reported where this approach was used to resect tuberculum sellae meningiomas (see Table 1) [1, 2, 5–35]. Gross total resections were possible in 67/78 (85.9%) cases. Complications included eight patients with worsening vision, seven with hyposmia/anosmia, one with a corneal abrasion, five with endocrinological problems, and two patients who died (one following ICH from a carotid artery injury, a second from unexplained cardiac arrest 40 days after surgery). There were three CSF leaks and no wound infections. These results are similar to the general open series discussed by Bohman et al., demonstrating no greater risk, with a similar rate of gross total resection, despite the smaller craniotomy [55].

4.7. Supraorbital Keyhole Approach for Olfactory Groove Meningiomas. The supraorbital keyhole approach has also been described for resection of olfactory groove meningiomas. In the literature, a MEDLINE search revealed a total of 81 cases reported in the literature where outcomes data were specific to the olfactory groove location of the tumor [1, 2, 5–22, 34]. 74 tumors were resected in a gross total fashion (91.4%). Complications reported included eight CSF leaks and five wound complications. This higher rate of CSF complications may be due to the midline anatomic location of olfactory groove meningiomas. Since the recessed cribriform plate is difficult to visualize with the microscope during a supraorbital keyhole approach, a higher CSF leak rate may occur. Other authors have described an endonasal endoscopic route to these lesions. However, a recent study compared traditional open craniotomy with endoscopic endonasal resection of tumors, concluding that better resections, and lower CSF leak rates, were possible through the open rather than the endoscopic approach [56]. Use of the endoscope for assistance in visualizing the cribriform plate may further permit complete resections of olfactory groove meningiomas while also helping with skull base reconstruction to prevent CSF leakage.

4.8. Supraorbital Keyhole Approach for Resection of Suprasellar Craniopharyngiomas in Comparison to Endoscopic Endonasal Extended Approaches. A case series of 43 patients was recently reported with either craniopharyngiomas or anterior skull base meningiomas resected through either an extended endoscopic endonasal route or through a keyhole supraorbital craniotomy and subfrontal approach [8]. Of the craniopharyngiomas treated, there were 18 treated through an extended endoscopic endonasal approach and 4 treated through a supraorbital route. There was one postoperative CSF leak in the endonasal cohort and none in the supraorbital cohort. There were two gross total resections in the endonasal cohort and none in the supraorbital cohort, although this was often not the goal of surgery. If there were dense adhesions to neurovascular structures, the authors noted they opted for a subtotal resection with planned postoperative radiation [8].

The location of the chiasm in relation to the tumor, along with the lateral extension of tumor, may determine whether a supraorbital keyhole or endoscopic endonasal approach is taken. Prechiasmatic craniopharyngiomas may be better accessed through a supraorbital keyhole approach especially if there is lateral or suprachiasmatic extension of tumor. Retrochiasmatic lesions, on the other hand, can pose a greater chance for injury to the visual apparatus through a supraorbital approach and may be better resected through an endoscopic endonasal approach [8].

4.9. Cosmetic Considerations of the Eyebrow Incision. Cosmesis has prevented many surgeons from attempting this approach or has led to their abandonment of this approach with its introduction early on. A number of modifications have led to what many now consider to be a superb cosmetic result with the supraorbital craniotomy and keyhole approach. A limited skin incision within the eyebrow, minimal temporalis muscle dissection, a small bone flap, and closure with the orbicularis oculi muscle/pericranium layers have contributed to the success of the eyebrow incision. Temporalis muscle atrophy, so common with standard frontotemporal and pterional craniotomies, can be avoided with the eyebrow incision [16]. Of course, orbicularis oculi muscle asymmetry can lead to less ideal cosmetic outcomes through this approach. This can occur through both muscle fiber and nerve injury [24, 25]. This can be avoided by first opening the incision only through the skin and dermis layers, and then opening the muscle more dorsally and cutting along the muscle fibers rather than across them.

There have been a number of ways to perform the incision including superciliary, transciliary, and even transpalpebral incisions in an attempt to improve cosmesis [6, 9, 24, 26, 29]. Superciliary incisions avoid depilating the hair follicles but leave a visible scar above the eyebrow. Transciliary incisions may lead to hair follicle depilation, but this typically does not occur if one avoids the use of cautery [48]. The transpalpebral approach places the incision through the folds of the eyelid, thus also avoiding depilation of the hair follicles, but typically requires the use of a second specialist with experience performing surgery through the eyelid [26]. All of these incisions can become problematic in the setting of infection, but thankfully infection risk is low with this approach (see Table 1).

Another important cosmetic consideration is performing the initial incision through the skin and dermis layers only. Cephalad dissection superficial to the orbicularis oculi, pericranium, and temporalis muscle is important for development of a separate tissue flap for covering the keyhole craniotomy during closure [2, 5, 13, 22, 46]. Additional considerations for a good cosmetic result include proper repositioning of the bone flap. Care must be taken to ensure that the outer cortex of the supraorbital ridge remains intact during the approach. Use of a burr hole cover and square titanium plates prevents the appearance or palpation of the gap between the bone flap and intact native bone following bone flap replacement in the patient. Final closure of the skin layer with a running subcuticular stitch (e.g., 5-0 Prolene) without any suture knots brings the edges of the eyebrow together for proper cosmesis as well.

5. Conclusions

The supraorbital craniotomy and keyhole approach through the eyebrow permit access to a number of lesions in the subfrontal corridor with minimal brain retraction and a much smaller area of potential injury of superficial structures. All minimally invasive techniques have a learning curve, and smaller, simpler lesions should be performed first through this approach before moving on to larger, more complicated lesions. Our experience is that midline and suprasellar lesions are more easily accessed through this approach than laterally based lesions. Endoscopy can play an important role in improving visualization through the keyhole corridor. Attention to detail can allow this approach to be performed with superb cosmetic results while still achieving surgical efficacy and limiting complications.

Acknowledgment

The authors have no disclosures. The authors would like to thank Eric Jablonowski for the illustrations in the paper.

References

[1] H.-C. Chen and W.-C. Tzaan, “Microsurgical supraorbital keyhole approach to the anterior cranial base,” *Journal of Clinical Neuroscience*, vol. 17, no. 12, pp. 1510–1514, 2010.

[2] R. Reisch and A. Perneczky, “Ten-year experience with the supraorbital subfrontal approach through an eyebrow skin incision,” *Neurosurgery*, vol. 57, no. 4, supplement, pp. 242–253, 2005.

[3] A. Perneczky, “Planning strategies for the suprasellar region: philosophy of approaches,” *Neurosurgeon*, vol. 11, pp. 343–348, 1992.

[4] A. Perneczky, W. Müller-Forell, E. van Lindert, and G. Fries, *Keyhole Concept in Neurosurgery*, Thieme Medical Publishers, Stuttgart, Germany, 1999.

[5] R. Reisch, A. Perneczky, and R. Filippi, “Surgical technique of the supraorbital key-hole craniotomy,” *Surgical Neurology*, vol. 59, no. 3, pp. 223–227, 2003.

[6] S. Czirják and G. T. Szeifert, “Surgical experience with frontolateral keyhole craniotomy through a superciliary skin incision,” *Neurosurgery*, vol. 48, no. 1, pp. 145–150, 2001.

[7] A. O. Dare, M. K. Landi, D. K. Lopes, and W. Grand, “Eyebrow incision for combined orbital osteotomy and supraorbital minicraniotomy: application to aneurysms of the anterior circulation: technical note,” *Journal of Neurosurgery*, vol. 95, no. 4, pp. 714–718, 2001.

[8] N. Fatemi, J. R. Dusick, M. A. De Paiva Neto, D. Malkasian, and D. F. Kelly, “Endonasal versus supraorbital keyhole removal of craniopharyngiomas and tuberculum sellae meningiomas,” *Neurosurgery*, vol. 64, no. 5, supplement, pp. 269–284, 2009.

[9] G. I. Jallo, I. Suk, and L. Bognár, “A superciliary approach for anterior cranial fossa lesions in children: technical note,” *Journal of Neurosurgery*, vol. 103, no. 1, pp. 88–93, 2005.

[10] H.-D. Jho, “Orbital roof craniotomy via an eyebrow incision: a simplified anterior skull base approach,” *Minimally Invasive Neurosurgery*, vol. 40, no. 3, pp. 91–97, 1997.

[11] Y. Ko, H. J. Yi, Y. S. Kim, S. H. Oh, K. M. Kim, and S. J. Oh, “Eyebrow incision using tattoo for anterior fossa lesions: technical case reports,” *Minimally Invasive Neurosurgery*, vol. 44, no. 1, pp. 17–20, 2001.

[12] I. Melamed, V. Merkin, A. Korn, and M. Nash, “The supraorbital approach: an alternative to traditional exposure for the surgical management of anterior fossa and parasellar pathology,” *Minimally Invasive Neurosurgery*, vol. 48, no. 5, pp. 259–263, 2005.

[13] P. Mitchell, R. R. Vindlacheruvu, K. Mahmood, R. D. Ashpole, A. Grivas, and A. D. Mendelow, "Supraorbital eyebrow minicraniotomy for anterior circulation aneurysms," *Surgical Neurology*, vol. 63, no. 1, pp. 47–51, 2005.

[14] J. Paladino, N. Pirker, D. Štimac, and R. Stern-Padovan, "Eyebrow keyhole approach in vascular neurosurgery," *Minimally Invasive Neurosurgery*, vol. 41, no. 4, pp. 200–203, 1998.

[15] G. Shanno, M. Maus, J. Bilyk et al., "Image-guided transorbital roof craniotomy via a suprabrow approach: a surgical series of 72 patients," *Neurosurgery*, vol. 48, no. 3, pp. 559–568, 2001.

[16] H.-J. Steiger, R. Schmid-Elsaesser, W. Stummer, and E. Uhl, "Transorbital keyhole approach to anterior communicating artery aneurysms," *Neurosurgery*, vol. 48, no. 2, pp. 347–352, 2001.

[17] R. Ramos-Zúñiga, H. Velázquez, M. A. Barajas, R. López, E. Sánchez, and S. Trejo, "Trans-supraorbital approach to supratentorial aneurysms," *Neurosurgery*, vol. 51, pp. 125–131, 2002.

[18] R. Ramos-Zúñiga, "The trans-supraorbital approach," *Minimally Invasive Neurosurgery*, vol. 42, no. 3, pp. 133–136, 1999.

[19] M. A. Sánchez-Vázquez, P. Barrera-Calatayud, M. Mejia-Villela et al., "Transciliary subfrontal craniotomy for anterior skull base lesions: technical note," *Journal of Neurosurgery*, vol. 91, no. 5, pp. 892–896, 1999.

[20] S. Telera, C. M. Carapella, F. Caroli et al., "Supraorbital keyhole approach for removal of midline anterior cranial fossa meningiomas: a series of 20 consecutive cases," *Neurosurgical Review*, vol. 35, pp. 67–83, 2012.

[21] E. Van Lindert, A. Perneczky, G. Fries, and E. Pierangeli, "The supraorbital keyhole approach to supratentorial aneurysms: concept and technique," *Surgical Neurology*, vol. 49, no. 5, pp. 481–490, 1998.

[22] X. Zheng, W. Liu, X. Yang et al., "Endoscope-assisted supraorbital keyhole approach for the resection of benign tumors of the sellar region," *Minimally Invasive Therapy and Allied Technologies*, vol. 16, no. 6, pp. 363–366, 2007.

[23] H. Wiedemayer, I. E. Sandalcioglu, H. Wiedemayer, and D. Stolke, "The supraorbital keyhole approach via an eyebrow incision for resection of tumors around the sella and the anterior skull base," *Minimally Invasive Neurosurgery*, vol. 47, no. 4, pp. 221–225, 2004.

[24] A. Perneczky, "Surgical results, complications and patient satisfaction after supraorbital craniotomy through eyebrow skin incision," in *Proceedings of the Joint Meeting mit der Ungarischen Gesellschaft für Neurochirurgie Deutsche Gesellschaft für Neurochirurgie (DGNC '04)*, Köln, Germany, April 2004.

[25] V. Lupret, T. Sajko, V. Beroš, N. Kudelić, and V. Lupret Jr., "Advantages and disadvantages of the supraorbital keyhole approach to intracranial aneurysms," *Acta Clinica Croatica*, vol. 45, no. 2, pp. 91–94, 2006.

[26] K. M. Abdel Aziz, S. Bhatia, M. H. Tantawy et al., "Minimally invasive transpalpebral "eyelid" approach to the anterior cranial base," *Neurosurgery*, vol. 69, no. 2, pp. 195–206, 2011.

[27] G. Fischer, A. Stadie, R. Reisch et al., "The keyhole concept in aneurysm surgery: results of the past 20 years," *Neurosurgery*, vol. 68, no. 1, pp. 45–51, 2011.

[28] H. L. Brydon, H. Akil, S. Ushewokunze, J. S. Dhir, A. Taha, and A. Ahmed, "Supraorbital microcraniotomy for acute aneurysmal subarachnoid haemorrhage: results of first 50 cases," *British Journal of Neurosurgery*, vol. 22, no. 1, pp. 40–45, 2008.

[29] S. Czirják, I. Nyáry, J. Futó, and G. T. Szeifert, "Bilateral supraorbital keyhole approach for multiple aneurysms via superciliary skin incisions," *Surgical Neurology*, vol. 57, no. 5, pp. 314–323, 2002.

[30] C. Hayhurst and C. Teo, "Tuberculum sella meningioma," *Otolaryngologic Clinics of North America*, vol. 44, no. 4, pp. 953–963, 2011.

[31] N. McLaughlin, L. F. S. Ditzel Filho, K. Shahlaie, D. Solari, A. B. Kassam, and D. F. Kelly, "The supraorbital approach for recurrent or residual suprasellar tumors," *Minimally Invasive Neurosurgery*, vol. 54, no. 4, pp. 155–161, 2011.

[32] R. Romani, A. Laakso, M. Kangasniemi, M. Lehecka, and J. Hernesniemi, "Lateral supraorbital approach applied to anterior clinoidal meningiomas: experience with 73 consecutive patients," *Neurosurgery*, vol. 68, no. 6, pp. 1632–1647, 2011.

[33] R. Romani, A. Laakso, M. Kangasniemi, M. Niemelä, and J. Hernesniemi, "Lateral supraorbital approach applied to tuberculum sellae meningiomas: experience with 52 consecutive patients," *Neurosurgery*, vol. 70, pp. 1504–1518, 2012.

[34] R. Romani, M. Lehecka, E. Gaal et al., "Lateral supraorbital approach applied to olfactory groove meningiomas: experience with 66 consecutive patients," *Neurosurgery*, vol. 65, no. 1, pp. 39–52, 2009.

[35] Y. B. Fernandes, D. Maitrot, P. Kehrli, O. I. De Tella Jr., R. Ramina, and G. Borges, "Supraorbital eyebrow approach to skull base lesions," *Arquivos de Neuro-Psiquiatria*, vol. 60, no. 2, pp. 246–250, 2002.

[36] G. Fries and A. Perneczky, "Endoscope-assisted brain surgery—part 2—analysis of 380 procedures," *Neurosurgery*, vol. 42, no. 2, pp. 226–232, 1998.

[37] E. Knosp, G. Müller, A. Perneczky, and A. L. Rhoton Jr., "The paraclinoid carotid artery: anatomical aspects of a microneurosurgical approach," *Neurosurgery*, vol. 22, no. 5, pp. 896–901, 1988.

[38] T. Menovsky, J. A. Grotenhuis, J. De Vries, and R. H. M. A. Bartels, "Endoscope-assisted supraorbital craniotomy for lesions of the interpeduncular fossa," *Neurosurgery*, vol. 44, no. 1, pp. 106–112, 1999.

[39] M.-Z. Zhang, L. Wang, W. Zhang et al., "The supraorbital keyhole approach with eyebrow incisions for treating lesions in the anterior fossa and sellar region," *Chinese Medical Journal*, vol. 117, no. 3, pp. 323–326, 2004.

[40] J. Park, D.-H. Kang, and B.-Y. Chun, "Superciliary keyhole surgery for unruptured posterior communicating artery aneurysms with oculomotor nerve palsy: maximizing symptomatic resolution and minimizing surgical invasiveness," *Journal of Neurosurgery*, vol. 115, no. 4, pp. 700–706, 2011.

[41] N. Chalouhi, P. Jabbour, I. Ibrahim et al., "Surgical treatment of ruptured anterior circulation aneurysms: comparison of pterional and supraorbital keyhole approaches," *Neurosurgery*, vol. 72, no. 3, pp. 437–441, 2013.

[42] M. E. Ivan and M. T. Lawton, "Mini supraorbital approach to inferior frontal lobe cavernous malformations: case series," *Journal of Neurological Surgery Part A*, vol. 74, no. 3, pp. 187–191, 2013.

[43] H. J. Kang, Y. S. Lee, S. J. Suh, J. H. Lee, K. Y. Ryu, and D. G. Kang, "Comparative analysis of the mini-pterional and supraorbital keyhole craniotomies for unruptured aneurysms with numeric measurements of their geometric configurations," *Journal of Cerebrovascular and Endovascular Neurosurgery*, vol. 15, no. 1, pp. 5–12, 2013.

[44] L. F. Ditzel Filho, N. McLaughlin, D. Bresson, D. Solari, A. B. Kassam, and D. F. Kelly, "Supraorbital eyebrow craniotomy for

removal of intraaxial frontal brain tumors: a technical note," *World Neurosurgery*, 2013.

[45] J. Park, T. D. Jung, D. H. Kang, and S. H. Lee, "Preoperative percutaneous mapping of the frontal branch of the facial nerve to assess the risk of frontalis muscle palsy after a supraorbital keyhole approach," *Journal of Neurosurgery*, vol. 118, no. 5, pp. 1114–1119, 2013.

[46] C. Cheng, A. Noguchi, A. Dogan et al., "Quantitative verification of the keyhole concept: a comparison of area of exposure in the parasellar region via supraorbital keyhole, frontotemporal pterional, and supraorbital approaches," *Journal of Neurosurgery*, vol. 118, pp. 264–269, 2013.

[47] R. C. Heros, "The supraorbital "keyhole" approach," *Journal of Neurosurgery*, vol. 114, no. 3, pp. 850–851, 2011.

[48] M. Berhouma, T. Jacquesson, and E. Jouanneau, "The fully endoscopic supraorbital trans-eyebrow keyhole approach to the anterior and middle skull base," *Acta Neurochirurgica*, vol. 153, no. 10, pp. 1949–1954, 2011.

[49] J. B. Delashaw Jr., H. Tedeschi, A. L. Rhoton, and J. A. Jane, "Modified supraorbital craniotomy: technical note," *Neurosurgery*, vol. 30, no. 6, pp. 954–956, 1992.

[50] J. B. Delashaw Jr., J. A. Jane, N. F. Kassell, and C. Luce, "Supraorbital craniotomy by fracture of the anterior orbital roof. Technical note," *Journal of Neurosurgery*, vol. 79, no. 4, pp. 615–618, 1993.

[51] J. A. Jane, T. S. Park, and L. H. Pobereskin, "The supraorbital approach: technical note," *Neurosurgery*, vol. 11, no. 4, pp. 537–542, 1982.

[52] O. Al-Mefty, "Supraorbital-pterional approach to skull base lesions," *Neurosurgery*, vol. 21, no. 4, pp. 474–477, 1987.

[53] Y. Lin, W. Zhang, Q. Luo, J. Jiang, and Y. Qiu, "Extracranial microanatomic study of supraorbital keyhole approach," *The Journal of Craniofacial Surgery*, vol. 20, no. 1, pp. 215–218, 2009.

[54] F. Beretta, N. Andaluz, C. Chalaala, C. Bernucci, L. Salud, and M. Zuccarello, "Image-guided anatomical and morphometric study of supraorbital and transorbital minicraniotomies to the sellar and perisellar regions: comparison with standard techniques," *Journal of Neurosurgery*, vol. 113, no. 5, pp. 975–981, 2010.

[55] L. Bohman, S. C. Stein, J. G. Newman et al., "Endoscopic versus open resection of tuberculum sellae meningiomas: a decision analysis," *Journal for Oto-Rhino-Laryngology and Its Related Specialties*, vol. 74, no. 5, pp. 255–263, 2012.

[56] R. J. Komotar, R. M. Starke, D. M. S. Raper, V. K. Anand, and T. H. Schwartz, "Endoscopic endonasal versus open transcranial resection of anterior midline skull base meningiomas," *World Neurosurgery*, vol. 77, no. 5-6, pp. 713–724, 2012.

7

Surgeons' Volume-Outcome Relationship for Lobectomies and Wedge Resections for Cancer Using Video-Assisted Thoracoscopic Techniques

Guy David,[1] Candace L. Gunnarsson,[2] Matt Moore,[3] John Howington,[4] Daniel L. Miller,[5] Michael A. Maddaus,[6] Robert Joseph McKenna Jr.,[7] Bryan F. Meyers,[8] and Scott J. Swanson[9]

[1] *Associate Professor of Health Care Management, The Wharton School, University of Pennsylvania, 202 Colonial Penn Center, 3641 Locust Walk, Philadelphia, PA 19104, USA*
[2] *S² Statistical Solutions, Inc., 11176 Main Street, Cincinnati, OH 45241, USA*
[3] *Healthcare Policy and Economics, Ethicon Endo-Surgery, 4545 Creek Road, Cincinnati, OH 45252, USA*
[4] *Division of Thoracic Surgery and Surgical Quality, NorthShore University Health System, 2650 Ridge Avenue, 3507 Walgreen Buliding, Evanston, IL 60201, USA*
[5] *Division of Thoracic Surgery, Emory University Healthcare, 1365 Clifton Rd NE, Atlanta, GA 30322, USA*
[6] *Division of Thoracic Surgery, University of Minnesota, 420 Delaware Street SE, Mayo Mail Code 195, Minneapolis, MN 55455, USA*
[7] *Division of Thoracic Surgery, Cedars Sinai Medical Center, 8635 West Third, Suite 675, Los Angeles, CA 90048, USA*
[8] *Division of Cardiothoracic Surgery, Barnes-Jewish Hospital Plaza, Washington University in St. Louis, Queeny Tower, Suite 3108, St. Louis, MO 63110-1013, USA*
[9] *Division of Minimally Invasive Thoracic Surgey, Brigham and Women's Hospital, Dana-Farber Cancer Institute, Harvard Medical School, 75 Francis Street, Boston, MA 02115, USA*

Correspondence should be addressed to Candace L. Gunnarsson, candaceg@s2stats.com

Academic Editor: Peng Hui Wang

This study examined the effect of surgeons' volume on outcomes in lung surgery: lobectomies and wedge resections. Additionally, the effect of video-assisted thoracoscopic surgery (VATS) on cost, utilization, and adverse events was analyzed. The Premier Hospital Database was the data source for this analysis. Eligible patients were those of any age undergoing lobectomy or wedge resection using VATS for cancer treatment. Volume was represented by the aggregate experience level of the surgeon in a six-month window before each surgery. A positive volume-outcome relationship was found with some notable features. The relationship is stronger for cost and utilization outcomes than for adverse events; for thoracic surgeons as opposed to other surgeons; for VATS lobectomies rather than VATS wedge resections. While there was a reduction in cost and resource utilization with greater experience in VATS, these outcomes were not associated with greater experience in open procedures.

1. Introduction

Lobectomies and wedge resections of the lung are performed using either open thoracotomy or minimally invasive techniques, particularly, video-assisted thoracoscopic surgery (VATS). The literature documents many purported benefits of VATS for major lung surgeries, such as smaller incisions, less pain, less blood loss, less respiratory compromise, faster recovery times translating into shortened hospital lengths of stay, and superior survival rates [1]. However, compared to open procedures, VATS has higher equipment costs, increased operating room times, and a learning curve for both surgeons and operating room personnel [2].

During the past three decades, a large body of empirical literature has established a positive relationship between provider volume and patient health outcomes across various medical and surgical procedures [3–10], with little attention paid to thoracic surgery. This is important, as the magnitude of the volume outcome effect was found to vary across health conditions and surgery procedures [8]. The reason that greater volume is associated with better throughput, clinical outcomes, and control over resources, is not well understood. This relationship may be the result of surgeons' "learning-by-doing" and/or the result of "selective referrals", where physicians with better outcomes command a higher demand for their services [3].

To date, most of the work on volume outcome relations was conducted at the hospital level, as opposed to the surgeon level. In the case of lung surgery, patients who received open lobectomy and other resections at high-volume hospitals were less likely to experience postoperative complications and enjoyed better long-term and short-term survival rates [11–13]. A similar relationship between hospital volume and patient outcomes has been observed across patients receiving minimally invasive procedures; for example, minimally invasive endovascular interventions for patients with abdominal aortic aneurysms [14–16].

Recently, there is some evidence that the associations between hospital volume and operative mortality are mediated by surgeon volume [14, 17]. The volume of the surgeon was found to have a greater influence on patient outcomes than hospital volume [18]. This should come as no surprise, as hospital volume is the aggregate of all participating surgeons' volumes. Surgeons make preoperative and intra-operative decisions, affect case selection, and determine the appropriate surgical technique to be used. Studies of the relationship between surgeon volume and outcomes for cancer patients are mixed. A majority of cancer studies find that high-volume surgeons have a lower rate of operative mortality, with the strength of the relationship varying by condition and procedure [14, 19]. Conclusions may be obscured by heterogenous definitions of high-volume across studies and procedures [18].

Few studies have examined the relationship between surgeon volume and operative mortality for lobectomies and wedge resections [18, 20, 21]. In one such study, high volume surgeons were found to have less locoregional recurrence of cancer, but no differences were observed for mortality [20]. While thoracic surgeons were more likely to perform lobectomies and wedge resections using VATS, adjusting for surgeon and hospital volume, lung cancer patients treated by general thoracic surgeons had a lower probability of death than those treated by cardiothoracic surgeons or general surgeons [21]. A number of case studies based on either a single center or a single surgeon found greater experience with VATS to improve such patient outcomes as blood loss, recurrence, operation time, surgeon-related thoracotomy conversions, and readmissions [22–24].

Understanding volume-outcome relationships is of considerable practical importance because it quantifies the effects of experience on clinical outcomes. However, experience must be relevant to performance. Even though surgeons often use different techniques (e.g., open procedure versus VATS), studies have not accounted for technique-specific experience in calculating volume. To our knowledge, this is the first study to accumulate experience with VATS separately from experience with open procedure, as the two techniques command different surgical skills. Information regarding skill development through practice is an important factor that may affect patient decisions of where to seek treatment and provider decisions about where to refer their patients. Furthermore, transitioning from open to VATS procedures is not trivial, hence it is important to study the degree of transferability of experience across the two procedures [25].

Volume-outcome studies of cancer patients have reported mortality, inpatient length-of-stay, readmissions, and several specific clinical indicators, such as blood loss and perioperative complications [26, 27]. However, greater experience can manifest itself in additional ways. Recent studies documented variations among physicians in their ability to shorten the length-of-stay for their patients, reduce resource utilization, improve quality, and reduce the likelihood of hospital-borne infections.

This current work aims to quantify the impact of a surgeon's volume on outcomes in lung surgery, adjusted for other potential explanatory variables. We studied performance on lobectomies and wedge resections separately and accounted for the experience of surgeons as represented by six-month case volumes using both VATS and open techniques. Also, we analyzed the effect of this technique-specific experience on inpatient costs, length of surgery, length of stay, as well as the likelihood and number of adverse surgical events.

2. Materials and Methods

A protocol describing the analysis objectives, criteria for patient selection, data elements of interest, and statistical methods was submitted to the New England Institutional Review Board (NEIRB), and exemption was obtained.The study was funded by Ethicon Endo-Surgery Inc. (Cincinnati, Ohio, USA).

2.1. Data Source. This study utilizes the Premier Hospital Database, which contains clinical and utilization information on patients receiving care in over 600 USA hospitals and ambulatory surgery centers across the nation. The database contains complete patient billing, hospital cost, and coding histories from more than 25 million inpatient discharges and 175 million hospital outpatient visits. Since VATS is a new technology, the analyzable dataset was restricted to procedures occurring in 2007-2008. Only data that were anonymized with regard to patient identifiers were used.

2.2. Patients and Procedures. Eligible patients were those of any age undergoing VATS lobectomy or wedge resection for cancer. International Classification of Diseases, 9th Revision (ICD-9) diagnosis codes and procedure codes for identifying lobectomy and wedge resection procedures, cancer diagnoses, comorbid conditions, and all adverse events are listed in Tables 7–10.

2.3. Volume Outcome Variable. The volume measure typically used in previous research utilized subsequent volume to predict outcomes. For example, many studies defined

TABLE 1: Patient characteristics.

Procedure*	VATS lobectomy		VATS wedge resection	
	All surgeons (including thoracic)	Thoracic surgeons (only)	All surgeons (including thoracic)	Thoracic surgeons (only)
Total N	716	546	1,982	1,350
(% of total N = 2,698)	(26.54%)	(20.24%)	(73.46%)	(50.04%)
Age average (SD)	66.68 (11.27)	66.51 (10.96)	61.09 (15.39)	61.37 (14.57)
<40	0.01	0.01	0.10	0.09
41–50	0.07	0.08	0.12	0.12
51–60	0.20	0.20	0.20	0.21
61–70	0.32	0.33	0.29	0.29
71–80	0.30	0.28	0.24	0.24
>80	0.10	0.10	0.06	0.06
Race				
Caucasian	0.79	0.84	0.74	0.79
African American	0.07	0.07	0.08	0.09
Other	0.13	0.10	0.18	0.13
Gender				
Female	0.55	0.55	0.53	0.53
Male	0.45	0.45	0.47	0.47
Marital status				
Married	0.59	0.62	0.54	0.58
Unmarried	0.41	0.38	0.46	0.42
Insurance type				
Commercial	0.07	0.07	0.07	0.07
Medicare	0.60	0.60	0.49	0.49
Medicaid	0.03	0.02	0.05	0.05
Managed care	0.28	0.30	0.35	0.35
Other	0.03	0.02	0.04	0.03
Malignancy indication**				
Primary neoplasm of the lung	0.96	0.95	0.86	0.85
Metastases from other primary malignancy	0.04	0.05	0.14	0.15
Illness severity level				
APR-DRG Severity Level (1, 2)	0.78	0.79	0.87	0.86
APR-DRG Severity Level (3, 4)	0.22	0.21	0.13	0.14

*All procedures are inpatient. CPT and ICD codes for resections in Table 7.
**ICD codes for lung cancer in Table 8.

physician volume as the number of surgeries done over a specific time period and used that measure to predict outcomes of each surgery performed within that same time period [8, 9, 12, 14, 28]. As a result, experience not yet acquired was used to describe current performance, which could potentially overestimate the influence of volume on surgeon outcomes.

For each outcome-surgeon combination, our measure of volume represented the aggregate experience level of the surgeon. Volume-accumulated experience over running six-month windows involved recording surgeons' volume at a given date as the number of procedures accumulated during the prior six months. This measure is more precise than fixed calendar periods and was used extensively in the literature, as it responds instantaneously to any changes in the surgeon's recent experience profile. Experience accumulation with moving, rather than fixed, windows can be viewed as smoothing the calendar step function and alleviating the imprecision that increases for observations occurring toward the end of the observation period [29].

2.4. Statistical Analyses. Initial counts, percentages, means, and standard deviations for patient demographics, comorbid conditions, hospital characteristics, as well as safety utilization and cost outcomes were summarized separately for VATS lobectomy versus VATS wedge resection and separately for thoracic surgeons versus all surgeons using descriptive statistics. Type of surgeon (thoracic versus general) was identified via physician identification codes provided in the database.

Table 2: Comorbid conditions*, **.

	VATS lobectomy		VATS wedge resection	
	All surgeons (including thoracic)	Thoracic surgeons (only)	All surgeons (including thoracic)	Thoracic surgeons (only)
Total *N* (2,698)	716	546	1,982	1,350
Myocardial infarction, acute or old	0.11	0.12	0.08	0.09
Congestive heart failure	0.07	0.07	0.07	0.08
Other chronic or unspecified heart failure	0.02	0.02	0.02	0.03
Peripheral vascular disease	0.10	0.10	0.08	0.08
Dementia	0.03	0.03	0.02	0.01
Chronic pulmonary disease	0.50	0.50	0.47	0.49
Connective tissue disease	0.03	0.03	0.05	0.05
Liver disease	0.05	0.05	0.06	0.06
Chronic viral hepatitis	0.01	0.01	0.01	0.01
Renal insufficiency, chronic	0.04	0.04	0.05	0.05
Diabetes mellitus	0.19	0.18	0.19	0.20

* Proportions of comorbid conditions existing for patients any time during or before procedure stay in Premier database (beginning in 2000).
**ICD codes for these variables are found in Table 10.

Table 3: Hospital characteristics.

	VATS lobectomy		VATS wedge resection	
	All surgeons (including thoracic)	Thoracic surgeons (only)	All surgeons (including thoracic)	Thoracic surgeons (only)
Total *N* (2,698)	716	546	1,982	1,350
Census region				
Northeast	0.22	0.22	0.21	0.17
Midwest	0.12	0.11	0.24	0.23
South	0.51	0.51	0.41	0.45
West	0.15	0.16	0.14	0.15
Location				
Urban	0.96	0.96	0.95	0.96
Nonurban	0.04	0.04	0.05	0.04
Type				
Teaching	0.63	0.62	0.57	0.57
Nonteaching	0.37	0.38	0.43	0.43
Bed count				
<200	0.05	0.04	0.06	0.05
200–400	0.20	0.21	0.26	0.25
400–600	0.29	0.31	0.30	0.35
>600	0.46	0.44	0.38	0.35

The safety outcomes of interest were pertinent adverse events occurring during or up to 30–60 days after surgery. A dichotomous variable was used indicating the existence of an adverse event as well as a continuous variable tallying the number of adverse events. Utilization outcomes were surgery duration (hours) and hospital length of stay (days). Cost outcomes were total hospital costs per patient, both fixed and variable. Since we only studied VATS procedures, we did not include costs for initial acquisition of the VATS equipment.

In addition, descriptive statistics for the volume explanatory variables are presented. The key explanatory variable was each surgeon's volume for lobectomy and wedge resection using VATS or open thoracotomy techniques. This measure of volume corresponded to the aggregate experience level of the surgeon over running six-month windows. Experience with open thoracotomy procedures may or may not contribute to performance with VATS, but it is certainly expected that experience specific to VATS will be the most relevant in explaining outcomes for patients treated with VATS.

Multivariable logistic regression analyses were estimated for the adverse event binary outcome: the presence or

TABLE 4: Volume and outcomes measures*.

	VATS lobectomy		VATS wedge resection	
	All surgeons (including thoracic)	Thoracic surgeons (only)	All surgeons (including thoracic)	Thoracic surgeons (only)
Total N (2,698)	716	546	1,982	1,350
Inpatient costs (dollars)	19,697	19,271	13,058	13,127
	[10,670]	[10,934]	[8,669]	[9,157]
Length of surgery (hours)	4.079	4.008	2.537	2.557
	[1.477]	[1.439]	[1.079]	[1.098]
Length of stay (days)	5.753	5.676	3.944	3.952
	[4.122]	[4.314]	[3.384]	[3.426]
Likelihood of adverse event	0.571	0.557	0.435	0.436
	[0.495]	[0.497]	[0.496]	[0.496]
Number of adverse events	1.126	1.092	0.722	0.740
	[1.361]	[1.347]	[1.062]	[1.094]
VATS six-month volume	28.42	31.64	22.30	24.59
	[30.80]	[33.57]	[27.11]	[30.56]
Open lobectomy six-month volume	5.27	5.46	5.52	5.38
	[4.54]	[4.51]	[5.48]	[4.85]
Open wedge Res six-month volume	3.66	3.73	4.02	3.97
	[3.11]	[2.89]	[3.75]	[3.43]

*Standard deviations are reported in brackets.
** ICD codes for these variables are found in Table 10.

TABLE 5: Multivariable results for cost, utilization, and adverse events.

	VATS lobectomy		VATS wedge resection	
	All surgeons (including thoracic)	Thoracic surgeons (only)	All surgeons (including thoracic)	Thoracic surgeons (only)
Total N (2,698)	716	546	1,982	1,350
Inpatient costs (dollars)				
Regression coefficient	−0.066***	−0.098***	−0.0436***	−0.0468***
	[0.0158]	[0.0170]	[0.00904]	[0.0104]
Length of surgery (hours)				
Regression coefficient	−0.045***	−0.074***	−0.0475***	−0.0317***
	[0.0135]	[0.0149]	[0.0077]	[0.0084]
Length of stay (days)				
Regression coefficient	−0.096***	−0.117***	−0.0778***	−0.0665***
	[0.0207]	[0.0237]	[0.0129]	[0.0141]
Likelihood of adverse events				
Regression coefficient	−0.002*	−0.002***	−0.0005	−0.00098
	[0.0009]	[0.0010]	[0.0006]	[0.0007]
Number of adverse events				
Regression coefficient	−0.083***	−0.142***	−0.0119	−0.0273
	[0.0396]	[0.0493]	[0.0269]	[0.0292]

Estimated marginal effects are reported, standard deviations are reported in brackets * and *** indicate significance at the 10% and 1% levels.

absence of specific individual events. Ordinary least squares (OLS) regression was used for all other continuous outcomes such as hospital costs, surgery time, length of stay, and number of adverse events. For all models, in addition to the volume measures, the following explanatory variables were included: age, gender, race, marital status, insurance type, diagnosis (metastasis versus primary cancer), comorbid conditions (e.g., diabetes), All Patient Refined-Diagnosis-Related Groups (APR-DRGs) severity index (an index of comorbidity unique to the Premier database that reflects

Table 6: Multivariable results for cost, utilization, and adverse events (including non-VATS volume).

	Lobectomy for all surgeons			Lobectomy for Thoracic Surgeons only			Wedge Resection for All Surgeons			Wedge Resection for Thoracic Surgeons only		
	VATS surgeon volume	Open lobectomy volume	Open wedge volume	VATS surgeon volume	Open lobectomy volume	Open wedge volume	VATS surgeon volume	Open lobectomy volume	Open wedge volume	VATS surgeon volume	Open lobectomy volume	Open wedge volume
Cost (dollars)												
Regression coefficient (marginal effects)	−0.062***	−0.014	0.044	−0.092***	0.006	−0.058***	−0.034***	−0.037***	−0.0043	−0.0474***	−0.0682***	−0.0077
Standard deviation	[0.0162]	[0.026]	[0.0287]	[0.0172]	[0.0277]	[0.0274]	[0.0093]	[0.0136]	[0.0163]	[0.0103]	[0.0149]	[0.0181]
Length of Surgery (Hours)												
Regression coefficient (marginal effects)	−0.043***	−0.003	−0.0195	−0.074***	−0.002	−0.0100	−0.032***	−0.083***	−0.017	−0.0339***	−0.089***	−0.022
Standard deviation	[0.0137]	[0.0239]	[0.0262]	[0.0152]	[0.0295]	[0.0277]	[0.0076]	[0.0100]	[0.0118]	[0.0084]	[0.0124]	[0.0251]
Length of Stay (Days)												
Regression coefficient (marginal effects)	−0.087***	0.022	−0.062*	−0.104***	0.048	−0.079***	−0.063***	−0.062***	−0.0005	−0.066***	−0.069***	0.0036
Standard deviation	[0.0162]	[0.027]	[0.0325]	[0.0234]	[0.0318]	[0.0361]	[0.0128]	[0.0214]	[0.0233]	[0.0141]	[0.0236]	[0.0123]
Likelihood of Adverse Events												
Regression coefficient (marginal effects)	−0.002*	−0.009	−0.005	−0.002***	−0.012	−0.009	−0.0002	−0.0035	−0.0009	−0.00085	−0.0033	−0.00595
Standard deviation	[0.0009]	[0.008]	[0.010]	[0.0010]	[0.011]	[0.011]	[0.0006]	[0.0034]	[0.0058]	[0.0007]	[0.0046]	[0.0061]
Number of Adverse Events												
Regression coefficient (marginal effects)	−0.005***	−0.032***	0.013	−0.163***	−0.180***	0.033	0.0022	−0.1005***	0.0398	−0.0289	−0.0998***	−0.0039
Standard deviation	[0.0019]	[0.0143]	[0.0208]	[0.0498]	[0.0732]	[0.0729]	[0.0278]	[0.0389]	[0.0455]	[0.0292]	[0.0428]	[0.0427]

Estimated marginal effects are reported, standard deviations are reported in brackets, * and *** indicate significance at the 10% and 1% levels.

Table 7

Pulmonary lobectomy CPT codes and ICD-9 codes sets	
Open procedures	
CPT 32480	Removal of lung, other than total pneumonectomy; single lobe (lobectomy)
ICD 32.49	Other lobectomy of lung
VATS procedures (i.e., via thoracoscopy)	
CPT 32663	Thoracoscopy, surgical; with lobectomy, total or segmental
ICD 32.41	Thoracoscopic lobectomy of lung
Wedge resection CPT codes and ICD-9 codes sets	
Open procedures	
CPT 32484	Removal of lung, other than total pneumonectomy; single segment (segmentectomy)
CPT 32500	Wedge resection
ICD 32.39*	Other and unspecified segmental resection of lung
ICD 32.29	Other local excision or destruction of lesion or tissue of lung (used for wedge resection)
VATS procedures (i.e., via thoracoscopy)	
CPT 32657	Thoracoscopy, surgical; with wedge resection of lung, single or multiple
ICD 32.30*	Thoracoscopic segmental resection of lung
ICD 32.20	Thoracoscopic excision of lesion or tissue of lung (used for thoracoscopic wedge resection)

*Codes 32.30 and 32.39 became effective on October 1, 2007. Prior to that date, the codes were simply 32.3 which did not differentiate between open and thoracoscopic excisions. Due to this lack of information in the ICD codes, data for this project was limited to discharges on or after October 1, 2007.

Table 8: ICD-9 codes for index diagnosis.

Indications for surgery	
Malignant	
Primary neoplasm of the lung	162.x, 209.21*
Metastatic site	197.0

*ICD code 209.21 (malignant carcinoid tumor of the lung) came into existence on October 1, 2008. Prior to October 1, 2008, this type of lung cancer was coded together with 162.x.

preoperative severity level), census region of hospital, rural versus urban hospitals, teaching versus nonteaching hospitals, and number of hospital beds.

Using these explanatory variables, multivariable models were estimated to isolate the effects of a surgeon's VATS volume on adverse events, hospital costs, surgery time, and length of stay. Because the cost and utilization variables were right skewed, they were converted to natural logarithms to normalize their distributions, although the results were not sensitive to this transformation. Missing data or values of zero were not included in the OLS regression models. Weights provided in the Premier database were used to transform the results in a manner that permitted generalizability to the USA population. All analyses were performed using Stata Version 10 (StataCorp LP, College Station, Texas, USA).

3. Results

Of 7,137 patients in the database with elective, inpatient resections for lung cancer, a total of 2,698 patients underwent lobectomy ($n = 716$) or wedge resection ($n = 1982$) using VATS. More than 70% of these procedures were performed by thoracic surgeons ($n = 1,896$). A patient attrition diagram is shown in Figure 1. Characteristics of eligible patients are summarized in Table 1. There were slightly more females than males in all four samples, and most patients in all samples were over 60 years of age and covered by Medicare. Most patients were Caucasian, with primary (as opposed to metastatic) neoplasm of the lung and only minimal to moderate illness severity level, as measured by the APR-DRG severity index. As expected, the severity index for patients undergoing lobectomy was higher than for patients undergoing wedge resection. Patient characteristics within procedure (lobectomy versus wedge resection) were similar across the thoracic surgeons sample and the all surgeons sample.

The distribution of specific patient comorbidities is shown in Table 2. The most frequent comorbidities reported were chronic obstructive pulmonary disease (COPD), diabetes mellitus, and heart disease. The distribution of these conditions is similar across all samples.

A total of 237 hospitals contributed data on VATS lobectomies and wedge resections. Patient-weighted hospital characteristics for the four samples are reported in Table 3. Compared with patients undergoing VATS wedge resection, patients undergoing VATS lobectomy were more likely to receive the procedure in a teaching hospital (63% versus 57%) and in a hospital with over 600 beds (46% versus 38%). All samples exhibit similar demographic distributions.

Average hospital costs, surgery time, length of hospital stay, the likelihood, and number of adverse events, as well as the surgeons' volume measures for each sample were examined prior to multivariable modeling. The data suggest that, on average, VATS lobectomies cost hospitals more than VATS wedge resections ($19,697 versus $13,058) are associated with both longer surgery time (four hours versus 2.5 hours) and longer lengths of hospital stay (5.7 days versus 3.9 days). Furthermore, patients undergoing lobectomy had a higher likelihood of experiencing an adverse

Table 9: Postoperative procedure-specific complications.

Postoperative procedure-specific complications*		Postoperative code
Pulmonary		
Acute respiratory failure	518.81, 518.84, 518.5	997.39
Spontaneous tension pneumothorax	512.0	997.39
Atelectasis/pulmonary collapse	518.0	997.39
Empyema	510.9	998.59
Bronchopleural fistula	510.0	998.59
Air leak and other pneumothorax	512.1, 512.8	
Chylothorax	457.8	
Pneumonia	480.x to 486, 507.0	997.39
Other pulmonary infections and inflammation	487.0, 490, 491.21–491.22, 511.0–511.1, 511.89, 511.9, 513.x, 519.01	997.39
Cardiac		
Arrhythmia	427.xx	997.1
Acute myocardial infarction	410.xx	997.1
Acute heart failure/pulmonary edema	428.1, 428.21, 428.23, 428.31, 428.33, 428.41, 428.43, 514, 518.4	997.1
Vascular/thromboembolic		
Acute pulmonary embolism/infarction	415.1x	
Acute deep venous thrombosis of extremities	453.4x, 453.8, 453.9	
Neurological		
Acute cerebrovascular accident (stroke)	433.x1, 434.x1, (997.02)	997.02
Transient cerebral ischemia/attack (TIA)	435.x, 437.1	997.09
Intracranial hemorrhage (includes hemorrhagic stroke)	430–432.x	997.02
Wound complications		
Dehiscence	998.30, 998.31, 998.32, 998.3	
Hematoma/seroma complicating a procedure	998.12–998.13, 998.51	
Cellulitis	998.59 plus 682.2	
Other postoperative infection, including other (noncellulitis) wound infection	998.59 when 510.9, 510.0, 038.xx, 790.7, 995.9x, 682.2 are NOT also present	
Other		
Perforations organ or vessels	998.2	
In-hospital deaths	Obtained from Premier variable	
Sepsis	038.xx, 790.7, 995.9x	998.59
Other postoperative complications	997.xx EXCEPT 997.02, 998.0, 998.11, 998.33, 998.4, 998.6, 998.7, 998.8*x*, and 998.9	
Conversion from /VATS to OPEN	V64.42	

*All procedures are inpatient.

event compared to patients undergoing wedge resection (0.57 versus 0.43) and had a higher number of adverse events on average (1.13 events versus 0.72 events).

This study tracks 575 surgeons performing lobectomies or wedge resections using VATS (366 of whom were thoracic surgeons). Patients treated by thoracic surgeons using VATS lobectomy had lower inpatient costs and shorter length of stay compared with patients seen by general and other surgeons. While these effects were statistically significant at the 1% level, they were evidently small. No other statistically meaningful differences between thoracic and other surgeons were found for patients treated using VATS wedge resection or for other outcomes (i.e., length of surgery, likelihood of adverse event, and number of adverse events).

Surgeons' six months experience with VATS varies by sample (Table 4). The most experienced surgeons, on average, are found in the sample of thoracic surgeons performing VATS lobectomies, 31.6 procedures. This average decreases to 22.3 procedures when considering all surgeons performing VATS wedge resections. Six months experience, for these

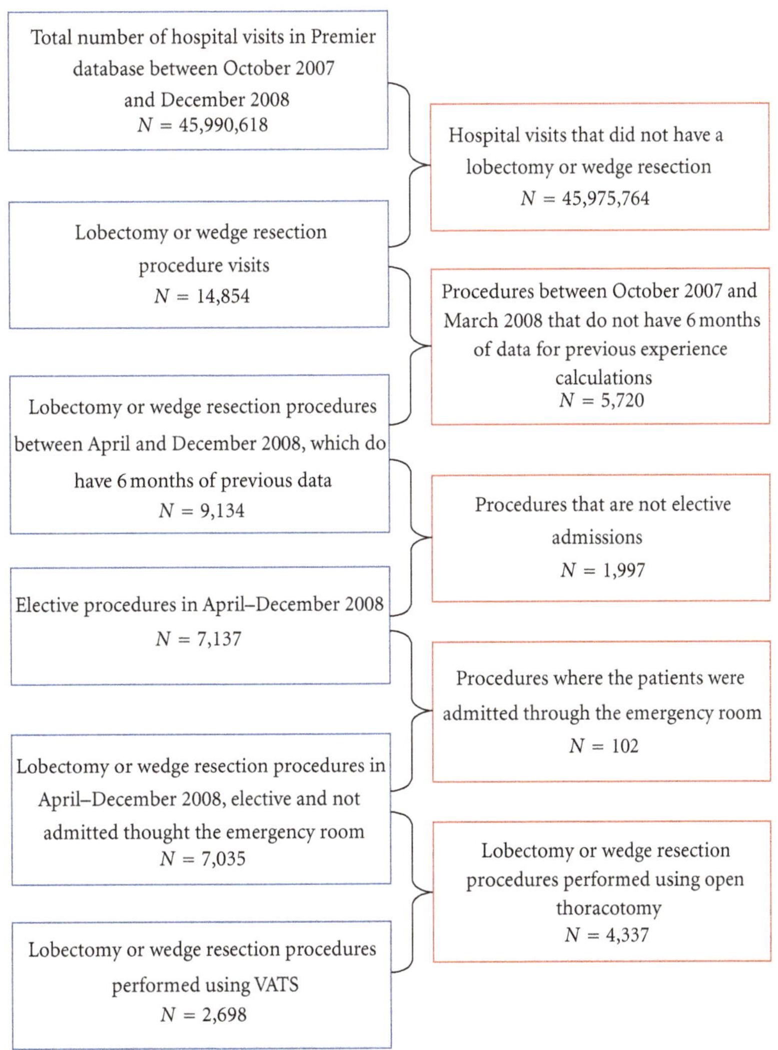

FIGURE 1: Attrition diagram. Thoracotomy: open versus VATS.

surgeons, with open lobectomies and open wedge resection was lower, 5.4 procedures and 3.9 procedures, respectively, for the entire sample.

3.1. Multivariable Findings. Given the possibility of confounders in these group comparisons of outcomes, we performed multivariable regression analyses, adjusting for a number of potential confounders, including patient demographics, metastatic versus primary cancer, comorbid conditions, APR-DRG severity index, and hospital characteristics. The results of these adjusted analyses of costs, surgery time, length of stay, likelihood of adverse event, and the number of adverse events are shown in Table 5. For ease of interpretation, we report the estimated marginal effects for each one of the 40 models presented in Table 5. The reported marginal effects measure the expected instantaneous change in each one of our five-outcome variables as a function of a change in surgeons' VATS volume, while keeping all the other covariates constant. Note that, for each outcome of interest, we compared the estimated marginal effects obtained from an unadjusted analysis with the estimated marginal effects from the multivariable analysis described above. (Note: only adjusted findings are reported in Table 5).

In the unadjusted analysis for the all surgeons lobectomy sample, doubling the average surgeon's volume was associated with a 10% reduction in inpatient cost ($2,029), a 5% reduction in surgery time (13 minutes), and a 15% reduction in length-of-stay (approximately one day). The effect of experience on the likelihood of an adverse event, while statistically significant, was small in magnitude. Increased surgeons' experience was associated with a reduction of one adverse event in one of every five patients. Even after adjusting for the variables detailed in Tables 1 through 3, all the findings above persist.

The first and second columns of Table 5 reports the analysis for lobectomies for all surgeons and then surgeries performed exclusively by thoracic surgeons. For the most part, the volume-outcome relationship for thoracic surgeons is stronger. Doubling of the thoracic surgeons experience was associated with a 13% reduction in inpatient cost ($2,409)

Table 10: Comorbid Conditions.

Comorbid conditions (existing for patient any time during or before procedure stay in Premier data)	
Myocardial infarction, acute or old	410.xx, 412
Congestive heart failure	428.0
Other chronic or unspecified heart failure	428.20, 428.22, 428.30, 428.32, 428.40, 428.42, 428.9
Peripheral vascular disease	440.xx, 443.8x, 443.9
Dementia	290.xx, 294.xx, 331.0, 331.11, 331.19, 331.2, 331.7, 331.82
Chronic pulmonary disease	490.xx–494.xx, 495.x, 496, 500–505
Connective tissue disease	710.xx, 714.xx
Liver disease	571.x, 572.*x*, 573.xx
Chronic viral hepatitis	070.22–070.23, 070.32–070.33, 070.44, 070.54
Renal insufficiency, chronic	585.xx
Diabetes mellitus	249.xx, 250.xx

and a 7% reduction in surgery time (18 minutes). All other results were similar to the ones obtained for all surgeons.

The second and third columns of Table 5 repeat the analysis for patients undergoing VATS wedge resection. Here, for most outcomes and specifications, the volume-outcome relationship appears much weaker. Doubling of the surgeon's experience was associated with a 3% reduction in inpatient cost ($389), a 2% reduction in surgery time (3 minutes), and an 8% reduction in hospital length of stay (a third of a day). The results were similar when considering the most saturated model and when limiting the sample to procedures performed solely by thoracic surgeons. The only exception was the reduction in cost for the thoracic surgeon sample, which was 5% ($659).

Table 6 reports results from models similar to those reported in Table 5, and includes two additional variables: the surgeon's six-months experience with open lobectomies and the surgeon's six-months experience with open wedge resections. The two additional volume measures allow for assessing the contribution of competing sources of learning. For example, for the VATS lobectomy sample, one may argue that any experience with lobectomy (open or VATS) may be an important contributor for performance. This is tested directly in Table 6. Overall we find the volume-outcome relationship for experience with VATS to be similar in sign, magnitude, and statistical significance to those described in Table 5. Experience with open lobectomy did not have an effect on outcomes for patients treated with VATS lobectomy, with the exception of the number of adverse events, where greater experience with open lobectomy was associated with a small reduction in the number of adverse events for VATS lobectomy. Similarly, experience with open wedge resection was associated with a reduction in inpatient cost and length of stay beyond the reductions associated with greater experience with VATS.

4. Discussion

An important strength of the Premier database is that it provides very large numbers of patients, surgeons, and procedures on a nationwide scale. Obtaining this extremely large sample size from a practical setting allows researchers to better understand processes such as the relationship between surgeons' volume and outcomes. In turn, this analysis provides hospitals, patients, and surgeons with a quantifiable measure of the benefits of surgeons' volume on outcomes in lung surgery. The sample size and large number of elements in the Premier database allows for analyzing the effect of experience with VATS on inpatient costs, length of surgery, length of stay, as well as the likelihood and number of adverse surgical events.

In this retrospective analysis, we find evidence of volume-outcome relationship. The relationship is stronger (1) for cost and utilization outcomes as opposed to adverse events, (2) for thoracic surgeons rather than other surgeons, and (3) for VATS lobectomy procedures more than for VATS wedge resection procedures. Finally, we find that while there was a reduction in cost and resource utilization associated with greater experience with VATS, these outcomes were not strongly linked with greater experience with open procedures. Thus, by and large, performance with VATS is associated primarily with experience with VATS.

The choice between VATS and open lobectomy has implications for the surgeon's learning profile, as the reduction in cost and resource utilization associated with greater experience with VATS were much larger than those associated with greater experience with open procedures. This finding reinforces the need for surgeons' specialization and centralization of delivery for VATS.

There were certain limitations of this study. This is a retrospective analysis from a transactional database (Premier) and not a prospective analysis where randomization and more detailed information about patients and procedures could be collected. For instance, it would have been of interest to examine the influence of additional patient characteristics, such as weight or BMI, and more procedure-related details. Nevertheless, we include numerous controls in our analysis, particularly, controls for patient characteristics [30] and hospital characteristics [12].

Another limitation, and a topic that can be the focus of future research, is the lack of information on surgeons' characteristics. In particular, data associated with surgeons' characteristics (e.g., years in practice, graduate of which medical school, completion of fellowship, etc.) would be of interest. This information may be important as surgeons do not randomly adopt VATS, and the results may therefore be biased if the most able surgeons are also the ones who adopt and utilize VATS extensively.

5. Conclusions

Our analysis of a large, nationally representative hospital database revealed three key findings: (1) there is a reduction in cost and resource utilization associated with greater experience with VATS, especially for VATS lobectomy for lung cancer; (2) thoracic surgeons have better VATS outcomes than non-thoracic surgeons; (3) greater experience with open procedures does not correlate with better VATS outcomes. These findings have implications for the organization of health care delivery of both minimally invasive and open procedures.

References

[1] A. Mahtabifard, C. B. Fuller, and R. J. McKenna Jr., "Video-assisted thoracic surgery sleeve lobectomy: a case series," *Annals of Thoracic Surgery*, vol. 85, no. 2, pp. S729–S732, 2008.

[2] R. O. Jones, G. Casali, and W. S. Walker, "Does failed video-assisted lobectomy for lung cancer prejudice immediate and long-term outcomes?" *Annals of Thoracic Surgery*, vol. 86, no. 1, pp. 235–239, 2008.

[3] H. S. Luft, S. S. Hunt, and S. C. Maerki, "The volume-outcome relationship: practice-makes-perfect or selective-referral patterns?" *Health Services Research*, vol. 22, no. 2, pp. 157–182, 1987.

[4] J. V. Tu, P. C. Austin, and B. T. B. Chan, "Relationship between annual volume of patients treated by admitting physician and mortality after acute myocardial infarction," *Journal of the American Medical Association*, vol. 285, no. 24, pp. 3116–3122, 2001.

[5] A. Elixhauser, C. Steiner, and I. Fraser, "Volume thresholds and hospital characteristics in the United States," *Health Affairs*, vol. 22, no. 2, pp. 167–177, 2003.

[6] A. Gandjour, A. Bannenberg, and K. W. Lauterbach, "Threshold volumes associated with higher survival in health care: a systematic review," *Medical Care*, vol. 41, no. 10, pp. 1129–1141, 2003.

[7] R. A. Dudley, K. L. Johansen, R. Brand, D. J. Rennie, and A. Milstein, "Selective referral to high-volume hospitals: estimating potentially avoidable deaths," *Journal of the American Medical Association*, vol. 283, no. 9, pp. 1159–1166, 2000.

[8] E. A. Halm, C. Lee, and M. R. Chassin, "Is volume related to outcome in health care? A systematic review and methodologic critique of the literature," *Annals of Internal Medicine*, vol. 137, no. 6, pp. 511–520, 2002.

[9] F. Hellinger, "Practice makes perfect: a volume-outcome study of hospital patients with HIV disease," *Journal of Acquired Immune Deficiency Syndromes*, vol. 47, no. 2, pp. 226–233, 2008.

[10] S. Sundaresan, B. Langer, T. Oliver, F. Schwartz, M. Brouwers, and H. Stern, "Standards for thoracic surgical oncology in a single-payer healthcare system," *Annals of Thoracic Surgery*, vol. 84, no. 2, pp. 693–701, 2007.

[11] P. B. Bach, L. D. Cramer, D. Schrag, R. J. Downey, S. E. Gelfand, and C. B. Begg, "The influence of hospital volume on survival after resection for lung cancer," *New England Journal of Medicine*, vol. 345, no. 3, pp. 181–188, 2001.

[12] M. C. Cheung, K. Hamilton, R. Sherman et al., "Impact of teaching facility status and high-volume centers on outcomes for lung cancer resection: an examination of 13,469 surgical patients," *Annals of Surgical Oncology*, vol. 16, no. 1, pp. 3–13, 2009.

[13] E. L. Hannan, M. Radzyner, D. Rubin, J. Dougherty, and M. F. Brennan, "The influence of hospital and surgeon volume on in-hospital mortality for colectomy, gastrectomy, and lung lobectomy in patients with cancer," *Surgery*, vol. 131, no. 1, pp. 6–15, 2002.

[14] J. D. Birkmeyer, T. A. Stukel, A. E. Siewers, P. P. Goodney, D. E. Wennberg, and F. L. Lucas, "Surgeon volume and operative mortality in the United States," *New England Journal of Medicine*, vol. 349, no. 22, pp. 2117–2127, 2003.

[15] J. B. Dimick and G. R. Upchurch, "Endovascular technology, hospital volume, and mortality with abdominal aortic aneurysm surgery," *Journal of Vascular Surgery*, vol. 47, no. 6, pp. 1150–1154, 2008.

[16] R. Ricciardi, H. P. Selker, N. N. Baxter, P. W. Marcello, P. L. Roberts, and B. A. Virnig, "Disparate use of minimally invasive surgery in benign surgical conditions," *Surgical Endoscopy and Other Interventional Techniques*, vol. 22, no. 9, pp. 1977–1986, 2008.

[17] A. P. Gutow, "Surgeon volume and operative mortality," *The New England Journal of Medicine*, vol. 350, no. 12, pp. 1256–1258, 2004.

[18] M. M. Chowdhury, H. Dagash, and A. Pierro, "A systematic review of the impact of volume of surgery and specialization on patient outcome," *British Journal of Surgery*, vol. 94, no. 2, pp. 145–161, 2007.

[19] R. L. Gruen, V. Pitt, S. Green, A. Parkhill, D. Campbell, and D. Jolley, "The effect of provider case volume on cancer mortality: systematic review and meta-analysis," *CA Cancer Journal for Clinicians*, vol. 59, no. 3, pp. 192–211, 2009.

[20] P. Hermanek and W. Hohenberger, "The importance of volume in colorectal cancer surgery," *European Journal of Surgical Oncology*, vol. 22, no. 3, pp. 213–215, 1996.

[21] F. Farjah, D. R. Flum, T. K. Varghese, R. G. Symons, and D. E. Wood, "Surgeon specialty and long-term survival after pulmonary resection for lung cancer," *Annals of Thoracic Surgery*, vol. 87, no. 4, pp. 995–1006, 2009.

[22] A. Iwasaki, S. Yamamoto, T. Shiraishi, and T. Shirakusa, "How much skill should we need for a VATS lobectomy in stage I lung cancer? An evaluation of surgeon groups," *International Surgery*, vol. 93, no. 3, pp. 169–174, 2008.

[23] A. Toker, S. Tanju, S. Ziyade, S. Kaya, and S. Dilege, "Learning curve in videothoracoscopic thymectomy: how many operations and in which situations?" *European Journal of Cardio-thoracic Surgery*, vol. 34, no. 1, pp. 155–158, 2008.

[24] J. Ferguson and W. Walker, "Developing a VATS lobectomy programme—can VATS lobectomy be taught?" *European Journal of Cardio-thoracic Surgery*, vol. 29, no. 5, pp. 806–809, 2006.

[25] T. Ng and B. A. Ryder, "Evolution to video-assisted thoracic surgery lobectomy after training: initial results of the first 30 patients," *Journal of the American College of Surgeons*, vol. 203, no. 4, pp. 551–557, 2006.

[26] H. Yasunaga, H. Yanaihara, K. Fuji, Y. Matsuyama, N. Deguchi, and K. Ohe, "Influence of hospital and surgeon volumes on operative time, blood loss and perioperative complications in radical nephrectomy," *International Journal of Urology*, vol. 15, no. 8, pp. 688–693, 2008.

[27] C. W. Seder, K. Hanna, V. Lucia et al., "The safe transition from open to thoracoscopic lobectomy: a 5-year experience," *Annals of Thoracic Surgery*, vol. 88, no. 1, pp. 216–226, 2009.

[28] J. D. Birkmeyer, J. B. Dimick, and D. O. Staiger, "Operative mortality and procedure volume as predictors of subsequent hospital performance," *Annals of Surgery*, vol. 243, no. 3, pp. 411–417, 2006.

[29] G. David and T. Brachet, "Retention, learning by doing, and performance in emergency medical services," *Health Services Research*, vol. 44, no. 3, pp. 902–925, 2009.

[30] R. W. Eppsteiner, N. G. Csikesz, J. P. Simons, J. F. Tseng, and S. A. Shah, "High volume and outcome after liver resection: surgeon or center?" *Journal of Gastrointestinal Surgery*, vol. 12, no. 10, pp. 1709–1716, 2008.

8

Management of Gastroesophageal Reflux Disease: A Review of Medical and Surgical Management

Nirali Shah and Sandhya Iyer

Department of General Surgery, Lokmanya Tilak Municpal Medical College and General Hospital, Sion, Mumbai 400022, India

Correspondence should be addressed to Nirali Shah; nirali1907@gmail.com

Academic Editor: Peng Hui Wang

Background. Gastroesophageal reflux disease currently accounts for the majority of esophageal pathologies. This study is an attempt to help us tackle the diagnostic and therapeutic challenges of this disease. This study specifically focuses on patients in the urban Indian setup. *Materials and Methods.* This study was a prospective interventional study carried out at a teaching public hospital in Mumbai from May 2010 to September 2012. Fifty patients diagnosed with gastroesophageal reflux disease (confirmed by endoscopy and esophageal manometry) were chosen for the study. *Results.* Fifty patients were included in the study. Twenty patients showed symptomatic improvement after three months and were thus managed conservatively, while 30 patients did not show any improvement in symptoms and were eventually operated. *Conclusion.* We suggest that all patients diagnosed to have gastroesophageal reflux disease should be subjected to 3 months of conservative management. In case of no relief of symptoms, patients need to be subjected to surgery. Laparoscopic Toupet's fundoplication is an effective and feasible surgical treatment option for such patients, associated with minimal side effects. However, the long-term effects of this form of treatment still need to be evaluated further with a larger sample size and a longer followup.

1. Introduction

Gastroesophageal reflux disease was not formerly a very significant problem but its incidence has shown an absolute increase in the last 20–30 years [1]. The diagnosis of gastroesophageal reflux disease is difficult to make on clinical grounds alone and relies on investigations like upper gastrointestinal endoscopy, esophageal manometry, and 24-hour pH studies. Apart from the physical symptoms attributed to the disease, the disease also has a profound effect on the quality of life of the patient [1].

Gastroesophageal reflux disease can be managed both medically as well as surgically. With the advances in minimally invasive laparoscopic surgery for gastroesophageal reflux, there has been an increasing trend towards surgical management of reflux in order to avoid long-term dependence on medications and to give a permanent cure. Laparoscopic surgery also has its own inherent risks related to the procedure. Currently there is no clear-cut consensus about which form of treatment is suited for which patient.

This study is an attempt to help us tackle this diagnostic and therapeutic challenge of gastroesophageal reflux disease. This study specifically focuses on patients in the urban Indian setup.

2. Materials and Methods

This study was a prospective interventional study carried out at a teaching public hospital in Mumbai from May 2010 to September 2012 after obtaining the institute's ethics committee approval. All patients with suspected gastroesophageal reflux disease were evaluated for their symptoms and quality of life. Diagnosis of gastroesophageal reflux disease was confirmed by endoscopy and esophageal manometry. 50 such patients (with the necessary inclusion and exclusion criteria and giving written informed consent) were chosen for the study.

Inclusion Criteria. Newly diagnosed cases of uncomplicated gastroesophageal reflux disease with hiatus hernia patients (aged between 20 and 60 years) with symptoms of gastroesophageal reflux disease whose diagnosis has been confirmed by endoscopy and manometry.

Exclusion Criteria. Presence of comorbid conditions like hypertension and diabetes mellitus as well as pregnancy.

A detailed history and physical examination was done for all the patients enrolled for the study. An inquiry was made for the presence of predisposing factors—alcohol consumption, tea/coffee drinking (more than two cups/day), smoking/tobacco chewing, sedentary lifestyle, and spicy, oily, and non-vegetarian food. All patients having symptoms of gastroesophageal reflux (heartburn, regurgitation, dysphagia, angina-like chest pain, and respiratory symptoms: cough and hoarseness) had their symptoms evaluated by the visual analogue scale (scored between 1 and 10) A score was given from 1 (worst possible symptom) to 10 (no symptom) [2].

The patients were subjected to upper gastrointestinal endoscopy (to look for presence of hiatal hernia and grade of esophagitis) and high resolution esophageal manometry (to look for pressure of lower esophageal sphincter, relaxation of lower esophageal sphincter, presence of hiatal hernia, and motility of esophageal body) to confirm the diagnosis. Hiatus hernia was diagnosed when the high pressure zone produced by the lower oesophageal sphincter gastroesophageal junction was at least 2 cm higher than the high pressure zone produced by the diaphragmatic crura (double high pressure zone or double hump). Only patients showing presence of hiatal hernia on both endoscopy and manometry were included in the study.

Patients diagnosed to have gastroesophageal reflux (with the necessary inclusion and exclusion criteria) were given a trial of conservative management (lifestyle changes and medications). Lifestyle changes included eating a low-fat, bland vegetarian diet, assuming an upright (head high/propped up) position while sleeping, abstaining from tea/coffee/alcohol, and avoiding a sedentary lifestyle.

Medications included a proton-pump inhibitor (tablet Pantoprazole 40 mg twice a day) and a prokinetic agent (tablet Levosulpiride 75 mg twice a day) given for a period of three months. Patients who improved symptomatically were continued on medical management. Those patients whose symptoms did not improve with conservative management and patients who required escalating doses of medications for symptom relief were subjected to laparoscopic Toupet's fundoplication. Pneumoperitoneum was created by closed technique via a supraumbilical port. Dissection was carried out at hiatus, and fundus of stomach was mobilised and passed through a window created behind the gastroesophageal junction (shoe-shine technique). A 270° posterior wrap was performed. Fundus was sutured to oesophagus by interrupted stitches. Crural stitches were placed in case the crura were far apart and the opening was too wide. Nasogastric tube was removed on postoperative day one and sips begun. Soft diet was begun on the evening of the first postoperative day and the patient was discharged the next day in case of an uneventful recovery. Medications (proton pump inhibitors and prokinetic drugs) were continued for one month postoperatively.

All patients were followed up for a period of 9 months after diagnosis (6 months after surgery for operated patients). Outcomes after treatment were evaluated by both subjective and objective criteria.

(1) Improvement in symptoms (assessed by visual analogue scale) at 3 and 9 months after diagnosis.

(2) Improvement in quality of life (assessed by SF-36 questionnaire) at 3 and 9 months after diagnosis. A score was obtained for eight specific areas of functional health status—physical functioning, role limitation due to physical health, role limitation due to emotional problems, energy/fatigue, emotional well-being, social functioning, pain, and general health [2].

(3) Changes in endoscopy findings at 9 months from diagnosis (6 months after surgery).

(4) Changes in manometry findings at 6 months after surgery.

Patients managed surgically were also evaluated for complications: intraoperative bleeding requiring blood transfusion, diaphragmatic injury, pleural breach, splenic injury, esophageal perforation, gastric perforation, postoperative dysphagia, and wound infection.

Results were analyzed using Student's t-test, chi-square test, and Wilcoxon sign rank test.

3. Results and Discussion

Fifty patients diagnosed to have gastroesophageal reflux disease (confirmed by endoscopy and esophageal manometry) were included in the study. 20 patients showed symptomatic improvement after three months and were thus managed conservatively, while 30 patients did not show any improvement in symptoms and were eventually operated.

88% of cases were in the age group of 20–40 years while 12% cases were in the age group of 41–50 years. Mean age of patients was 32.20 years. 50% of the total cases were females in this study. Mean height, weight, and BMI of the patients were within normal limits. These findings are comparable to those found in the study by Lal et al. [3], where mean age was 37.38 years and 35.33 years for the groups treated by laparoscopic Nissen's and laparoscopic Toupet's fundoplication, respectively [3]. They had also found that gastroesophageal reflux disease had equal sex distribution (50% for males and females) [3]. Nagpal et al. [4] found that 57.14% of the patients were males and 42.86% were females [4].

72% cases had daily intake of tea or coffee (more than 2 cups per day) and 68% cases had sedentary life style, whereas 50% cases had spicy and oily food and 46% had non-vegetarian diet. 32% cases had alcohol consumption and smoking/tobacco chewing, respectively. This is in accordance with the study by Somi et al. [5], where drinking excess amount of tea was associated with symptoms of gastroesophageal reflux disease [5].

Heartburn (94%) and regurgitation (92%) were the most common symptoms at the time of diagnosis. Dysphagia (16%) was uncommon. Angina like chest pain and respiratory symptoms (cough and hoarseness) were not seen (Table 1). In the study done by Nagpal et al. [4], the most common symptom was heartburn, followed by regurgitation and constipation [4]. In a study of 107 patients done by Balsara

Table 1: Symptomatology at presentation.

Symptom	Present (VAS score 1–5)	Absent (VAS > 5)
Heartburn	47 (94%)	3 (6%)
Regurgitation	46 (92%)	4 (8%)
Dysphagia	8 (16%)	42 (84%)
Angina like chest pain	0 (0%)	50 (0%)
Respiratory symptoms	0 (0%)	50 (0%)

VAS: visual analogue scale.

Table 2: Comparison of changes in endoscopy findings in operated cases.

Endoscopy findings	Baseline (N = 30)	3 months after surgery (N = 30)
Hiatal hernia present	30 (100%)	1 (3.33%)*
Esophagitis Grade A	10 (33.33%)	1 (3.33%)*
Esophagitis Grade B	11 (36.66%)	0 (0%)
Esophagitis Grade C	1 (3.33%)	0 (0%)
Esophagitis Grade D	0 (0%)	0 (0%)
No abnormality detected	0 (0%)	29 (96.6%)

By chi-square test; * significant.

et al. [6], the symptoms on presentation were heartburn in all (100%), regurgitation in 43 (50.59%), and volume reflux in 39 (45.88%) patients [6].

On endoscopy, hiatal hernia was present in 100% of the cases at diagnosis. All the patients had type I (sliding) hiatal hernia. Esophagitis was present in 66% patients (mainly Grade A and Grade B) at diagnosis (Table 2).

On esophageal manometry, there was a hypotensive lower esophageal sphincter with complete relaxation and presence of hiatal hernia in 100% of the cases. Esophageal body motility was normotensive in the majority of cases (88%) and was hypotensive in only 12% (Table 3). No studies have documented manometric findings in such detail.

Barium studies were not done as they are outdated now. 24-hour pH studies could not be done as they are expensive and not available in our public setup.

After three months of conservative management (with lifestyle changes, tablet Pantoprazole 40 mg twice a day, and tablet Levosulpiride 75 mg twice a day), heartburn (54%) and regurgitation (50%) were the persistent symptoms. Overall, there were 30 patients who were still symptomatic (60% cases) after three months of conservative management. This is in accordance with the findings of Sifrim and Zerbib [7], who noted that approximately a third of patients with suspected gastroesophageal reflux disease are resistant or partial responders to proton pump inhibitors [7]. These patients were subjected to surgery, that is, laparoscopic Toupet's fundoplication. Nissen's fundoplication was not preferred due to the greater incidence of postoperative dysphagia [3]. Also, most patients were poor and hailed from the rural interiors and would not be able to follow up regularly and afford repeated dilatations if required.

Transient postoperative dysphagia was the commonest complication, seen in 46.66% of the cases. However, it was only temporary and subsided within 6 weeks in all cases without any treatment, except for reassurance and adjustment of food habits. The rare complications of pleural breach, splenic injury, and esophageal perforation occurred in 1 case each and these 3 cases required conversion to open surgery. These complications occurred in the initial period of the study, demonstrating that there is a learning curve in laparoscopic surgery. Wound infection was seen in 30% of the cases; however, it was always a minor infection requiring removal of a single skin suture. None of the patients with wound infection developed fever or required incision and drainage or increase in duration of hospital stay. No patient developed a major infection that persisted for 10 or more days. This is in accordance with the study of 10 patients by Parshad et al. [8], where one patient (10%) required reexploration due to bleeding from a short gastric vessel. The most frequent postoperative complication was temporary dysphagia in 60% of patients, which improved with conservative management over 2 to 3 weeks [8].

After 3 months of medical management, mean score of heartburn showed statistically significant rise of 1.17 times (117%) in 20 patients. These patients were continued on conservative management while the other 30 were operated. At 9 months, mean score of heartburn showed significant increase of 1.50 times (150%) among the operative group and 1.30 times (130%) in the conservative group from baseline. After 3 months of medical management, mean score of regurgitation showed statistically significant increase of 1.07 times (107%) in 20 patients. Thus these patients were continued on conservative management while the other 30 patients were operated. At 9 months, mean score of regurgitation showed significant increase of 1.08 times (108%) among the operative group and 1.11 times (111%) in the conservative group from baseline. These findings were similar to those obtained in the review of four trials by Wileman et al. [9].

On endoscopy, 100.0% cases had hiatal hernia at baseline. At 3 months after surgery, 96.66% cases did not have hiatal hernia as compared to baseline. This difference was statistically significant. Overall, though 22 patients (73.33%) had esophagitis before surgery, only 1 patient had persistent esophagitis after surgery. Thus 70% patients showed improvement in esophagitisafter surgery. These findings are similar to those obtained by Parshad et al. [8], where 8 out of 9 patients (88%) had endoscopic resolution of esophagitis [8].

At 6 months after surgery, 96.6% patients showed a normotensive lower esophageal sphincter compared to all patients showing hypotensive sphincter before surgery and this change was statistically significant. There was a statistically significant increase in the distance of lower esophageal sphincter from central incisors after surgery. Lower esophageal sphincter relaxation remained complete both pre- and postoperatively in 100% cases. Hiatal hernia which was present in all cases (100%) pre-operatively was totally absent postoperatively (100%) and this difference was statistically significant. These findings were in accordance with those obtained by Wileman et al. [9]. Seven patients needed to continue the medications for three weeks after surgery to control symptoms. None of the patients required medications on a long-term basis.

Table 3: Comparison of changes in manometry findings in operated cases.

Parameter	Finding	Baseline (N = 30)	6 months after surgery (N = 30)
Pressure of lower esophageal sphincter	Hypotensive	30 (100%)	1 (33.33%)*
	Normotensive	0 (0%)	29 (96.66%)*
	Hypertensive	0 (0%)	0 (0%)
Relaxation of lower esophageal sphincter	Present	30 (100%)	30 (100%)
	Absent	0 (0%)	0 (0%)
Hiatal hernia	Present	30 (100%)	0 (0%)*
	Absent	0 (0%)	30 (100%)*
Motility of esophageal body (type of peristalsis)	Hypotensive	6 (20%)	2 (6.66%)
	Normotensive	24 (80%)	26 (86.66%)
	Hypertensive	0 (0%)	2 (6.66%)

By chi-square test; *significant.

Table 4: Table showing changes in mean score of quality of life in operated patients.

Parameter	Mean score (N = 30)		
	Baseline	3 months	9 months
Physical functioning	60.90	61.40	83.70
Role limitation due to physical health	63.60	64.00	84.30
Role limitation due to emotional problems	66.00	67.10	85.30
Energy/fatigue	71.10	71.10	86.30
Emotional well-being	67.90	68.80	84.80
Social functioning	73.60	73.70	88.70*
Pain	62.50	64.90	83.80*
General health	71.80	71.90	87.30*

By Student's t-test; *significant.

Quality of life was assessed using the SF-36 questionnaire. Among the patients who were operated, the SF-36 score for quality of life did not show statistically significant change in all the eight parameters after 3 months of conservative management. The mean score for all the 8 parameters of quality of life showed improvement at 6 months after surgery. This increase was statistically significant in the areas of social functioning, pain, and general health. Among the patients who were managed conservatively, there was statistically significant improvement in score for physical functioning, role limitation due to physical health, role limitation due to emotional problems, emotional well-being, social functioning, and general health at 3 months. Mean score for these 6 parameters improved further at 9 months from diagnosis. Increase in mean score for pain was statistically insignificant at 3 months; however, it was statistically significant at 9 months (Table 4). In the review done by Wileman et al. [9], there were statistically significant improvements in the health-related quality of life at three months and one year after surgery compared to medical therapy.

4. Conclusion

The conclusions of our prospective study of 50 patients of gastroesophageal reflux disease can be summarized as follows.

(1) In the urban Indian setup, gastroesophageal reflux disease was the most common in the age group of 20 to 40 years and both sexes were equally affected.

(2) Lifestyle related factors like daily intake of tea or coffee, sedentary life style, spicy and oily food, nonvegetarian diet, alcohol consumption and smoking/tobacco chewing may be associated with gastroesophageal reflux disease.

(3) Heartburn and regurgitation were the most common presenting symptoms in patients with gastroesophageal reflux disease.

(4) The majority of patients with gastroesophageal reflux disease had hiatal hernia and esophagitis on endoscopy.

(5) On esophageal manometry, all patients had hiatal hernia with hypotensive lower esophageal sphincter and complete relaxation of lower esophageal sphincter. The majority of the patients had normal esophageal motility. Findings of hiatal hernia on endoscopy were confirmed by manometry; therefore, endoscopy is a good method for screening for hiatal hernia.

(6) After 3 months of medical management, 40% patients showed significant improvement in symptoms and quality of life and thus were continued on conservative management. The remaining 60% patients underwent surgery (laparoscopic Toupet's fundoplication).

(7) Both the conservative and the operative groups of patients showed significant improvement in symptoms with treatment.

(8) Endoscopy and manometry findings also showed significant improvement in the operative group.

(9) Quality of life (evaluated by SF-36 score) also showed significant improvement in both groups.

Thus all patients diagnosed to have gastroesophageal reflux disease should be subjected to 3 months of conservative management. In case of no relief of symptoms, patients need to be subjected to surgery. laparoscopic Toupet's fundoplication is an effective and feasible surgical treatment option for such patients, associated with minimal side effects. However, the long-term effects of this form of treatment still need to be evaluated further with a larger sample size and a longer followup.

References

[1] F. C. Brunicardi, D. K. Andersen, T. R. Billiar et al., Eds., *Schwartz's Principles of Surgery*, McGraw-Hill, New York, NY, USA, 9th edition, 2010.

[2] P. Bytzer, "Assessment of reflux symptom severity: methodological options and their attributes," *Gut*, vol. 53, no. 4, pp. iv28–iv34, 2004.

[3] P. Lal, N. Leekha, J. Chander, R. Dewan, and V. K. Ramteke, "A prospective nonrandomized comparison of laparoscopic Nissen fundoplication and laparoscopic Toupet fundoplication in Indian population using detailed objective and subjective criteria," *Journal of Minimal Access Surgery*, vol. 8, no. 2, pp. 39–44, 2012.

[4] A. P. Nagpal, H. Soni, and S. P. Haribhakti, "Retrospective evaluation of patients of gastroesophageal reflux disease treated with laparoscopic Nissen's fundoplication," *Journal of Minimal Access Surgery*, vol. 6, no. 2, pp. 42–45, 2010.

[5] M. H. Somi, S. Farhang, S. Nasseri-Moghaddam et al., "Prevalence and risk factors of gastroesophageal reflux disease in Tabriz, Iran," *Iranian Journal of Public Health*, vol. 37, no. 3, pp. 85–90, 2008.

[6] K. P. Balsara, C. R. Shah, and M. Hussain, "Laparoscopic fundoplication for gastro-esophageal reflux disease: an 8 year experience," *Journal of Minimal Access Surgery*, vol. 4, no. 4, pp. 99–103, 2008.

[7] D. Sifrim and F. Zerbib, "Diagnosis and management of patients with reflux symptoms refractory to proton pump inhibitors," *Gut*, vol. 61, no. 9, pp. 1340–1354, 2012.

[8] R. Parshad, M. V. Kumar, S. Bal, A. Saraya, and M. P. Sharma, "Laparoscopic Nissen fundoplication; results of a prospective pilot study.," *Tropical Gastroenterology*, vol. 24, no. 3, pp. 152–156, 2003.

[9] S. M. Wileman, S. McCann, A. M. Grant, Z. H. Krukowski, and J. Bruce, "Medical versus surgical management for gastrooesophageal reflux disease (GORD) in adults," *Cochrane Database of Systematic Reviews*, vol. 3, Article ID CD003243, 2010.

9

Two Ports Laparoscopic Inguinal Hernia Repair in Children

Medhat M. Ibrahim

Pediatric Surgery Unit, Faculty of Medicine, Al-Azhar University, Nasr City, Cairo 11884, Egypt

Correspondence should be addressed to Medhat M. Ibrahim; dr_medhat_ibrahem@yahoo.com

Academic Editor: Peng Hui Wang

Introduction. Several laparoscopic treatment techniques were designed for improving the outcome over the last decade. The various techniques differ in their approach to the inguinal internal ring, suturing and knotting techniques, number of ports used in the procedures, and mode of dissection of the hernia sac. *Patients and Surgical Technique.* 90 children were subjected to surgery and they undergone two-port laparoscopic repair of inguinal hernia in children. Technique feasibility in relation to other modalities of repair was the aim of this work. 90 children including 75 males and 15 females underwent surgery. Hernia in 55 cases was right-sided and in 15 left-sided. Two patients had recurrent hernia following open hernia repair. 70 (77.7%) cases were suffering unilateral hernia and 20 (22.2%) patients had bilateral hernia. Out of the 20 cases 5 cases were diagnosed by laparoscope (25%). The patients' median age was 18 months. The mean operative time for unilateral repairs was 15 to 20 minutes and bilateral was 21 to 30 minutes. There was no conversion. The complications were as follows: one case was recurrent right inguinal hernia and the second was stitch sinus. *Discussion.* The results confirm the safety and efficacy of two ports laparoscopic hernia repair in congenital inguinal hernia in relation to other modalities of treatment.

1. Introduction

During recent years, the trend toward laparoscopic approach for hernia repair in children has been increasingly justified. The ability to detect and repair the contralateral opening of internal rings simultaneously, along with safe high ligation of the hernia sac without injury of the vas deference or the spermatic vessels, make laparoscopic approach a reliable alternative to the conventional open techniques [1].

The universally known limitations of the laparoscopic surgery are as follows. (1) Most of these methods employ a laparoscope inserted via an umbilical incision and two lateral ports for instruments to ligate the hernia defect [2]. The necessity for intra-abdominal skills, such as intracorporeal suturing, knot tying, and manipulation of the suture on a needle may be time-consuming and cumbersome. (2) Recurrence rate after laparoscopic surgery is generally known to be higher than after open surgery [2].

With the increase in laparoscopic inguinal hernia repair, several treatment techniques have developed over the past two decades, aimed at improving the outcome [3]; the various techniques differ in their approach to the inguinal internal ring, suturing and knotting techniques, number of ports used in the procedures, endoscopic instruments used, mode of dissection of the hernia sac, and extracorporeal and intracorporeal suturing and knotting techniques [4].

This study is an early experience of two ports laparoscopic repair of inguinal hernia. I used two 5 mm ports which reduce the port numbers and size, the purse string suturing, and extracorporeal knotting of the hernia sac.

2. Materials and Surgical Technique

This study was conducted from April 2009 to April 2013. 90 children with inguinal hernia were subjected to full clinical evaluation and routine investigations. The main outcome measurements were correlation between clinical diagnosis, abdominal ultrasound results and the laparoscopic evaluation of contralateral hernia, feasibility of two ports laparoscopic repair of the inguinal hernia, conversion rate, need for additional port, operative time, postoperative pain and requirement of analgesia, hospital stay, recurrence rate, and fat of nonexcised hernia sac and development of post-operative hydrocele. The ethical committee approved the technique. Written consent was obtained from the family

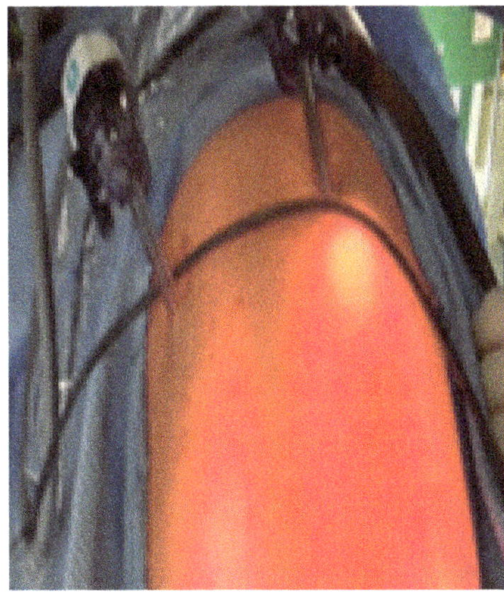

Figure 1: Port position used in right congenital inguinal hernia.

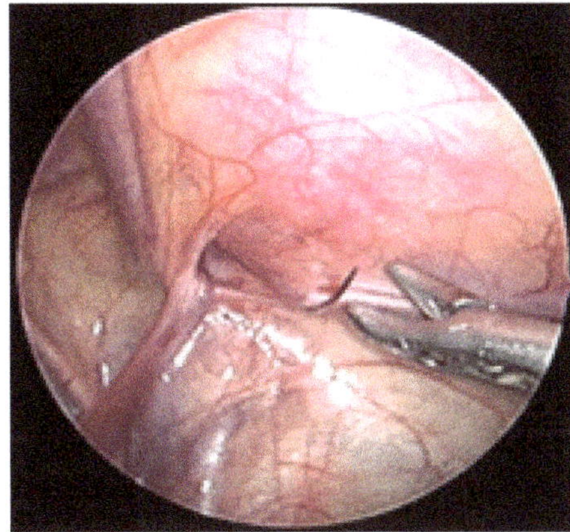

Figure 2: Needle passing to the peritoneal cavity.

after getting full information about the surgery and the postoperative squeal. All patients received one dose of antibiotic prophylaxis in the form of ceftriaxone 50 mg/kg at the time of induction of anesthesia. Under general endotracheal anesthesia, patients were scraped and draped. The surgeon position was at the child head. ENDOPATH XCEL port (5 mm) with 00 scope inserted supra umbilical by close technique. Pneumo-peritoneum pressure adjusted at 8–12 mm Hg according to child condition. Initial visualization of both internal rings was done for the bilateral hernia diagnosis. Seconded working port 5 mm was inserted according to the unilaterally and bilaterally hernia under visualization (Figure 1). Patient position was changed to trendelenburg position 45° which helped in reduction of the hernia contents and gave better visualization of the rings. Proline 3/0 suture mounted needle was passed from the outside through skin and abdominal wall muscles to the peritoneal cavity under visualization (Figure 2). Laparoscopic needle holder grasps the needle inside the abdominal cavity.

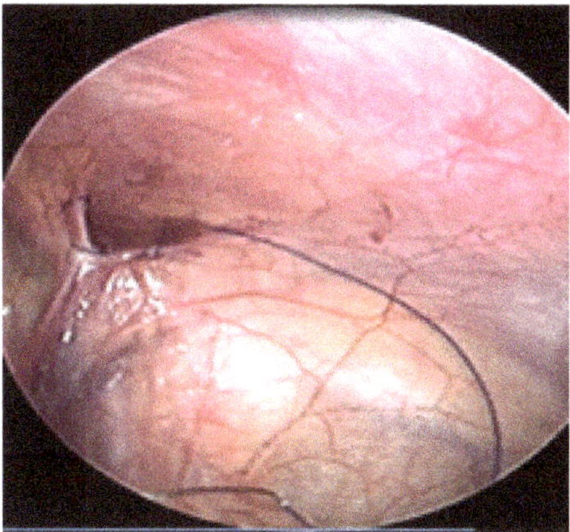

Figure 3: Proline purse string suture around the hernia neck.

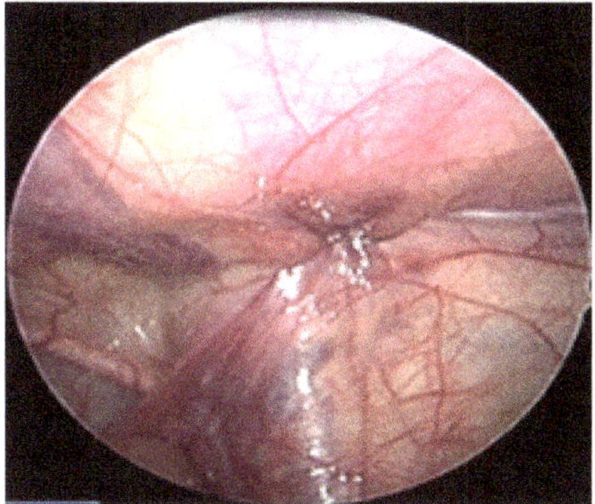

Figure 4: Closed hernia sac neck.

The hernial sac neck was closed by purse string 3/0 non- absorbable proline suture as high as possible (Figure 3). The suture was placed between the peritoneum and the fascia with preservation of the testicular vessels and the vas deference. The needle pushed out the abdomen by the laparoscopic needle holder until it appears outside the abdomen. Extracorporeal knot tying was done. The knot was fixed deep in the abdominal wall by small snip skin incision by number 11 knife. Full inspection of the abdominal wall and the closed defect was done (Figure 4). Laparoscopic abdominal exploration was done in all cases. All patients were asked to come for follow-up at outpatient clinic after 7 days, 2 weeks, 6 months, and 1 year. 90 children including 75 males and 15 females underwent two ports laparoscopic inguinal hernia repair. Hernia in 55 cases was right-sided and in 15 left-sided. Two patients had recurrence following previous hernia repair through groin incision. 70 (77.7%) cases were suffering unilateral inguinal hernia and 20 (22.2%) patients had bilateral inguinal hernia. Out of the 20 cases 5 cases were diagnosed by laparoscopic exploration (25%). These cases were diagnosed as left congenital inguinal hernia by clinical and ultrasound examinations while the laparoscope shows the metachronous hernia at the time of surgery.

The age of the patients ranged from 6 months to 8 years. The median age was 18 months. The mean operative time for unilateral repairs was (15 to 20 minutes) and bilateral hernia repair was (21 to 30 minutes). The scars on the abdominal wall were small and minute (5 mm incision for umbilical port, 5 mm working port and stitch site). There was no conversion or third port insertion. During follow-up there was one patient who got noncomplicated right recurrent inguinal hernia after two weeks from surgery. This patient underwent open right herniotomy where the hernia sac was not closed and proline stitch did not surround all the circumferences of the sac. Another case gets stitch sinuses at the proline knot site, which required open surgical removal of the stitch and open herniotomy at the same time. In this case the hernia sac was closed completely by the proline stitch. Once the proline stitch removed the sac opened, so, herniotomy and Trans fixation was done. There were no other complications such as testicular atrophy or secondary hydrocele. All patients were recovered smoothly from anesthesia and there was no need for analgesia. All patients were discharged home two hours after full recovery from anesthesia.

3. Discussion

Inguinal hernia in pediatric age group is a common problem and all the pediatric surgeons are fully familiar with the various aspects of its traditional surgical repair through the groin incision which has a high success rate and acceptable cosmetic results with few complications [4].

By far one of the drawbacks of this conventional technique is inability to rule out the contralateral patent processes vaginalis and synchronous hernia. With the advent of minimal access surgery, many pediatric surgeons accepted it, as a suitable and reliable alternative to the open techniques, considering its superiority for handling tissues during repair of recurrent inguinal hernias and also for its capabilities in regard to justifying and managing the synchronous subtle contralateral hernia [5]. However, there are still some issues regarding the introduction of laparoscopic inguinal hernia repair as the gold standard method, especially taking into consideration the possible longer operative time and the inevitable need for three separate ports which is the case in routine laparoscopic herniotomy techniques. In these works only two ports were used to do laparoscopic hernia repair in children, which increases the benefit of the laparoscopic herniotomy. The modified, new laparoscopic technique improved the diagnosis of ipsilateral hernia, using extracorporeal tying, that yields excellent cosmetic result.

Out of the 20 cases 5 (25%) case were diagnosed by laparoscopic exploration. These cases were diagnosed as left congenital inguinal hernia clinically and ultrasound examinations cannot detect the metachronous hernia in the right side prior to surgery. Laparoscope was superior to ultrasound in diagnosis of the metachronous hernia, while in other studies significant number of children (20%) presenting with unilateral hernias have contralateral patent processes vaginalis [5, 6]. The options for detection of contralateral patent processes vaginalis are many, namely, routine bilateral open surgery explorations [7], use of ultrasonography [8], laparoscopy [9], and the wait and watch policy [10].

Although laparoscopy proves advantageous over open surgery by precise detection and simultaneous repair of contralateral patent processes vaginalis, its management remains a contentious issue. The current consensus amongst surgeons practicing open surgery favors operating on the symptomatic side alone [9] as the rate of metachronous hernia is significant that it necessitates subsequent surgery in a twentieth of patients [11]. Therefore, this advantage of laparoscopic hernia repair may be significant in clinical practice as it gives good diagnosis and also repair for the metachronous hernia.

In open surgery, time is consumed in gaining access, obtaining adequate exposure, identification of the hernia sac, and dissection of the cord structures from the sac without harming the important cord structures [10]. In laparoscopic surgery, approaching from within makes the area of interest bloodless, and the magnification renders anatomy splendidly clear, making surgery precise [12]. But the time limiting step remains intracorporeal suturing that places considerable demands on the requirement of hand eye coordination, especially while negotiating the posterior and medial hemicircumference of the internal ring, over the iliac and inferior epigastric vessels [11]. With growing experience [11] and in this study the subfascia purse string suture and extracorporeal subcutaneous knotting with two ports markedly reduce the operative time over the traditional three ports laparoscopic hernia repair with intracorporeal suture ligation. In this study the mean operative time for unilateral repairs was (15 to 20 minutes) and bilateral hernia repair was (21 to 30 minutes); the mean duration of surgery was markedly less than the operative time noted in Lukong study [3]. The extracorporeal suturing was effective easy not need for special tool or surgical skills which also proved by other studys [11, 12].

The difference in postoperative pain following open surgery and laparoscopic surgery is subject to controversy. Some report less pain while others report greater pain in the immediate postoperative period following laparoscopic surgery compared with open surgery [13]. Bharathi R. found pain perception following either procedure to be similar. Parietal pain predominates in open surgery can well be controlled by caudal analgesia. On the other hand, pain perception is multimodal and multifactorial in laparoscopic surgery [14]. In addition to parietal pain caused by port placement, capnoperitoneum causes visceral pain due to stretching (peritoneal and diaphragmatic) and acidosis [14]. Neither the use of smaller ports nor the use of caudal analgesia would completely obliterate pain following laparoscopy [14]. Therefore, the decrease in the size of the incision does not necessarily translate into a proportionate decrease in pain. Hence, the difference in postoperative pain between laparoscopic surgery and open surgery is not significant enough to rate either surgery superior. In this study, the intraperitoneal gas pressure was located less than in other studies [14] due to the less number of ports and no need for intra-abdominal surgical maneuvers. Which reduced the post-operative pain. All patient was not need for post-operative analgesia.

Many new techniques have recently taken place in pediatric laparoscopic inguinal hernia surgery. Lee and Liang

[15] introduced the Endo-needle designed specifically for laparoscopic extraperitoneal closure of the patent processus vaginalis. Endo and Ukiyama performed microlaparoscopic high ligation in 450 patients with good results. They reported no complications related to the procedure and a remarkably low recurrence rate (0.88%) [16]. Prasad et al. used a stainless steel curved awl and a 1.7 mm telescope to safely perform needlescopic inguinal herniorrhaphy [17]. Shalaby et al. used RN for closure of IIR in 150 patients successfully with excellent cosmetic results without any recurrence [18]. Chan and Tam [19] introduced the saline injection and needle sign to reduce the recurrence rate in his series. Bharathi et al. [20] used the TNH technique in 67 repairs, and 146 repairs were performed using the SEAL technique. They stated that SEAL resulted in marked reduction of operative time when compared to the TNH technique (unilateral: 15 versus 25 minutes; bilateral: 25 versus 40 minutes). They added that avoiding the vas deferens and gonadal vessels during the SEAL repair in boys may leave a small gap at the internal ring as well as leaving the hernia sac in situ, which has the potential to contribute to a higher incidence of recurrence in male patients. They believe that ligation of the internal ring leads to scarring and obliteration of the space distally. This would explain the relatively low incidence of postoperative hydrocele. Fluid accumulating in the distal sac postoperatively often reabsorbs spontaneously and does not necessitate additional intervention [20]. In this study there was no hydrocele detected as a postoperative complication in spite of no excision of the sac and the recurrence rate was 1% recurrence. Several piercings of the peritoneum by RN around the neck of the sac may add fixation of the suture at this level that prevents migration of the suture distally initiating recurrence. It may result in creation of adhesions of the sac preventing hydrocele formation. This may explain the high incidence of recurrence in the series of Manoharan et al. [9] and Bharathi et al. [20] that apply the subcutaneous suture around the internal ring without piercing the peritoneum. However, Chan and Tam [19] reported a very low recurrence rate (1%) after refinement of the technique by using TNH and injecting saline around the vas and vessels and using the needle sign to avoid damage to the testicular vessel and vas. They claimed that presence of a complete ring around IIR prevents recurrence. Prasad et al. reported no recurrence in their early small series of 8 cases [17]. Shalaby et al. reported no recurrence in their series [18]. The results of this study confirm the safety and efficacy of laparoscopic hernia repair with two ports in congenital inguinal hernia in children. It resulted in good diagnosis and management of metachronous hernia and marked reduction of operative time, less recurrence, no hydrocele formation, excellent cosmetic, and no postoperative pain results.

References

[1] R. Saranga Bharathi, *Comparative study of laparoscopic versus conventional surgery for congenital inguinal hernia in children [M.S. thesis]*, University of Pune, 2008.

[2] Y.-T. Chang, "Technical refinements in single-port laparoscopic surgery of inguinal hernia in infants and children," *Diagnostic and Therapeutic Endoscopy*, vol. 2010, Article ID 392847, 6 pages, 2010.

[3] C. S. Lukong, "Surgical techniques of laparoscopic inguinal hernia repair in childhood: a critical appraisal," *Journal of Surgical Technique and Case Report*, vol. 4, no. 1, pp. 1–5, 2012.

[4] P. Kapur, M. G. Caty, and P. L. Glick, "Pediatric hernias and hydroceles," *Pediatric Clinics of North America*, vol. 45, no. 4, pp. 773–789, 1998.

[5] F. Schier, P. Montupet, and C. Esposito, "Laparoscopic inguinal herniorrhaphy in children: a three-center experience with 933 repairs," *Journal of Pediatric Surgery*, vol. 37, no. 3, pp. 395–397, 2002.

[6] D. Ozgediz, K. Roayaie, H. Lee et al., "Subcutaneous endoscopically assisted ligation (SEAL) of the internal ring for repair of inguinal hernias in children: report of a new technique and early results," *Surgical Endoscopy*, vol. 21, no. 8, pp. 1327–1331, 2007.

[7] F. Rathauser, "Historical overview of the bilateral approach to pediatric inguinal hernias," *The American Journal of Surgery*, vol. 150, no. 5, pp. 527–532, 1985.

[8] D. M. Miltenburg, J. G. Nuchtern, T. Jaksic, C. Kozinetiz, and M. L. Brandt, "Laparoscopic evaluation of the pediatric inguinal hernia—a meta-analysis," *Journal of Pediatric Surgery*, vol. 33, no. 6, pp. 874–879, 1998.

[9] S. Manoharan, U. Samarakkody, M. Kulkarni, R. Blakelock, and S. Brown, "Evidence-based change of practice in the management of unilateral inguinal hernia," *Journal of Pediatric Surgery*, vol. 40, no. 7, pp. 1163–1166, 2005.

[10] C. Esposito, L. Montinaro, F. Alicchio, A. Savanelli, T. Armenise, and A. Settimi, "Laparoscopic treatment of inguinal hernia in the first year of life," *Journal of Laparoendoscopic and Advanced Surgical Techniques*, vol. 20, no. 5, pp. 473–476, 2010.

[11] F. Schier, "Laparoscopic inguinal hernia repair-a prospective personal series of 542 children," *Journal of Pediatric Surgery*, vol. 41, no. 6, pp. 1081–1084, 2006.

[12] P. Chinnaswamy, V. Malladi, K. V. Jani et al., "Laparoscopic inguinal hernia repair in children," *Journal of the Society of Laparoendoscopic Surgeons*, vol. 9, no. 4, pp. 393–398, 2005.

[13] P. Ekstein, A. Szold, B. Sagie, N. Werbin, J. M. Klausner, and A. A. Weinbroum, "Laparoscopic surgery may be associated with severe pain and high analgesia requirements in the immediate postoperative period," *Annals of Surgery*, vol. 243, no. 1, pp. 41–46, 2006.

[14] V. L. Wills and D. R. Hunt, "Pain after laparoscopic cholecystectomy," *British Journal of Surgery*, vol. 87, no. 3, pp. 273–284, 2000.

[15] Y. Lee and J. Liang, "Experience with 450 cases of microlaparoscopic herniotomy in infants and children," *Pediatric Endosurgery and Innovative Techniques*, vol. 6, no. 1, pp. 25–28, 2002.

[16] M. Endo and E. Ukiyama, "Laparoscopic closure of patent processus vaginalis in girls with inguinal hernia using a specially devised suture needle," *Pediatric Endosurgery & Innovative Techniques*, vol. 5, no. 2, pp. 187–191, 2001.

[17] R. Prasad, H. N. Lovvorn III, G. M. Wadie, and T. E. Lobe, "Early experience with needleoscopic inguinal herniorrhaphy

in children," *Journal of Pediatric Surgery*, vol. 38, no. 7, pp. 1055–1058, 2003.

[18] R. Y. Shalaby, M. Fawy, S. M. Soliman, and A. Dorgham, "A new simplified technique for needlescopic inguinal herniorrhaphy in children," *Journal of Pediatric Surgery*, vol. 41, no. 4, pp. 863–867, 2006.

[19] K. L. Chan and P. K. H. Tam, "Technical refinements in laparoscopic repair of childhood inguinal hernias," *Surgical Endoscopy and Other Interventional Techniques*, vol. 18, no. 6, pp. 957–960, 2004.

[20] R. S. Bharathi, A. K. Dabas, M. Arora, and V. Baskaran, "Laparoscopic ligation of internal ring—three ports versus single-port technique: are working ports necessary?" *Journal of Laparoendoscopic and Advanced Surgical Techniques*, vol. 18, no. 6, pp. 891–894, 2008.

A New Proposal for Learning Curve of TEP Inguinal Hernia Repair: Ability to Complete Operation Endoscopically as a First Phase of Learning Curve

Mustafa Hasbahceci,[1] Fatih Basak,[2] Aylin Acar,[3] and Orhan Alimoglu[4]

[1] *Department of General Surgery, Faculty of Medicine, Bezmialem Vakif University, Vatan Street, Fatih, 34093 Istanbul, Turkey*
[2] *Department of General Surgery, Umraniye Education and Research Hospital, Umraniye, 34766 Istanbul, Turkey*
[3] *Department of General Surgery, Lutfi Kirdar Kartal Education and Research Hospital, Kartal, 34890 Istanbul, Turkey*
[4] *Department of General Surgery, Faculty of Medicine, Istanbul Medeniyet University, Kadikoy, 34722 Istanbul, Turkey*

Correspondence should be addressed to Mustafa Hasbahceci; hasbahceci@yahoo.com

Academic Editor: Steve Ramcharitar

Background. The exact nature of learning curve of totally extraperitoneal inguinal hernia and the number required to master this technique remain controversial. *Patients and Methods.* We present a retrospective review of a single surgeon experience on patients who underwent totally extraperitoneal inguinal hernia repair. *Results.* There were 42 hernias (22 left- and 20 right-sided) in 39 patients with a mean age of 48.8 ± 15.1 years. Indirect, direct, and combined hernias were present in 18, 12, and 12 cases, respectively. The mean operative time was 55.1 ± 22.8 minutes. Peritoneal injury occurred in 9 cases (21.4%). Conversion to open surgery was necessitated in 7 cases (16.7%). After grouping of all patients into two groups as cases between 1–21 and 22–42, it was seen that the majority of peritoneal injuries (7 out of 9, 77.8%, $P = 0.130$) and all conversions ($P = 0.001$) occurred in the first 21 cases. *Conclusions.* Learning curve of totally extraperitoneal inguinal hernia repair can be divided into two consequent steps: immediate and late. At least 20 operations are required for gaining anatomical knowledge and surgical pitfalls based on the ability to perform this operation without conversion during immediate phase.

1. Introduction

Totally extraperitoneal (TEP) inguinal hernia repair has gained popularity in the recent two decades since the first introduction in 1992 by Dulucq [1]. It offers a hernia repair of minimal incisions with more favorable postoperative course including less pain and quicker return to work especially more pronounced in bilateral inguinal hernia [2]. However, this technique requires specialized anatomical knowledge, two-hand manipulation for reduction of hernia sac, and mesh placement within a limited working space. Therefore, acceptance and implementation of this technique have been slow compared to the adoption of other minimal invasive procedures such as cholecystectomy [3, 4].

In addition to the technical dexterity, there are some drawbacks for the common adoption of this technique including increased operative times, complications during the early learning curve, and almost absolute necessity for general anesthesia [5, 6]. Consequently, the learning curve of TEP inguinal hernia repair for the inexperienced surgeons carries paramount importance. However, the exact nature of learning curve and the number required to master the technique are still focus of a debate.

There are a limited number of studies evaluating the learning curve for TEP inguinal hernia repair [2, 3, 7, 8]. Although there were some numerical suggestions beginning from 20 cases, the required number of operation to fulfill the learning curve has been reported even 250 repairs to fully master all aspects of the TEP approach [2, 3, 6, 9]. However, instead of recognizing the learning curve as a solid piece, it could be separated into two phases in order to ease the implementation and evaluation: *immediate* as an initial phase of ability to complete the operation and *late* as a latter phase of performing TEP with good outcomes.

In the present study, we try to evaluate the minimum required number of cases from the beginning of the learning curve to complete the operation as TEP inguinal hernia repair without conversion in the absence of supervision from an experienced endoscopic hernia surgeon.

2. Patients and Methods

A retrospective demographic, clinical, and operative data collection of adult patients who underwent TEP inguinal hernia repair between December 2011 and May 2012 was performed from a prospectively held database. Written consent was taken from each patient for both TEP and Lichtenstein inguinal hernia repairs for the cases in which conversion might be required. The patients with American Society of Anesthesiologists (ASA) classes IV and V, who had contraindications for general anesthesia, previous open, or laparoscopic lower abdominal surgery except open inguinal hernia repair, with emergency admission for complicated inguinal hernia, with femoral hernia diagnosed by imaging techniques, and who were unwilling to be operated by TEP inguinal hernia repair, were excluded.

All TEP repairs were performed under general anesthesia by a single surgeon (MH) who had a satisfactory experience with laparoscopic cholecystectomy and who performed more than 500 Lichtenstein inguinal hernia repair previously. For TEP inguinal hernia repair, active participation to the operations ($n > 10$) performed by an experienced surgeon was done.

Patients' demographics, body mass index (kg/m^2), ASA class, features of the hernias, operative findings including time, presence of peritoneal injury, conversion to open surgery, and cause for the conversion, complications within the postoperative 30 days, and length of hospital stay were documented prospectively into a computerized database.

Operation time was calculated as the time from the first incision to the last suture. Complications were grouped as intraoperative including bleeding from epigastric or testicular arteries, peritoneal, testicular, or nerve injuries, and postoperative including hematoma or seroma formation, urinary retention treated by catheterization, neuralgia, wound infection, and early recurrence during the first 30 days. Hematoma or seroma was defined as an accumulation of blood or fluid in the subcutaneous tissues from the umbilicus to the scrotum. Neuralgia was defined as a pain in the inguinal region and medial aspect of the thigh occurred after the operation. Wound infection was defined as occurrence of redness with or without drainage from the incisions. In the absence of hematoma and seroma, any swelling in the inguinal region verified by clinical examination and imaging techniques was defined as early recurrence. Length of stay was calculated as the number of days in the hospital after the surgery. Patients were seen within the fourth week postoperatively.

2.1. Operative Technique. Patients were asked to empty their urinary bladder just before the operation. No prophylactic antibiotics were administered. Under general anesthesia, anterior rectus sheath on the side of inguinal hernia was incised via infraumbilical incision. Then, a space was created below the rectus without incising the posterior rectus sheath. In case of bilateral inguinal hernia, the entrance was done on the dominant side. After formation of a tunnel with the help of blunt-tipped instruments, 10 mm trocar was introduced and carbon dioxide insufflation was started with a maximum pressure of 15 mmHg. Balloon dissectors were not used.

The optical telescope with 0 degree was inserted and blunt dissection by gentle side-to-side movements was performed until the symphysis pubis was clearly seen. The inferior epigastric vessels were clearly visualized laterally on the posterior surface of the rectus muscle. The retropubic space of Retzius and the space of Bogros were easily expanded by this telescopic approach. Two 5 mm trocars were introduced between the umbilicus and the symphysis pubis. The hernia defect was identified. Dissection of the peritoneal sac from the cord structures in cases of laterally placed indirect inguinal hernia or retraction from the abdominal wall defect in cases of medially placed direct inguinal hernia or both in cases of combined inguinal hernia were performed. Dissection of indirect inguinal hernia sac was completed either by reduction or transection in which it was closed by metallic clips. Peritoneal defects were closed either by metallic clips or suturing. After appropriate dissection of all potential hernia spaces medially from the symphysis pubis laterally to the psoas muscle and reduction of the hernia sac(s), a polypropylene mesh (Prolene, Ethicon, LCC) with a diameter of 15×10 cm was inserted and placed over the entire musculopectineal orifice with sufficient overlap at the medial and lateral borders. No keyhole over the mesh or no fixation of the mesh was being used. After the complete desufflation under permanent visual control of the operative area, removal of the trocars was performed. One fascial suture to subumbilical incision was applied. Skin incisions were closed in an appropriate manner. In case of difficulty or in the event of a complication, the operation was converted to Lichtenstein inguinal hernia repair in all cases.

2.2. Statistical Analysis. Statistical calculations were performed using NCSS (Number Cruncher Statistical System, 2007) and PASS (Power Analysis and Sample Size) Statistical software (Utah, USA, 2008). Normally distributed continuous variables were expressed as mean ± standard deviation (SD). The range including minimum and maximum values was also added. Categorical variables were expressed as frequencies and percentages of an appropriate denominator. The Student's t-test was used for analysis of normally distributed, descriptive continuous variables, which were expressed as mean ± SD. The Chi-Square Test and Fischer's Exact Test were used to compare qualitative variables. Differences were considered statistically significant, if the P value was equal to or less than 0.05.

3. Results

The study group included 38 male and one female patient with 42 hernias. The mean age and body mass index of

Table 1: Causes for conversion.

Reason	Number
Peritoneal injury causing loss of exposure	2
Difficulty to determine the anatomy	2
Adhesions caused by previous hernia repair	2
Sliding hernia	1

Table 2: Demographic and operative data of the groups.

Parameter	Groups		P
	Group I (numbers 1–21)	Group II (numbers 22–42)	
Age$^{\beta}$ (years)	47.0 ± 18.0 (19–73)	50.6 ± 11.6 (27–69)	0.434
BMI$^{\beta}$ (kg/m^2)	25.9 ± 3.8 (19–32)	26.4 ± 2.8 (21–30)	0.606
Operation time$^{\beta,¥}$ (min)	58.6 ± 28.3 (20–110)	52.8 ± 18.7 (25–90)	0.476
Peritoneal injury (n/%)	7 (33.3)	2 (9.5)	0.130
Conversion (n/%)	7 (33.3)	0 (0)	0.009*

*Statistical significance.
$^{\beta}$Mean ± SD.
¥Operation times excluding converted operations.

the patients were 48.8 ± 15.1 years (range from 19 to 73 years) and 26.2±3.4 kg/m^2 (range from 19 to 32 kg/m^2), respectively. ASA classes I, II, and III distribution of the patients was 25, 15, and 2, respectively.

There were 22 left- and 20 right-sided hernias. Indirect, direct, and combined hernias were present in 18, 12, and 12 cases, respectively. Hernias with previous repairs were detected only in 4 cases. Peritoneal injury occurred in 9 cases (21.4%). Conversion to open surgery was necessitated in 7 cases (16.7%). There was no bleeding and testicular or nerve injury intraoperatively. The mean operative times were 55.1 ± 22.8 minutes (range from 20 to 110 minutes) excluding the patients with conversion to open surgery. The causes for conversion were summarized in Table 1.

Occurrence of peritoneal injury was not related with the age and BMI of the patient, type and side of hernia, and presence of previous repair ($P > 0.05$ for all). Conversion occurred significantly in right-sided ($P = 0.041$) and recurrent hernias ($P = 0.011$). No significant differences were detected between age and BMI of the patients and type of the hernia and conversion ($P > 0.05$ for all).

All patients were grouped into two groups: Groups I and II consisted of the cases between 1–21 and 22–42, respectively (Table 2). Two groups were similar with regard to age, BMI, and operation time. Although peritoneal injury occurred more frequently in Group I (33.3% versus 9.5%), it did not reach statistical significance ($P = 0.130$). However, all conversions were seen in Group I ($P = 0.009$).

All patients were discharged at the first day postoperative. Postoperative urinary retention, neuralgia, and wound infection were not seen. However, in three patients, two in Group I and one in Group II, seroma formation was detected and managed conservatively. There was one early recurrence in Group I. No mortality was seen.

4. Discussion

The learning curve has been defined as the minimum number of operations required for gaining adequate knowledge of pitfalls and technical factors leading stabilization of operation times and complication rates [3, 9]. In literature, there were several cut-off values for the learning period of endoscopic hernia repair up to 250 cases which was regarded as comfort zone [6, 10]. In a Cochrane review, it was suggested to perform at least between 30 and 100 operations as a critical threshold level to become an experienced surgeon [10, 11]. It is generally accepted that for a recurrence rate of less than 1%, more than 60 cases under supervision were recommended [2, 10, 12]. Lau et al. reported that at least 80 operations were required for the mean operation time of less than 1 hour [3]. It was also shown that even after more than 400 individually performed TEP procedures, there was a progress in reducing the conversion rate, the incidence of short-term complications, and the operative times [10]. These findings suggested the necessity of a rather long learning curve for TEP procedures.

In previous studies, operation time less than 1 hour has been regarded as one of the parameters used to state the learning curve precisely [3, 4]. However, it is possible to perform this operation in a time period of less than one hour even in the beginning period, as in the present study. Gaining experience to use the minimal invasive techniques in other aspects of surgery might help to implement the technique in short time with greater efficiency. However, mastering the technique mandates not only finishes the operation in short time without conversion but also performs the operation with low recurrence rates. It could be helpful to separate two phases of learning curve as *immediate* and *late*. Therefore, we and others propose that an inexperienced beginner surgeon should perform at least 20 cases in accordance with the principles of endoscopic TEP inguinal hernia repair to become a familiar surgeon [9]. The exact number for becoming an experienced surgeon which is most probably more than 20 cases should be evaluated with future prospective studies.

Perceived pressure of the surgeons to complete the operations expediently was thought to be responsible for the high conversion rate which has been frequently experienced during endoscopic TEP inguinal hernia repair with an incidence of 2%–17% [8, 13]. Although our conversion rate during the first 21 cases was higher, we did not encounter any conversion during the second part of this study in accordance with Lal's findings [7]. Some authors have mentioned that more than 50 cases were required for the surgeons who were unfamiliar with preperitoneal space [7]. However, adequate perception of the preperitoneal anatomy with careful dissection can be gathered during the first 20 cases without causing any morbidity according to the present study.

Appropriate patient selection has been shown to be an important parameter for the success of the operation during early period. Irreducible hernias, hernias in patients with previous lower quadrant surgery, have been excluded in several early TEP series [3, 14]. Certain patient characteristics including female gender, higher BMI, previous history of abdominal surgery, and scrotal and bilateral hernias were also shown to be important for the high risk of conversion and intraoperative complications even for experienced surgeons. However, liberal inclusion of the patients in to the study including recurrent and sliding hernias was applied during the learning curve of this study which might affect our high conversion rate. It could be possible to diminish the conversion rate in our study, if the strict inclusion criteria were used. Indeed, it is recommended to select relatively younger and slender male patients less than 60 years of age with unilateral, nonscrotal primary inguinal hernia during the learning period for TEP inguinal hernia repair [8, 14].

It has been also shown that the presence of an experienced endoscopic hernia surgeon or performance of previous Stoppa's procedures prevents unnecessary recurrences caused by surgical errors and helps overcome the difficulty which has been experienced during the learning period [7, 8]. Experience with preperitoneal space anatomy is the most important factor for performing the posterior approaches either through open or endoscopic approaches [7, 15]. Therefore, performance of previous Stoppa's procedure might also be unhelpful for a surgeon who is unfamiliar to this space. Therefore, it is believed that active participation to endoscopic TEP inguinal hernia repairs performed by an experienced surgeon can facilitate the transition to TEP procedures [4, 9, 12].

Peritoneal injury has been regarded as the most important operative complication to cause the loss of exposure in a limited preperitoneal area [8]. It has been reported that the occurrence of this complication can be seen in almost half of the cases [16]. In the present study, peritoneal injury occurred in 21.4% of the cases and was regarded as the reason for conversion in two out of seven conversions. Thus, use of nontraumatic graspers and scissors with cautery is advised to avoid such complication during dissection of the operative area and reduction of the indirect hernia sac.

Preperitoneal dissection can be performed by disposable balloon dissectors or by the help of 0° telescopes [17]. The balloon dissector has been known to decrease the operation time and to reduce conversion rates [13, 18]. Therefore, it is recommended to use such instruments especially during the early period in the learning curve besides its high cost. However, these instruments were not favored in the present study because of the financial considerations though their beneficial effect. Blunt dissection by using 0° telescopes can be easy, if the entrance to the preperitoneal space can be succeeded through cleavage of the posterior lamina of transversalis fascia. We recommend dissecting the preperitoneal space by using telescopes only in accordance with the precautions published before [15].

During endoscopic TEP inguinal hernia repair, it is important to dissect all possible hernia sites to prevent the recurrences. The short-term recurrences were most likely due to technical errors causing improper identification of the indirect hernia sac [3, 8]. Although there was only one short-term recurrence in our series, inadequate dissection causing missed indirect hernia was thought to be responsible for early recurrence. Therefore, it is advised to isolate the cord structures at least for a distance of 4 cm to dissect the all defective areas and to deflate the air under direct vision to overcome such technical problems. For prevention of the direct recurrences, extensive lateral preperitoneal dissection and good positioning of the mesh with sufficient size covering the Hasselbach triangle is recommended [3, 7, 8].

This study has some limitations including its retrospective design with small number of cases and lack of the long-term follow-up. The main objective of this study was to measure the minimum number of endoscopic TEP inguinal hernia repairs to complete the operation without any conversion for a beginner surgeon. Therefore, we did not include several operative outcomes including long-term recurrence and postoperative pain into the aims of this study, although these parameters are the most important endpoints for a successful evaluation of an endoscopic hernia repair [8].

Our results were derived from a single teaching hospital and from a single surgeon experience. Although there may be some difficulty to generalize our findings because of the individual differences based on skill set and training structure, they can be regarded as a baseline level for the minimum requirement for TEP inguinal hernia repair.

5. Conclusion

The learning curve of TEP inguinal hernia repair can be divided in two consequent steps: the *immediate* which shows the technical experience to accomplish endoscopic surgery without complications and conversions and the *late* to become an experienced surgeon with a late recurrence rate of less than 1%. At least 20 operations are required for gaining anatomical knowledge of preperitoneal space and surgical pitfalls based on the ability to perform the operation without conversion.

Acknowledgments

This study was performed at Umraniye Education and Research Hospital, Department of General Surgery, Umraniye, Istanbul, Turkey. This study was presented at XVI. Annual Meeting of the European Society of Surgery, Istanbul, Turkey, November 22–24, 2012.

References

[1] J. L. Dulucq, "Treatment of inguinal hernias by inserting a subperitoneal prosthetic patch using pre-peritoneoscopy (with a video film)," *Chirurgie: Memoires de l'Academie de Chirurgie*, vol. 118, no. 1-2, pp. 83–85, 1992 (French).

[2] J. Haidenberg, M. L. Kendrick, T. Meile, and D. R. Farley, "Totally extraperitoneal (TEP) approach for inguinal hernia: the favorable learning curve for trainees," *Current Surgery*, vol. 60, no. 1, pp. 65–68, 2003.

[3] H. Lau, N. G. Patil, W. K. Yuen, and F. Lee, "Learning curve for unilateral endoscopic totally extraperitoneal (TEP) inguinal hernioplasty," *Surgical Endoscopy and Other Interventional Techniques*, vol. 16, no. 12, pp. 1724–1728, 2002.

[4] Y. Y. Choi, Z. Kim, and K. Y. Hur, "Learning curve for laparoscopic totally extraperitoneal repair of inguinal hernia," *Canadian Journal of Surgery*, vol. 55, no. 1, pp. 33–36, 2012.

[5] B. Zendejas, D. A. Cook, J. Bingener et al., "Simulation-based mastery learning improves patient outcomes in laparoscopic inguinal hernia repair: a randomized controlled trial," *Annals of Surgery*, vol. 254, no. 3, pp. 502–511, 2011.

[6] L. Neumayer, A. Giobbie-Hurder, O. Jonasson et al., "Open mesh versus laparoscopic mesh repair of inguinal hernia," *The New England Journal of Medicine*, vol. 350, no. 18, pp. 1819–1922, 2004.

[7] P. Lal, R. K. Kajla, J. Chander, and V. K. Ramteke, "Laparoscopic total extraperitoneal (TEP) inguinal hernia repair: overcoming the learning curve," *Surgical Endoscopy and Other Interventional Techniques*, vol. 18, no. 4, pp. 642–645, 2004.

[8] M. S. L. Liem, C. J. van Steensel, R. U. Boelhouwer et al., "The learning curve for totally extraperitoneal laparoscopic inguinal hernia repair," *American Journal of Surgery*, vol. 171, no. 2, pp. 281–285, 1996.

[9] A. D. G. Lamb, A. J. Robson, and S. J. Nixon, "Recurrence after totally extra-peritoneal laparoscopic repair: implications for operative technique and surgical training," *Surgeon*, vol. 4, no. 5, pp. 299–307, 2006.

[10] N. Schouten, R. K. Simmermacher, T. van Dalen et al., "Is there an end of the "learning curve" of endoscopic totally extraperitoneal (TEP) hernia repair?" *Surgical Endoscopy*, vol. 27, no. 3, pp. 789–794, 2013.

[11] B. L. Wake, K. McCormack, C. Fraser, L. Vale, J. Perez, and A. M. Grant, "Transabdominal pre-peritoneal (TAPP) vs totally extraperitoneal (TEP) laparoscopic techniques for inguinal hernia repair," *Cochrane Database of Systematic Reviews*, no. 1, Article ID CD004703, 2005.

[12] B. Zendejas, E. O. Onkendi, R. D. Brahmbhatt, C. M. Lohse, S. M. Greenlee, and D. R. Farley, "Long-term outcomes of laparoscopic totally extraperitoneal inguinal hernia repairs performed by supervised surgical trainees," *American Journal of Surgery*, vol. 201, no. 3, pp. 379–384, 2011.

[13] B. J. Leibl, C. Jäger, B. Kraft et al., "Laparoscopic hernia repair—TAPP or/and TEP?" *Langenbeck's Archives of Surgery*, vol. 390, no. 2, pp. 77–82, 2005.

[14] N. Schouten, J. W. Elshof, R. K. Simmermacher et al., "Selecting patients during the "learning curve" of endoscopic totally extraperitoneal (TEP) hernia repair," *Hernia*, vol. 17, no. 6, pp. 737–743, 2013.

[15] J. F. Lange, P. P. G. M. Rooijens, S. Koppert, and G. J. Kleinrensink, "The preperitoneal tissue dilemma in totally extraperitoneal (TEP) laparoscopic hernia repair: an anatomo-surgical study," *Surgical Endoscopy and Other Interventional Techniques*, vol. 16, no. 6, pp. 927–930, 2002.

[16] Z. Haitian, L. Jian, L. Qinghua et al., "Totally extraperitoneal laparoscopic hernioplasty: the optimal surgical approach," *Surgical Laparoscopy, Endoscopy and Percutaneous Techniques*, vol. 19, no. 6, pp. 501–505, 2009.

[17] J.-L. Dulucq, P. Wintringer, and A. Mahajna, "Laparoscopic totally extraperitoneal inguinal hernia repair: lessons learned from 3,100 hernia repairs over 15 years," *Surgical Endoscopy and Other Interventional Techniques*, vol. 23, no. 3, pp. 482–486, 2009.

[18] S. Bringman, Å. Ek, E. Haglind et al., "Is a dissection balloon beneficial in totally extraperitoneal endoscopic hernioplasty (TEP)? A randomized prospective multicenter study," *Surgical Endoscopy*, vol. 15, no. 3, pp. 266–270, 2001.

11

Laparoscopic-Assisted Single-Port Appendectomy in Children: It Is a Safe and Cost-Effective Alternative to Conventional Laparoscopic Techniques?

Sergio B. Sesia and Frank-Martin Haecker

Department of Pediatric Surgery, University Children's Hospital Basel, Spitalstrasse 33, 4056 Basel, Switzerland

Correspondence should be addressed to Sergio B. Sesia; sergio.sesia@ukbb.ch

Academic Editor: Peng Hui Wang

Aim. Laparoscopic-assisted single-port appendectomy (SPA), although combining the advantages of open and conventional laparoscopic surgery, is still not widely used in childhood. The aim of this study was to evaluate the safety and the cost effectiveness of SPA in children. *Methods.* After institutional review board approval, we retrospectively evaluated 262 children who underwent SPA. The appendix was dissected outside the abdominal cavity as in open surgery. For stump closure, we used two 3/0 vicryl RB-1 sutures. *Results.* We identified 146 boys (55.7%) and 116 girls (44.3%). Median age at operation was 11.4 years (range, 1.1–15.9). Closure of the appendiceal stump using two sutures (cost: USD 15) was successful in all patients. Neither a stapler (cost: USD 276) nor endoloops (cost: USD 89) were used. During a follow-up of up to 69 months (range, 30–69), six obese children (2.3%, body mass index >95th percentile) developed an intra-abdominal abscess after perforated appendicitis. No insufficiency of the appendiceal stump was observed by ultrasound. Five of them were treated successfully by antibiotics, one child required drainage. *Conclusion.* The SPA technique with conventional extracorporal closure of the appendiceal stump is safe and cost effective. In our unit, SPA is the standard procedure for appendectomy in children.

1. Introduction

Since the first description of laparoscopic appendectomy by Semm in 1983 [1], several laparoscopic techniques have evolved to attain stump closure. Surgeons can choose between clip, stapler, endoloops [2, 3], or simple sutures as in open surgery. Commonly, endoloops or endostaplers are used for closing the stump of the appendix [3, 4]. We report about the cost of appendiceal stump closure using only sutures in laparoscopic-assisted single-port appendectomy (SPA) in children.

2. Materials and Methods

After institutional review board approval, we retrospectively reviewed the medical records of children who underwent SPA between August 2005 and December 2008 at the University Children's Hospital of Basle (UKBB). According to the World Organization of Gastroenterology Research Committee [5], diagnosis of acute appendicitis was made by comprehensive anamnesis, physical examination with particular attention of rebound tenderness on the right lower abdominal quadrant, supporting laboratory tests such as white blood cell count (WBC) and C-reactive protein (CRP), and ultrasound scan of the abdomen. All children admitted on our emergency room with suspected acute appendicitis were considered for SPA and included in this study. The only exclusion criterion was appendectomy performed by an open surgical approach. Surgery was performed under the supervision of five board-certified pediatric surgeons. Extracorporal sutures closed the stumps of all appendices, including perforated appendicitis. Neither endoloops nor endostaples were used. The SPA with extracorporal stump closure represented the standard technique for appendectomy. The main purpose of this retrospective single-center study was to analyze the cost for closing the appendiceal stump. Other material and personnel costs for surgery, anesthesia, and costs for operating room and for hospital stay were not considered. Data were stored in an Excel database (Microsoft Corporation, Redmond, WA).

3. Surgical Technique

As previously described [6], SPA was performed using one 12-mm single-use balloon-trocar (Auto Suture, United States Surgical/Tyco Healthcare, Type OMS-T10BT, Norwalk, CT) with one conventional laparoscopic forceps (COMEG, Endoskopie GmbH & Co., Type PAJUNK 12929410). After introducing the trocar through a subumbilical incision, the appendix was grasped and exteriorized through the umbilicus. Dissection and appendectomy were performed in the standard open fashion. After ligature of the basis of the appendix, one purse-string suture and one z-shaped absorbable suture 3/0 vicryl RB-1 placed through the sero-muscular base of the caecum closed the appendiceal stump.

All operations were accomplished on emergency basis. All children with suspected appendicitis were managed according to a standard preoperative protocol such as mechanical cleaning of the umbilicus with noncolored octenidine dihydrochloride (Octenisept) and a loading i.v.-dose of metronidazole and of cefuroxime within 15 minutes before starting surgery [6].

4. Results

Between August 2005 and December 2008, 262 children underwent SPA, including 146 males (55.7%) and 116 females (44.3%). Median age at operation was 11.4 years (range, 1.1–15.9). Closure of the appendiceal stump using two vicryl RB-1 sutures at a cost of USD 7.5 each was successful in all patients. Conversion to open appendectomy occurred in 35 children (13.4%) and to conventional 3-trocar laparoscopic appendectomy in 9 children (3.4%). In a previous study, we reported about complications and main outcomes in correlation to histological results [6]. No insufficiency of the appendiceal stump was observed by ultrasound. During a followup of 69 months (range, 30–69), six obese children (2.3%, body mass index > 95th percentile) developed an intraabdominal abscess after perforated appendicitis. One child (0.4%) required surgical drainage, and the other five children (1.1%) responded to conservative treatment. No recurrence of intraabdominal abscess was noted to date. Neither a stapler (cost: USD 276) nor endoloops (cost: USD 89) were used. There was no mortality related to SPA in this series. Median operating time was 55 minutes (range, 15.0–160.0). The median length of hospital stay was 4 days (range, 3.0–18.0). As referred earlier [6], the operating surgeon was in 71.7% a resident under the direct supervision of a board certified senior pediatric surgeon.

5. Discussion

The increasing pressure of national healthcare insurance to contain costs of inpatient hospitalization aroused our interest in performing this cost-benefit analysis of SPA. Since this year, diagnosis-related group (DRG) was introduced in Switzerland. Now, a flat rate reimbursement replaced the traditional cost-based reimbursement system called TARMED (Tarif médical) [7, 8].

Appendicitis is the most common cause of acute abdominal disease in children [9]. Despite several advantages of laparoscopic appendectomy (LA) such as less pain, earlier discharge, better cosmesis, and earlier return to normal activities [10], open appendectomy (OA) still represents a standard surgical technique [11, 12]. In particular, SPA has not yet evolved as gold standard for the treatment of acute appendicitis. Compared to OA, LA using the three-trocar technique has been shown to induce less postoperative pain and faster recovery of the bowel function but seems to be associated with a higher rate of intraabdominal abscess formation, especially in perforated appendicitis [13], and with higher costs [14].

The different manner of closing the appendiceal stump may play a role in developing an intraabdominal abscess [13] and influence substantially the cost of LA. The technique of closure of the appendiceal stump in LA varies greatly. Usually, a noninversion of the appendiceal stump is performed in conventional three-trocar LA. This circumstance could explain a higher rate of intraabdominal abscess in conventional LA. Since the introduction of SPA in mid-2005 at our department, the appendiceal stump is ligated, inverted, and closed by one z-shaped suture. As reported earlier [6], we encountered 6 cases of intraabdominal abscess after SPA. All of them occurred in obese children (BMI > 95th percentile) with perforated appendicitis. In four of them, the surgeon carried out a lavage of the peritoneal cavity with saline. Despite a controversial discussion in the literature [15, 16], we hypothesize that the saline lavage may be responsible for bacterial spread throughout the abdomen and the cause of intraabdominal abscess. Due to this experience, we only perform suction of the abdominal fluid collections and no more lavage. A review of the literature shows no significant difference in the incidence of intraabdominal abscess when comparing the suture technique with endoloop and stapler to endoloop only for appendiceal stump closure [17]. But there is a noteworthy difference with regards to the cost.

The decision as to which LA-technique to use depends on its safety and cost. In our opinion, SPA joins the safety of OA (i.e., dissection under direct view) and the advantages of conventional LA (i.e., small skin incision and visibility of the entire abdominal cavity). Different ways to close the appendiceal stump exist such as stapler, clips, endoloop, or endobag [18]. In contrast to several reports of single-port or single-incision laparoscopic appendectomy [19], techniques that involve special trocar, and multiple instruments [20], our SPA-technique requires only one trocar (USD 172) and one conventional laparoscopic instrument and does not necessitate the use of expensive equipment such as retrieval pouch. Regarding these facts, our SPA-technique is less expensive than conventional three-trocar LA reported elsewhere [21, 22]. Closing the appendiceal stump using two 3/0 vicryl RB-1 sutures (USD 15) is 5.9 times less costly than by endoloop and 18.4 times less costly than by stapler.

Table 1: Recents reports of transumbilical laparoscopic-assisted single-port appendectomy.

Author, year	n	Journal	Intraoperative complications	Postoperative complications	Conversions to OA	Conversions to LA
D'Alessio et al., 2002 [25]	150	Eur J Pediatr Surg	5 (bleeding, rupture appendix)	5 (2 WI, 2 IAA, and 1 omphalitis)	6	6
Pappalepore et al., 2002 [26]	58	Eur J Pediatr Surg	0	0	1	1
Meyer et al., 2004 [27]	163	Zentralbl Chir	0	4 WI, 3 IAA	3	6
Koontz et al., 2006 [22]	111	J Pediatr Surg	0	8 (7 WI, 1 IAA)	2	2
Visnjic 2008 [9]	29	Surg Endosc	n.s.	4 WI	0	0
Sesia et al., 2010 [6]	262	J Laparoendosc Adv Surg Tech	1 serosa lesion	7 (1 WI, 6 IAA)	35	9
Guanà et al., 2010 [28]	231	Afr J Paediatr Surg	n.s.	4 (2 WI)	2	2
Stanfill et al., 2010 [29]	48	J Laparoendosc Adv Surg Tech	0	5 (1 ileus, 1 WI, and 3 IAA)	0	0
Lee et al., 2011 [24]	152	Surg Endosc	0	7 (7 IAA)	0	0
Cobellis et al., 2007 [30]	182	J Laparoendosc Adv Surg Tech	0	2 WI	31	0
Kagawa et al., 2012 [31]	158	Int J Colorectal Dis	0	8 (1 WI, 4 IAA, and 3 ileus)	7	26
Ohno et al., 2012 [21]	416	Surg Endosc	21 (2 serosa lesions, 16 tears of appendix, and 3 bleeding)	77 (31 WI, 21 intestinal obstruction, 15 IAA, 8 enterocolitis, 1 leakage, and 1 stitch abscess)	70	14
Shekherdimian and DeUgarte 2011 [32]	18	Am Surg	n.s.	0	0	0

IAA: intraabdominal abscess, WI: wound infection, n.s.: not specified, OA: open appendectomy, LA: laparoscopic appendectomy.

Our median operating time of 55 min. was slightly higher than those reported in the literature [22], which is related to our learning curve. Especially in complicated appendicitis, the operative time was higher than 55 min., as reported in the literature [23]. Safety of surgical techniques is one of the primary concerns in the literature; the safety of a surgical technique is characterized by its rate of complications. Table 1 displays the main outcomes of a review of the literature concerning laparoscopic-assisted single-port appendectomy.

The low rate of perioperative complications and of conversions to OA by extension of the subumbilical incision or to conventional LA by the introduction of 2 or more trocars, corroborate the finding that SPA remains a safe operative technique. The safety of OA is commonly accepted, and there are numerous studies underlining the reliability and the safety of LA also in complicated appendicitis in children [15]. However, SPA combines the advantages of both open and laparoscopic surgery and allows for use of both skills in open surgical and laparoscopy techniques. The need for only one single umbilical incision, one conventional laparoscopic instrument without any highly technical devices such as stapler, endoloop, and endobag reduce the time and the mean cost of the SPA-operation. Furthermore, the SPA-technique is extensible allowing additional trocars or devices such as stapler. Notably, SPA can be converted to conventional LA at any time for the treatment of additional pathologies.

6. Conclusion

SPA represents an expeditious and reliable technique for appendicitis in pediatric populations. In our opinion, SPA is a safe and cost-effective technique. The main negative features of conventional LA, that are longer operative time and operating room cost compared to OA [24], seem to be not attributable to SPA. Additional randomized trials are needed to verify this hypothesis. In our unit, SPA is the standard procedure for appendectomy in children.

References

[1] K. Semm, "Endoscopic appendectomy," *Endoscopy*, vol. 15, no. 2, pp. 59–64, 1983.

[2] A. Hanssen, S. Plotnikov, and R. Dubois, "Laparoscopic appendectomy using a polymeric clip to close the appendicular stump," *Journal of the Society of Laparoendoscopic Surgeons*, vol. 11, no. 1, pp. 59–62, 2007.

[3] G. Beldi, K. Muggli, C. Helbling, and R. Schlumpf, "Laparoscopic appendectomy using endoloops: a prospective, randomized clinical trial," *Surgical Endoscopy and Other Interventional Techniques*, vol. 18, no. 5, pp. 749–750, 2004.

[4] M. Wagner, D. Aronsky, J. Tschudi, A. Metzger, and C. Klaiber, "Laparoscopic stapler appendectomy: a prospective study of 267 consecutive cases," *Surgical Endoscopy*, vol. 10, no. 9, pp. 895–899, 1996.

[5] F. T. de Dombal, "The OMGE acute abdominal pain survey. Progress report, 1986," *Scandinavian Journal of Gastroenterology. Supplement*, vol. 23, no. 144, pp. 35–42, 1988.

[6] S. B. Sesia, F.-M. Haecker, R. Kubiak, and J. Mayr, "Laparoscopy-assisted single-port appendectomy in children: is the post-operative infectious complication rate different?" *Journal of Laparoendoscopic & Advanced Surgical Techniques*, vol. 20, no. 10, pp. 867–871, 2010.

[7] J.-F. Boudry, J.-P. Studer, and G. Villard, "Reflections on Tarmed's one year of operation," *Revue Medicale Suisse*, vol. 1, no. 17, pp. 1173–1174, 2005.

[8] E. Greer Gay and J. J. Kronenfeld, "Regulation, retrenchment—the DRG experience: problems from changing reimbursement practice," *Social Science and Medicine*, vol. 31, no. 10, pp. 1103–1118, 1990.

[9] S. Visnjic, "Transumbilical laparoscopically assisted appendectomy in children: high-tech low-budget surgery," *Surgical Endoscopy and Other Interventional Techniques*, vol. 22, no. 7, pp. 1667–1671, 2008.

[10] Y. S. Lee, J. H. Kim, E. J. Moon et al., "Comparative study on surgical outcomes and operative costs of transumbilical single-port laparoscopic appendectomy versus conventional laparoscopic appendectomy in adult patients," *Surgical Laparoscopy, Endoscopy and Percutaneous Techniques*, vol. 19, no. 6, pp. 493–496, 2009.

[11] L. I. Partecke, W. Kessler, W. von Bernstorff, S. Diedrich, C.-D. Heidecke, and M. Patrzyk, "Laparoscopic appendectomy using a single polymeric clip to close the appendicular stump," *Langenbeck's Archives of Surgery*, vol. 395, no. 8, pp. 1077–1082, 2010.

[12] C. Reißfelder, B. M. Cafferty, and M. von Frankenberg, "Open appendectomy. When do we still need it?" *Chirurg*, vol. 80, no. 7, pp. 602–607, 2009.

[13] A. Rickert, R. Bönninghoff, S. Post, M. Walz, N. Runkel, and P. Kienle, "Appendix stump closure with titanium clips in laparoscopic appendectomy," *Langenbeck's Archives of Surgery*, vol. 397, no. 2, pp. 327–331, 2012.

[14] E. Sporn, G. F. Petroski, G. J. Mancini, J. A. Astudillo, B. W. Miedema, and K. Thaler, "Laparoscopic appendectomy—is it worth the cost? Trend analysis in the US from 2000 to 2005," *Journal of the American College of Surgeons*, vol. 208, no. 2, pp. 179–185, 2009.

[15] M. Menezes, L. Das, M. Alagtal, J. Haroun, and P. Puri, "Laparoscopic appendectomy is recommended for the treatment of complicated appendicitis in children," *Pediatric Surgery International*, vol. 24, no. 3, pp. 303–305, 2008.

[16] S.-Y. Lee, H.-M. Lee, C.-S. Hsieh, and J.-H. Chuang, "Transumbilical laparoscopic appendectomy for acute appendicitis: a reliable one-port procedure," *Surgical Endoscopy*, vol. 25, no. 4, pp. 1115–1120, 2011.

[17] G. Kazemier, K. H. in't Hof, S. Saad, H. J. Bonjer, and S. Sauerland, "Securing the appendiceal stump in laparoscopic appendectomy: evidence for routine stapling?" *Surgical Endoscopy and Other Interventional Techniques*, vol. 20, no. 9, pp. 1473–1476, 2006.

[18] M. Sahm, R. Kube, S. Schmidt, C. Ritter, M. Pross, and H. Lippert, "Current analysis of endoloops in appendiceal stump closure," *Surgical Endoscopy and Other Interventional Techniques*, vol. 25, no. 1, pp. 124–129, 2011.

[19] Y. H. Tam, K. H. Lee, J. D. Y. Sihoe, K. W. Chan, S. T. Cheung, and K. K. Y. Pang, "A surgeon-friendly technique to perform single-incision laparoscopic appendectomy intracorporeally in children with conventional laparoscopic instruments," *Journal of Laparoendoscopic & Advanced Surgical Techniques*, vol. 20, no. 6, pp. 577–580, 2010.

[20] S. Horgan, K. Thompson, M. Talamini et al., "Clinical experience with a multifunctional, flexible surgery system for endolumenal, single-port, and NOTES procedures," *Surgical Endoscopy and Other Interventional Techniques*, vol. 25, no. 2, pp. 586–592, 2011.

[21] Y. Ohno, T. Morimura, and S.-I. Hayashi, "Transumbilical laparoscopically assisted appendectomy in children: the results of a single-port, single-channel procedure," *Surgical Endoscopy and Other Interventional Techniques*, vol. 26, no. 2, pp. 523–527, 2012.

[22] C. S. Koontz, L. A. Smith, H. C. Burkholder, K. Higdon, R. Aderhold, and M. Carr, "Video-assisted transumbilical appendectomy in children," *Journal of Pediatric Surgery*, vol. 41, no. 4, pp. 710–712, 2006.

[23] C. Esposito, A. I. Calvo, M. Castagnetti et al., "Open versus laparoscopic appendectomy in the pediatric population: a literature review and analysis of complications," *Journal of Laparoendoscopic & Advanced Surgical Techniques*, vol. 22, no. 8, pp. 834–839, 2012.

[24] T. H. Hong, H. L. Kim, Y. S. Lee et al., "Transumbilical single-port laparoscopic appendectomy (TUSPLA): scarless intracorporeal appendectomy," *Journal of Laparoendoscopic & Advanced Surgical Techniques*, vol. 19, no. 1, pp. 75–78, 2009.

[25] A. D'Alessio, E. Piro, B. Tadini, and F. Beretta, "One-trocar transumbilical laparoscopic-assisted appendectomy in children: our experience," *European Journal of Pediatric Surgery*, vol. 12, no. 1, pp. 24–27, 2002.

[26] N. Pappalepore, S. Tursini, N. Marino, G. Lisi, and P. Lelli Chiesa, "Transumbilical laparoscopic-assisted appendectomy (TULAA): a safe and useful alternative for uncomplicated appendicitis," *European Journal of Pediatric Surgery*, vol. 12, no. 6, pp. 383–386, 2002.

[27] A. Meyer, M. Preuß, S. Roesler, M. Lainka, and G. Omlor, "Transumbilical laparoscopic-assisted "one-trocar" appendectomy—TULAA—as an alternative operation method in the treatment of appendicitis," *Zentralblatt für Chirurgie*, vol. 129, no. 5, pp. 391–395, 2004.

[28] R. Guanà, R. Gesmundo, E. Maiullari et al., "Treatment of acute appendicitis with one-port transumbilical laparoscopic-assisted appendectomy: a six-year, single-centre experience," *African Journal of Paediatric Surgery*, vol. 7, no. 3, pp. 169–173, 2010.

[29] A. B. Stanfill, D. K. Matilsky, K. Kalvakuri, R. H. Pearl, L. J. Wallace, and R. K. Vegunta, "Transumbilical laparoscopically assisted appendectomy: an alternative minimally invasive technique in pediatric patients," *Journal of Laparoendoscopic and Advanced Surgical Techniques*, vol. 20, no. 10, pp. 873–876, 2010.

[30] G. Cobellis, A. Cruccetti, L. Mastroianni, G. Amici, and A. Martino, "One-trocar transumbilical laparoscopic-assisted management of Meckel's diverticulum in children," *Journal of Laparoendoscopic and Advanced Surgical Techniques*, vol. 17, no. 2, pp. 238–241, 2007.

[31] Y. Kagawa, S. Hata, J. Shimizu, M. Sekimoto, and M. Mori, "Transumbilical laparoscopic-assisted appendectomy for children and adults," *International Journal of Colorectal Disease*, vol. 27, no. 3, pp. 411–413, 2012.

[32] S. Shekherdimian and D. DeUgarte, "Transumbilical laparoscopic-assisted appendectomy: an extracorporeal single-incision alternative to conventional laparoscopic techniques," *American Surgeon*, vol. 77, no. 5, pp. 557–560, 2011.

12

Laparoscopic Primary Colorrhaphy for Acute Iatrogenic Perforations during Colonoscopy

Eric M. Haas,[1,2] Rodrigo Pedraza,[1,2] Madhu Ragupathi,[1,2] Ali Mahmood,[1,2] and T. Bartley Pickron[1,2]

[1] *Division of Minimally Invasive Colon and Rectal Surgery, Department of Surgery, The University of Texas Medical School at Houston, Houston, TX 77030, USA*
[2] *Colorectal Surgical Associates, LLP, Ltd., Houston, TX, USA*

Correspondence should be addressed to Eric M. Haas; ehaasmd@houstoncolon.com

Academic Editor: Peng Hui Wang

Purpose. We present our experience with laparoscopic colorrhaphy as definitive surgical modality for the management of colonoscopic perforations. *Methods.* Over a 17-month period, we assessed the outcomes of consecutive patients presenting with acute colonoscopic perforations. Patient characteristics and perioperative parameters were tabulated. Postoperative outcomes were evaluated within 30 days following discharge. *Results.* Five female patients with a mean age of 71.4 ± 9.7 years (range: 58–83), mean BMI of 26.4 ± 3.4 kg/m^2 (range: 21.3–30.9), and median ASA score of 2 (range: 2-3) presented with acute colonoscopic perforations. All perforations were successfully managed through laparoscopic colorrhaphy within 24 hours of development. The perforations were secondary to direct trauma ($n = 3$) or thermal injury ($n = 2$) and were localized to the sigmoid ($n = 4$) or cecum ($n = 1$). None of the patients required surgical resection, diversion, or conversion to an open procedure. No intra- or postoperative complications were encountered. The mean length of hospital stay was 3.8 ± 0.8 days (range: 3–5). There were no readmissions or reoperations. *Conclusion.* Acute colonoscopic perforations can be safely managed via laparoscopic primary repair without requiring resection or diversion. Early recognition and intervention are essential for successful outcomes.

1. Introduction

Iatrogenic perforation represents an uncommon yet potentially life-threatening complication during colonoscopy [1, 2]. Traditionally, patients have required open surgery with either primary repair of the perforation or bowel resection with or without ostomy creation [1, 3, 4]. Although these procedures are an effective approach, they often require large open incisions and may be associated with high complication rates, such as wound infection and hernias [1, 4]. In addition, the open approach usually results in slower recovery with longer hospital stay [5–7].

Minimally invasive colorectal surgery represents an efficacious alternative to the open approach, utilizing smaller incisions and resulting in diminished postoperative pain, earlier recovery, and lower postoperative morbidity [5–9]. Laparoscopic intervention has more recently been reported for the definitive treatment of acute colonoscopic perforations. This approach has shown to be a viable option, resulting in enhanced recovery in comparison to open primary colorrhaphy [5–7]. We began utilizing minimally invasive surgical (MIS) technique for repair of colonoscopic perforations in an effort to provide a safe and efficacious alternative to an open procedure. Our aim was to assess and report our initial experience with laparoscopic primary repair of acute colonic perforations during colonoscopy.

2. Patients and Methods

Between October 2008 and March 2010, consecutive patients presenting with acute iatrogenic colonic perforation during colonoscopy were evaluated. Laparoscopic surgical repair of the perforations was performed by one of three board-certified colorectal surgeons (A. Mahmood, T. B. Pickron, and E. M. Hass) with extensive experience in minimally invasive procedures. Preoperative data including age, gender, body mass index (BMI), American Society of Anesthesiologists (ASA) score, indication for colonoscopy, and time interval between perforation and surgery were assessed. Intraoperative parameters including estimated blood loss (EBL), conversion to open surgery, and complications were collected. With respect to postoperative data, return of bowel function, resumption of oral intake, complications, length of stay (LOS), secondary interventions, and readmissions within 30 days after discharge were evaluated.

2.1. Operative Technique. Initial entry into the peritoneal cavity was achieved under direct visualization using an Optiview trocar (Ethicon Endo-Surgery Inc., Cincinnati, OH, USA). An additional two or three 5 mm trocars were utilized with placement dependent on the suspected location of the perforation. Laparoscopic exploration was performed and followed by identification and isolation of the site of the colonic perforation. Any bowel spillage was aspirated, and the area was irrigated. The necrotic edges of the perforation were debrided, and colorrhaphy was performed with interrupted 3-0 Vicryl (Ethicon Inc., Somerville, NJ, USA) suture in a single layer technique. An air insufflation test was performed in all cases to confirm the integrity of the repair.

3. Results

Five female patients presented with acute iatrogenic colonic perforation, which occurred during screening colonoscopy. The mean age, mean BMI, and median ASA of the patients were 71.4 ± 9.7 years (range: 58–83 years), 26.4 ± 3.4 kg/m^2 (range: 21.3–30.9 kg/m^2), and 2 (range: 2-3), respectively (Table 1). Three perforations were secondary to mechanical trauma and recognized during the colonoscopy, while two perforations occurred due to thermal injury and were identified within 24 hours of the colonoscopy. The perforations were located in the sigmoid ($n = 4$) and cecum ($n = 1$). While in 3 cases the time interval between perforation and surgery was 3-4 hours, in 2 cases surgery was performed following 18 and 20 hours of perforation.

All procedures were successfully performed using pure laparoscopic technique. There was no significant blood loss (range: 0–50 mL) or intraoperative complications during the procedures, and none required conversion to open surgery. Surgical resection and diversion were not required for any of the perforations. Mean resumption of oral intake and return of bowel function, as evidenced by passage of flatus, were 1.4 ± 0.5 and 1.6 ± 0.9 days, respectively (range: 1-2 days). The average length of hospital stay (LOS) was 3.8 ± 0.8 days (range: 3–5 days). There were no postoperative complications, and none of the patients required readmission or secondary operative intervention (Table 2).

4. Discussion

Although complications during colonoscopy are uncommon, colonic perforation represents a potentially life-threatening event that may result in peritonitis, sepsis, and multiorgan failure, thus demanding prompt diagnosis and intervention [1]. While colonic perforations have traditionally been managed through emergent laparotomy with segmental resection and possible diversion, MIS techniques, including laparoscopic segmental resection or primary suture repair and endoscopic suturing or clipping, have more recently been implemented [1, 3–7, 10–12]. The utilization of laparoscopic modalities has demonstrated to result in diminished surgical trauma, lower conversion rates, reduced complication rates, and quicker recovery with shorter length of hospital stay compared with open surgery [5–7].

Four main mechanisms have been hypothesized in the pathogenesis of colonoscopic perforation: direct penetration of the bowel wall, barotrauma, thermal abrasion, and traction injury [3, 13, 14]. The selection of an appropriate approach for the management of a colonoscopic perforation must be individualized on a case-by-case basis. A history of previous colonic pathology requiring partial colectomy, such as recurrent diverticulitis or neoplastic disease, may preclude consideration of primary repair. Lack of optimal bowel preparation prior to colonoscopy or a prolonged interval between perforation and intervention may increase the risk of fecal contamination of the peritoneal cavity. In such cases, resection with diversion may be considered [6, 13]. However, preservation of a minimally invasive platform may be accomplished through laparoscopic segmental resection [6]. Furthermore, some colonoscopic perforations may be managed with endoscopic clipping or with conservative measures [11, 15–17]. When identified during the index colonoscopy, endoscopic clipping may be successfully accomplished, avoiding any further intervention and its potential complications [11, 17]. Delayed colonoscopic perforations are typically due to thermal injury, which are in most cases small perforations. These minor perforations represent the main indication for conservative treatment, which consists of intravenous hydration, antibiotics, and bowel rest [16].

Laparoscopic surgery represents an efficient technique for primary colonic repair. During this MIS technique, laparoscopic exploration is performed to visualize the perforation and assess the bowel content spillage into the peritoneal cavity. It is important to examine the entire large bowel in order to identify and repair secondary perforations. Occasionally, the proper identification of the perforation is not readily achieved; in such cases, colonoscopic assistance may be required. In this scenario, colonoscopic insufflation with CO_2 is preferred over air insufflation, as the former is avidly absorbed through the colonic mucosa, avoiding substantial increment in the intraluminal pressure. Minimization of spillage is achieved by clamping the proximal bowel and using steep Trendelenburg for right colon perforations or reverse-Trendelenburg for left colon perforations. Once the colonic wall injury is identified, the edges of the perforation must be debrided if necrotic. This maneuver is challenging when performed laparoscopically, as the surrounding mesentery may be damaged resulting in considerable bleeding. Most colonic perforations occur in the antimesenteric bowel border; however, when the mesenteric

TABLE 1: Preoperative and intraoperative parameters.

Patient	Gender	Age (years)	BMI (kg/m^2)	ASA	Perforation site	Mechanism of perforation	Time between perforation and surgery (hours)	Conversion to open procedure	Intraoperative complications
1	F	67	26.3	2	Sigmoid	Direct trauma	4	No	No
2	F	83	21.3	3	Sigmoid	Direct trauma	3	No	No
3	F	58	30.9	2	Sigmoid	Thermal injury¶	18	No	No
4	F	78	26.1	3	Sigmoid	Direct trauma	3	No	No
5	F	71	27.5	2	Cecum	Thermal injury¥	20	No	No
Overall$	Female 100%	71.4 ± 9.7	26.4 ± 3.4	2	Sigmoid: 80%; Cecum: 20%	Direct trauma: 60%; Thermal injury: 40%	9.6 ± 9.3	0%	0%

ASA: American College of Anesthesiologists Score; BMI: Body Mass Index.
$Mean ± standard deviation, except ASA, which is represented as median.
¶Thermal injury following anterior rectosigmoid polypectomy.
¥Thermal injury following ablation of two incidentally found large cecal angiodysplasias.

TABLE 2: Postoperative outcomes.

Patient	Return of oral intake (days)	Bowel function recovery (days)	Length of Hospital stay (days)	Complications	Reoperation	Readmission
1	2	1	5	No	No	No
2	1	2	4	No	No	No
3	2	1	4	No	No	No
4	1	1	3	No	No	No
5	1	1	3	No	No	No
Overall$	1.4 ± 0.5	1.6 ± 0.9	3.8 ± 0.8	0%	0%	0%

$Mean ± standard deviation.

bowel border is involved in the perforation, it must be sutured initially to avoid a residual unrepaired wall defect in the mesenteric commissure of the perforation. The colorrhaphy itself consists of interrupted stitches with absorbable suture, usually in one layer to avoid narrowing of the lumen, especially in the sigmoid, and to minimize stretching of the serosal layer (Figure 1). Prior to the completion of the procedure, an air insufflation test is recommended to evaluate the integrity of the repair.

In our series, the majority of perforations ($n = 3$) were secondary to direct penetrating trauma from the tip or shaft of the endoscope. They were recognized during the colonoscopy, and the patients were taken to the operating room within 4 hours of occurrence. Laparoscopic exploration revealed absence of significant spillage or peritonitis and presence of viable tissue at the edges of the perforation. Primary colorrhaphy was successfully completed for management in all three cases. Two patients developed delayed perforation due to thermal injury. In the first case (patient 3), the perforation was secondary to polypectomy with argon-plasma coagulation, whereas in the second case (patient 5), the perforation occurred following ablation of 2 large cecal angiodysplasias. Both patients presented to the emergency department within 20 hours of their respective colonoscopies with mild generalized abdominal pain and absence of peritoneal signs on physical exam. Free air was noted on abdominal radiologic studies (Figure 2). Laparoscopic exploration revealed perforation with necrotic edges in both cases. Following debridement, laparoscopic primary colorrhaphy was successfully performed.

Our postoperative outcomes compared favorably with those reported in the published literature. We encountered a mean length of hospitalization of 3.8 days, and there were no postoperative complications. In 2007, Hansen et al. [10] evaluated their experience with laparoscopic primary repair in 7 cases of colonic perforation. The overall mean LOS was 7.6 days, and they encountered two (28.6%) postoperative complications. One patient developed new onset atrial fibrillation, which resolved spontaneously. The remaining complication consisted of an intraabdominal abscess secondary to leakage at the site of the colorrhaphy, requiring sigmoid resection and end colostomy creation. In 2008, Rumstadt et al. [5] reported a case series that evaluated 13 cases of primary colon repair for free colonic perforations following colonoscopy. Laparoscopic approach was initially attempted in 10 patients; however, 2 cases required conversion to open technique due to severe peritonitis. The average LOS for the laparoscopic group was 7.1 days. This rather prolonged LOS was in part due to the discouragement of early discharge in the institutions in which the procedures were performed. Despite this, the authors reported significantly shorter LOS for the laparoscopic approach in comparison to the open

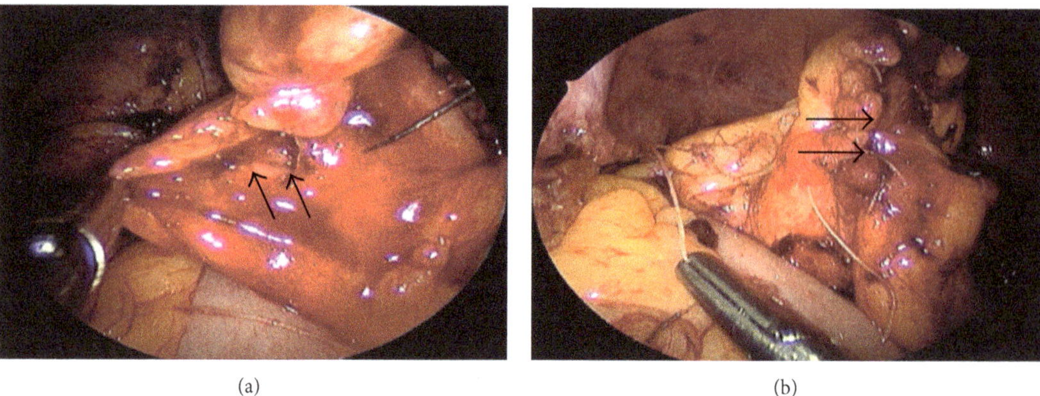

(a) (b)

Figure 1: (a) Intraoperative image showing the colonic perforation (arrows) during laparoscopic exploration. (b) Intraoperative image showing the successful laparoscopic primary repair of the colonic perforation (arrows).

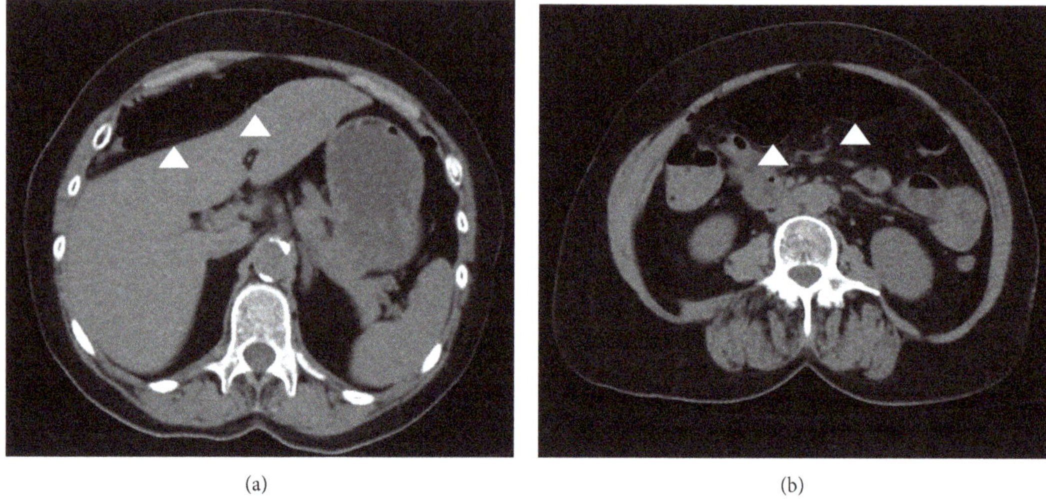

(a) (b)

Figure 2: Abdominal CT scan images of a patient with colonoscopic perforation. The images show intraabdominal free air (arrowheads).

technique (7.1 versus 14.3 days, $P = 0.019$). In the same year, Bleier et al. [6] published a study comparing outcomes following open and laparoscopic primary repair for the management of iatrogenic colonic perforations. Patient demographics were similar between both groups. The LOS was significantly shorter for the laparoscopic group (5 versus 9 days, $P = 0.01$). Furthermore, the complication rate was lower in the laparoscopic group (2/12 versus 5/7, resp., $P = 0.01$). In this comparative study, the authors concluded that the laparoscopic primary repair, when performed by experienced laparoscopic surgeons, is advantageous over the open technique.

The present study evaluated the outcomes of our initial experience utilizing laparoscopic primary repair for the treatment of acute iatrogenic colonic perforations during colonoscopy. We found this minimally invasive approach to be safe and feasible for such cases. Accordingly, we currently consider this modality as an initial approach for the management of such perforations. If favorable conditions exist (e.g., minimal spillage, absence of sepsis), we could primarily repair. Otherwise, laparoscopic resection with ostomy creation should be entertained. None of our cases required conversion to open surgery; however, if the minimally invasive platform proves unsuccessful, a conversion to laparotomy can be readily performed.

5. Conclusion

Laparoscopic primary colorrhaphy is a safe and feasible approach for the management of acute colonoscopic perforations. Conventional laparoscopic suture repair facilitates a minimally invasive procedure with minimal surgical trauma, rapid postoperative recovery, and low complication rate. Early comparative studies have demonstrated comparable efficacy with open techniques for repair of perforations. Consequently, laparoscopic primary colon repair may increasingly play an important role as a therapeutic option in the future management of various perforations. Additional prospective comparative studies will be necessary to further elicit the benefits and limitations of this approach.

References

[1] C. W. Iqbal, Y. S. Chun, and D. R. Farley, "Colonoscopic perforations: a retrospective review," *Journal of Gastrointestinal Surgery*, vol. 9, no. 9, pp. 1229–1236, 2005.

[2] G. Arora, A. Mannalithara, G. Singh, L. B. Gerson, and G. Triadafilopoulos, "Risk of perforation from a colonoscopy in adults: a large population-based study," *Gastrointestinal Endoscopy*, vol. 69, no. 3, pp. 654-664, 2009.

[3] D. V. Avgerinos, O. H. Llaguna, A. Y. Lo, and I. M. Leitman, "Evolving management of colonoscopic perforations," *Journal of Gastrointestinal Surgery*, vol. 12, no. 10, pp. 1783–1789, 2008.

[4] A. Y. B. Teoh, C. M. Poon, J. F. Y. Lee et al., "Outcomes and predictors of mortality and stoma formation in surgical management of colonoscopic perforations: a multicenter review," *Archives of Surgery*, vol. 144, no. 1, pp. 9–13, 2009.

[5] B. Rumstadt, D. Schilling, and J. Sturm, "The role of laparoscopy in the treatment of complications after colonoscopy," *Surgical Laparoscopy, Endoscopy and Percutaneous Techniques*, vol. 18, no. 6, pp. 561–564, 2008.

[6] J. I. Bleier, V. Moon, D. Feingold et al., "Initial repair of iatrogenic colon perforation using laparoscopic methods," *Surgical Endoscopy and Other Interventional Techniques*, vol. 22, no. 3, pp. 646–649, 2008.

[7] C. Coimbra, L. Bouffioux, L. Kohnen et al., "Laparoscopic repair of colonoscopic perforation: a new standard?" *Surgical Endoscopy*, vol. 25, pp. 1514–1517, 2011.

[8] M. R. S. Siddiqui, M. S. Sajid, K. Khatri, E. Cheek, and M. K. Baig, "Elective open versus laparoscopic sigmoid colectomy for diverticular disease: a meta-analysis with the sigma trial," *World Journal of Surgery*, vol. 34, no. 12, pp. 2883-2901, 2010.

[9] Clinical Outcomes of Surgical Therapy Study G, "A comparison of laparoscopically assisted and open colectomy for colon cancer," *The New England Journal of Medicine*, vol. 350, pp. 2050–2059, 2004.

[10] A. J. Hansen, D. J. Tessier, M. L. Anderson, and R. T. Schlinkert, "Laparoscopic repair of colonoscopic perforations: indications and guidelines," *Journal of Gastrointestinal Surgery*, vol. 11, no. 5, pp. 655–659, 2007.

[11] R. Magdeburg, P. Collet, S. Post, and G. Kaehler, "Endoclipping of iatrogenic colonic perforation to avoid surgery," *Surgical Endoscopy and Other Interventional Techniques*, vol. 22, no. 6, pp. 1500–1504, 2008.

[12] A. Trecca, F. Gaj, and G. Gagliardi, "Our experience with endoscopic repair of large colonoscopic perforations and review of the literature," *Techniques in Coloproctology*, vol. 12, no. 4, pp. 315–322, 2008.

[13] L. Miranda, A. Settembre, D. Piccolboni, P. Capasso, and F. Corcione, "Iatrogenic colonic perforation: repair using laparoscopic technique," *Surgical Laparoscopy Endoscopy & Percutaneous Techniques*, vol. 21, pp. 170–174, 2011.

[14] L. J. Damore II, P. C. Rantis, A. M. Vernava III, and W. E. Longo, "Colonoscopic perforations: etiology, diagnosis, and management," *Diseases of the Colon and Rectum*, vol. 39, no. 11, pp. 1308–1314, 1996.

[15] W. Heldwein, M. Dollhopf, T. Rösch et al., "The Munich Polypectomy Study (MUPS): prospective analysis of complications and risk factors in 4000 colonic snare polypectomies," *Endoscopy*, vol. 37, no. 11, pp. 1116–1122, 2005.

[16] T. Sagawa, S. Kakizaki, H. Iizuka et al., "Analysis of colonoscopic perforations at a local clinic and a tertiary hospital," *World Journal of Gastroenterology*, vol. 18, pp. 4898–4904, 2012.

[17] D. Y. Won, I. K. Lee, Y. S. Lee et al., "The indications for nonsurgical management in patients with colorectal perforation after colonoscopy," *The American Journal of Surgery*, vol. 78, pp. 550–554, 2012.

13

Laparoscopic versus Open Surgery for Colorectal Cancer: A Retrospective Analysis of 163 Patients in a Single Institution

Abdulkadir Bedirli, Bulent Salman, and Osman Yuksel

Department of General Surgery, Gazi University Medical Faculty, Besevler, 06510 Ankara, Turkey

Correspondence should be addressed to Abdulkadir Bedirli; bedirlia@gazi.edu.tr

Academic Editor: Chin-Jung Wang

Background. The present study aimed to compare the clinical outcomes of laparoscopic versus open surgery for colorectal cancers. *Materials and Methods.* The medical records from a total of 163 patients who underwent surgery for colorectal cancers were retrospectively analyzed. Patient's demographic data, operative details and postoperative early outcomes, outpatient follow-up, pathologic results, and stages of the cancer were reviewed from the database. *Results.* The patients who underwent laparoscopic surgery showed significant advantages due to the minimally invasive nature of the surgery compared with those who underwent open surgery, namely, less blood loss, faster postoperative recovery, and shorter postoperative hospital stay ($P < 0.05$). However, laparoscopic surgery for colorectal cancer resulted in a longer operative time compared with open surgery ($P < 0.05$). There were no statistically significant differences between groups for medical complications ($P > 0.05$). Open surgery resulted in more incisional infections and postoperative ileus compared with laparoscopic surgery ($P < 0.05$). There were no differences in the pathologic parameters between two groups ($P < 0.05$). *Conclusions.* These findings indicated that laparoscopic surgery for colorectal cancer had the clear advantages of a minimally invasive surgery and relative disadvantage with longer surgery time and exhibited similar pathologic parameters compared with open surgery.

1. Introduction

Colorectal cancer remains the third most common cancer diagnosed and the third most common cause of cancer death in both sexes in industrialized nations [1]. Although many studies have suggested that laparoscopic surgery is superior to open surgery, the acceptance of this technique for colorectal cancer has been rather slow in clinical practice [2, 3]. One of the reasons for the low penetration of this procedure is laparoscopic colon resections which are technically demanding procedures and as such were initially prohibitive for the majority of surgeons [4]. To successfully complete each component of the operation (mobilization of colon, dissection and division of major vessels, removing the specimen, and anastomosis), the surgeon must possess advanced laparoscopic skills, including the ability to operate and recognize anatomy from multiple viewpoints [5].

Concerning the oncologic safety of the laparoscopic approach to colorectal cancers, multiple randomized controlled studies demonstrated that oncological outcomes of laparoscopic surgery were similar to open surgery [6, 7]. The benefits of laparoscopic colorectal surgery are seen in terms of reduced blood loss, less postoperative pain, better pulmonary function, faster return of bowel function, fewer complications, and shorter hospital stay [3, 8]. However, despite the theoretical short-term advantages and equivalent cancer outcomes, adoption rates of laparoscopic colorectal surgery remain low in Europe and USA. The aim of this retrospective review is to assess the feasibility and oncologic adequacy of laparoscopic surgery comparing the operative characteristics and short-term oncological outcomes for laparoscopic surgery with conventional open surgery in patients with colorectal cancer over a period of 3 years in our center.

2. Materials and Methods

Between January 2011 and January 2014, we retrospectively analyzed a database containing information about who underwent laparoscopic or open surgery for stage I–III colorectal cancer at Gazi University Hospital, Ankara. Patient's demographic data, operative details and postoperative early outcomes, outpatient follow-up, pathologic results, and stages of the cancer were reviewed from the database. All patients had histologically verified carcinoma of the colon or rectum. The definitive staging in all patients was established via pathological examination of the resected specimens. Operative time was calculated as the time between laparotomy and skin suture for open surgery and pneumoperitoneum induction and port-site closure for laparoscopic surgery.

For this study, we analyzed 65 patients who underwent laparoscopic colorectal surgery (LCRS group) and their results with those of matched 98 patients from our colorectal resection database who had undergone conventional open colorectal surgery (OCRS group) during the same period. Patients with synchronous tumors, tumors located in the transverse colon, stage 0 and IV tumors, and previous malignant tumor and those requiring total colectomy, abdominoperineal resections, or urgent surgery were excluded. All patients and their families were correctly informed and gave their full consent before surgery.

2.1. Operation Technique. All operations were performed by the same surgical team that had wide experience with open and laparoscopic colorectal surgery. All patients had bowel preparation with polyethylene glycol, low molecular weight heparin, and intravenous gentamicin plus metronidazole. For laparoscopic resections, pneumoperitoneum with an intra-abdominal pressure between 12 and 14 mmHg was maintained throughout the operation. The first step of the laparoscopic operation is dissection of the colon from medial to lateral and vessel ligation. In right colon operations, specimen is taken out from the incision and the anastomosis is performed extracorporeally with linear stapler. In the left colon and rectum operations, distal resection is performed laparoscopically and proximal end is taken out from the suprapubic incision. After placing the anvil outside, anastomosis is performed intracorporeally. In all patients, a port wound was extended to deliver the specimen under the protection of a plastic ring. A no-touch technique was also used in the open group. Anterior or low anterior resection is performed in rectum tumors according to the localization. Temporary ileostomy is mostly performed in low anterior resection cases. Patients in both groups underwent routine operation according to the complete mesocolic or mesorectal excision principles.

A low-vacuum drainage system was left at the resection site at the end of all operations. Postoperative ileus was defined when insertion of a nasogastric tube was needed and/or there were nausea and vomiting that delayed oral intake for more than 2 days. Patients were discharged when a soft diet was tolerated and they were ambulatory.

2.2. Outcome Measures and Statistical Analyses. Clinicopathological characteristics, postoperative outcomes, hospital stay, postoperative morbidity and mortality, and short-term oncological outcomes, including the number of lymph nodes retrieved, the distal margin, radial margin, and pathological staging, were compared. The mean values were compared using paired and unpaired Student's t-test. The frequency and distribution were compared using chi-squared test. Statistical significance was assumed when the P value was <0.05. These analyses were performed using SPSS 10.0 software (SPSS, Chicago, IL, USA).

3. Results

Ninety-eight patients in the OCRS group were compared with 65 patients in the LCRS group. The patient demographic and pathologic characteristics are described in Table 1. Baseline characteristics, including age, sex, surgical risks as assessed by the American Society of Anesthesiologists (ASA), tumor location, and surgical procedures, were similar between the two groups. Protective ileostomy was performed in 23 patients (23%) in OCRS group and 19 patients (29%) in LCRS group. The proportion of patients submitted to neoadjuvant chemoradiotherapy was also similar between the two groups.

The operation time was significantly longer in LCRS group (216 ± 53 min) when compared with OCRS group (172 ± 48 min) ($P < 0.05$). Total amount of blood loss was significantly higher in OCRS group (220 ± 45 mL) when compared with LCRS group (140 ± 35 mL) ($P < 0.05$). There is no conversion to open surgery in LCRS group. Patients in the LCRS group showed a significantly faster postoperative recovery, including faster first flatus time, onset time of the liquid, and normal diet ($P < 0.05$). Despite the similar stay in intensive care unit, total hospital stay was significantly longer for OCRS group than LCRS group (Table 2).

Postoperative details are given in Table 3. No intraoperative complications were reported in both groups. One postoperative death was observed in OCRS group due to a severe pneumosepsis. No significant difference was seen between groups for medical complications ($P > 0.05$). One patient in LCRS group and 9 patients in OCRS group have incisional infections ($P < 0.05$). As for major complications, anastomotic leaks were observed in two patients in LCRS group (one right hemicolectomy and one low anterior resection) and three patients in OCRS (one right hemicolectomy and two low anterior resections) ($P > 0.05$). Two patients in LCRS group and 5 patients in OCRS group suffered postoperative ileus ($P < 0.05$).

All the resections in both groups were performed to remove a malignancy. Most frequent histologic types were moderately differentiated adenocarcinoma in both groups. The mean number of lymph nodes harvested was comparable between LCRS and OCRS groups, 19 ± 7 versus 23 ± 8, respectively. The ratio of patients with stage III tumors was relatively higher in the OCRS group. However, none of these pathologic parameters showed statistical differences between two groups ($P > 0.05$) (Table 4).

Table 1: Patient and tumor characteristics.

	LCRS group ($n = 65$)	OCRS group ($n = 98$)	P^*
Age (y), mean ± SD	57.7 ± 9.2	62.3 ± 11.1	NS
Gender (male/female)	38/27	56/42	NS
ASA (%)			NS
I	16 (25)	22 (22)	
II	29 (44)	45 (46)	
III	20 (31)	31 (32)	
Tumor distribution (%)			NS
Right colon	17 (26)	31 (32)	
Left colon	6 (9)	7 (7)	
Sigmoid colon	13 (20)	24 (24)	
Rectum	29 (45)	36 (37)	
Operation (%)			NS
Right hemicolectomy	17 (26)	31 (32)	
Left hemicolectomy	6 (9)	7 (7)	
Sigmoid resection	11 (17)	10 (10)	
Anterior resection	9 (14)	21 (21)	
Low anterior resection	22 (34)	29 (30)	
Protective ileostomy: yes (%)	19 (29)	23 (23)	NS
Neoadjuvant chemoradiotherapy: yes (%)	17 (26)	22 (22)	NS

NS: not significant. ASA: American Society of Anesthesiologist.
*Chi-square test.

Table 2: Operative and postoperative results of the two patient groups.

	LCRS group ($n = 65$)	OCRS group ($n = 98$)	P
Operation time (min), mean ± SD	216 ± 53	172 ± 48	0.039†
Operative blood loss (mL), mean ± SD	140 ± 35	220 ± 45	0.040†
Time to flatus (d), mean ± SD	1.6 ± 1.4	2.3 ± 1.7	0.014†
Time to liquid diet (d), mean ± SD	2.3 ± 1.9	2.9 ± 2.3	0.032†
Time to normal diet (d), mean ± SD	3.4 ± 2.2	4.2 ± 2.8	0.030†
Stay in ICU (d), mean ± SD	2.3 ± 2.7	2.4 ± 4.4	NS
Total hospital stay (d), mean ± SD	4.5 ± 4.0	6.2 ± 5.3	0.028†

NS: not significant. ICU: intensive care unit.
†Student's t-test.

4. Discussion

This study compares the short-term surgical outcomes of 163 consecutive patients undergoing open or laparoscopic surgery for colorectal cancer. Compared with open surgery, laparoscopic surgery at our institution was associated with slightly longer operative time, significantly faster postoperative recovery, lower incisional infections and postoperative ileus, and similar pathologic results.

Laparoscopic colorectal surgery in particular has raised the last decade after multiple, large, randomized, controlled trials in colorectal cancer have displayed that this approach is safe and with equal oncological results as open surgery [6, 9, 10]. Despite similar cancer outcomes and postoperative advantages in laparoscopic surgery, most colorectal cancers are treated by open surgery. The main barrier to widespread adoption has been the technical difficulty of these operations [4]. Laparoscopic colorectal surgery demands not only the experiences in open surgery of colon and rectum but also skills in advanced laparoscopic techniques. At the beginning, operation time is the one of the much discussed subjects in laparoscopic surgery. When 4125 cases which were collected from the related randomised clinical studies were evaluated, it was seen that the operation time in laparoscopic surgery is significantly longer than open surgery [11]. When we look at the progress of the laparoscopic surgery teams, it is clearly seen that the operation time is significantly decreased with the experience [12]. In our study, the mean

TABLE 3: Postoperative morbidity and mortality.

	LCRS group (n = 65)	OCRS group (n = 98)	P
Incision infection	1 (2)	9 (9)	0.021[†]
Anastomotic leakage	2 (3)	3 (3)	NS
Postoperative ileus	2 (3)	5 (5)	0.021[†]
Major medical complication (%)			NS
Pneumonia	3 (5)	3 (3)	
Cardiac decompensation	1 (2)	—	
Myocardial infarction	1 (2)	1 (1)	
Renal failure	—	1 (1)	
Cerebrovascular accident	—	1 (1)	
Death in hospital	—	1 (1)	NS

NS: not significant.
[†]Student's t-test.

TABLE 4: Comparison of the pathological parameters in two groups.

	LCRS group (n = 65)	OCRS group (n = 98)	P
Number of lymph nodes, mean ± SD	19 ± 7	23 ± 8	NS
Histology (%)			NS
Well-differentiated adenocarcinoma	16 (25)	20 (20)	
Moderately differentiated adenocarcinoma	29 (45)	41 (42)	
Poorly differentiated adenocarcinoma	17 (26)	31 (32)	
Others	3 (4)	6 (6)	
Tumor stage (TNM) (%)			NS
I	7 (11)	7 (7)	
II-A	14 (21)	17 (17)	
II-B	17 (26)	27 (28)	
III-A	9 (14)	19 (20)	
III-B	11 (17)	16 (16)	
III-C	7 (11)	12 (12)	

NS: not significant.

time difference between laparoscopy and open surgery was around 40 minutes. In previous studies, it was found that intraoperatively the amount of blood loss in laparoscopic surgery was significantly less than in the open surgery [2, 11]. Although measurement of intraoperative blood loss is hard to standardize, it is obvious that blood loss is minimal because of high definition and large view and fine dissection in laparoscopic surgery. Similar to the previous studies, the amount of blood loss in OCRS group was significantly higher than the LCRS group in our study.

As being a difficult operation, conversion to open surgery can be an option during laparoscopic colorectal surgery in some instances. The rate of conversion to open surgery has been reported between 10 and 15% in different series [13, 14]. Restrictive factors for the reasons to conversion to open surgery are obesity, type of surgery, ASA scores of the patients, large tumor, intra-abdominal adhesions, technical problems, organ injuries, being unable to see the operation area, being unable to free the structures, unsafe tumor resection site, and difficulties in anastomosis. There has not been any conversion to open surgery in our study. Surgical experience and careful patient selection can be accepted as the reasons for the lack of conversion to open surgery. In our study, anastomotic leak rate was low overall (3%), with two patients in the LCRS group and three patients in the OCRS group. Leak rates for open surgery were from 2.4% to 6.8% [15, 16]. In meta-analyses comparing outcomes in laparoscopic colorectal surgery by Kelly and colleagues, the overall rate of anastomotic leak rate was 2.7% [17]. It is well documented that postoperative complications are decreasing with the increased surgical experience especially anastomosis leakage, intra-abdominal infection, and mortality [4, 5].

Large number of randomized controlled trials comparing laparoscopic to open surgery for colon cancer have established better short-term results, less pain, shorter length of stay, faster return of bowel function, and equivalent oncological outcomes [2, 3]. Laparoscopic rectal surgery is still developing with promising short-term benefit, although depending on the skills and techniques of the surgeon [5]. According to the COLOR study, the increased number of the patients treated with laparoscopy at an institution closely related with the improved short-term results of the operations [8]. In our study, the benefits of laparoscopic colorectal surgery are seen in terms of reduced blood loss, faster return of bowel function, fewer surgical complications, and shorter hospital stay.

After the initial description in 1991, several reports of laparoscopic colectomy for colorectal cancer were described. Significant concerns regarding this approach surfaced when minimally invasive techniques applied to colorectal malignancy lead to increased surgical complications and worse cancer outcomes compared to conventional open approaches. Although well-defined method of laparoscopic surgery for colorectal cancer, surgery should be performed by expert surgeons in selected patients. One of the important parameters in oncological surgery is dissected lymph nodes. At least 12 lymph nodes should be resected for a sufficient lymph node dissection. The status of lymph nodes is closely related with prognosis and the adjuvant treatment protocol. For this reason, the number of resected lymph nodes is an important oncological parameter in laparoscopy also. In our study, mean 19 and 23 lymph nodes were resected from the patients in the LCRS and OCRS groups, respectively. Sufficient number of resected lymph nodes shows appropriate mesorectum and mesocolic dissection in our study. In several previous studies, the number of resected lymph nodes is found to be increased with the increased experience [18, 19]. Similarly in our study the number of resected lymph nodes significantly increased after the learning curve period. In the COST and COLOR studies, it is advised to operate the patients with small tumors (T1, T2) or easy cases like sigmoid tumors in learning curve periods and then operate big tumors (T3, T4) and difficult cases like low anterior resections when more experience has been gained [20, 21].

5. Conclusion

It has been demonstrated in the literature that laparoscopic colorectal surgery is safe and feasible, with an oncological adequacy comparable to the open approach. But apart from these published data, open surgery is still performed more frequently worldwide. So we believe that it is important to share clinics own experiences on laparoscopic colorectal surgery. Supporting the literature results of this study showed that laparoscopic colorectal surgery is convenient and less invasive and probably could be the first choice of intervention for colorectal cancers. In our series, the operating time represents a disadvantage for laparoscopic surgery; however, we think that this might be overcome with increased experience.

References

[1] R. Siegel, D. Naishadham, and A. Jemal, "Cancer statistics, 2013," *CA: A Cancer Journal for Clinicians*, vol. 63, no. 1, pp. 11–30, 2013.

[2] J. D. Rea, M. M. Cone, B. S. Diggs, K. E. Deveney, K. C. Lu, and D. O. Herzig, "Utilization of laparoscopic colectomy in the United States before and after the clinical outcomes of surgical therapy study group trial," *Annals of Surgery*, vol. 254, no. 2, pp. 281–288, 2011.

[3] G. D. McKay, M. J. Morgan, S.-K. C. Wong et al., "Improved short-term outcomes of laparoscopic versus open resection for colon and rectal cancer in an area health service: a multicenter study," *Diseases of the Colon and Rectum*, vol. 55, no. 1, pp. 42–50, 2012.

[4] L. L. Swanström and N. J. Soper, Eds., *Mastery of Endoscopic and Laparoscopic Surgery*, Lippincott Williams & Wilkins, Philadelphia, Pa, USA, 4th edition, 2014.

[5] N. T. Nguyen and C. E. H. Scott-Conner, Eds., *The SAGES Manual*, Springer, New York, NY, USA, 3rd edition, 2012.

[6] J. Fleshman, D. J. Sargent, E. Green et al., "Laparoscopic colectomy for cancer is not inferior to open surgery based on 5-year data from the COST Study Group trial," *Annals of Surgery*, vol. 246, no. 4, pp. 655–662, 2007.

[7] E. Kuhry, W. Schwenk, R. Gaupset, U. Romild, and J. Bonjer, "Long-term outcome of laparoscopic surgery for colorectal cancer: a cochrane systematic review of randomised controlled trials," *Cancer Treatment Reviews*, vol. 34, no. 6, pp. 498–504, 2008.

[8] M. H. van der Pas, E. Haglind, M. A. Cuesta et al., "Laparoscopic versus open surgery for rectal cancer (COLOR II): short-term outcomes of a randomised, phase 3 trial," *The Lancet Oncology*, vol. 14, no. 3, pp. 210–218, 2013.

[9] D. G. Jayne, P. J. Guillou, H. Thorpe et al., "Randomized trial of laparoscopic-assisted resection of colorectal carcinoma: 3-Year results of the UK MRC CLASICC trial group," *Journal of Clinical Oncology*, vol. 25, no. 21, pp. 3061–3068, 2007.

[10] M. Buunen, R. Veldkamp, W. C. Hop et al., "Survival after laparo-scopic surgery versus open surgery for colon cancer: long-term outcome of a randomised clinical trial," *The Lancet Oncology*, vol. 10, no. 1, pp. 44–52, 2009.

[11] T. Lourenco, A. Murray, A. Grant, A. McKinley, Z. Krukowski, and L. Vale, "Laparoscopic surgery for colorectal cancer: safe and effective?—A systematic review," *Surgical Endoscopy and other Interventional Techniques*, vol. 22, no. 5, pp. 1146–1160, 2008.

[12] J. C. M. Li, A. W. I. Lo, S. S. F. Hon, S. S. M. Ng, J. F. Y. Lee, and K. L. Leung, "Institution learning curve of laparoscopic colectomy-a multi-dimensional analysis," *International Journal of Colorectal Disease*, vol. 27, no. 4, pp. 527–533, 2012.

[13] C. A. Vaccaro, G. L. Rossi, G. O. Quintana, E. R. Soriano, H. Vaccarezza, and F. Rubinstein, "Laparoscopic colorectal resections: a simple predictor model and a stratification risk for conversion to open surgery," *Diseases of the Colon & Rectum*, vol. 57, no. 7, pp. 869–874, 2014.

[14] R. R. Cima, I. Hassan, V. P. Poola et al., "Failure of institutionally derived predictive models of conversion in laparoscopic colorectal surgery to predict conversion outcomes in an independent data set of 998 laparoscopic colorectal procedures," *Annals of Surgery*, vol. 251, no. 4, pp. 652–658, 2010.

[15] C. Platell, N. Barwood, G. Dorfmann, and G. Makin, "The incidence of anastomotic leaks in patients undergoing colorectal surgery," *Colorectal Disease*, vol. 9, no. 1, pp. 71–79, 2007.

[16] C. E. Reinke, S. Showalter, N. N. Mahmoud, and R. R. Kelz, "Comparison of anastomotic leak rate after colorectal surgery using different databases," *Diseases of the Colon and Rectum*, vol. 56, no. 5, pp. 638–644, 2013.

[17] M. Kelly, A. Bhangu, P. Singh, J. E. F. Fitzgerald, and P. P. Tekkis, "Systematic review and meta-analysis of trainee—*versus* expert surgeon-performed colorectal resection," *British Journal of Surgery*, vol. 101, no. 7, pp. 750–759, 2014.

[18] F. Köckerling, M. A. Reymond, C. Schneider et al., "Prospective multicenter study of the quality of oncologic resections in patients undergoing laparoscopic colorectal surgery for cancer," *Diseases of the Colon and Rectum*, vol. 41, no. 8, pp. 963–970, 1998.

[19] K. Prakash, N. Kamalesh, K. Pramil, I. Vipin, A. Sylesh, and M. Jacob, "Does case selection and outcome following laparoscopic colorectal resection change after initial learning curve? Analysis of 235 consecutive elective laparoscopic colorectal resections," *Journal of Minimal Access Surgery*, vol. 9, no. 3, pp. 99–103, 2013.

[20] The Clinical Outcomes of Surgical Therapy Study Group, "A comparison of laparoscopically assisted and open colectomy for colon cancer," *The New England Journal of Medicine*, vol. 350, no. 20, pp. 2050–2059, 2004.

[21] R. Veldkamp, M. Gholghesaei, H. J. Bonjer et al., "Laparoscopic resection of colon cancer: consensus of the European Association of Endoscopic Surgery (E.A.E.S.)," *Surgical Endoscopy and other Interventional Techniques*, vol. 18, no. 8, pp. 1163–1185, 2004.

14

Transforaminal Approach in Thoracal Disc Pathologies: Transforaminal Microdiscectomy Technique

Sedat Dalbayrak,[1] Onur Yaman,[2] Kadir Öztürk,[1] Mesut Yılmaz,[1] Mahmut Gökdağ,[1] and Murat Ayten[1]

[1] *Neurospinal Academy, Neurosurgery, 34940 Istanbul, Turkey*
[2] *Tepecik Education and Training Hospital, Clinic of Neurosurgery, 35120 Izmir, Turkey*

Correspondence should be addressed to Onur Yaman; dronuryaman@yahoo.com

Academic Editor: Peng Hui Wang

Objective. Many surgical approaches have been defined and implemented in the last few decades for thoracic disc herniations. The endoscopic foraminal approach in foraminal, lateral, and far lateral disc hernias is a contemporary minimal invasive approach. This study was performed to show that the approach is possible using the microscope without an endoscope, and even the intervention on the discs within the spinal canal is possible by having access through the foramen. *Methods.* Forty-two cases with disc hernias in the medial of the pedicle were included in this study; surgeries were performed with transforaminal approach and microsurgically. Extraforaminal disc hernias were not included in the study. Access was made through the Kambin triangle, foramen was enlarged, and spinal canal was entered. *Results.* The procedure took 65 minutes in the average, and the mean bleeding amount was about 100cc. They were mobilized within the same day postoperatively. No complications were seen. Follow-up periods range between 5 and 84 months, and the mean follow-up period is 30.2 months. *Conclusion.* Transforaminal microdiscectomy is a method that can be performed in any clinic with standard spinal surgery equipment. It does not require additional equipment or high costs.

1. Introduction

Symptomatic thoracic disc herniation is one of the rare degenerative diseases of the spine. Its share among other similar pathologies can be indicated as 0,25 to 1%. Studies conducted on the general population revealed its incidence rate as approximately 1/1000000 patient in one year [1–3]. This rate applies to both women and men, and it is usually observed at ages 30 to 50 [4]. The pathology usually localizes at the medial or mediolateral region and rarely can one see a real lateral localization of the pathology [3, 5]. The rate of incidence for calcified pathologies is 30 to 70% [6, 7].

Decision for the surgical indication is controversial, due to the limited amount of information obtained so far on the natural course of thoracic disc herniation [8, 9]. On the one hand, the necessity of surgical treatment is not a matter of debate in the presence of progressive myelopathy symptoms, but on the other, it is still not clear whether the surgery can fix the symptoms in patients presenting radicular pain.

Wood et al. followed up 20 patients, who were randomly diagnosed with thoracic disc pathology, for an average duration of 26 months and reported that the patients were still asymptomatic at the end of this follow-up period [10]. Brown et al. assessed 55 symptomatic patients with thoracic disc pathology and reported that 77% of the 40 patients (73%) who were given nonsurgical treatment had complete recovery from their symptoms [11].

Although the decision for the eligible surgical approach is still controversial, the search is ongoing to find an effective, safe, and simple surgical approach especially for thoracic disc pathologies with medial localization.

2. Material and Method

Forty-two cases with disc hernias in the medial of the pedicle and foraminal disc hernias were included in this study and surgeries were performed with transforaminal

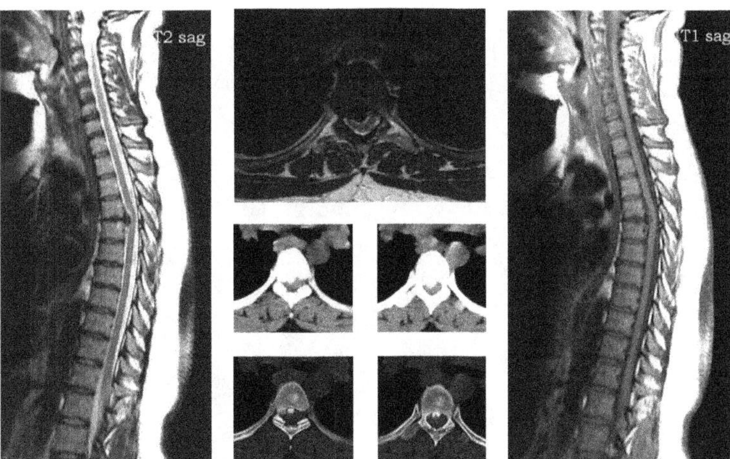

FIGURE 1: 35-year-old female. Back pain and also in both legs. Progressive weakness in lower extremities. Preoperative VAS was 5. In the neurological examination there was paraparesis in low extremities (Case 1). Preoperative views of the patient revealed a thoracic 4-5 disc herniation.

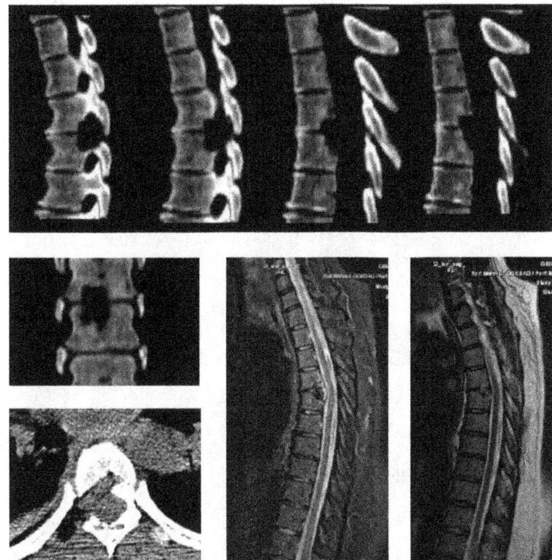

FIGURE 2: Early postoperative images of the patient after the performance of right transforaminal approach (Case 1).

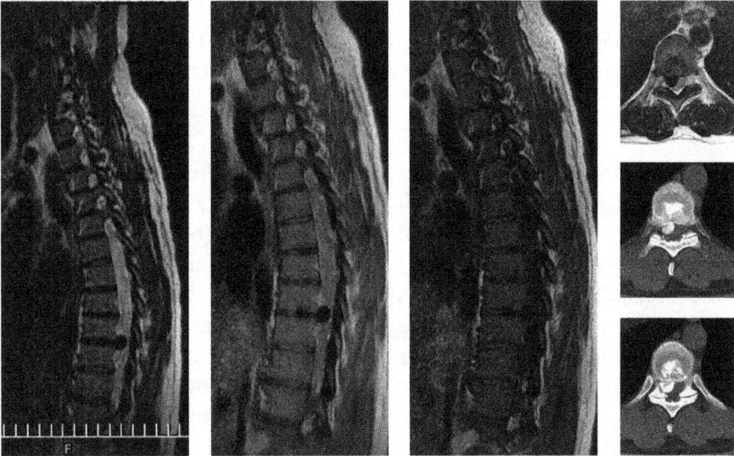

FIGURE 3: 36-year-old female. Weakness in lower extremities. Preoperative ASIA was C (Case 5). Preoperative CT and MRI revealed a thoracic 8-9 disc herniation.

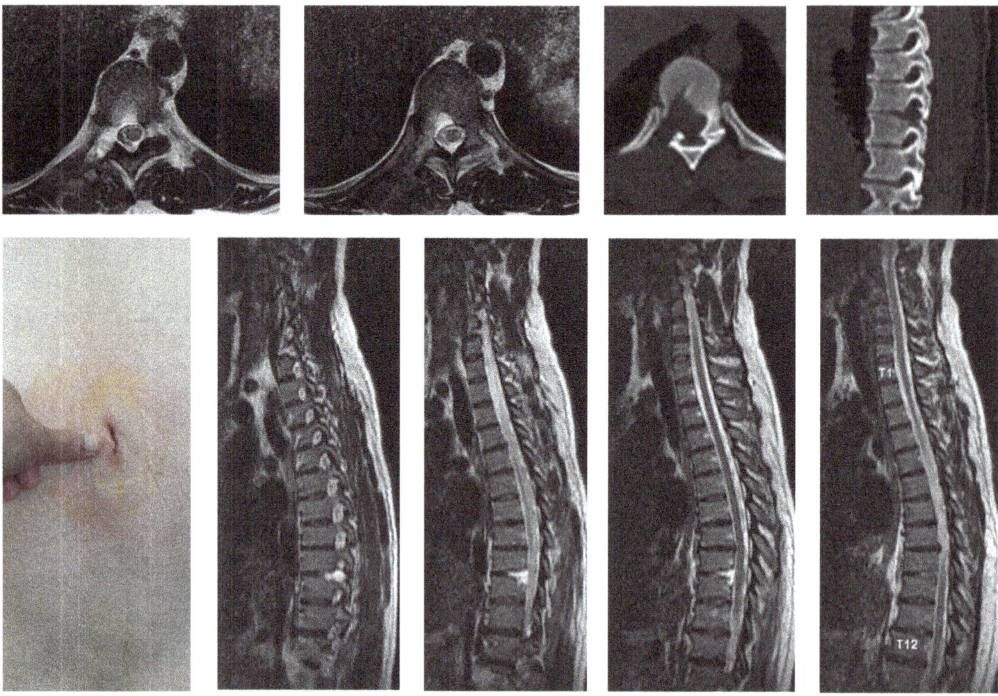

Figure 4: Postoperative CT, MRI images of Case 5. View of the incision.

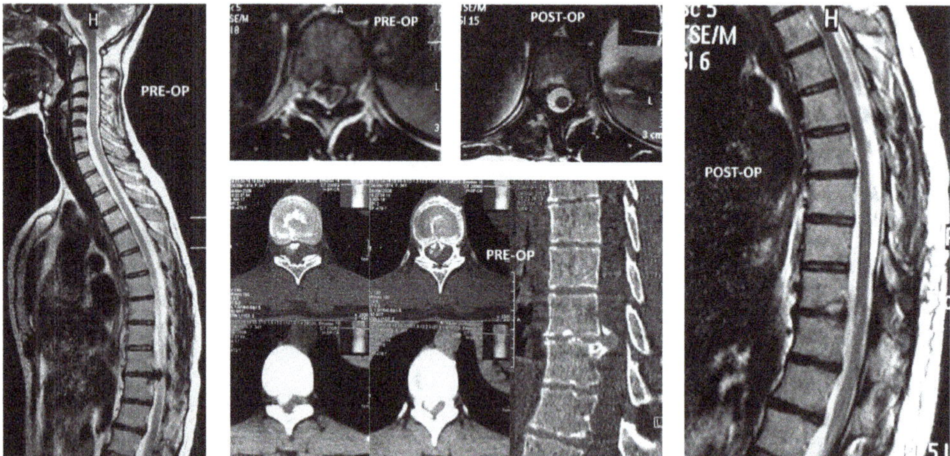

Figure 5: 34-year-old female. In the neurological examination there was paraparesis in lower extremities (ASIA C). Cord compression of a thoracic 9-10 disc herniation (Case 10). Preoperative CT and MR images at the left side and postoperative images at the right side.

approach and microsurgically. Extraforaminal disc hernias were not included in the study. Access was established with the patient in flexed prone position through an incision of 2–2.5 cm in length made 6 to 10 cm away from the midline (mean 8 cm). After opening the fascia, digital dissection was used to advance in the intermuscular space to expose the transverse process and the lateral of the superior articular process (lateral of the facet joint junction). The planned disc level was accessed after the control of the distance with scopy. Access was made through the Kambin triangle, foramen was enlarged, and spinal canal was entered (Figure 2). Transforaminal microdiscectomy (TFMD) was performed using standard instruments.

2.1. Surgical Technique. The materials we use in this procedure are those available in any center where microneurosurgery is performed: surgical microscope, radiolucent operation table, C-arm scopy, microsurgical instruments, Landolt separators used in pituitary surgery, Meyerding separators used in lumbar microdiscectomy, separators used in anterior cervical approach (Caspar, Clovard, etc.), or nasal speculum whichever is found or convenient.

We perform the procedure with patient in prone position under spinal or general anesthesia. The table can be tilted to the lateral. The level is determined using C-arm scopy and AP and lateral scopy. Later, depending on the anatomy of the area, type of the pathology, and depth of the pathology, a skin

TABLE 1: Preoperative and postoperative features of the patients.

Cases	Gender/age	Level	Preop. VAS	Preop. ODI	Preop. ASIA	Side	Time	Postop. VAS	Postop. ODI	Postop. ASIA
Case 1	F/35	T4-T5	5	82	C	Right	135	0	0	E
Case 2	M/52	T6-T7	5	66	D	Left	130	1	24	D
Case 3	F/54	T8-T9	6	86	C	Right	90	1	22	D
Case 4	M/57	T9-10	6	86	C	Right	120	1	26	D
Case 5	F/36	T9-T10	6	80	C	Right	115	0	0	E
Case 6	F/46	T9-T10	6	68	D	Right	95	1	8	E
Case 7	F/48	T10-T11	5	64	D	Right	85	1	14	E
Case 8	M/62	T10-T11	6	90	C	Left	105	2	64	C
Case 9	F/55	T10-T11	6	86	C	Right	85	1	34	D
Case 10	F/34	T10-T11	6	84	C	Right	130	2	26	D
Case 11	F/45	T11-T12	5	68	D	Left	110	1	14	E
Case 12	F/40	T11-T12	7	66	D	Right	95	1	28	D
Case 13	F/56	T11-T12	6	62	D	Left	100	1	10	E
Case 14	M/20	T11-T12	7	50	E	Right	90	0	0	E
Case 15	M/25	T12-L1	8	46	Ê	Left	90	0	0	E

incision of 2–2.5 cm in length is made at 6 to 10 cm lateral of the midline (Figure 3). After cutting the fascia, access will be with digital dissection between the paraspinal muscles and the lateral side of the facet and transverse processes and the intertransverse ligament. Following the repeat scopy control, the separator is placed and the required distance is reached. The disc is reached directly from the inferior of the foramen if the disc has no cranial or caudal extensions. Dissection is started on the transverse process-pedicle junction in the superior of the foramen. The root is exposed first, and then discectomy is performed. The pedicle of the lower vertebra prevents exploration in discs with caudal extension.

3. Findings

5 of the cases were males, while 10 were females. Ages ranged between 20 and 62 (average 44.3). There was thoracal (Th) 4-5 disc hernia in 1 case, Th (6-7) in 1 case, Th (8-9) in 1 case, Th (9-10) in 3 cases, Th (10-11) in 4 cases, Th11-12 in 4 cases, and Th (12)-Lumbar (L)1 in 1 case.

They were mobilized within the same day postoperatively and were discharged the next day. No complications were seen except for mild radicular paresthesia in 1 case that lasted for about 8 weeks. Follow-up periods ranged between 10 and 72 months, and the mean follow-up period is 34.8 months.

Preoperative pain score in cases was changing between 5 and 8 (mean 6) according to VAS (Visual Analogue Scale). Pain score was marked between 0 and 1 (mean 0.87) by the patients, according to VAS, postoperatively.

At ODI (Oswestry Disability Index) questioned form that was filled preoperatively, score was between 46% to 90% (mean 72.27%) (daily life completely restricted because of pain), and postoperatively it was 0% to 64% (mean 18%) (pain is not a serious problem in daily life).

Compared with preoperative results, postoperative VAS and ODI results have significant improvement ($P < 0.001$). Patients' pathology levels, preoperative and postoperative VAS, ODI, and neurological statues are summarized in Table 1.

41 of patients answered "Yes" when 1 patient answered "Undecided, maybe" to the question "If you knew the result before, would you have taken this treatment anyway?" at a postoperatively filled patient satisfaction form.

4. Sample Cases

See Figures 1, 2, 3, 4, and 5.

5. Discussion

Indications of thoracic disc herniation and the surgical method of selection have long been under discussion. There are no absolute factors to help one take a decision on the surgical treatment, as the clinical natural course of thoracic disc herniation is still not fully discovered. Many surgical approaches have been defined and implemented in the last few decades. The best method for thoracic disc herniation is still controversial. Except for the laminectomy method that has been abandoned lately, a comparison of the results obtained by studies on various surgical methods indicates that 60 to 80% of the patients recover from the pain or improve their neurological picture.

Posterior laminectomy and/or discectomy is the first method used in surgical treatment of thoracic disc herniation [12]. By using this method, it is difficult to decompress midline disc pathologies attached to the dura. The risk of morbidity is high, and even paraplegia may develop. Furthermore, it contains the risk of late kyphotic deformity development [13, 14]. This method has now become historic, and it is not anymore used as a surgical treatment approach for thoracic disc herniation [15].

Transpedicular approach, transfacet pedicle sparing approach, costotransversectomy, and transfacet/transforaminal approach are listed among posterolateral approaches [16–23].

Perot Jr. and Munro [14] described the transthoracic approach in 1969 and in 1988 Bohlman and Zdeblick recapitulated this approach. This technique provides access to all levels under T4. It provides direct visibility in central, paracentral, and lateral pathologies [24]. The method proves to be effective in soft and hard pathologies, and it has high efficacy in multilevel pathologies [25]. The method presents high rates of complications such as atelectasis, pleural effusion, and pneumonia, which is a disadvantage. If the surgeon has to free the diaphragm, hernia may develop. Large arteries or venous structures may be damaged, and left-side approaches bear the risk of infarct and impaired blood supply to the spinal cord due to the obstruction of Adamkiewicz artery. However, Mulier and Debois indicated that even though pulmonary complications may be observed unlike lateral and posterolateral approaches, this approach yielded better neurological improvement [26]. Otani et al. described transthoracic extrapleural approach to reduce the risk of pulmonary complications [27].

The advantages of anterior video-assisted thoracoscopic approach include minimal dissection, low morbidity, no need to retract for rib resection, short hospital stay, and short rehabilitation period. The biggest disadvantage is that the surgeon should be particularly trained to perform this approach. In their study involving 29 patients, Regan et al. reported 76% satisfactory results [25].

Transforaminal endoscopic discectomy is among the methods applicable for thoracic disc disease. It may be used not only for far lateral and foraminal discs but also in midline discs [28]. Transforaminal endoscopic discectomy (TFD) has increased success rates in eligible patients. Computed Tomography helps to discover the bone structure at the preoperative stage.

Transforaminal microdiscectomy (TFMD) saved the surgeons from the two-dimensional limitation of endoscopy and offered them a three-dimensional view. Compared to classical surgery, TFMD reduced the rate of instability and muscle denervation. Early postoperative mobilization of the patient and short hospital stay are the other advantages of this system. It offers a safer surgery by providing better microscopic view and light, which neurosurgeons are more accustomed to. Furthermore, TFMD does not require additional equipment, which is a cost-reducing factor.

6. Conclusion

Transforaminal microdiscectomy can be performed by using standard neurosurgery equipment and it does not require additional surgical equipment. TFMD can be performed without causing neurologic deficits and wide decompressions leading to instability.

References

[1] R. Bransford, F. Zhang, C. Bellabarb, M. Konodi, and J. R. Chapman, "Early experience treating thoracic disc herniations using a modified transfacet pedicle-sparing decompression and fusion: clinical article," *Journal of Neurosurgery: Spine*, vol. 12, no. 2, pp. 221–231, 2010.

[2] C. B. Stillerman, T. C. Chen, J. D. Day, W. T. Couldwell, and M. H. Weiss, "The transfacet pedicle-sparing approach for thoracic disc removal: cadaveric morphometric analysis and preliminary clinical experience," *Journal of Neurosurgery*, vol. 83, no. 6, pp. 971–976, 1995.

[3] J. S. Ross, N. Perez-Reyes, T. J. Masaryk, H. Bohlman, and M. T. Modic, "Thoracic disk herniation: MR imaging," *Radiology*, vol. 165, no. 2, pp. 511–515, 1987.

[4] C. Arseni and F. Nash, "Thoracic intervertebral disc protrusion: a clinical study," *Journal of Neurosurgery*, vol. 17, pp. 418–430, 1960.

[5] J. S. Uribe, W. D. Smith, L. Pimenta et al., "Minimally invasive lateral approach for symptomatic thoracic disc herniation: initial multicenter clinical experience—clinical article," *Journal of Neurosurgery: Spine*, vol. 16, no. 3, pp. 264–279, 2012.

[6] A. Landi, N. Marotta, C. Mancarella, D. E. Dugoni, and R. Delfini, "Management of calcified thoracic disc herniation using ultrasonic bone curette SONO-PET: technical description," *Journal of Neurosurgical Sciences*, vol. 55, no. 3, pp. 283–288, 2011.

[7] H. Sheikh, D. Samartzis, and M. J. Perez-Cruet, "Techniques for the operative management of thoracic disc herniation: minimally invasivethoracic microdiscectomy," *Orthopedic Clinics of North America*, vol. 38, no. 3, pp. 351–361, 2007.

[8] E. M. J. Cornips, M. L. F. Janssen, and E. A. M. Beuls, "Thoracic disc herniation and acute myelopathy: clinical presentation, neuroimaging findings, surgical considerations, and outcome: clinical article," *Journal of Neurosurgery: Spine*, vol. 14, no. 4, pp. 520–528, 2011.

[9] M. K. Kasliwal and H. Deutsch, "Minimally invasive retropleural approach for central thoracic disc herniation," *Minimally Invasive Neurosurgery*, vol. 54, no. 4, pp. 167–171, 2011.

[10] K. B. Wood, J. M. Blair, D. M. Aepple et al., "The natural history of asymptomatic thoracic disc herniations," *Spine*, vol. 22, no. 5, pp. 525–529, 1997.

[11] C. W. Brown, P. A. Deffer Jr., J. Akmakjian, D. H. Donaldson, and J. L. Brugman, "The natural history of thoracic disc herniation," *Spine*, vol. 17, no. 6, supplement, pp. S97–S102, 1992.

[12] V. Logue, "Thoracic intervertebral disc prolapse with spinal cord compression," *Journal of Neurology, Neurosurgery, and Psychiatry*, vol. 15, no. 4, pp. 227–241, 1952.

[13] J. G. Love and E. J. Kieffer, "Root pain and paraplegia due to protrusions of thoracic intervertebral disks," *Journal of Neurosurgery*, vol. 7, no. 1, pp. 62–69, 1950.

[14] P. L. Perot Jr. and D. D. Munro, "Transthoracic removal of midline thoracic disc protrusions causing spinal cord compression," *Journal of Neurosurgery*, vol. 31, no. 4, pp. 452–458, 1969.

[15] K. H. Abbott and R. H. Retter, "Protrusions of thoracic intervertebral disks," *Neurology*, vol. 1, pp. 1–10, 1956.

[16] R. H. Patterson Jr. and E. Arbit, "A surgical approach through the pedicle to protruded thoracic discs," *Journal of Neurosurgery*, vol. 48, no. 5, pp. 768–772, 1978.

[17] P. D. Le Roux, M. M. Haglund, and A. B. Harris, "Thoracic disc disease: experience with the transpedicular approach in twenty

consecutive patients," *Neurosurgery*, vol. 33, no. 1, pp. 58–66, 1993.

[18] C. B. Stillerman, T. C. Chen, J. D. Day, W. T. Couldwell, and M. H. Weiss, "The transfacet pedicle-sparing approach for thoracic disc removal: cadaveric morphometric analysis and preliminary clinical experience," *Journal of Neurosurgery*, vol. 83, no. 6, pp. 971–976, 1995.

[19] R. G. Fessler, D. D. Dietze Jr., M. M. Millan, and D. Peace, "Lateral parascapular extrapleural approach to the upper thoracic spine," *Journal of Neurosurgery*, vol. 75, no. 3, pp. 349–355, 1991.

[20] A. Hulme, "The surgical approach to thoracic intervertebral disc protrusions," *Journal of Neurology, Neurosurgery, and Psychiatry*, vol. 23, pp. 133–137, 1960.

[21] E. G. Singounas, E. M. Kypriades, A. J. Kellerman, and N. Garvan, "Thoracic disc herniation. Analysis of 14 cases and review of the literature," *Acta Neurochirurgica*, vol. 116, no. 1, pp. 49–52, 1992.

[22] V. Menard, "Causes de la paraplegia dans la maladie de Pott, son traitement chirurgical par l'ouverture directe du foyer tuberculeaux des vertebras," *Orthopedic Reviews*, pp. 47–64, 1894.

[23] M. MacHino, Y. Yukawa, K. Ito, H. Nakashima, and F. Kato, "A new thoracic reconstruction technique "transforaminal Thoracic Interbody Fusion": a preliminary report of clinical outcomes," *Spine*, vol. 35, no. 19, pp. E1000–E1005, 2010.

[24] H. H. Bohlman and T. A. Zdeblick, "Anterior excision of herniated thoracic discs," *Journal of Bone and Joint Surgery A*, vol. 70, no. 7, pp. 1038–1047, 1988.

[25] J. J. Regan, A. Ben-Yishay, and M. J. Mack, "Video-assisted thoracoscopic excision of herniated thoracic disc: description of technique and preliminary experience in the first 29 cases," *Journal of Spinal Disorders*, vol. 11, no. 3, pp. 183–191, 1998.

[26] S. Mulier and V. Debois, "Thoracic disc herniations: transthoracic, lateral, or posterolateral approach? A review," *Surgical Neurology*, vol. 49, no. 6, pp. 599–608, 1998.

[27] K. Otani, M. Yoshida, E. Fujii, S. Nakai, and K. Shibasaki, "Thoracic disc herniation. Surgical treatment in 23 patients," *Spine*, vol. 13, no. 11, pp. 1262–1267, 1988.

[28] P. Kambin and M. D. Brager, "Percutaneous posterolateral discectomy: anatomy and mechanism," *Clinical Orthopaedics and Related Research*, no. 223, pp. 145–154, 1987.

15

Single-Access Laparoscopic Rectal Surgery Is Technically Feasible

Siripong Sirikurnpiboon and Paiboon Jivapaisarnpong

Colorectal Division, General Surgery Department, Rajavithi Hospital, Rangsit University, Bangkok 10400, Thailand

Correspondence should be addressed to Siripong Sirikurnpiboon; laizan99@hotmail.com

Academic Editor: Peng Hui Wang

Introduction. Single-access laparoscopic surgery (SALS) has been successfully introduced for colectomy surgery; however, for mid to low rectum procedures such as total mesorectal excision, it can be technically complicated. In this study, we introduced a single-access technique for rectum cancer operations without the use of other instruments. *Aims*. To show the short-term results of single-access laparoscopic rectal surgery in terms of pathologic results and immediate complications. *Settings and Design*. Prospective study. *Materials and Methods*. We selected middle rectum to anal canal cancer patients to undergo single-access laparoscopic rectal resection for rectal cancer. All patients had total mesorectal excisions. An umbilical incision was made for the insertion of a single multichannel port, and a mesocolic window was created to identify the inferior mesenteric artery and vein. Total mesorectal excision was performed. There were no perioperative complications. The mean operative time was 269 minutes; the median hospital stay was 7 days; the mean wound size was 5.5 cm; the median number of harvested lymph nodes was 15; and all patients had intact mesorectal capsules. *Statistical Analysis Used*. Mean, minimum–maximum. *Conclusion*. Single-access laparoscopic surgery for rectal cancer is feasible while oncologic principles and patient safety are maintained.

1. Introduction

Single-access laparoscopic surgery (SALS) has been successfully introduced for colectomy [1]. But for mid to low rectum procedures, such as total mesorectal excision, it can be technically complicated. Only a few reports have been published about single-access laparoscopic low anterior resection [2–6]. The usual techniques used to maintain an adequate operative field for TME are lifting the rectum with a second forceps or suspending the rectum with transparietal sutures. In this study, however, we introduced a single-access technique for rectal surgery without the use of other instruments.

2. Materials and Methods

The study took place from December, 2011 to December, 2012 in the Tertiary Care Unit of Rajavithi Hospital. All operations were performed by a colorectal surgeon.

The inclusion criteria were (1) patients who had been diagnosed with cancer at the middle or low rectum or the anal canal and (2) patients who had rejected neoadjuvant chemotherapy.

The exclusion criteria were (1) patients who were unfit for surgery; (2) patients who did not attend for followup; (3) patients for whom anesthesia was contraindicated; and (4) patients with asymptomatic stage IV disease.

The study was approved by the Ethical Committee of Rajavithi Hospital.

3. Operative Technique

All the procedures were performed by the same colorectal surgeon. All of the patients underwent bowel preparation 1 day preoperatively either with 4 litres of polyethylene glycol electrolyte solution or 90 mL of sodium phosphate solution depending on their comorbid disease.

Surgical procedures were performed through a 5-6 cm single umbilical incision using a single-access multiport device (Glove Port-Single Port, Nelis Ltd., Gyeonggi-do, Korea) (Figure 1) that allows three additional trocars (two

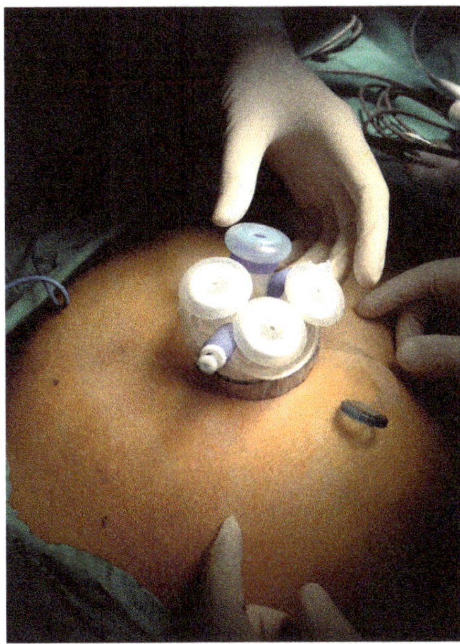

FIGURE 1: Port position.

5 mm and one 10–12 mm) to be inserted and has a CO_2 connection for insufflations (Figure 1). The camera was a flexible videolaparoscope (Olympus Medical Systems Corp., Tokyo, Japan).

The reverse Trendelenburg semiright lateral position was used. The surgeon and cameraman stood on the right side of the patient.

Operations were performed using a surgical technique similar to the standard laparoscopic (medial-to-lateral) approach. The inferior mesenteric artery and the inferior mesenteric vein were both skeletonized and clipped by Hem-o-lok (Teleflex Medical, Durham, NC, USA) or Liga clip (Johnson and Johnson, New York, NY, USA) and divided with scissors. Then, we dissected downwards in a semicircular motion from the mesenteric window to the pelvis on the right side of the rectum. For posterior dissection, the rectum was grasped and pushed anteriorly using Endo grasp forceps or a flexible Endo clinch and dissection was performed from the promontory of the sacrum in a semicircular motion deep down to the coccyx. The next step was to mobilize the sigmoid colon up to the splenic flexure. The descending colon was grasped by Endo grasp forceps or flexible Endo clinch and pulled anteromedially to clearly identify the lateral peritoneal attachment, and it was then severed by cauterization up to the splenic attachment (Figure 2). At this point downward, medial traction was applied to the colon to expose the splenic attachment and then divided with cautery. The flexible tip videolaparoscope proved helpful for changing the angle and operative view in this phase. To facilitate the process of dissecting deep into the pelvis, we used the force of gravity by moving the patient into the reverse Trendelenburg position, and we also utilised a port that allowed two Endo grasps or Endo clinches to push the rectum anteriorly. For anterior dissection, the peritoneal attachment was pulled up anteriorly, and the mobilized rectum was

TABLE 1: Demographic data.

Age (mean, years)	69 ± 11.76 (52–86)
BMI (mean, min–max)	21.77 ± 4.48 (15.00–30.00)
Sex (male/female)	6/4
ASA classification (median, min–max)	2 (1–3)
Location of tumor	
Anal canal/lower rectum	9
Middle rectum	1
Clinical stage	
Stage II	2
Stage III	8

dissected (Figure 3). In the low anterior resection, the rectum was transected using 2 endoscopic linear staplers (Endo GIA, Covidien plc, Dublin, Ireland). The position of the applied stapler is shown in Figure 4. Due to limitations in Endo stapler angulation and pelvis diameter, the proximal colon was extracted through the umbilical incision. Resection was achieved following extracorporealization, and anastomosis was performed with the double stapling technique using a transanally inserted circular stapler (CDH29, Ethicon Endo-Surgery Inc., Cincinnati, OH, USA). Diverting stoma was not usually performed. A pelvic drainage tube was inserted at a new stab incision at the right lower quadrant under laparoscopic view. In the APR cases, we started the perineal resection phase after finishing the intraperitoneal phase using the standard AP resection technique. In our hospital, cylindrical abdominoperineal resection is not routinely used.

4. Data Collection

Demographic data including patients' age, gender, and body mass index (BMI) were tabulated together with their history of prior abdominal surgery. Intraoperative parameters including operative time, estimated blood loss, and intraoperative complications were analyzed.

Pathologic characteristics such as depth invasion, lymph node retrieval, circumferential margin, distal margin, and mesorectal capsule status were reviewed, and postoperative outcomes including length of stay in hospital and complication rates were collected.

5. Results

Between December, 2011 and December, 2012, 10 patients (4 females and 6 males, mean age 69 years, range 52–86) underwent SALS for middle rectal, low rectal, and anal canal cancer. The operations comprised 9 abdominoperineal resections and 1 low anterior resection. All patients had stage II or III disease preoperatively. None received preoperative neoadjuvant therapy because they had rejected it. The average body mass index was 21.77 (range 15 to 30 kg/m^2) (Table 1). In all cases, the patients' consent for single-access laparoscopic surgery was obtained.

The median total surgical time was 269 minutes (range 200–300 min). The average intraoperative blood loss was

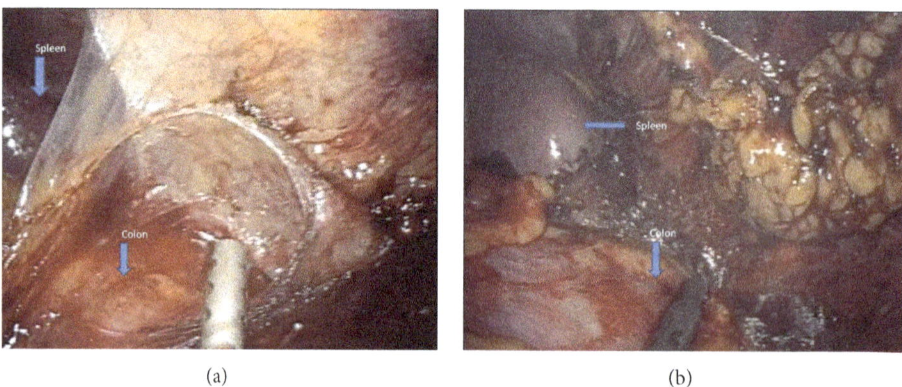

(a) (b)

FIGURE 2: Splenic flexure mobilization.

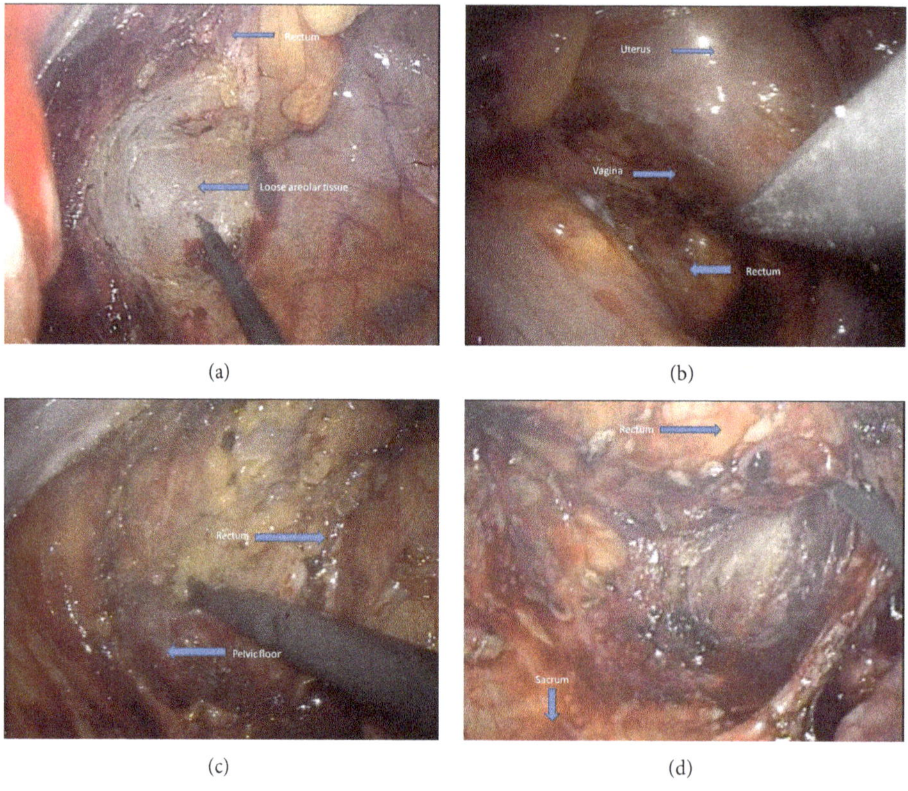

(a) (b) (c) (d)

FIGURE 3: Pelvic dissection.

145 mL (range 50–300 mL). In the LAR case, the anastomosis was 6 cm from the anal verge (Table 2). Intraoperatively, there were no complications, but postoperatively, there were 6 problems: 2 cases of lung atelectasis; 2 instances of nonorganic cause delirium; 1 case of thrombophlebitis on the forearm; and 1 case of perineal wound infection. None of the patients developed neurogenic bladder (Table 3), and none of the male patients developed any sexual disorders.

The median number of harvested lymph nodes was 15 (range 8–30 nodes). Postoperatively, all patients were oncologic stage II or III (4 patients were stage II, and the other 6 were stage III), and all patients received adjuvant chemoradiation therapy. Surgical margins were negative in all patients, with a distal margin of at least 2 cm and circumferential margin of at least 2 mm in all cases (Figure 5). And the mean wound size was 5.5 cm (Figure 6). All patients were allowed oral fluid on the first postoperative day; bowel movement median occurrence was on the third postoperative day; free light diet was allowed on the subsequent day; and patients were discharged when they were able to return to a regular diet with the exception of one patient who developed a perineal wound infection. He was discharged on postoperative day 10 in good condition. There were no readmissions postoperatively.

6. Discussion

Nowadays, the use of minimally invasive surgery is widely accepted. NOTES (natural orifice translumenal endoscopic surgery) and SALS are at the cutting edge of these techniques.

TABLE 2: Operation and pathologic result.

Operation	
APR	9
LAR	1
Surgical time (minutes)	269 ± 41.75 (200–300)
Blood loss (mL)	145 ± 76.19 (50–300)
Pathologic result	
T stage	T3—7 patients T2—3 patients
Lymph node retrieval (median, min–max)	15 (8–30)
Quirk mesorectal grading [7, 8]	Grade 3—9 patients Grade 2—1 patients
CRM	All negative
Pathologic staging	
Stage II	4
Stage III	6

TABLE 3: Postoperative details and complications.

Immediate postoperative complication	
Postoperative lung atelectasis	2
Perineal wound infection	1
Thrombophlebitis	1
Postoperative delirium	2
Hospital stay (day) (median, min–max)	7 (5–10)
30-day mortality	0
Postoperative first bowel movement (day) (median, min–max)	3 (2-3)
Port site wound length (cm) (mean, range)	5.5 ± 0.44 (5-6)

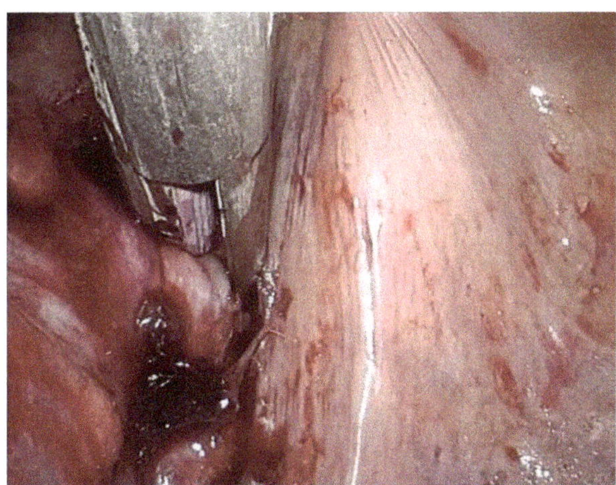

FIGURE 4: Position of placed Endo articulating linear stapler.

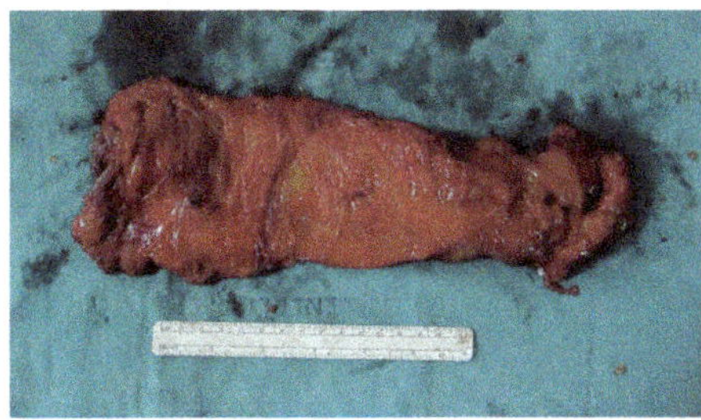

FIGURE 5: Specimen in LAR.

SALS has some significant advantages over NOTES, in particular its facilitation of the use of all common laparoscopic instruments such as laparoscopes, straight and articulating instruments, and the full range of commercially available energy-based dissecting devices [13]. The first report of single-access laparoscopic surgery was a right hemicolectomy in 2008 [14]. Recently, a report from Egi et al. [15] showed no difference in oncologic results between single-port laparoscopic techniques and conventional ones. However, the major problem from a surgical point of view is that the concept of "triangulation," to which laparoscopic surgeons have grown accustomed to in terms of both the instruments and scope, is lacking [16]. Examples of this are the laparoscope's view and articulating instruments. With regard to rectum surgery, the major technical problems are (1) the difficulty in obtaining TME and (2) the limitations of Endo staple instrument use in the pelvis.

A report from Leroy et al. [17] showed that laparoscopic surgery achieved good long-term oncologic results in TME. In single-access laparoscopic surgery, the first report from Hamzaoglu et al. [9] shows promising preliminary pathologic results in 4 cases of LAR with the introduction of a sutured sigmoid hung into the abdominal wall as a way of attaining adequate exposure for TME. In 2010, Uematsu et al. [18] reported a novel single-access port for use in a sigmoidectomy, and in 2011 there was a report of the use of a suspending bar to lift up the sigmoid for TME [10] with excellent pathologic results. Another 2 reports [11, 12] also showed good pathologic results (Table 4). Our study attempted to share our initial experience of performing single-port laparoscopic surgery of rectal cancer in which we achieved equally good pathologic results. From our results, we believe that (1) a bigger port was helpful in reducing instrument collision during operations and enlarged the working channel to manipulate operative field; (2) articulating instruments, especially Endo clinches or graspers, are useful as they help to maintain "triangulation"; (3) a flexible videolaparoscope is necessary or even essential because of its adjustable tip which helps to provide an adequate operative field in rectal dissection; and lastly (4) the reverse Trendelenburg position is useful in helping to pull the rectum in a cranial direction using the force of gravity. With regard to the pelvic diameter and the limited articulation of Endo linear staplers, we had only limited experience; however, Kim et al. [19] reported that the use of multiple stapler firings was a significant risk factor for anastomotic leakage, and they concluded that a reduction in the number of linear stapler firings is necessary to avoid anastomotic leakage after laparoscopic colorectal anastomosis with a double stapling technique. In the LAR case in our study, we used 2 laparoscopic staples to transect

Table 4: Previous results in Single access rectal cancer surgery.

Author, year	Patient number	Operation	Special Technique or Instrument	Port type	Mean operative time (minutes)	Staging	Mean wound length	Quirke's mesorectal fascia grade
Hamzaoglu et al., 2011 [9]	4	3 LAR 1 TAE	Suture-hung sigmoid with abdominal wall	Triport	347	2 stage III 2 stage I	3.5 cm	3
Uematsu et al., 2011 [10]	7	LAR	Suspending bar and extracorporeal magnet	Self innovation	205	2, stage II 5 stage III	3 cm	NA
Hirano et al., 2012 [11]	15	AR	NA	EZ lap protector + 12 mm port	276	0 stage 0 3 stage I 3 stage II 7 stage III 2 stage IV	2.8 cm	NA
Hua-Feng et al., 2012 [12]	20	APR	Start from perineal resection phase	Self-innovation	138	NA	NA	NA

LAR: low anterior resection, TAE: transabdominal anal excision, AR: anterior resection, APR: abdominoperineal resection.

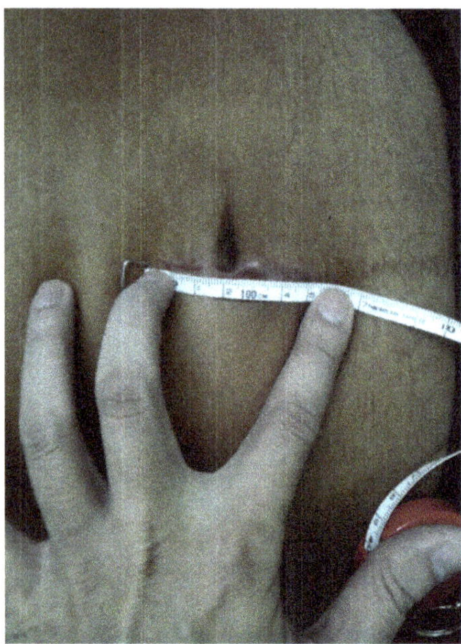

Figure 6: Postoperative wound length.

the rectum vertically, and we did not create a protective ileostomy.

7. Conclusion

The single-access laparoscopic technique is gaining favour with surgeons around the world with the evolution of minimally invasive techniques and instruments. Our results show that the single-access technique for rectal surgery seems to be safe and effective with potentially reproducible oncologic results. In the future, randomized clinical trials should be carried out to confirm our preliminary results showing the benefits of single-access procedures.

Key Messages

Single-access laparoscopic surgery (SALS)for rectal cancer showed that it could be adopted as a feasible option for the management of rectal cancer. Our preliminary results showed acceptable pathologic results and a low level of complications in comparison with previous studies.

References

[1] B. P. Jacob and B. Salky, "Laparoscopic colectomy for colon adenocarcinoma: an 11-year retrospective review with 5-year survival rates," *Surgical Endoscopy*, vol. 19, no. 5, pp. 643–649, 2005.

[2] D. P. Geisler, E. T. Condon, and F. H. Remzi, "Single incision laparoscopic total proctocolectomy with ileopouch anal anastomosis," *Colorectal Disease*, vol. 12, no. 9, pp. 941–943, 2010.

[3] W. M. Chambers, M. Bicsak, M. Lamparelli, and A. R. Dixon, "Single-incision laparoscopic surgery (SILS) in complex colorectal surgery: a technique offering potential and not just cosmesis," *Colorectal Disease*, vol. 13, no. 4, pp. 393–398, 2011.

[4] A. Nagpal, H. Soni, and S. Haribhakti, "Single-incision laparoscopic restorative proctocolectomy with ileal pouch anal anastomosis for ulcerative colitis: first Indian experience and literature review," *International Journal of Colorectal Disease*, vol. 26, no. 4, pp. 525–526, 2011.

[5] R. A. Cahill, I. Lindsey, O. Jones, R. Guy, N. Mortensen, and C. Cunningham, "Single-port laparoscopic total colectomy for medically uncontrolled colitis," *Diseases of the Colon and Rectum*, vol. 53, no. 8, pp. 1143–1147, 2010.

[6] O. Bulut and C. B. Nielsen, "Single-incision laparoscopic low anterior resection for rectal cancer," *International Journal of Colorectal Disease*, vol. 25, no. 10, pp. 1261–1263, 2010.

[7] P. Quirke, P. Durdey, M. F. Dixon, and N. S. Williams, "Local recurrence of rectal adenocarcinoma due to inadequate surgical resection. Histopathological study of lateral tumour spread and surgical excision," *Lancet*, vol. 2, no. 8514, pp. 996–999, 1986.

[8] S. Maslekar, A. Sharma, A. MacDonald, J. Gunn, J. R. T. Monson, and J. E. Hartley, "Mesorectal grades predict recurrences after curative resection for rectal cancer," *Diseases of the Colon and Rectum*, vol. 50, no. 2, pp. 168–175, 2007.

[9] I. Hamzaoglu, T. Karahasanoglu, B. Baca, A. Karatas, E. Aytac, and A. S. Kahya, "Single-port laparoscopic sphincter-saving mesorectal excision for rectal cancer: report of the first 4 human cases," *Archives of Surgery*, vol. 146, no. 1, pp. 75–81, 2011.

[10] D. Uematsu, G. Akiyama, M. Narita, and A. Magishi, "Single-access laparoscopic low anterior resection with vertical suspension of the rectum," *Diseases of the Colon and Rectum*, vol. 54, no. 5, pp. 632–637, 2011.

[11] Y. Hirano, M. Hattori, K. Douden et al., "Single-incision plus one port laparoscopic anterior resection for rectal cancer as a reduced port Surgery," *Scandinavian Journal of Surgery*, vol. 101, no. 4, pp. 283–286, 2012.

[12] P. Hua-Feng, J. Zhi-Wei, W. Gang, L. Xin-Xin, and L. Feng-Tao, "A novel approach for the resection of low rectal cancer," *Surgical Laparoscopy Endoscopy & Percutaneous Techniques*, vol. 22, no. 6, pp. 537–541, 2012.

[13] P. W. Dhumane, M. Diana, J. Leroy, and J. Marescaux, "Minimally invasive single-site surgery for the digestive system: a technological review," *Journal of Minimal Access Surgery*, vol. 7, no. 1, pp. 40–51, 2011.

[14] A. M. Merchant and E. Lin, "Single-incision laparoscopic right hemicolectomy for a colon mass," *Diseases of the Colon and Rectum*, vol. 52, no. 5, pp. 1021–1024, 2009.

[15] H. Egi, M. Hattori, T. Hinoi et al., "Single-port laparoscopic colectomy versus conventional laparoscopic colectomy for colon cancer: a comparison of surgical results," *World Journal of Surgical Oncology*, vol. 10, article 61, 2012.

[16] J. R. Romanelli and D. B. Earle, "Single-port laparoscopic surgery:an overview," *Surgical Endoscopy*, vol. 23, pp. 1419–1427, 2009.

[17] J. Leroy, F. Jamali, L. Forbes et al., "Laparoscopic total mesorectal excision (TME) for rectal cancer surgery: long-term outcomes," *Surgical Endoscopy*, vol. 18, no. 2, pp. 281–289, 2004.

[18] D. Uematsu, G. Akiyama, M. Matsuura, and K. Hotta, "Single-access laparoscopic colectomy with a novel multiport device in sigmoid colectomy for colon cancer," *Diseases of the Colon and Rectum*, vol. 53, no. 4, pp. 496–501, 2010.

[19] J. S. Kim, S. Y. Cho, B. S. Min, and N. K. Kim, "Risk factors for anastomotic leakage after laparoscopic intracorporeal colorectal anastomosis with a double stapling technique," *Journal of the American College of Surgeons*, vol. 209, no. 6, pp. 694–701, 2009.

16

In Silico Investigation of a Surgical Interface for Remote Control of Modular Miniature Robots in Minimally Invasive Surgery

Apollon Zygomalas,[1] Konstantinos Giokas,[2] and Dimitrios Koutsouris[2]

[1] *Life Science Informatics-Medical Informatics, Department of Surgery, University of Patras, Rio, 26500 Patras, Greece*
[2] *Biomedical Engineering Laboratory, School of Electrical and Computer Engineering, National Technical University of Athens, 15780 Zografou, Athens, Greece*

Correspondence should be addressed to Apollon Zygomalas; azygomalas@upatras.gr

Academic Editor: Peng Hui Wang

Aim. Modular mini-robots can be used in novel minimally invasive surgery techniques like natural orifice transluminal endoscopic surgery (NOTES) and laparoendoscopic single site (LESS) surgery. The control of these miniature assistants is complicated. The aim of this study is the in silico investigation of a remote controlling interface for modular miniature robots which can be used in minimally invasive surgery. *Methods.* The conceptual controlling system was developed, programmed, and simulated using professional robotics simulation software. Three different modes of control were programmed. The remote controlling surgical interface was virtually designed as a high scale representation of the respective modular mini-robot, therefore a modular controlling system itself. *Results.* With the proposed modular controlling system the user could easily identify the conformation of the modular mini-robot and adequately modify it as needed. The arrangement of each module was always known. The in silico investigation gave useful information regarding the controlling mode, the adequate speed of rearrangements, and the number of modules needed for efficient working tasks. *Conclusions.* The proposed conceptual model may promote the research and development of more sophisticated modular controlling systems. Modular surgical interfaces may improve the handling and the dexterity of modular miniature robots during minimally invasive procedures.

1. Introduction

Minimally invasive surgery is nowadays a consolidated alternative to the traditional open surgery for a number of operations. Minimally invasive surgical techniques include laparoscopy, single site surgery, and natural orifice transluminal endoscopic surgery. Laparoscopy has proved to be less traumatic for the patient, with minimal operative blood loss, less postoperative pain, accelerated recovery, and excellent cosmesis. A new promising minimally invasive approach is the laparoendoscopic single site (LESS) surgery, also known by a variety of other names (e.g., single incision laparoscopic surgery (SILS) and reduced port surgery (RPS)). LESS has become popular among surgeons as an alternative to standard laparoscopic surgery for a variety of operations [1]. The evolution of minimally invasive surgery to the natural orifice transluminal endoscopic surgery (NOTES) began in 2004 when Kalloo et al. published his study on the transgastric surgery [2]. NOTES is very fascinating in terms of surgical technique but its evolvement seems to be strictly connected to technology [3].

Informatics and robotics offer novel tools to the modern surgeon. The development of in vivo miniature robots for use in surgery is nowadays a reality with potential advantages and possible application in minimally invasive surgery in the future [4, 5]. A revolutionary idea is the development of modular miniature robots. Modular miniature robots are composed of small subunits (modules) which could be assembled and construct a functional mini-robot [6]. Controlling modular mini-robots is rather complicated. It is essential therefore to develop appropriate software and hardware technology that will provide the surgeon with all necessary information and give him an easy and precise control of his miniature assistants. Using robotic simulation

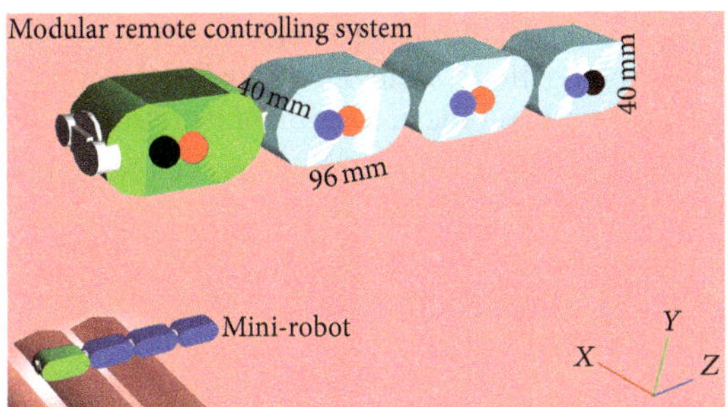

FIGURE 1: The modular remote controlling system (MCS) is identical to the modular miniature robot but in large scale, thus four times larger.

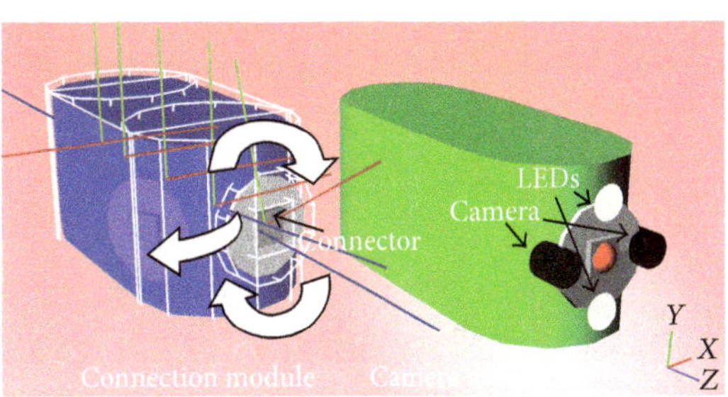

FIGURE 2: A connection module and a camera module. A servomotor gives motion on an arc of 180° on axis Y, (90° left and 90° right). A second motor gives a 360° motion on Z (or X) axis.

software, we can virtually develop mini-robots and investigate their capabilities in silico.

The aim of this study is the experimental in silico investigation of a conceptual model of a surgical remote control interface for modular miniature robots that can be used in minimally invasive surgery.

2. Materials and Methods

The development of our conceptual model is based on the idea that the user-surgeon could handle a modular remote controller similar, but in large scale, to the intra-abdominal modular mini-robot that he wants to control. He then could move the controller's modules as he tries to find a suitable configuration for his miniature assistant. We therefore designed a simple modular snake-like miniature robot consisting of four subunits and its respective modular remote controller and simulated them (Figure 1).

For the development and simulation of the controller and the respective mini-robot, we used the Webots version 6.0.0 (Cyberbotics, Switzerland) [7]. All modules were designed using simple 3D basic geometry objects. One cube and two cylinders construct the body of each module. The dimension of a mini-robot module is 24 mm × 10 mm × 10 mm. The modular remote controlling system (MCS) subunits have the same structure as those of the mini-robot but with dimensions of 96 mm × 40 mm × 40 mm, thus four times larger. This size should be rather handy for a surgeon.

We designed two different types of modules: a connection module and a camera module (Figure 2). All modules are symmetrical in Z axis and are equipped with four active rotational servomotors which provide the assembled mini-robot with motion. Two servomotors are positioned on the front side and two on the rear side. In this way, one motor gives a 180° arc motion on axis Y, so as to have a motion of 90° left and 90° right and the other motor gives a 360° motion on axis Z (or X) for a complete rotation of the module when connected (Figure 2). Electromagnetic symmetrical connectors with controlled connection/disconnection are positioned on the front and rear sides of each subunit. The camera subunit of the mini-robot is equipped with two color cameras and two white light-emitting diodes (LEDs). The camera module of the controlling system does not have functioning cameras. Finally, each subunit is provided with an emitter and a receiver to achieve a wireless bidirectional module ID-based communication between the MCS and the mini-robot.

One red and one blue LED are mounted on each MCS subunit. These LEDs provide the user with visible information regarding the connection state. The blue LED is activated when the front connector is inside the magnetic field of the paired connector of another module and red LED is activated when the rear connector is inside the field. Detailed electromechanic robotic components were not designed. This was out of the aims of this study.

Three different controlling modes of the modular mini-robot were programmed. (A) The first is an absolute master-slave mapping mode where the configuration of the MCS is transmitted in real time to the modular mini-robot. For example, when the second module of the MCS is rotating, simultaneously the second module of the mini-robot performs an identical motion. (B) The second is a postaction mode (delayed master-slave mapping) in which the surgeon can move the modules of the MCS to achieve a preferred conformation and then transmit the new arrangement to the modular mini-robot when he desires (e.g., by pressing an appropriate button). (C) In the third mode, the user can select a preprogrammed simple motion or configuration from a list of actions. The MCS and the miniature robot execute simultaneously the command. Snake-like sinusoidal motions were programmed to achieve robot locomotion. Motion scaling was incorporated for accurate manipulation during the surgical procedure.

The C programming language with special libraries was used for the development of the simulation's programmable controllers using the built-in editor and compiler of Webots. All connection modules use a programmatically identical controller that positions the servomotors using a module ID-based control table. Camera modules use another controller which in addition implements the control of the video camera.

A number of physics parameters were defined using the physics nodes of Webots. Mass distribution, gravity force, and friction parameters were set, allowing the physics simulation engine to compute realistic forces.

Intra-abdominal structures like the intestine, the liver, and the gallbladder were designed using simple 3D objects

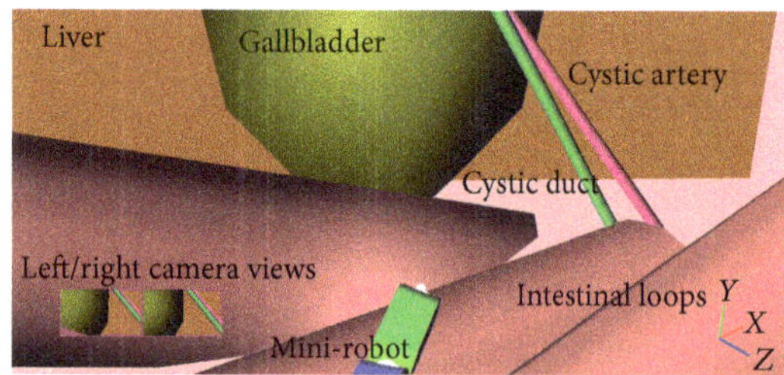

FIGURE 3: The intra-abdominal environment was simulated by simple 3D structures representing the intestine, the liver, and the gallbladder. On the lower left corner of the figure, the mini-robot's onboard camera views are shown. The gallbladder is suspended by a grasper like mini-robot (refer to [15]).

(Figure 3). The intraperitoneal environment was simulated in order to investigate vision and motion of the modular mini-robot in relationship to the controlling capabilities of the MCS.

Remote control was investigated regarding configuration, kinematics, coordination, localization, and user interaction.

3. Results

The modular controlling system allowed the user to immediately determine the conformation of the modular mini-robot. Real-time mode allowed for a standard use of the mini-robot executing pair commands as needed. This was the simplest way to control the miniature robot when it was stationary, thus while operating on tissues, for example. It seems to be impossible to provoke locomotion of the mini-robot using the real-time mode, as this procedure needs a quick and precise coordination of all the subunits. Fast changes of the conformation using rotational movements with over 0.25 rad/sec resulted in unpredictable positioning of the robot mainly due to moment of forces (Table 1). The actuation speed is user-dependent. An actuation speed limiter resolved the problem but restricted the user performance. It was easier to operate in real-time mode when the rear subunit of the system was fixed, thus a configuration similar to an external magnetic anchoring system (MAGS) [8]. It was difficult to control more than four subunits in real-time mode. The larger number of subunits complicated the behavior of the mini-robot because of additional forces like moment forces and friction which the user has to consider mentally in real-time.

The postaction mode helped to find different conformations without synchronous modification of the micro-robot. The user was able to find the most suitable configuration for his activity. However, in many occasions, using this mode significantly changed the arrangement and orientation of the intra-abdominal robot in an unpredictable way. This fact is caused by the torque which was developed during high speed (>0.25 rad/sec) rotational motions of the modules and subsequently due to collisions with some surrounding structures. For that reason, the postaction mode speed was set to 0.1 rads/sec. This mode proved useful when it was used to predict a stable configuration for operation. The postaction mode is by default ineffective for locomotion. It seems that there is no limit in the number of subunits that can be handled by this controlling mode, although the higher the number, the harder the control and the prediction of its result.

The preprogrammed action mode proved to be the only one to provide an acceptable locomotion of the mini-robot and a quick rearrangement of its subunits. During the execution of commands under this mode, the MCS was accessible to the operator. However, the operator could only start and stop a preprogrammed action and not modify it. There seems to be no limit in the number of subunits that can be handled using this mode. Regarding robot locomotion, the more the subunits used, the better the results were. High rotational speed (>0.25 rad/sec) of the servomotors gave acceptable locomotion of the robot. Nevertheless, if a preprogrammed conformation without locomotion was desirable, then the high rotational speed of the servomotors resulted in some occasions to unpredictable positioning of the robot mainly due to torque. A speed limit of 0.1 rad/sec was set for all the preprogrammed actions except for the sinusoidal locomotion.

The configuration of the modular mini-robot was always identified only by observing the MCS conformation. However, its positioning and orientation were not predictable all the time. This principally occurred due to collisions with the surrounding structures or slippage (i.e., on intestine) (Figure 4). Another reason for the unpredictable positioning was the development of considerable torque during high speed rotational motions (>0.25 rad/sec). The mini-robot executed all the commands sent by the MCS but its modules motion depended on their interaction with the surrounding structures which in some occasions blocked a motion or even forced a disconnection of a module.

The LEDs of the MCS provided visual information regarding the connection state of the miniature modules. This proved to be useful while constructing the modular mini-robot. It was also helpful when accidental or voluntary disconnection occurred. All the commands sent by the MCS were logged in order to let the user read information regarding his actions.

4. Discussion

Surgery is historically connected with scars and pain. This aspect can be eliminated by minimally invasive surgery and especially with LESS and NOTES. However, software, hardware, novel surgical tools, and approaches should be evolved. Miniature robots can be equipped with surgical tools and sensors in order to provide information from the abdominal cavity and the possibility of remotely controlled surgical operations [9]. Miniature robots could be handled even by nonspecialized personnel and remote-controlled by surgeons miles away from the patient [10].

The use of modular mini-robots for minimally invasive surgery poses difficulties to surgeons related to the coordinative controlling of the robotic subunits. A single module by itself cannot operate, but modules arranged together can achieve complex tasks and controlling such a system could be rather difficult. The surgical robots are commonly controlled

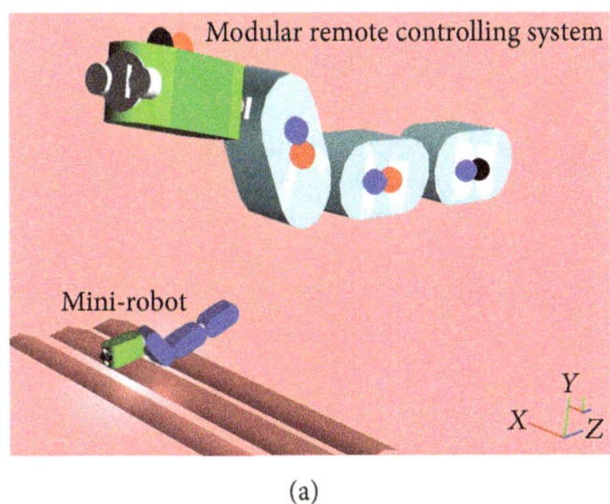

(a)

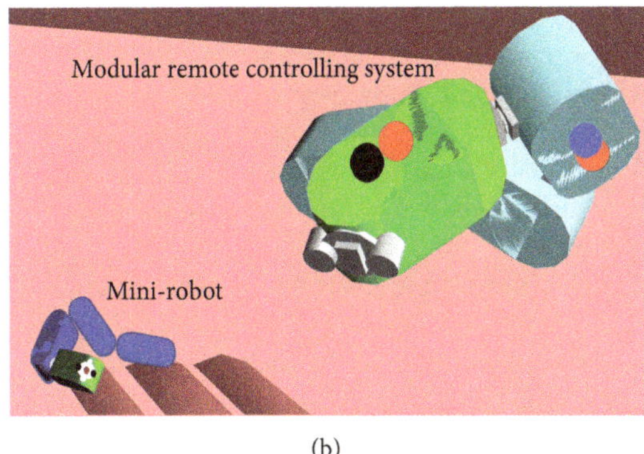

(b)

FIGURE 4: (a) Identical conformation between MCS and mini-robot with slightly different (acceptable) positioning of the second. (b) Identical conformation but very different orientation and positioning.

TABLE 1: Modular remote controlling system operating modes.

Operating mode	Actuation speed	Ideal number of modules	Pros	Cons
Absolute master-slave mapping	User-dependent	4	Natural operation	User dependent action speed control
Delayed master-slave mapping	Set to 0.1 rad/sec	4–6	Predictable conformation	Unpredictable positioning and orientation
Preprogrammed	Set according to the desired action	4–6	Locomotion	No user interaction

from outside the patient's body under indirect video assisted vision with the use of a joystick-like surgical interface [4, 11, 12]. Snake-like modular mini-robots can be in some cases compared to flexible endoscopes. Having this in mind, we should consider the study of Allemann et al. who proved that the use of robotized endoscopes with joystick interface is insufficient to enhance immediate intuitiveness of flexible endoscopy for NOTES [13]. Because of the complexity of locomotion and the precision of the task that modular mini-robots should perform, novel remote controlling systems should be developed in order to make the surgeon, and not the engineer, operate. The surgeon who will use modular miniature robots should feel safe and relaxed; therefore, a remote controlling system should be simple and accurate.

Wortman et al. presented a miniature robot prototype in which surgical interface is a kinematically matched master-slave configuration scaled model of the robot's arms [14]. This master system allows the surgeon to control the robot by directly mapping each joint. The scale of master-slave is 1.8 : 1 in length. Our conceptual model has the same basic idea of pairing master-slave configuration but is proposed for totally intracorporeal modular miniature robots (internal robots) [15]. The system of Wortman et al. provides the user with direct control over each joint of the mini-robot, allowing for a better sense of control. However, because none of the joints is provided with motors, the master arm cannot be held in place when the robot arm is locked. The master must be returned to an orientation similar to the robot before it can be unlocked. Our conceptual model of controller is equipped with motors and by default its configuration is always the same as that of the intra-abdominal miniature robot.

Our experimental investigation gave some useful information regarding the type of control, the working speed of the servomotors, and the number of modules that a modular robot can have in order to be efficiently controlled (Table 1). Although the real-time control of the mini-robot is the most natural to be utilized during a surgical operation, it is difficult to control more than four subunits and it is impossible to induce locomotion of the whole robotic system. On the other hand, the usefulness of postaction mode resulted in doubt. This situation was created because of the unpredictable interaction of the robotic subunits with the surrounding structures during rearrangement. Furthermore, if the rotational speed of the servomotors was high during the rearrangements, then the torque was considerable. This fact should be taken into consideration in such a miniature scale. However, using this type of control, it was easier to find an appropriate conformation for a stable operational robot. The preprogrammed mode was the only one that provided the robot with locomotion. However, when activated, the robot conformation changes as the preprogrammed commands need, and this sometimes may have unpredictable results regarding the interactions with the surrounding structures and the modules moment forces as mentioned above.

The positioning of the subunits on the modular mini-robot was always known and in the case of the real world the surgeon could virtually "touch" his mini-robot through his twin big brother remote controller. Slow and steady motion of the modules is desirable in order to minimize torque and achieve desirable conformation, positioning, and orientation. However, a more detailed study by a team of robotics specialists and the use of more sophisticated simulation libraries that take into account all the characteristics of the robot and the environment in which it operates are required. It is essential to construct and study in vivo such a mini-robot and its surgical interface. Effective cooperation between surgeons, robotics specialists, and informatics specialists is fundamental for a successful use of miniature robots in minimally invasive surgery.

Although this was a simple and basic simulation, it may be useful for a future construction of remote controlling surgical interfaces that can be used in order to control modular miniature robots during minimally invasive surgical procedures. Another idea is to modify this conceptual model as a "hand glove" which a surgeon can wear and control with it his miniature assistants (every module could be a phalange or a part of the upper limb, e.g., the front camera module paired to a finger, the second module paired to the hand, the third module paired to the forearm, and the fourth module paired to the arm). The present work represents only a conceptual in silico experimental study with no intention to solve mechanical, electrical, and robotic engineering problems in general.

5. Conclusions

The design of the proposed conceptual model may facilitate the development of more sophisticated and complex modular controlling systems. Modular surgical interfaces may improve the handling and the dexterity of modular miniature robots during minimally invasive procedures.

Acknowledgments

This work represents a part of the study conducted as a Master of Science Thesis in Medical Informatics-Life Science Informatics during 2008 and 2010 at the University of Patras, Greece. Thanks are due to Professor Hatziligeroudis and Professor Papatheodorou (Department of Computer Engineering and Informatics, University of Patras) for their help on computer programming and thesis correction. Thanks are due to Dr. Drosou (Biologist) for her indications on tissue behavior and snakes locomotion.

References

[1] J. R. Romanelli and D. B. Earle, "Single-port laparoscopic surgery: an overview," *Surgical Endoscopy and Other Interventional Techniques*, vol. 23, no. 7, pp. 1419–1427, 2009.

[2] A. N. Kalloo, V. K. Singh, S. B. Jagannath et al., "Flexible transgastric peritoneoscopy: a novel approach to diagnostic and therapeutic interventions in the peritoneal cavity," *Gastrointestinal Endoscopy*, vol. 60, no. 1, pp. 114–117, 2004.

[3] D. W. Rattner, R. Hawes, S. Schwaitzberg, M. Kochman, and L. Swanstrom, "The second SAGES/ASGE white paper on natural orifice transluminal endoscopic surgery: 5 Years of progress," *Surgical Endoscopy and Other Interventional Techniques*, vol. 25, no. 8, pp. 2441–2448, 2011.

[4] A. C. Lehman, N. A. Wood, S. Farritor, M. R. Goede, and D. Oleynikov, "Dexterous miniature robot for advanced minimally invasive surgery," *Surgical Endoscopy and Other Interventional Techniques*, vol. 25, no. 1, pp. 119–123, 2011.

[5] A. Zygomalas, I. Kehagias, K. Giokas, and D. Koutsouris, "Miniature surgical robots in the era of NOTES and LESS: dream or reality?" *Surgical Innovation*, 2014.

[6] Z. Nagy, R. Oung, J. J. Abbott, and B. J. Nelson, "Experimental investigation of magnetic self-assembly for swallowable modular robots," in *Proceedings of the IEEE/RSJ International Conference on Intelligent Robots and Systems (IROS '08)*, pp. 1915–1920, Nice, France, September 2008.

[7] Webots: robot simulator—about [Internet], http://www.cyberbotics.com/about.

[8] D. J. Scott, S.-J. Tang, R. Fernandez et al., "Completely transvaginal NOTES cholecystectomy using magnetically anchored instruments," *Surgical Endoscopy and Other Interventional Techniques*, vol. 21, no. 12, pp. 2308–2316, 2007.

[9] A. C. Lehman, K. A. Berg, J. Dumpert et al., "Surgery with cooperative robots," *Computer Aided Surgery*, vol. 13, no. 2, pp. 95–105, 2008.

[10] J. A. Hawks, M. E. Rentschler, S. Farritor, D. Oleynikov, and S. R. Platt, "A modular wireless in vivo surgical robot with multiple surgical applications," *Studies in Health Technology and Informatics*, vol. 142, pp. 117–121, 2009.

[11] A. C. Lehman, J. Dumpert, N. A. Wood et al., "Natural orifice cholecystectomy using a miniature robot," *Surgical Endoscopy and Other Interventional Techniques*, vol. 23, no. 2, pp. 260–266, 2009.

[12] G. Petroni, M. Niccolini, S. Caccavaro et al., "A novel robotic system for single-port laparoscopic surgery: preliminary experience," *Surgical Endoscopy and Other Interventional Techniques*, vol. 27, no. 6, pp. 1932–1937, 2013.

[13] P. Allemann, L. Ott, M. Asakuma et al., "Joystick interfaces are not suitable for robotized endoscope applied to NOTES," *Surgical Innovation*, vol. 16, no. 2, pp. 111–116, 2009.

[14] T. D. Wortman, A. Meyer, O. Dolghi et al., "Miniature surgical robot for laparoendoscopic single-incision colectomy," *Surgical Endoscopy and Other Interventional Techniques*, vol. 26, no. 3, pp. 727–731, 2012.

[15] A. Zygomalas, K. Gkiokas, and D. D. Koutsouris, "In silico development and simulation of a modular reconfigurable assembly micro-robot for use in natural orifice transluminal endoscopic surgery," *Hellenic Journal of Surgery*, vol. 83, no. 4, pp. 190–196, 2011.

17

Adnexal Masses Treated Using a Combination of the SILS Port and Noncurved Straight Laparoscopic Instruments: Turkish Experience and Review of the Literature

Polat Dursun,[1] Tugan Tezcaner,[2] Hulusi B. Zeyneloglu,[1] Irem Alyazıcı,[1] Ali Haberal,[1] and Ali Ayhan[1]

[1] *Department of Obstetrics and Gynecology, Baskent University, School of Medicine, Ankara, Turkey*
[2] *Department of Surgery, Baskent University, School of Medicine, Ankara, Turkey*

Correspondence should be addressed to Polat Dursun; pdursun@yahoo.com

Academic Editor: Peng Hui Wang

Objective. To report our experience treating adnexal masses using a combination of the SILS port and straight nonroticulating laparoscopic instruments. *Study Design.* This prospective feasibility study included 14 women with symptomatic and persistent adnexal masses. Removal of adnexal masses via single-incision laparoscopic surgery using a combination of the SILS port and straight nonroticulating laparoscopic instruments was performed. *Results.* All of the patients had symptomatic complex adnexal masses. Mean age of the patients was 38.4 years (range: 21–61 years) and mean duration of surgery was 71 min (range: 45–130 min). All surgeries were performed using nonroticulating straight laparoscopic instruments. Mean tumor diameter was 6 cm (range: 5–12 cm). All patient pathology reports were benign. None of the patients converted to laparotomy. All the patients were discharged on postoperative d1. Postoperatively, all the patients were satisfied with their incision and cosmetic results. *Conclusion.* All 14 patients were successfully treated using standard, straight nonroticulating laparoscopic instruments via the SILS port. This procedure can reduce the cost of treatment, which may eventually lead to more widespread use of the SILS port approach. Furthermore, concomitant surgical procedures are possible using this approach. However, properly designed comparative studies with single port and classic laparoscopic surgery are urgently needed.

1. Introduction

Adnexal masses are one of the most common indications for surgery in gynecology clinics, and laparoscopy is generally accepted as the gold standard treatment. Classical laparoscopic surgery for adnexal masses is generally performed using ≥3 trocars. On the other hand, single-port access surgery (SPAS), also known as laparoendoscopic single-site surgery (LESS) and single-incision laparoscopic surgery (SILS), is an evolving endoscopic approach for minimal access surgery. Various surgical procedures, including appendectomy, cholecystectomy, nephrectomy, oophorectomy, hysterectomy, adrenalectomy, gastric bypass, Nissen fundoplication, hernia repair, splenectomy, and colon resection, have been performed via SILS. SILS can result in better cosmesis, shorter recovery time, and less pain than conventional laparoscopy, which requires use of multiple trocar incisions [1, 2].

It was recently reported that adnexal masses could also be treated via SILS [3, 4]. Endoscopic surgery conducted via 3 special luminal ports, including the SILS port (Covidien, Norwalk, CT), GelPort (Applied Medical Resources, Rancho Santa Margarita, CA), and X-cone (Karl Storz, Tuttlingen, Germany), as well as others, is frequently referred to as SILS. SILS requires a 2-3 cm incision on the umbilicus for the placement of the special port. Furthermore, nonconventional roticulating and articulated laparoscopic instruments are necessary for SILS in order to ensure that the instruments do not collide during SILS [5, 6].

SILS performed using conventional laparoscopic instruments for appendectomy and cholecystectomy has been reported; however, to the best of our knowledge, the combined use of the SILS port (Covidien, Norwalk, CT) and conventional laparoscopic instruments has not been reported in the gynecology literature [6, 7]. Herein we report on 14 patients with adnexal masses that were treated using the SILS port and conventional straight laparoscopic instruments.

2. Materials and Methods

2.1. Participants. The study included 14 women with symptomatic and persistent adnexal masses. Inclusion criteria were as follows: a persistent adnexal mass, a growing adnexal mass on follow-up, an adnexal mass that cannot exclude surgical emergencies, cystic rupture with acute abdomen, and an adnexal mass with intractable pelvic pain. Patients with imaging studies strongly suggesting a malignant adnexal mass were excluded from the study.

2.2. Surgical Technique. Each patient was placed in the modified lithotomy position under general anesthesia. Initially, the surgeon stood on the left side of each patient. The lateral sides of the umbilicus were everted using 2 clamps. Then, a 2 cm vertical intraumbilical skin incision was made (Figure 1). Sharp and blunt dissection was performed on the subcutaneous fatty tissue; the fascia was exposed and cut using number 11 scalpel blade, and the peritoneum was incised using Metzenbaum scissors. The incision was then extended by an additional 0.5 cm via stretching of the skin. No other extraumbilical skin incisions were used.

A SILS port (Covidien, Norwalk, CT) with 3 access inlets was inserted into the abdominal cavity using a Heaney clamp, and a carbon dioxide pneumoperitoneum was created. A 10 mm rigid video laparoscope was used together with 2 classical nonroticulating straight laparoscopic instruments (Figure 1). One bipolar and 1 monopolar cautery, 1 dissection forceps, and suction-irrigation devices were used sequentially as indicated during surgery. If collision of the instruments resulted in inadequate surgical movement for dissection, cutting, or coagulation, the surgeon changed the placement of the instruments, his position from the lateral side of the patient to the patient's head, or the placement of the endoscope in order to perform the necessary movements (Figure 2). Specimens were retracted from the umbilical incision at the end of each surgery. If there was a suspicious mass for malignancy, specimen was retracted using endobag via umbilical incision (Figure 3).

The fascia was then closed using number 1 vicryl interrupted sutures. After surgery all patients reported that they are very satisfied with their incision. All surgical procedures were performed by 1 surgeon (PD), except for appendectomy and cholecystectomy, which were performed by a general surgeon (TT).

3. Results

Patient characteristics are shown in Table 1. Briefly, all 14 patients had symptomatic complex adnexal masses. Mean age of the patients was 38.4 years and mean duration of surgery was 71 min. All patients were treated using straight, nonroticulating laparoscopic instruments. Mean tumor diameter was 6 cm (range: 5–12 cm). In total, 5 patients underwent cystectomy, 3 unilateral salpingo-oopherectomies (USO), 1 bilateral salpingo-oopherectomy (BSO), 1 USO + intraligamentary myomectomy, and 2 salpingectomies. In 2 of the patients, cholecystectomy (USO + cholecystectomy) and appendectomy (cystectomy + appendectomy) were performed concomitantly. All patient pathology reports were benign. None of the patients converted to laparotomy. All patients were discharged on postoperative d1. None of the patients required readmission to hospital. After surgery all patients reported that they were satisfied with their incision and cosmetic results, and none of the patients experienced any wound problem (Figures 4 and 5).

4. Discussion

SILS is a promising form of minimally invasive surgery and is currently in the initial stages of clinical use. There is growing interest in and enthusiasm for SILS among surgeons, patients, and the medical industry [1, 2]. The first single-port appendectomy was performed in 2005, followed by the first single-port cholecystectomy in 2007. Today, complex urological, gynecological, colorectal, and bariatric surgical procedures have been performed using the SILS technique and equipment. Use of SILS has been facilitated by the introduction of rotating and curved instruments into clinical practice [11–14]. On the other hand, new surgical devices, including expensive single ports, roticulating devices, and curved instruments, may limit the widespread use of SILS. If the technical difficulties associated with SILS could be overcome using less expensive conventional laparoscopic instruments, this novel surgical approach may become more common, without extra cost or lesser cost [15].

Following the introduction of SILS, some surgeons modified the approach and produced their own single-port access devices using surgical gloves. Hayashi et al. proved the effectiveness of a self-made surgical glove port for SILS in 23 patients. They made a 1.5 cm skin incision on the umbilicus, and then a small wound retractor was installed in the umbilical wound. Next, a nonpowdered surgical glove was placed on the wound retractor through which three 5 mm slim trocars were inserted via the fingertips. Surgery in all 23 cases was successful without the occurrence of intra- or postoperative complications [16]. Moreover, other studies reported an approach using a single port in the umbilicus and triangular classical trocars [1, 2, 17].

In relative terms, there are currently only a small number of reports of adnexal masses treated via SILS using straight classical laparoscopic instruments. Herein we described a modification of SILS surgery that eliminates the necessity of using expensive roticulating devices. In the present study, we used the SILS port and conventional, straight laparoscopic instruments. SILS is associated with some limitations, such as the close proximity of the working instruments, limited triangulation of the instruments, limited range of motion, an unstable camera platform, and often a small number of

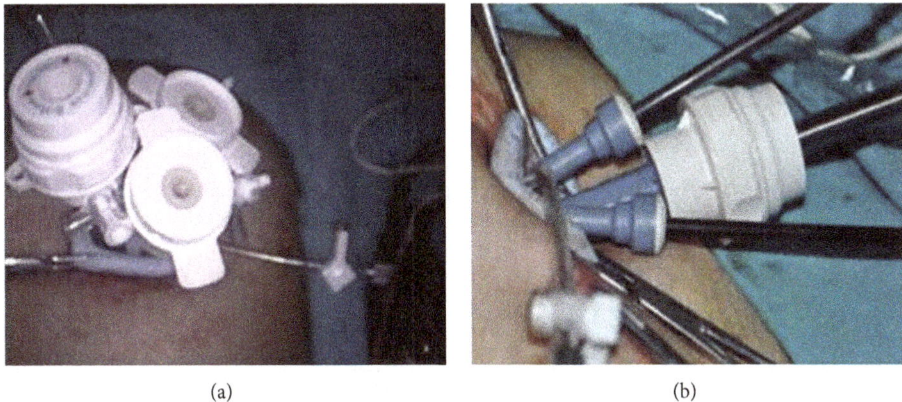

(a) (b)

FIGURE 1: SILS port and instruments positions.

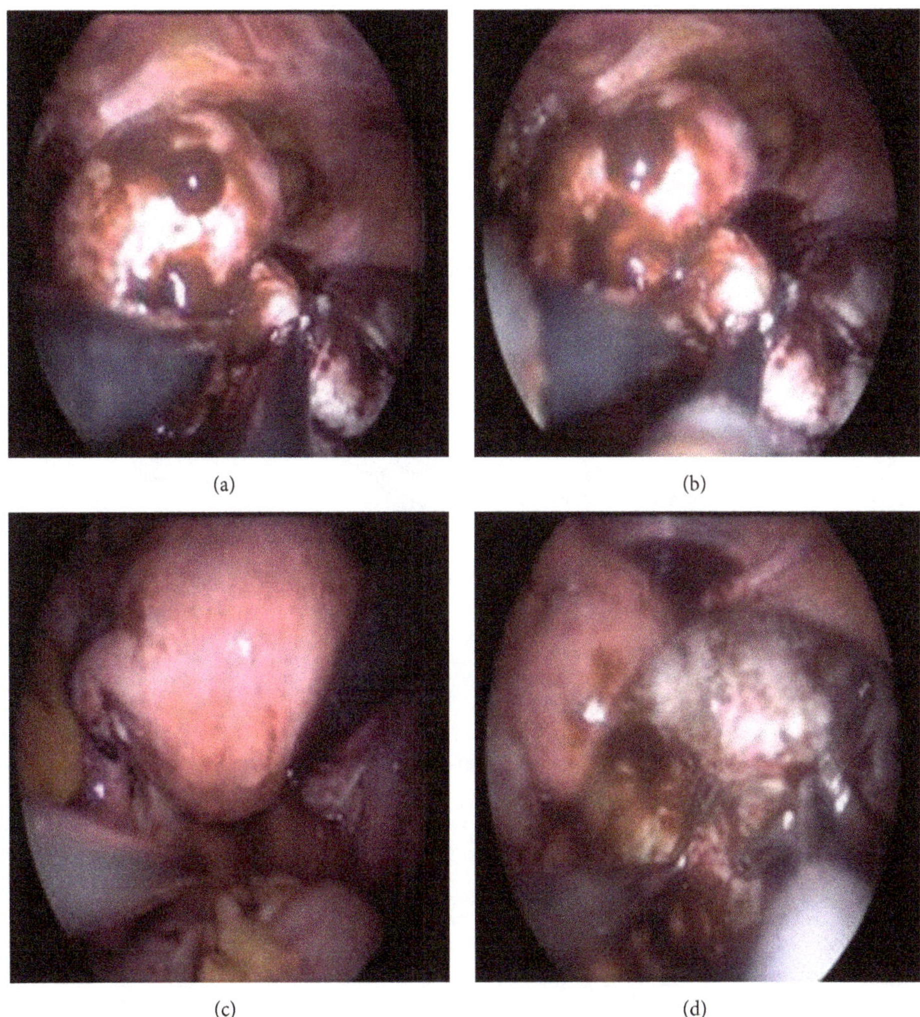

(a) (b)

(c) (d)

FIGURE 2: Intraoperative positions of different straight nonroticulating instruments during operations.

ports. In fact, the term "sword fighting" was used to describe instrument collision during SILS. Such limitations make SILS difficult and are associated with prolonged surgical duration, as compared to conventional laparoscopy [15, 17]. Paek et al. used a special Alexis wound retractor and a homemade single multichannel port access system for SILS hysterectomy. They reported that collision between the camera and surgical instruments was a major problem during the procedure and

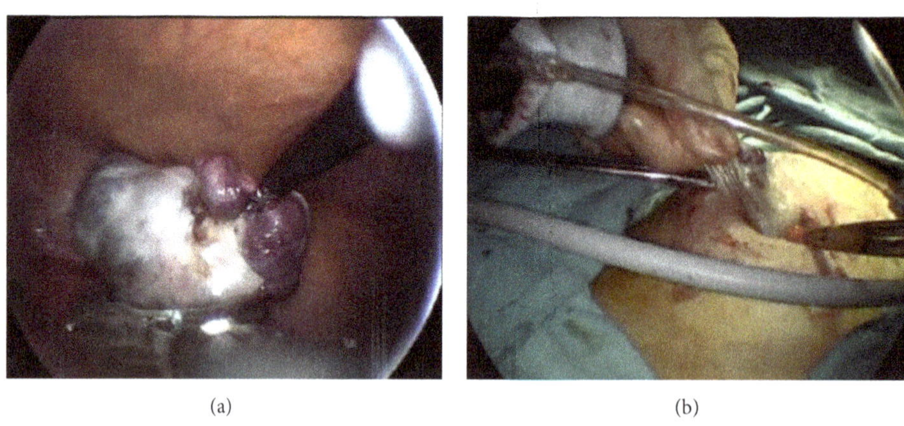

(a) (b)

FIGURE 3: (a) USO material inserted into endobag. (b) Specimen extraction using endobag.

TABLE 1: Characteristics of the patients.

Patients no	Age (years)	Menopausal status	Size and features of adnexal mass	Type of operation	Duration of operation (minutes)	Pathology
1	61	Postmenopausal	7 cm trilobulated and septated ovarian cyst	BSO	85	Serous cystadenoma
2	52	Postmenopausal	7 cm solid cystic ovarian cyst	USO	70	Serous cystadenoma
3	42	Postmenopausal	5 cm complex ovarian cysts on left ovary	USO + Adhesiolysis	60	Serous cystadenoma
4	39	Premenopausal	12 cm endometrioma	Cystectomy + Adhesiolysis	130	Endometrioma
5	34	Premenopausal	5 cm ruptured ovarian cysts with massive hemoperitoneum	Cystectomy	55	Corpus hemorhagicum
6	28	Premenopausal	5 cm complex ovarian cysts	Cystectomy	60	Endometrioma
7	21	Premenopausal	5 cm ruptured ovarian cysts with massive hemoperitoneum	Cystectomy	60	Corpus hemorhagicum
8	28	Premenopausal	5 cm ruptured ovarian endometrioma	Cystectomy	80	Endometrioma
9	33	Premenopausal	4 cm adnexal mass	Salpingectomy	50	Ectopic pregnancy
10	36	Premenopausal	6 cm Tubo-ovarian abscess	Salpingectomy	45	Tubo-ovarian abscess
11	46	Premenopausal	8 cm complex adnexal mass	USO + Intraligamentary myomectomy	50	Serous cyst + leiomyoma
12	66	Postmenopausal	7 cm complex ovarian cysts	USO	130	Mucinous cystadenoma + Cholecystitis
13	28	Premenopausal	5 cm ruptured ovarian cysts with massive hemoperitoneum	Cystectomy + appendectomy	90	Corpus hemorhagicum + appendicitis
14	24	Premenopausal	9 cm endometrioma	Cystectomy	65	Endometrioma

BSO: bilateral salpingo-oopherectomy.
USO: unilateral salpingo-oopherectomy.

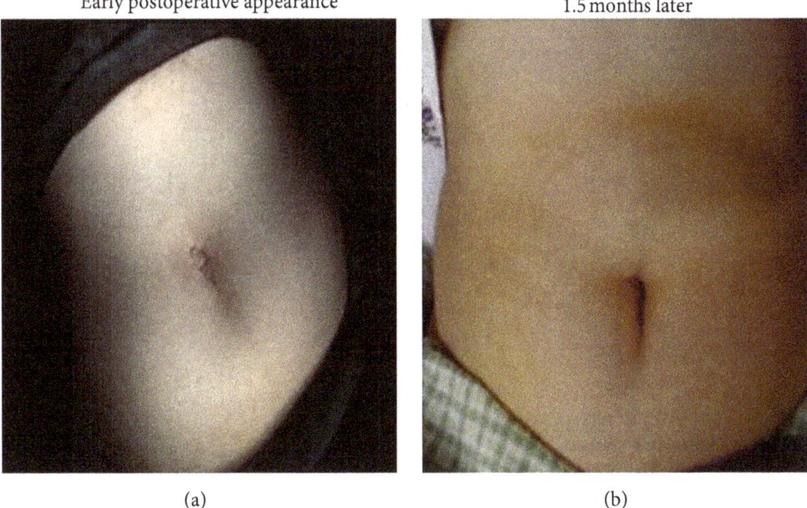

FIGURE 4: Final appearance at the end of the operation and 1–5 months later.

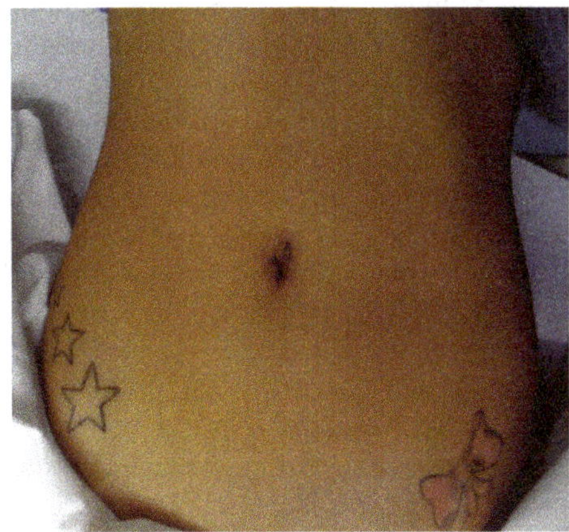

FIGURE 5: Scar of SILS cystectomy, appearance at 6 months.

suggested using a 5 mm endoscope with an angle of 30 degrees, as it provides a wider field of vision [17].

In the present study, we used a 10 mm endoscope with an angle of 0 degrees and did not encounter any serious problems, although we do acknowledge having some difficulty due to collision of the instruments and camera. The most important problem we encountered during surgery was the collision of the conventional laparoscopic device and limited space for instrument movements; however, these difficulties never resulted in an aborted or cancelled procedure. Although instrument collision was a major problem during this procedure, it was overcome by repositioning the instruments and/or the surgeon; positioning the surgeon at the patient's head rather on the lateral side was an effective solution to instrument collision, making this procedure much easier. However, to prevent any intra- and postoperative complications related to instrument collision, surgeons should carefully perform these operations.

The most important part of the usage of the straight laparoscopic instrument in SILS surgery was the easy transfer of the oldest experience with these surgical devices. In the present study, laparoscopic treatment of adnexal masses using the SILS port and standard, straight laparoscopic instruments was successful in all 14 patients. Garcia-Henriquez et al. reported that SILS cholecystectomy is feasible using standard, straight surgical instruments and that use of the SILS port decreased back end instrument collisions and facilitated better separation between the trocar heads and platform, as compared to using 3 individual ports in a single incision [17]. Akgür et al. described single-port incisionless intracorporeal conventional equipment endoscopic appendectomy (SPICES). The researchers used an 11 mm conventional port (that did not require an incision beyond the umbilicus) and conventional working instruments [6]. Supraumbilical, infraumbilical, or transumbilical incisions can be used for SILS. It is generally accepted that a transumbilical incision, rather than a supra- or infraumbilical incision, results in a more cosmetically pleasing scar and an almost normal-looking umbilicus [14]. In the present study, the transumbilical approach was used, and in all 14 patients the incision was 2.0–2.5 cm, as previously reported [14].

Tam et al. reported that SILS appendectomy using conventional instruments in children was feasible. They concluded that use of conventional instruments in SILS is technically possible in children undergoing simple to complex procedures and may have the potential to popularize this approach by eliminating the mandatory demand for specially designed instruments [5]. SILS was initially performed by crossing roticulating and articulating laparoscopic instruments. Some researchers suggested using 1 roticulating instrument and 1 straight instrument for dissection [5, 18, 19]. Use of roticulating and articulating devices is complicated due to the difficult hand-eye coordination and limited surgical space, and use of conventional straight instruments may overcome this difficulty; however, use of conventional instruments also has some drawbacks, including instrument collision, limited instrument triangulation, limited range of motion, and often a small number of ports [17].

Table 2: Review of the literature of single port laparoscopy in the management of adnexal masses.

Author	Country, year	n	Type of port	Size of the adnexal mass, size (range)	Duration of operation, minutes (range)	Complication	Conclusion
Kim et al. [4]	Korea, 2009	24	Homemade glove port	5 cm (3–10)	70 (40–128)	—	Feasible
Escobar et al. [3]	USA, 2010	8	Multichannel port	—	—	—	Additional investigation is needed
Lee et al. [8]	Korea, 2010	17	Homemade glove port	—	—	—	Comparable operative outcomes
Jung et al. [9]	Korea, 2011	86	Homemade glove port	6	64 (21–176)	—	Feasible
Kim et al. [10]	Korea, 2011	94	Homemade glove port	6	50	—	Safe and feasible
Current	Turkey, 2012	14	SILS Port	6 (5–12)	71 (45–130)	—	Feasible

Tam et al. reported that crossing 2 straight instruments was not significantly different than conventional laparoscopic skills and that the instruments may need to be moved between hands during surgery. In the present study, we also frequently changed the placement of surgical instruments, which we think may have helped in overcoming the problem of instrument collision [5]. Podolsky and Curcillo II reported their 2-year experience with more than 100 SILS procedures; their major technical refinement was the transition from special roticulating instruments to conventional straight instruments [20].

In the present study, we performed 1 cholecystectomy and 1 appendectomy concomitantly with ovarian cystectomy and unilateral salpingo-oopherectomy, respectively, via the same umbilical incision; the ability to perform multiple procedures via a single incision is an advantage which SILS has over the classical laparoscopic approach. Surico et al. reported concomitant ovarian cystectomy and cholecystectomy using a multi-instrument access port and concluded that single-port surgery eliminates the problem of multiple site placement of accessory ports [21]. On the other hand, Hart et al. reported concomitant SILS cholecystectomy and hysterectomy for the treatment of a symptomatic fibroid uterus and symptoms of cholelithiasis in a 37-year-old woman. They concluded that complex concomitant procedures could be performed using the SILS approach [22]. SILS reduces the number of trocars used in classical multiport laparoscopic surgery [20].

The significance and importance of any new surgical approach are dependent upon its widespread acceptance and use in a large number of patients. The cost and availability of new instruments, the need surgeon retraining, and efficacy and safety are all important factors that determine the level of acceptance of any new technique [5]. This approach may help increase the popularity of SILS for adnexal masses.

Umbilical hernia is a concern about SILS surgery due to the relatively large umbilical incision. Gunderson et al. retrospectively reviewed the 211 women who underwent SILS surgery for a benign or malignant gynecologic indication via a single 1.5 to 2.0 cm umbilical incision. After a median postoperative follow-up time of 16 months, 2.4% of the patients developed umbilical hernia. However, majority of these women (4/5) had some significant risk factors for fascial weakening independent of LESS, like requirement for a second abdominal surgery and a cancer diagnosis with postoperative chemotherapy administration. When these subjects deemed "high risk" for incisional disruption were excluded from the analysis, the umbilical hernia rate was 0.5% (1/207). The authors concluded that the overall umbilical hernia rate was 2.4% and was lower (0.5%) in subjects without significant comorbidities [23]. However, further studies with larger sampler size and longer follow-up are needed to reach clear conclusions on this debate.

Another important concern is the prolongation of the operative time in SILS surgery. Lee et al. compared perioperative outcomes of single port access laparoscopic adnexal surgery versus conventional laparoscopic adnexal surgery. In this study, there were no differences between SPA and conventional groups in median operation time (64 min versus 57.5 min, $P = 0.252$) [8]. Park et al. reported that operative time was 60 minutes (27–245), 105 minutes (50–185), and 60 minutes (30–115) for an oophorectomy, cystectomy, and salpingectomy, respectively [24]. Also, Jung et al. reported that mean duration of single port adnexal surgery was 64.5 min (range 21–176 min) similar to our experience [9]. However, it has been also reported that duration of operation decreases by the end of the learning curve and that in an experienced hands duration of operation will not increase too much [25].

Although we did not perform a comparative study, we observed that single port incision has a better cosmetic outcome compared with traditional laparoscopic surgery Also, patients satisfaction was very good in patients who underwent SILS surgery. However, further comparative studies between classical laparoscopic surgery and SILS surgery with larger sample size are needed to reach clear conclusion about the cosmetic outcome.

Review of the literature in Table 2 showed that single port management of benign adnexal masses is feasible without increasing complication rates. A relatively increased duration of operation might be related to learning curve and instrument collision. However, umbilical incision might reduce the risk of tumor spillage related to cyst rupture. However, of properly designed comparative studies with single port and classic laparoscopic surgery are urgently needed.

5. Conclusion

We think that this procedure described herein is feasible for the treatment of adnexal masses and is more cost effective than standard SILS; however, it is associated with some difficulties, including the collision of straight laparoscopic instruments. The present study is limited by its retrospective design and limited samples size, and further prospective studies with larger sample size are needed to reach more clear conclusions. Additional research is needed to more clearly discern the safety and benefit of this approach. Also, confirmation of SILS superiority to other minimal invasive laparoscopic approaches needs to be confirmed in prospective randomized studies. Furthermore, this approach should also be validated for other commercial ports.

Condensation. Removal of adnexal masses via single-incision laparoscopic surgery using a combination of the SILS port and straight nonroticulating laparoscopic instruments is feasible.

References

[1] A. Y. Tsai and D. J. Selzer, "Single-port laparoscopic surgery," *Advances in Surgery*, vol. 44, no. 1, pp. 1–27, 2010.

[2] D. Canes, M. M. Desai, M. Aron et al., "Transumbilical single-port surgery: evolution and current status," *European Urology*, vol. 54, no. 5, pp. 1020–1030, 2008.

[3] P. F. Escobar, M. A. Bedaiwy, A. N. Fader, and T. Falcone, "Laparoendoscopic single-site (LESS) surgery in patients with benign adnexal disease," *Fertility and Sterility*, vol. 93, no. 6, pp. 2074-e7–2074-e10, 2010.

[4] T. J. Kim, Y. Y. Lee, M. J. Kim et al., "Single port access laparoscopic adnexal surgery," *Journal of Minimally Invasive Gynecology*, vol. 16, no. 5, pp. 612–615, 2009.

[5] Y. H. Tam, K. H. Lee, J. D. Y. Sihoe, K. W. Chan, S. T. Cheung, and K. K. Pang, "Initial experience in children using conventional laparoscopic instruments in single-incision laparoscopic surgery," *Journal of Pediatric Surgery*, vol. 45, no. 12, pp. 2381–2385, 2010.

[6] F. M. Akgür, M. Olguner, G. Hakgüder, and O. Ateş, "Appendectomy conducted with single port incisionless-intracorporeal conventional equipment-endoscopic surgery," *Journal of Pediatric Surgery*, vol. 45, no. 5, pp. 1061–1063, 2010.

[7] M. J. Colon, D. Telem, C. M. Divino, and E. H. Chin, "Laparoendoscopic single site surgery can be performed completely with standard equipment," *Surgical Laparoscopy, Endoscopy and Percutaneous Techniques*, vol. 21, no. 4, pp. 292–294, 2011.

[8] Y. Y. Lee, T. J. Kim, C. J. Kim et al., "Single port access laparoscopic adnexal surgery versus conventional laparoscopic adnexal surgery: a comparison of peri-operative outcomes," *European Journal of Obstetrics Gynecology and Reproductive Biology*, vol. 151, no. 2, pp. 181–184, 2010.

[9] Y. W. Jung, Y. M. Choi, C. K. Chung et al., "Single port transumbilical laparoscopic surgery for adnexal lesions: a single center experience in Korea," *European Journal of Obstetrics Gynecology and Reproductive Biology*, vol. 155, no. 2, pp. 221–224, 2011.

[10] W. C. Kim, J. E. Lee, Y. S. Kwon, Y. J. Koo, I. H. Lee, and K. T. Lim, "Laparoendoscopic single-site surgery (LESS) for adnexal tumors: one surgeon's initial experience over a one-year period," *European Journal of Obstetrics & Gynecology and Reproductive Biology*, vol. 158, no. 2, pp. 265–268, 2011.

[11] G. Navarra, G. L. Malfa, L. Salvatore, U. Gabriele, and C. Giuseppe, "SILS and NOTES cholecystectomy: a tailored approach," *Journal of Laparoendoscopic and Advanced Surgical Techniques*, vol. 20, no. 6, pp. 511–514, 2010.

[12] T. E. Langwieler, T. Nimmesgern, and M. Back, "Single-port access in laparoscopic cholecystectomy," *Surgical Endoscopy and Other Interventional Techniques*, vol. 23, no. 5, pp. 1138–1141, 2009.

[13] H. C. Tai, C. D. Lin, C. C. Wu, Y. C. Tsai, and S. S. Yang, "Homemade transumbilical port: an alternative access for laparoendoscopic single-site surgery (LESS)," *Surgical Endoscopy and Other Interventional Techniques*, vol. 24, no. 3, pp. 705–708, 2010.

[14] R. Sinha, "Single-incision laparoscopic transabdominal preperitoneal inguinal hernia repair using only conventional instruments: an initial report," *Journal of Laparoendoscopic and Advanced Surgical Techniques*, vol. 21, no. 4, pp. 335–340, 2011.

[15] J. Paek, E. J. Nam, Y. T. Kim, and S. W. Kim, "Overcoming technical difficulties with single-port access laparoscopic surgery in gynecology: using conventional laparoscopic instruments," *Journal of Laparoendoscopic and Advanced Surgical Techniques*, vol. 21, no. 2, pp. 137–141, 2011.

[16] M. Hayashi, M. Asakuma, K. Komeda, Y. Miyamoto, F. Hirokawa, and N. Tanigawa, "Effectiveness of a surgical glove port for single port surgery," *World Journal of Surgery*, vol. 34, no. 10, pp. 2487–2489, 2010.

[17] N. Garcia-Henriquez, S. R. Shah, and T. D. Kane, "Single-incision laparoscopic cholecystectomy in children using standard straight instruments: a surgeon's early experience," *Journal of Laparoendoscopic and Advanced Surgical Techniques*, vol. 21, no. 6, pp. 555–559, 2011.

[18] K. E. Roberts, D. Solomon, A. J. Duffy, and R. L. Bell, "Single-incision laparoscopic cholecystectomy: a surgeon's initial experience with 56 consecutive cases and a review of the literature," *Journal of Gastrointestinal Surgery*, vol. 14, no. 3, pp. 506–510, 2010.

[19] Y. Bayazit, I. A. Aridogan, D. Abat, N. Satar, and S. Doran, "Pediatric transumbilical laparoendoscopic single-site nephroureterectomy: initial report," *Urology*, vol. 74, no. 5, pp. 1116–1119, 2009.

[20] E. R. Podolsky and P. G. Curcillo II, "Single port access (SPA) surgery—a 24-month experience," *Journal of Gastrointestinal Surgery*, vol. 14, no. 5, pp. 759–767, 2010.

[21] D. Surico, S. Gentilli, A. Vigone, E. Paulli, L. Leo, and N. Surico, "Laparoendoscopic single-site surgery for treatment of concomitant ovarian cystectomy and cholecystectomy," *Journal of Minimally Invasive Gynecology*, vol. 17, no. 5, pp. 656–659, 2010.

[22] S. Hart, S. Ross, and A. Rosemurgy, "Laparoendoscopic single-site combined cholecystectomy and hysterectomy," *Journal of Minimally Invasive Gynecology*, vol. 17, no. 6, pp. 798–801, 2010.

[23] C. C. Gunderson, J. Knight, J. Ybanez-Morano et al., "The risk of umbilical hernia and other complications with laparoendoscopic single-site surgery," *Journal of Minimally Invasive Gynecology*, vol. 19, no. 1, pp. 40–45, 2012.

[24] H. S. Park, T. J. Kim, T. Song et al., "Single-port access (SPA) laparoscopic surgery in gynecology: a surgeon's experience with an initial 200 cases," *European Journal of Obstetrics Gynecology and Reproductive Biology*, vol. 154, no. 1, pp. 81–84, 2011.

[25] P. F. Escobar, D. C. Starks, A. N. Fader, M. Barber, and L. Rojas-Espalliat, "Single-port risk-reducing salpingo-oophorectomy with and without hysterectomy: surgical outcomes and learning curve analysis," *Gynecologic Oncology*, vol. 119, no. 1, pp. 43–47, 2010.

18

3D Printing Applications in Minimally Invasive Spine Surgery

Megan R. Hsu,[1] Meraaj S. Haleem,[2] and Wellington Hsu[2]

[1]Department of Orthopedic Surgery, Beaumont Hospital Research Institute, 3811 West 13 Mile Road, Suite #404, Royal Oak, MI 48073, USA
[2]Department of Orthopedic Surgery, Northwestern University Feinberg School of Medicine, 676 Saint Clair St. Suite #1350, Chicago, IL 60611, USA

Correspondence should be addressed to Wellington Hsu; wkhsu@yahoo.com

Academic Editor: Brian J. Dlouhy

3D printing (3DP) technology continues to gain popularity among medical specialties as a useful tool to improve patient care. The field of spine surgery is one discipline that has utilized this; however, information regarding the use of 3DP in minimally invasive spine surgery (MISS) is limited. 3D printing is currently being utilized in spine surgery to create biomodels, hardware templates and guides, and implants. Minimally invasive spine surgeons have begun to adopt 3DP technology, specifically with the use of biomodeling to optimize preoperative planning. Factors limiting widespread adoption of 3DP include increased time, cost, and the limited range of diagnoses in which 3DP has thus far been utilized. 3DP technology has become a valuable tool utilized by spine surgeons, and there are limitless directions in which this technology can be applied to minimally invasive spine surgery.

1. Introduction

Additive manufacturing (AM) techniques such as 3D printing (3DP) have been recently used in many disciplines of medicine including the field of spine surgery. More specifically, 3DP pertains to several possible applications in the field of minimally invasive spine surgery including use as biomodels, surgical guides, and implants. 3DP biomodels have the potential to improve preoperative planning and to be used as a valuable teaching tool; surgical guides can increase hardware placement accuracy and precision; implants can be custom designed to fit patient anatomy as well as improve upon the biologic characteristics compared to existing manufacturing methods. This review will delineate the potential for 3DP technology to optimize patient outcomes during minimally invasive spine surgery, as well as current challenges limiting widespread implementation.

2. Background

Additive manufacturing such as 3DP utilizes a digital computer-aided design to build a 3-dimensional model by adding successive layers of material rather than through subtractive manufacturing, potentially leading to decreased manufacturing waste (Figure 1) [1].

The idea of using 2D imaging modalities to construct a 3D anatomical model was first described in 1979, and the technology has expanded widely in the medical field since that time [2]. Oral and maxillofacial surgery and orthopedic surgery were two of the first subspecialties to report the use of 3D printing [3]. Its use in the field of spine surgery was first described in 1999 to print models of the entire spine to assist in visualization of complex deformity cases [4].

Since the advent of rapid prototyping (RP), 3DP has become an increasingly valuable adjunct for surgical specialties by facilitating the creation of a wide variety of surgical tools including patient-specific anatomic models, hardware, and cutting guides, as well as implants and prosthetics. As this technology becomes more prevalent, costs are expected to decrease while ease of use will simultaneously increase, and together these factors have the potential to fuel a rapid growth in its adoption [3].

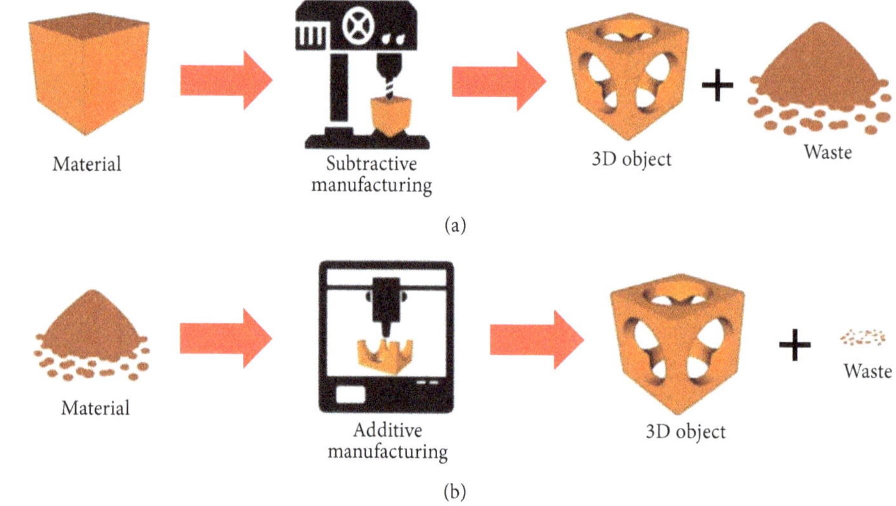

FIGURE 1: (a) Subtractive manufacturing versus (b) additive manufacturing (source: reproduced and adapted with permission from Ambrosi et al.).

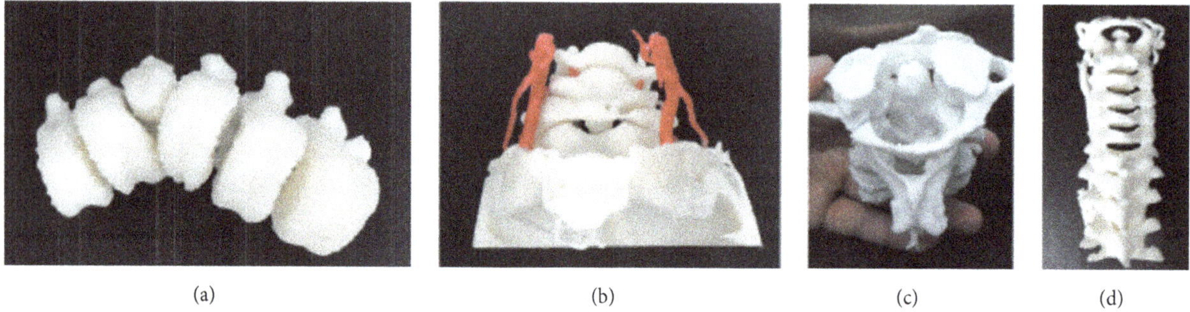

FIGURE 2: (a) Scoliosis. (b) Atlas neoplasm. (c) and (d) Cervical fracture-dislocation (source: reproduced and adapted with permission from Wang et al.).

3. Biomodels

3DP biomodeling involves the translation of traditional 2D images into a patient-specific anatomic model, which offers several advantages over standard imaging modalities. Izatt et al. quantified orthopedic spinal surgeons' perceptions of the usefulness of biomodels compared to standard 2D imaging modalities in treating patients with either complex spinal deformities or spinal tumors. The biomodels were used both for preoperative planning and intraoperative anatomical reference, and it was reported that anatomical details were more visible on the biomodel in 65% of cases and exclusively visible on the biomodel in 11% of cases [5]. Furthermore, use of a 3D biomodel preoperatively led to alternative decision-making regarding the choice of materials used in over half of the cases and the implantation site in 74% of cases and reduced operating time by an average of 22% [5]. These data support biomodeling as a useful, and sometimes essential, imaging tool used for complex spinal surgery.

Biomodeling in spine surgery has the potential to play a significant role in preoperative planning. The ability to interact with a patient's anatomy in a tactile manner prior to the procedure itself produces several tangible benefits including reduced operative time, lower blood loss, and reduced transfusion volumes [6–8]. Furthermore, the creation of such biomodels allows surgeons to optimize their intraoperative hardware placement prior to the time of surgery, especially in patients with complex anatomical pathologies including rheumatoid arthritis and complex scoliosis [6, 9, 10]. A retrospective review compared 50 patients who had 3DP spinal biomodels composed of polystyrene created prior to surgical correction of Lenke Type 1 adolescent idiopathic scoliosis with 76 patients who received the standard of care (no biomodeling) and showed that the treatment group had a significantly ($p = 0.02$) decreased rate of pedicle screw misplacement in patients with a Cobb angle of >50 degrees [6]. Additionally, 4 complex patients who had congenital scoliosis, an atlas neoplasm, atlantoaxial dislocation, and an atlantoaxial fracture-dislocation were treated with the aid of 3D printed photosensitive resin biomodels created prior to surgery (Figure 2) [11].

Postoperative imaging in these 4 patients demonstrated that no pedicle penetration or screw misplacement took place, again demonstrating the use of biomodels to assist surgeons in treating patients suffering from complex anatomical pathologies.

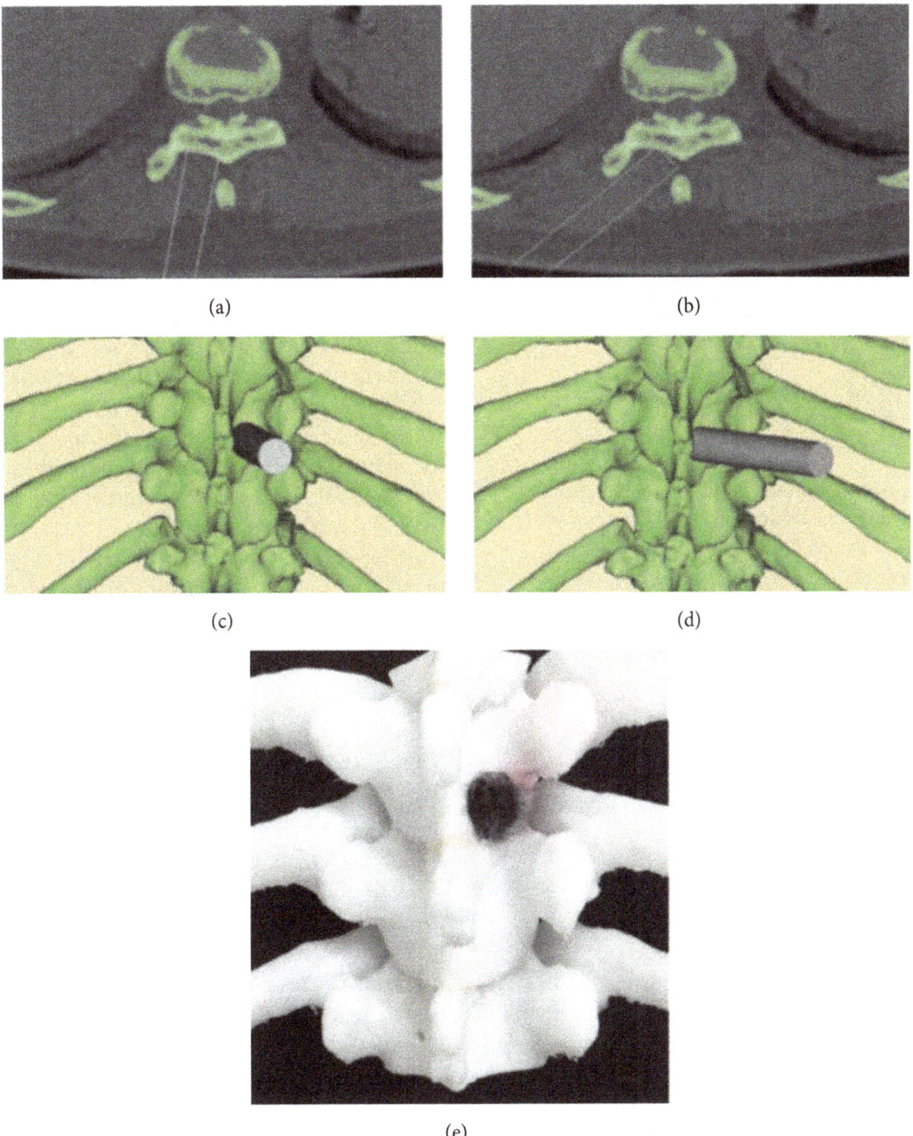

FIGURE 3: Surgical simulation demonstrating virtual channel placement (a–d). 3DP thoracic vertebra for preoperative planning (e) (source: reproduced and adapted with permission from Zhao et al.).

Minimally invasive spine surgery (MISS) has unique clinical challenges surgeons encounter on a daily basis, such as small exposure corridors, difficult visualization, minute working spaces, and a steep learning curve paired with low tolerability for error [12]. In response, biomodels can provide MIS surgeons with tactile feedback and facilitate the means to understand complex patient anatomy during the preoperative planning phase. One example of this application is treatment of thoracic ossification of the ligamentum flavum (TOLF) using biomodel assisted MISS. This approach was utilized in a study of 13 patients who each had 3D biomodels of their spinal anatomy created prior to microsurgical decompression of TOLF (Figure 3) [13]. The biomodel was utilized to determine anatomical variations between patients, preoperatively optimize the angle of insertion of percutaneous tubular retractors, and delineate the location and size of the relevant bony spaces to reduce damage to adjacent muscles, tendons, and bones.

A similar approach was taken to assist in the case of a 66-year-old man with T10-T12 OLF in whom a biomodel was printed during the preoperative planning phase. The surgeons utilized this model to verify their osteotomy angle, as well as confirm the size, location, and boundaries of the OLF [14].

Because the successful mastery of MISS skills requires a thorough understanding of 3D spinal architecture, there is a steep learning curve for these procedures [12]. Potential complications include durotomy, implant malpositioning, and neural injury. 3DP biomodels have the potential to play an important role in the training of new surgeons by illuminating the intricate anatomy and architecture of the spine that cannot be simulated using alternate modalities. By providing real-time, tactile feedback, these models can

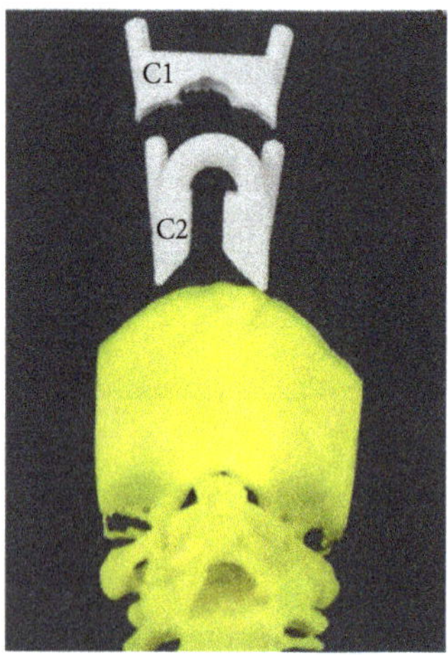

FIGURE 4: 3DP drill guide custom designed to fit a biomodel of 57-year-old male with atlantoaxial dislocation (source: reproduced and adapted with permission from Guo et al.).

accelerate the comfort and familiarity of early adopting surgeons in working within this space. For example, published experiences in the use of 3DP models in other diagnoses such as aortic aneurysms have led to better scores on a preoperative assessment compared to counterparts who used traditional CT imaging [15].

4. Guides and Templates

3DP can facilitate the creation of patient-specific guides and templates, which can aid preoperative planning thereby increasing the accuracy and precision of hardware placement intraoperatively. The mechanism for this usually utilizes a computed tomography scan of the spine that can then be translated into a 3DP guide or template. Potential benefits include shorter operating room times and reduction of radiation exposure to the patient and the surgical team [8, 16–18]. Also, 3D-printed screw placement guides have demonstrated superior accuracy in the placement of pedicle and laminar screws in several studies, thereby increasing patient safety and clinical outcomes [17, 19, 20]. In one study by Merc et al., the incidence of cortex perforation was found to be significantly reduced in the group utilizing a 3DP template versus freehand screw placement under fluoroscopic guidance [21]. Furthermore, a study by Lu et al. utilized a reverse engineered biomodel and 3DP lumbar pedicle drill guide, which was used to place screws in 6 patients [22]. The drill template precisely fit over all patients' anatomy, allowing for rapid template positioning, drilling, and screw placement. Postoperative CT imaging demonstrated a high degree of precision and accuracy as all drill trajectories and screw placements were found to be in their optimal locations. Another study by Guo et al. compared the efficacy of using 3DP guided screw placement in the upper cervical spine (atlas and axis) versus traditional placement under fluoroscopy (Figures 4 and 5) [23].

Screws placed using the 3DP guide demonstrated increased placement accuracy with reduced pedicle cortex perforation and reduced operation time and fluoroscopic frequency when compared with traditional placement. Together, these studies demonstrate the benefits of 3DP templates, which include efficient, accurate, and precise drill trajectories and screw placement, which can lead to faster surgery times and improved patient outcomes.

3DP templates and guides have a number of applications to minimally invasive spine procedures. Specific examples of such applications include minimizing exposure sites and incision size, navigating variable patient anatomy, and patient-specific instrumentation. First, 3DP may allow for smaller templates and guides, which in conjunction with optimized drill trajectories would promote smaller incisions and exposures. The ultimate goal in this arena would be the construction of a device that fits externally on the patient's body that guides drill trajectories and screw placement without the need for invasive exposures. However, drawbacks do exist with the use of smaller, more precise instruments. For example, although smaller guides and templates minimize native tissue disruption, there is the simultaneous risk that smaller exposures and instrumentation may preclude proper hardware fit and placement. Surgeons utilizing minimally invasive techniques should be aware of the tradeoffs that exist in using these tools.

Another critical application to MISS is within the arena of craniocervical surgery, where anatomical structures can be highly variable between patients [24]. Drill templates and trajectories that can be optimized prior to surgery would be invaluable in navigating within this intricate anatomical space and could mitigate the risks of vertebral artery injury, a potentially life threatening complication. A future application of 3DP guides and templates may be patient-specific instrumentation to work specifically within the unique architecture of each patient's anatomy. One possible example would be the introduction of biologics in a small posterior interbody space, where a surgeon could use 3DP instruments that are unique to the size of that patient's disc and opening space. The specificity of such instruments may facilitate the use of MISS in cases where patient anatomy precluded the use of such techniques beforehand. In all of these examples, the use of 3DP can ease the difficulty of placing hardware or biologics in compressed spaces and under limited visibility.

5. Implants

3D printing can also contribute to MISS by creating custom-designed and patient-specific implants for insertion. Furthermore, these processes allow for fine tuning of material characteristics and can serve as a platform for tissue engineered scaffolds to promote bone healing [25, 26].

Examples include a custom printed spinal prosthesis for a posterior C1-C2 fusion in a 65-year-old female patient as well as a prosthesis to reconstruct the C2 vertebrae in a pediatric patient with ewing sarcoma (Figures 6 and 7) [27, 28].

In another case, investigators created a custom spinal fusion cage with patient-specific dimensions using the patient's CT scan data [29]. The goal was to create an implant that was custom fit to the patient's vertebral body endplates. Researchers first made a 3D reconstruction of the patient's spine from their CT DICOM and subsequently restored sagittal balance by adjusting the lordotic angle of the proposed

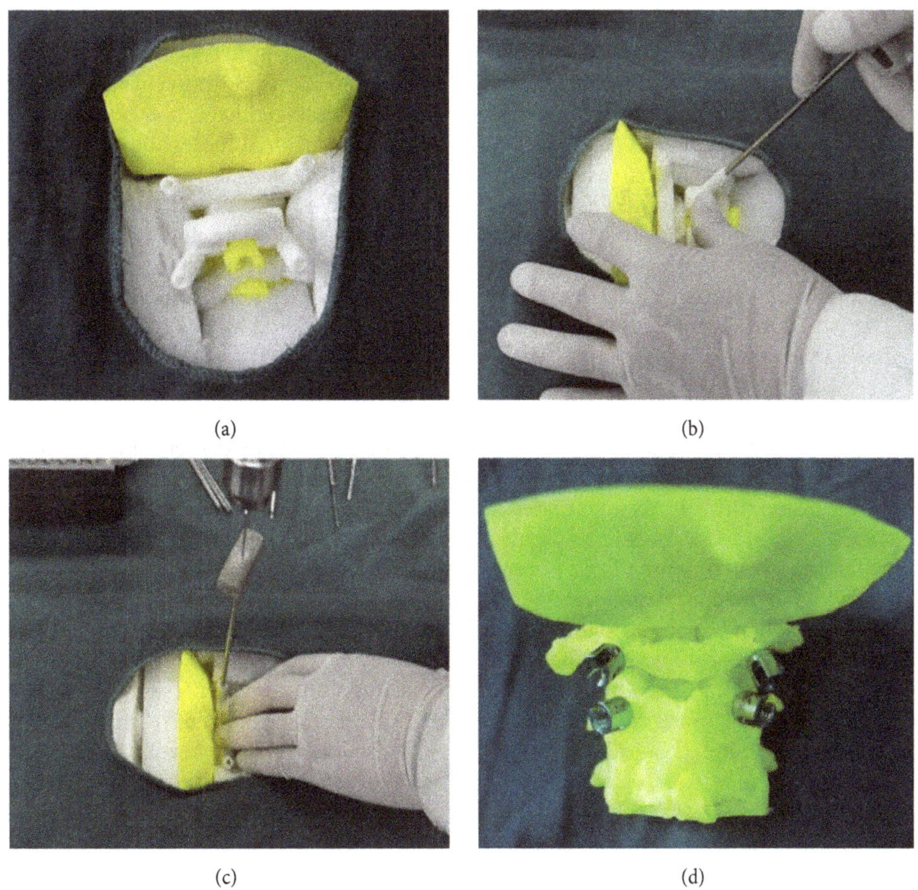

FIGURE 5: Navigation template-assisted pedicle screw fixation in upper cervical spine. (a) Navigation template pressed to fit with vertebra. (b) Placement of navigation protective sleeve. (c) Kirschner wire perforated along protective sleeve. (d) Pedicle screw fixation (source: reproduced and adapted with permission from Guo et al.).

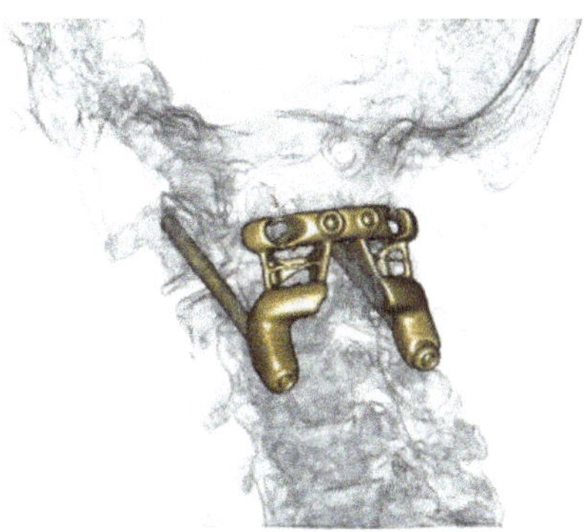

FIGURE 6: CT with proposed 3DP titanium C1-C2 prosthesis overlaid (source: reproduced and adapted with permission from Phan et al.).

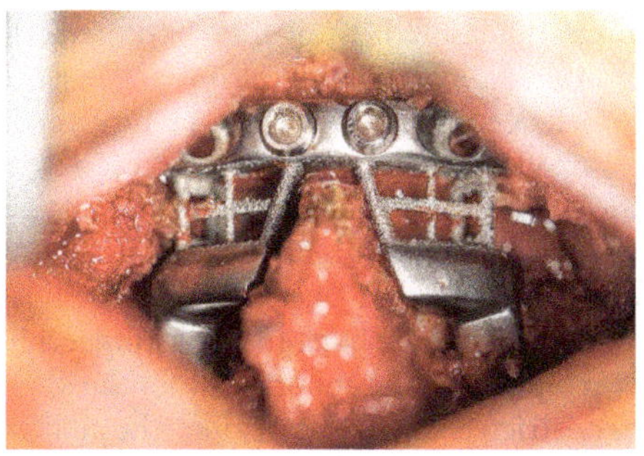

FIGURE 7: Intraoperative implantation of 3DP custom printed spinal prosthesis for a posterior C1-C2 fusion (source: reproduced and adapted with permission from Phan et al.).

implant. The 3D model also allowed for simulated osteophyte removal and implant placement preoperatively. The custom-designed titanium cage was manufactured using additive manufacturing direct metal printing (DMP) technology. In all cases, patient-specific implant rendering can maximize anatomic fit of the device and minimize the chance of implant drift or subsidence.

3DP implants can also be created from different materials with customizable stiffness and porosity, allowing them to maximize bony ingrowth and osseointegration [30]. McGilvray et al. directly compared the bony ingrowth potential and biomechanical properties of a novel 3DP porous titanium alloy (PTA) interbody cage with commercially available polyetheretherketone (PEEK) and plasma sprayed porous titanium coated PEEK (PSP) interbody cages in an ovine lumbar interbody fusion model [31]. Investigators reported a statistically significant decrease in flexion-extension range of motion upon biomechanical testing, and a statistically significant increase in stiffness in the PTA cages compared to PEEK and PSP cages ($p = 0.02$ and $p \leq 0.01$, resp.). MicroCT revealed a statistically significant increase in bone volume ($p < 0.01$) of PTA cages compared to PEEK and PSP cages at 8-week and 16-week time points. Authors attribute these findings to increased peri-implant osteogenesis evident on histomorphometric analysis, theorizing that increased ingrowth across the osteoconductive surface provided by the 3DP PTA cage contributes to increased implant stability and fusion-promotion.

Investigative 3DP spinal implants have been applied to fusion, artificial disc, and SI joint implants. In a proof of concept model with the goal of reducing reoperation rates in minimally invasive SI joint fusion, investigators compared a 3D-printed, additive manufactured (AM), porous triangular implant with a solid titanium plasma spray (TPS) porous coated implant in a bilateral ovine distal femoral defect model. They found that AM implants displayed significantly more bony ingrowth into the device's core versus superficial ingrowth with the TPS coated implant. Authors suggest the increased porosity of AM implants more closely mimics native bone and may enhance the biomechanical stability in MIS SI joint fusion [32].

Finally, this manufacturing technology has been used to promote bone regeneration without the need for autografts, allografts, or exogenous factors such as BMP-2. The use of autografts and allografts is limited due to donor site pain, increased morbidity, limited availability, and the potential for disease transmission, while rh-BMP2 can cause significant complications at supraphysiologic doses [33–35]. Jakus et al. utilized 3DP to produce hyperelastic "bone" (HB) which is a synthetic biomimetic with similar elastic properties to native bone. In this study, HB not only supported cell growth, but also promoted differentiation of BMSCs *in vitro* without the aid of osteogenic factors in the culture media. Jakus et al. additionally found higher mean fusion scores with a HB scaffold in a rat PL fusion model versus a collagen scaffold control [36]. The ability to 3D-print a synthetic, growth-factor-free material may represent a superior and safer method to regenerate bone than existing techniques.

These examples provide opportunity for the MIS surgeon. Given the constricted working corridors, the ability to create hardware and biologics specific to the patient's anatomy could prove invaluable. The capacity to fine-tune the osteoinductive nature of implantable materials would decrease pseudarthrosis rates, which is a known complication from these types of procedures. The reduction of operative times, the need to retract surrounding neural structures, and nonunion rates are all exciting potential benefits of this technology for the MIS surgeon.

5.1. "Off-the-Shelf" Implants. In addition to its uses to develop custom, patient-specific implants, 3DP technology is also being used to optimize the geometric properties of premade "Off-the-Shelf" (OTS) implants [37]. As described previously by McGilvray et al., the customizable porosity and stiffness of 3DP materials can more closely mimic native bone and facilitate bony ingrowth [30–32]. OTS products are created by premanufacturing implants with a wide variety of sizes and fits, thus reducing the additional time required for additional imaging studies and custom implant printing [37]. Therefore, the core appeal of 3DP implants, namely, their customizable porosity and dimensions, is maintained, while also making 3DP technology more cost-effective and less time intensive. In all, this process would make 3DP implants more widely available, while still conferring the unique structural advantages offered by this emerging technology.

6. Limitations

Despite the benefits conferred by the use of 3DP in surgery, barriers remain that have precluded its widespread adoption. Among the most significant of these barriers appears to be the additional cost incurred in utilizing 3DP technology (including start-up, cleaning, and maintenance), the time required to develop the 3DP device, and the lack of data supporting the use of 3DP for routine procedures [38, 39]. 3DP remains a highly specialized process that requires significant capital investments in complex design software, cameras, and the 3D printing machine itself [39]. The price of such an investment may reduce a hospital's willingness to adopt 3DP as well as inflicting a prohibitive cost burden upon the patient. By reducing the demand for such technology from both the hospital and patient side, the financial burdens of 3DP have severely curtailed its adoption on a wider scale.

Additionally, the amount of time required to develop 3DP devices is not insignificant. The process for creating a single device for a patient may involve additional imaging procedures, development in the 3D modeling space, and the printing of the device itself [39]. These lengthy time requirements may deter patients who cannot or will not tolerate additional time spent in a clinical environment.

Lastly, the benefits for 3DP in spine surgery have thus far been limited to complex cases that are handled by a very limited number of specialized surgeons [38]. This technology has provided surgeons with an unparalleled ability to provide patient-specific interventions in such cases. However, not all spine surgery cases possess the complexity to require this degree of specificity, and the benefits provided by 3DP are not always translatable. As such, 3D printing technology currently exists in relatively niche cases, which reduces its market potential and generalizability and limits its overall use.

7. Conclusion

The use of 3D printing in the field of spine surgery is rapidly evolving, including its emerging use to enhance the field of minimally invasive spine surgery. Potential applications are myriad and include biomodels, surgical guides, and implants. Biomodels can assist with preoperative planning, mitigate the complications incurred during the initial learning curve associated with MISS, and serve to increase patient understanding and satisfaction. 3D printed surgical guides can improve accuracy and specificity in hardware placement. Lastly, 3D-printed implants promote superior fit and osteoinductivity, which work synergistically with the principles of minimal disruption that underlies MISS. Although cost, time, and the relatively specialized market are currently inhibiting widespread adoption of 3DP technology, it is nonetheless a valuable area that merits ongoing research.

References

[1] J. Alcisto, A. Enriquez, H. Garcia et al., "Tensile properties and microstructures of laser-formed Ti-6Al-4V," *Journal of Materials Engineering and Performance*, vol. 20, no. 2, pp. 203–212, 2011.

[2] C. Alberti, "Three-dimensional CT and structure models.," *British Journal of Radiology*, vol. 53, no. 627, pp. 261-262, 1980.

[3] D. Hoang et al., "Surgical applications of three-dimensional printing: a review of the current literature & how to get started," *Annals of Translational Medicine*, vol. 4, no. 23, 2016.

[4] P. S. D'Urso, O. D. Williamson, and R. G. Thompson, "Biomodeling as an aid to spinal instrumentation," *The Spine Journal*, vol. 30, no. 24, pp. 2841–2845, 2005.

[5] M. T. Izatt, P. L. P. J. Thorpe, R. G. Thompson et al., "The use of physical biomodelling in complex spinal surgery," *European Spine Journal*, vol. 16, no. 9, pp. 1507–1518, 2007.

[6] M. Yang, C. Li, Y. Li et al., "Application of 3D rapid prototyping technology in posterior corrective surgery for Lenke 1 adolescent idiopathic scoliosis patients," *Medicine*, vol. 94, no. 8, 2015.

[7] J. Guarino, S. Tennyson, G. McCain, L. Bond, K. Shea, and H. King, "Rapid prototyping technology for surgeries of the pediatric spine and pelvis: Benefits analysis," *Journal of Pediatric Orthopaedics*, vol. 27, no. 8, pp. 955–960, 2007.

[8] P. Tack, J. Victor, P. Gemmel, and L. Annemans, "3D-printing techniques in a medical setting: A systematic literature review," *Biomedical Engineering Online*, vol. 15, no. 1, p. 115, 2016.

[9] K. Mao, Y. Wang, S. Xiao et al., "Clinical application of computer-designed polystyrene models in complex severe spinal deformities: A pilot study," *European Spine Journal*, vol. 19, no. 5, pp. 797–802, 2010.

[10] J. Mizutani, T. Matsubara, M. Fukuoka et al., "Application of full-scale three-dimensional models in patients with rheumatoid cervical spine," *European Spine Journal*, vol. 17, no. 5, pp. 644–649, 2008.

[11] Y.-T. Wang, X.-J. Yang, B. Yan, T.-H. Zeng, Y.-Y. Qiu, and S.-J. Chen, "Clinical application of three-dimensional printing in the personalized treatment of complex spinal disorders," *Chinese Journal of Traumatology (English Edition)*, vol. 19, no. 1, pp. 31–34, 2016.

[12] Z. A. Smith and R. G. Fessler, "Paradigm changes in spine surgery-evolution of minimally invasive techniques," *Nature Reviews Neurology*, vol. 8, no. 8, pp. 443–450, 2012.

[13] W. Zhao, C. Shen, R. Cai et al., "Minimally invasive surgery for resection of ossification of the ligamentum flavum in the thoracic spine," *Wideochirurgia i Inne Techniki Maloinwazyjne*, vol. 12, no. 1, pp. 96–105, 2017.

[14] Q. Ling, E. He, H. Ouyang, J. Guo, Z. Yin, and W. Huang, "Design of mulitlevel OLF approach ("V"-shaped decompressive laminoplasty) based on 3D printing technology," *European Spine Journal*, pp. 1–7, 2017.

[15] C. Wilasrusmee, J. Suvikrom, J. Suthakorn et al., "Three-dimensional aortic aneurysm model and endovascular repair: An educational tool for surgical trainees," *International Journal of Angiology*, vol. 17, no. 3, pp. 129–133, 2008.

[16] Y. Kawaguchi, M. Nakano, T. Yasuda, S. Seki, T. Hori, and T. Kimura, "Development of a new technique for pedicle screw and magerl screw insertion using a 3-dimensional image guide," *The Spine Journal*, vol. 37, no. 23, pp. 1983–1988, 2012.

[17] S. Lu, Y. Q. Xu, W. W. Lu et al., "A novel patient-specific navigational template for cervical pedicle screw placement," *The Spine Journal*, vol. 34, no. 26, pp. E959–E964, 2009.

[18] T. Sugawara, N. Higashiyama, S. Kaneyama et al., "Multistep pedicle screw insertion procedure with patient-specific lamina fit-and-lock templates for the thoracic spine: Clinical article," *Journal of Neurosurgery: Spine*, vol. 19, no. 2, pp. 185–190, 2013.

[19] S. Kaneyama, T. Sugawara, and M. Sumi, "Safe and accurate midcervical pedicle screw insertion procedure with the patient-specific screw guide template system," *The Spine Journal*, vol. 40, no. 6, pp. E341–E348, 2015.

[20] S. Lu, Y. Q. Xu, Y. Z. Zhang, L. Xie, H. Guo, and D. P. Li, "A novel computer-assisted drill guide template for placement of C2 laminar screws," *European Spine Journal*, vol. 18, no. 9, pp. 1379–1385, 2009.

[21] M. Merc, I. Drstvensek, M. Vogrin, T. Brajlih, and G. Recnik, "A multi-level rapid prototyping drill guide template reduces the perforation risk of pedicle screw placement in the lumbar and sacral spine," *Archives of Orthopaedic and Trauma Surgery*, vol. 133, no. 7, pp. 893–899, 2013.

[22] S. Lu, Y. Q. Xu, Y. Z. Zhang et al., "Rapid prototyping drill guide template for lumbar pedicle screw placement," *Chinese Journal of Traumatology*, vol. 12, no. 3, pp. 177–180, 2009.

[23] F. Guo, J. Dai, J. Zhang et al., "Individualized 3D printing navigation template for pedicle screw fixation in upper cervical spine," *PLoS ONE*, vol. 12, no. 2, Article ID e0171509, 2017.

[24] P. H. Maughan, A. F. Ducruet, A. M. Elhadi et al., "Multimodality management of vertebral artery injury sustained during cervical or craniocervical surgery," *Neurosurgery*, vol. 73, no. suppl_2, pp. ons271–ons282, 2013.

[25] E. Provaggi, J. J. H. Leong, and D. M. Kalaskar, "Applications of 3D printing in the management of severe spinal conditions," *Proceedings of the Institution of Mechanical Engineers, Part H: Journal of Engineering in Medicine*, vol. 231, no. 6, pp. 471–486, 2017.

[26] A. E. Jakus and R. N. Shah, "Multi and mixed 3D-printing of graphene-hydroxyapatite hybrid materials for complex tissue engineering," *Journal of Biomedical Materials Research Part A*, vol. 105, no. 1, pp. 274–283, 2017.

[27] K. Phan, A. Sgro, M. M. Maharaj, P. D'Urso, and R. J. Mobbs, "Application of a 3D custom printed patient specific spinal implant for C1/2 arthrodesis," *Journal of Spine Surgery*, vol. 2, no. 4, pp. 314–318, 2016.

[28] N. Xu, F. Wei, X. Liu et al., "Reconstruction of the upper cervical spine using a personalized 3D-printed vertebral body in an adolescent with ewing sarcoma," *The Spine Journal*, vol. 41, no. 1, pp. E50–E54, 2016.

[29] U. Spetzger, M. Frasca, and S. A. König, "Surgical planning, manufacturing and implantation of an individualized cervical fusion titanium cage using patient-specific data," *European Spine Journal*, vol. 25, no. 7, pp. 2239–2246, 2016.

[30] X. Wang, S. Xu, S. Zhou et al., "Topological design and additive manufacturing of porous metals for bone scaffolds and orthopaedic implants: a review," *Biomaterials*, vol. 83, no. 6, pp. 127–141, 2016.

[31] K. McGilvray, J. Easley, H. B. Seim et al., "Bony ingrowth potential of 3D printed porous titanium alloy: a direct comparison of interbody cage materials in an in vivo ovine lumbar fusion model," *The Spine Journal*, 2018.

[32] R. F. MacBarb, D. P. Lindsey, S. A. Woods, P. A. Lalor, M. I. Gundanna, and S. A. Yerby, "Fortifying the bone-implant interface part 2: An in vivo evaluation of 3D-printed and TPS-coated triangular implants," *International Journal of Spine Surgery*, vol. 11, no. 3, pp. 116–128, 2017.

[33] C. A. Tannoury and H. S. An, "Complications with the use of bone morphogenetic protein 2 (BMP-2) in spine surgery," *The Spine Journal*, vol. 14, no. 3, pp. 552–559, 2014.

[34] A. Gupta, N. Kukkar, K. Sharif, B. J. Main, C. E. Albers, and S. F. El-Amin, "Bone graft substitutes for spine fusion: A brief review," *World Journal of Orthopedics*, vol. 6, no. 6, pp. 449–456, 2015.

[35] S. D. Boden, "The ABCs of BMPs," *Orthopaedic Nursing*, vol. 24, no. 1, pp. 49–52, quiz 53-54, 2005.

[36] A. E. Jakus, A. L. Rutz, S. W. Jordan et al., "Hyperelastic "bone": A highly versatile, growth factor-free, osteoregenerative, scalable, and surgically friendly biomaterial," *Science Translational Medicine*, vol. 8, no. 358, Article ID 358ra128, p. 358ra127, 2016.

[37] B. Wilcox, R. J. Mobbs, A. Wu, and K. Phan, "Systematic review of 3D printing in spinal surgery: the current state of play," *Journal of Spine Surgery*, vol. 3, no. 3, pp. 433–443, 2017.

[38] C. A. Grant, M. T. Izatt, R. D. Labrom, G. N. Askin, and V. Glatt, "Use of 3D Printing in Complex Spinal Surgery: Historical Perspectives, Current Usage, and Future Directions," *Techniques in Orthopaedics*, vol. 31, no. 3, pp. 172–180, 2016.

[39] N. Martelli, C. Serrano, H. Van Den Brink et al., "Advantages and disadvantages of 3-dimensional printing in surgery: A systematic review," *Surgery*, vol. 159, no. 6, pp. 1485–1500, 2016.

19

The Role of VATS in Lung Cancer Surgery: Current Status and Prospects for Development

Dariusz Dziedzic and Tadeusz Orlowski

Department of Thoracic Surgery, National Research Institute of Chest Diseases, Warsaw, Poland

Correspondence should be addressed to Dariusz Dziedzic; drdariuszdziedzic@gmail.com

Academic Editor: Stephen Kavic

Since the introduction of anatomic lung resection by video-assisted thoracoscopic surgery (VATS) 20 years ago, VATS has experienced major advances in both equipment and technique, introducing a technical challenge in the surgical treatment of both benign and malignant lung disease. The demonstrated safety, decreased morbidity, and equivalent efficacy of this minimally invasive technique have led to the acceptance of VATS as a standard surgical modality for early-stage lung cancer and increasing application to more advanced disease. Formerly there was much debate about the feasibility of the technique in cancer surgery and proper lymph node handling. Although there is a lack of proper randomized studies, it is now generally accepted that the outcome of a VATS procedure is at least not inferior to a resection via a traditional thoracotomy.

1. Introduction

The concept of thoracoscopy was first described in 1910 by Jacobaeus, an internist, for the management of pleural effusion with a urological cystoscope [1]. A simple cystoscope was used, with a rigid working channel and an illumination source at its end, with which the pleural space could be directly visualised. The procedure was performed under local anaesthesia. In the years to follow, thoracoscopy has become a common therapeutic procedure for the lysis of pleural pulmonary adhesions caused by tuberculosis during collapse therapy to create a pneumothorax. The number of thoracoscopy procedures in tuberculosis has decreased with the introduction of streptomycin in 1945 as the first effective antituberculosis chemotherapy. In the following years, thoracoscopy has been mainly used for diagnosis. New methods of diagnostic imaging utilizing improved light delivery system and the newly developed diagnostic imaging devices combining a hollow tube and a camera to transmit image to a screen to capture images of the operating field have prompted the development of thoracoscopic techniques. The notion of video-assisted thoracoscopic surgery (VATS) has emerged. VATS continued to evolve in close connection with technical advancements in imaging techniques and the refinement of surgical instruments, which made room for new indications for VATS. The introduction of a "cold" halogen light source was another major step in enhancing the visualization of anatomical structures. This was a major development in VATS since the blood in the operation field would absorb up to 50% of the light [2]. Angled lens were another improvement that helped visualize anatomic structures that are difficult to access. Another milestone in VATS development was the introduction of endostaplers. Presenting endostaplers guided by VATS opened the way for effective and safe lung parenchyma through a tiny incision. From then on, video-assisted thoracoscopy (VATS) has been gaining popularity in thoracic surgery not only in diagnosis, but also in the management of pneumothorax, resection of small pulmonary nodules, or in the treatment of thoracic injuries. This is how VATS (video-assisted thoracic surgery) emerged and evolved, which many surgeons believe is clearly distinct from traditional thoracoscopy. The first ever large-scale symposium dedicated to VATS was staged by the Society of Thoracic Surgeons in San Antonio, Texas, in January 1992 [3].

Also in 1992, the first anatomic resection was performed with VATS [4]. The main idea behind popularization of VATS was to significantly reduce procedure-related injury and complications that frequently accompanied traditional open thoracotomies.

2. Definition

VATS has no universally recognised definition. In general, a variety of different VATS techniques is used. The procedure of lung resection in cancer patients is referred to as VATS lobectomy. The essential assumptions of VATS lobectomy are to make 1.5–2 cm access incisions for 2 to 4 thoracoscopic ports, and 2–6 cm access incisions in the anterior part of the thorax for a minithoracotomy (utility incision). Number of ports (with 1, 2, or 3) through which surgical instruments are inserted varies and depends on the experience of the surgeon. The VATS approach does not require any rib spreading, resulting in a less invasive injury in the intercostal space. The length of the access incision was observed to have no significant effect on the rates of procedure-related complications. In international literature, there are two types of VATS procedures distinguished: c-VATS (complete VATS) and a-VATS (assisted VATS). In completely video-assisted thoracoscopic surgery (cVATS), the procedure is done under control of a video camera and with instruments inserted through the thoracoscopic access ports. In assisted video-assisted thoracoscopic surgery (aVATS), the procedure is performed through video-assisted minithoracotomy [5]. The development of both c-VATS and a-VATS has been closely linked with technological advancements. State-of-the-art high-definition visualization, including 3D techniques, and the continuous refinement of instruments, with a focus on endostaplers with rotational member, promote the development of VATS lobectomy and its widespread introduction in clinical practice. According to STS (STS-GTD, Society of Thoracic Surgeons General Thoracic Database) data, the percentage of VATS lobectomy procedures has increased progressively as compared to traditional open approach surgeries, from 10% in 2002 to 29% in 2007 [6]. In 2014, the database included records of 56,656 patients who underwent VATS [7, 8]. The highest percentage of VATS lobectomy versus thoracotomy procedures was reported for Denmark (55%). In Copenhagen, VATS lobectomy was used in 80% of patients [9]. The percentage rates of VATS lobectomy versus open approach surgeries increased from 2% in 1993 to 14% in 2011 in UK and Ireland [10]. In Poland, the KRRP registry (national lung cancer registry) includes data of 305 VATS, accounting for 10.8% of lobectomies in patients with stage I and II nonsmall cell lung cancer. VATS lobectomy is defined as

(i) 4–6 cm incision made between the ribs,

(ii) no rib spreading,

(iii) procedure performed under control of VATS camera.

3. Indications and Contraindications

Indications for VATS lobectomy remain controversial, even more so as the traditional open chest surgery is a broadly recognised and well-established approach. VATS is generally recognised as a modality dedicated to the management of early stage cancer (stages I and II) with no signs of lymph node invasion [11]. Pulmonary function values are an important eligibility criterion; that is, single-lung ventilation is considered mandatory for VATS lobectomy. However, VATS lobectomy procedures in patients with predicted postoperative FEV1 < 30% have been reported as well. Although some authors suggest that in this group of patient VATS- segmentectomy is more favourable. Zhong et al. [12] presented that VATS-segmentectomy is a safe option and provides comparable oncologic results to VATS-lobectomy specially in stage IA nonsmall cell lung cancer. The essential condition is to carefully qualify patients based on the findings of imaging procedures and invasive diagnostic tests (bronchoscopy, EBUS-TBNA, EUS-FNA, and mediastinoscopy). The dynamic development of diagnostic imaging techniques has been inextricably linked with the increasingly common application of VATS in clinical practice. For example, local stage of tumour progression can be now examined with PET-CT scanning. However, sceptics argue that these diagnostic procedures have considerable limitations. Herth et al. [13] reported that EBUS-TBNA was detected as much as 19% of lymph node involvement in a group of 100 patients with <10 mm lymph nodes in CT and absence of metabolically active lesions in PET-CT. This is particularly important in the context of VATS lobectomy since lymph node involvement is considered one of contraindications to VATS. Still, with the increasing experience and technical advancement, the eligibility criteria for VATS lobectomy have been progressively extended to include more advanced stages of cancer. According to the previous updates in eligibility criteria, patients with >6 cm or T3 tumours are considered ineligible for VATS lobectomy [14]. Here is a list of relative contraindications:

(i) dense pleural adhesions (especially for less experienced surgeons);

(ii) tumours visible by bronchoscopy (where the lesion is directly adjacent to the origin of the lobe and a possible sleeve resection might be needed);

(iii) lymphadenopathy (related to a benign tumour or the underlying condition);

(iv) preoperative radiation therapy or chemotherapy;

(v) tumour infiltration to the chest wall.

4. Conversion to Thoracotomy and VATS Complications

An open thoracotomy remains the gold standard approach to thoracic procedures in lung cancer and should be considered whenever individual surgeon's experience is too limited for a safe and effective VATS lobectomy, or if any life-threatening perioperative complications emerge. The causes of intraoperative conversions to thoracotomy during VATS lobectomy can be divided into the following groups: perioperative complications, technical reasons, anatomy, and tumour related causes. In clinical studies, nearly 30% of all conversions were not related to the tumour [15]. In a study by Krasna et al. [15], 37% of conversions were due to bleeding, 30% for local advancement, 23% for dense pleural adhesions, 7% for technical problems with the stapler, and 3% for pneumothorax on the opposite side (3%).

The percentage of complications following VATS lobectomy varies from 6% to 34.2%, estimated on a large volume of clinical data [16–18]. The risk of complications in traditional open thoracotomy can be as high as 58% [16]. Whitson et al. [17] reported the following common postoperative complications: prolonged air leak of >7 days (56%), atrial fibrillation (32%), massive pleural drainage (14%), pneumonia (13%), and myocardial infarction (10%). Bronchopleural fistula was present in 3% of patients. In studies by Sakuraba et al. [19], the rates of atelectasis requiring bronchoscopy were lower in VATS group as compared to patients undergoing open thoracotomy (0% versus 6.3%, resp.). Moreover, chest tube drainage >7 days (1.5 versus 10.8%, resp.) and hospital length of stay (5 versus 7 days, resp.) scores were better in VATS versus open.

5. Benefits of VATS versus Open Thoracotomy

Major benefits of VATS relate to reduced pain following surgery. Pain was demonstrated to occur in up to 50–70% of patients at two months or more after thoracotomy procedures using a retractor, and over 40% of patients may still have some degree of pain at one year after surgery, with 5% of patients experiencing significant levels of pain. Pain can cause a number of peri- and postoperative complications both immediately and long after the surgery [19]. Less pain, reduced chest drain durations, and shorter lengths of stay and recovery period are highlighted as the main advantages of VATS. In a study by Sakuraba et al. [19], statistically significant differences were demonstrated in 752 patients who underwent either video-assisted thoracoscopic or open lobectomy: shorter median operative time (video-assisted thoracoscopy 117.5 minutes versus open 171.5 minutes), lower chest tubes drainage (987 mL in video-assisted thoracoscopy versus 1504 mL in open lobectomy), and shorter length of stay (4.5 days versus 7 days). A statistically significant difference was also found in perioperative blood loss to the advantage of VATS.

There is no objective method to measure pain intensity, and the perception of pain intensity is difficult to analyse. Interesting to note is that according to some reports there are no significant differences between the intensity and duration of pain following VATS lobectomy and open thoracotomy. In a study by Scott et al. [20] from the renown Memorial Sloan Kettering Cancer Center, the percentage of patients experiencing intensive postoperative pain at 4, 8, and 12 months after VATS and open thoracotomy was comparable (14%, 16%, 14%, and 10%,7 for VATS and 11%, 23%, 18%, 12%, and 6% for open thoracotomy). Postoperative respiratory parameters (FEV1 and FVC) were demonstrated to be significantly higher after VATS as compared to open thoracotomy in a number of studies [17]. The latest studies investigate the patterns of postoperative immunosuppression. VATS was associated with a less significant reduction in lymphocyte T (CD4), CRP, and interleukin 6 counts. These data may be indicative of a lower degree of invasiveness of VATS, an important precondition for shorter postsurgery recovery and recuperation period [21]. However, better immune system parameters do not translate directly into lower risk of postoperational infection complications in patients after VATS versus open thoracotomy.

6. Oncologic Aspect

Oncologic aspect of video-assisted thoracic surgery remains controversial. Sceptics argue that the decreased invasiveness of VATS affects the radicality of tumour resection, which translates into poorer long-term outcomes of cancer treatment as compared to open thoracotomy. On the other hand, those in favour of VATS lobectomy claim that the principles of surgical treatment remain unaffected by the use of a different surgical access technique. The first step is to assess patient eligibility for VATS lobectomy as this technique should be essentially used in patients with early stage lung cancer. Verifying patient eligibility should preferably involve all diagnostic methods (diagnostic imaging techniques: CT, PET-CT, and NMR and endoscopic methods bronchoscopy, EBUS-TBNA, and EUS-FNA) and in cases of doubt, invasive methods as well (mediastinoscopy). The learning curve is another important factor. Many studies on VATS lobectomy include a separate analysis of VATS lobectomy in early and late phase of a surgeon's learning curve. A lot of attention is devoted to the correct evaluation of the condition of lymph nodes and changes in the mediastinum. In one of the latest studies, the findings seem to support the arguments in favour of open thoracotomy [22]. The mean number of nodes dissected in the VATS group was significantly lower (9.9/patient) as compared to the open group (14.7/patient, p value 0.003). Particularly significant differences were reported for N2 group: 4.7 and 8.5/patient in VATS and open groups, respectively (p value 0.002). The differences were insignificant in N1 group. In the open lobectomy group, 24.6% of patients were upstaged from N0 to N1 and from N1 to N2 compared with 10% in the VATS group. These findings may fuel scepticism for VATS. However, the 3-year survival was similar between the groups (89.9% for VATS versus 84.7% for open lobectomy). Also, comparable effectiveness of both methods has been reported in a number of papers. Merritt et al. [23] demonstrated that the number of lymph nodes removed per patient was 24 and 25.1 in VATS on the left and the right side, respectively, and was comparable to the number of lymph nodes removed in an open chest procedure: 21.1 and 25.2, respectively. These are the findings of a prospective and randomized study. In a study by Whitson et al. [17], 5-year survival rate in VATS patients of 75% was comparable to lobectomy with thoracotomy. In Palade et al. [24], the 5-year overall survival rate in the VATS patients of 95% was higher than in the open group. Another issue related to VATS is the rate of recurrences following videothoracoscopic treatment. Of particular concern are local recurrences and minithoracotomy site recurrences associated with the very narrow access space. Walker et al. [25] demonstrated a lower recurrence rate in VATS versus open thoracotomy group of 18% and 29%, respectively. In patients after thoracotomy, the percentage of distant metastases was higher (63% versus 32% in VATS). Surprising was the fact that the percentage of synchronous primary tumours confirmed perioperatively in the open group was higher than in VATS (12% versus 7%, resp.). The risk of minithoracotomy site recurrences could not be confirmed in a number of studies, which is likely to result from the current prevention measures (surgical field protection and retrieval bags).

7. Learning Curve

VATS lobectomy is a relatively young technique and is still evolving. The majority of thoracic surgeons are extensively trained in traditional open chest surgery. Training in traditional thoracic surgery is the essential precondition for later training in VATS and makes surgeons ready for emergency conversion to open thoracotomy. Obligatory education in VATS lobectomy is not broadly used and is only beginning to emerge in Poland. Being skillful in anatomical pulmonary resection accompanied by thoracotomy for transthoracic access does not necessarily translate into the ability to perform VATS. This is possibly due to the specific visualization of the operating field (highly enlarged 2D images) and the use of different instruments. Effective identification of anatomic structures may be difficult in the initial phase of the learning curve. Flores et al. [26] compared different surgical aspects of VATS in the first 20 patients (group A) and patients operated in late phase of the surgeon's learning curve (group B). The study covered all VATS lobectomies performed by a single experienced thoracic surgeon over a 3-year period. The conversion rate was 25% in group A and only 5% in group B. The median operative time was significantly shorter in group B (150 min versus 192.5 min in group A). Initially, 25% of all lobectomies were performed with the VATS technique, which has increased to 75% in late stage of the learning curve. The authors argue that a surgeon can acquire the VATS lobectomy technique with minimum 20 cases. Other authors claim that surgeons have to overcome a learning curve of at least 25 cases and previous 100 cases of "smaller" VATS procedures [27]. Patient selection is particularly important in early stage of the learning curve. Small peripheral lesions are preferred instead of central tumours. Inexperienced surgeons should avoid cases with noncancer lymphadenopathy. The choice of the resected lobe is also important. Lower lobe resection is considered easier due to the limited number of blood vessels.

8. New Trends

Minimally invasive pulmonary resection techniques have been evolving to achieve improved radicality and to significantly reduce perioperative injury. A single-port or "uniport" access performed with only one incision has been described in a number of recent papers [28]. If used for diagnostic or limited resection purposes, the uniport technique and traditional videothoracoscopy proved comparable in terms of effectiveness. Wang et al. [29] investigated the uniport VATS surgery in patients with early stage cancer (group A) and T3 or T4 tumors (group B). The conversion rate was significantly lower in group A than in group B (1.1 versus 6.5%). Surgical time was longer (144 versus 183 minutes) in group B. The majority of patients from both groups did not experience any significant pain (82.8% in group A and 86% in group B). 65.5% of patients in group A were discharged in the first 72 hours versus 51.2% of patients in group B. The 30-month survival was 90.4% for group A and 73.7% for group B. Based on the above findings, it can be concluded that the uniportal VATS lobectomy will be soon broadly used in clinical practice. The progress in VATS lobectomy is closely linked with the development of new instruments. Needlescopic video-assisted thoracic surgery is where traditional intercostal ports are avoided. Another trend is robot-assisted minimally invasive techniques. Gonzalez-Rivas et al. [30] performed a series of robot-assisted approaches to lung cancer resection in 54 patients using a four-arm Vinci Robotic System. The conversion rate was 13%. Postoperative complications were observed in 20% of patients. The median number of lymph nodes removed was compared in the 2 groups (17.5 versus 17/patient). Postoperative hospitalization was significantly shorter after robotic than after open operations (4.5 versus 6 days). However, the cost of four-arm robotic lobectomy may be considered a significant disadvantage. Robot-assisted resection is by around EUR 2,000 more expensive than VATS lobectomy and thoracotomy. New developments also emerge in anaesthesia for thoracic surgery to limit side effects. Thoracoscopic surgery with regional anaesthesia and without endotracheal intubation was described in a number of papers. Lung collapse occurs naturally on introduction of the first port to the pleura. In a study by Veronesi et al. [31], 446 patients were treated by nonintubated thoracoscopic surgery, with lobectomy performed in 189 patients. 3.6% of patients required conversion to thoracotomy. Anaesthetic side effects were noted in 6.3% of patients; 3.6% of patients required conversion to tracheal intubation. Nonintubated thoracoscopic surgery may be considered in patients with decreased respiratory reserve, at risk of serious perioperative complications associated with traditional anaesthesia and one lung ventilation.

9. Summary

The evolution of VATS lobectomy is driven by technological advancement and refinement of surgical instruments. It is increasingly used worldwide. In some medical centres, this approach has become the dominant method of lung cancer surgery. The effectiveness of VATS lobectomy is a controversial matter. The only way to address these controversies is to perform large-scale clinical studies covering large population of patients. The eligibility criteria for VATS lobectomy have been progressively extending to accommodate advanced stages of cancer. Proper patient selection is considered of paramount importance, also in terms of surgeon's experience. Research shows that minimally invasive treatment methods are as effective as traditional methods but are accompanied by less suffering. In the coming years, we will perhaps be able to objectively assess the benefits of VATS by learning more about this thoracic surgery technique.

References

[1] H. C. Jacobaeus, "Ueber die moglichkeit die zystoskopie bei untersuchung seroser Honlungen anzuwenden," *Münchener Medizinische Wochenschrift*, vol. 57, pp. 2090–2092, 1910.

[2] E. Berber and A. E. Siperstein, "Understanding and optimizing laparoscopic videosystems," *Surgical Endoscopy*, vol. 15, no. 8, pp. 781–787, 2001.

[3] M. J. Mack, S. R. Hazelrigg, R. J. Landreneau, and K. S. Naunheim, "The first international symposium on thoracoscopic surgery," *The Annals of Thoracic Surgery*, vol. 56, pp. 605–806, 1993.

[4] G. Roviaro, F. Varoli, C. Vergani, O. Nucca, M. Maciocco, and F. Grignani, "Long-term survival after videothoracoscopic lobectomy for stage I lung cancer," *Chest*, vol. 126, no. 3, pp. 725–732, 2004.

[5] N. Shigemura, A. Akashi, S. Funaki et al., "Long-term outcomes after a variety of video-assisted thoracoscopic lobectomy approaches for clinical stage IA lung cancer: a multi-institutional study," *Journal of Thoracic and Cardiovascular Surgery*, vol. 132, no. 3, pp. 507–512, 2006.

[6] S. Paul, N. K. Altorki, S. Sheng et al., "Thoracoscopic lobectomy is associated with lower morbidity than open lobectomy: a propensity-matched analysis from the STS database," *Journal of Thoracic and Cardiovascular Surgery*, vol. 139, no. 2, pp. 366–378, 2010.

[7] E. H. J. Belgers, J. Siebenga, A. M. Bosch, E. H. J. Van Haren, and E. C. M. Bollen, "Complete video-assisted thoracoscopic surgery lobectomy and its learning curve. A single center study introducing the technique in The Netherlands," *Interactive Cardiovascular and Thoracic Surgery*, vol. 10, no. 2, pp. 176–180, 2010.

[8] S. Begum, H. J. Hansen, and K. Papagiannopoulos, "VATS anatomic lung resections—the European experience," *Journal of Thoracic Disease*, vol. 6, supplement 2, pp. S203–S210, 2014.

[9] H. J. Hansen and R. H. Petersen, "Video-assisted thoracoscopic lobectomy using a standardized three-port anterior approach—the Copenhagen experience," *Annals of Cardiothoracic Surgery*, vol. 1, no. 1, pp. 70–76, 2012.

[10] J. M. Richards, J. Dunning, and J. Oparka, "Video-assisted thoracoscopic lobectomy: the Edinburgh posterior approach," *Annals of Cardiothoracic Surgery*, vol. 1, pp. 61–69, 2012.

[11] M. Congregado, R. J. Merchan, G. Gallardo, J. Ayarra, and J. Loscertales, "Video-assisted thoracic surgery (VATS) lobectomy: 13 Years' experience," *Surgical Endoscopy*, vol. 22, no. 8, pp. 1852–1857, 2008.

[12] C. Zhong, W. Fang, T. Mao, F. Yao, W. Chen, and D. Hu, "Comparison of thoracoscopic segmentectomy and thoracoscopic lobectomy for small-sized stage IA lung cancer," *Annals of Thoracic Surgery*, vol. 94, no. 2, pp. 362–367, 2012.

[13] F. J. F. Herth, A. Ernst, R. Eberhardt, P. Vilmann, H. Dienemann, and M. Krasnik, "Endobronchial ultrasound-guided transbronchial needle aspiration of lymph nodes in the radiologically normal mediastinum," *European Respiratory Journal*, vol. 28, no. 5, pp. 910–914, 2006.

[14] W. R. Burfeind and T. A. D'Amico, "Thoracoscopic lobectomy," *Operative Techniques in Thoracic and Cardiovascular Surgery*, vol. 9, no. 2, pp. 98–114, 2004.

[15] M. J. Krasna, S. Deshmukh, and J. S. McLaughlin, "Complications of thoracoscopy," *The Annals of Thoracic Surgery*, vol. 61, no. 4, pp. 1066–1069, 1996.

[16] R. O. Jones, G. Casali, and W. S. Walker, "Does failed video-assisted lobectomy for lung cancer prejudice immediate and long-term outcomes?" *Annals of Thoracic Surgery*, vol. 86, no. 1, pp. 235–239, 2008.

[17] B. A. Whitson, S. S. Groth, S. J. Duval, S. J. Swanson, and M. A. Maddaus, "Surgery for early-stage non-small cell lung cancer: a systematic review of the video-assisted thoracoscopic surgery versus thoracotomy approaches to lobectomy," *Annals of Thoracic Surgery*, vol. 86, no. 6, pp. 2008–2018, 2008.

[18] R. J. McKenna Jr., W. Houck, and C. B. Fuller, "Video-assisted thoracic surgery lobectomy: experience with 1,100 cases," *Annals of Thoracic Surgery*, vol. 81, no. 2, pp. 421–426, 2006.

[19] M. Sakuraba, H. Miyamoto, S. Oh et al., "Video-assisted thoracoscopic lobectomy vs. conventional lobectomy via open thoracotomy in patients with clinical stage IA non-small cell lung carcinoma," *Interactive Cardiovascular and Thoracic Surgery*, vol. 6, no. 5, pp. 614–617, 2007.

[20] W. J. Scott, M. S. Allen, G. Darling et al., "Video-assisted thoracic surgery versus open lobectomy for lung cancer: a secondary analysis of data from the American College of Surgeons Oncology Group Z0030 randomized clinical trial," *The Journal of Thoracic and Cardiovascular Surgery*, vol. 139, no. 4, pp. 976–983, 2010.

[21] N. P. Rizk, A. Ghanie, M. Hsu et al., "A prospective trial comparing pain and quality of life measures after anatomic lung resection using thoracoscopy or thoracotomy," *Annals of Thoracic Surgery*, vol. 98, no. 4, pp. 1160–1166, 2014.

[22] H. A. Leaver, S. R. Craig, P. L. Yap, and W. S. Walker, "Lymphocyte responses following open and minimally invasive thoracic surgery," *European Journal of Clinical Investigation*, vol. 30, no. 3, pp. 230–238, 2000.

[23] R. E. Merritt, C. D. Hoang, and J. B. Shrager, "Lymph node evaluation achieved by open lobectomy compared with thoracoscopic lobectomy for N0 lung cancer," *Annals of Thoracic Surgery*, vol. 96, no. 4, pp. 1171–1176, 2013.

[24] E. Palade, B. Passlick, T. Osei-Agyemang, J. Günter, and S. Wiesemann, "Video-assisted vs open mediastinal lymphadenectomy for Stage I non-small-cell lung cancer: results of a prospective randomized trial," *European Journal of Cardio-Thoracic Surgery*, vol. 44, no. 2, pp. 244–249, 2013.

[25] W. S. Walker, M. Codispoti, S. Y. Soon, S. Stamenkovic, F. Carnochan, and G. Pugh, "Long-term outcomes following VATS lobectomy for non-small cell bronchogenic carcinoma," *European Journal of Cardio-thoracic Surgery*, vol. 23, no. 3, pp. 397–402, 2003.

[26] R. M. Flores, U. N. Ihekweazu, N. Rizk et al., "Patterns of recurrence and incidence of second primary tumors after lobectomy by means of video-assisted thoracoscopic surgery (VATS) versus thoracotomy for lung cancer," *Journal of Thoracic and Cardiovascular Surgery*, vol. 141, no. 1, pp. 59–64, 2011.

[27] A. Brunswicker, M. Berman, M. van Leuven, F. van Tornout, and W. R. Bartosik, "Video assisted lobectomy learning curve—what is the magic number?" *Journal of Cardiothoracic Surgery*, vol. 8, supplement 1, article O221, 2013.

[28] R. H. Petersen and H. J. Hansen, "Learning curve associated with VATS lobectomy," *Annals of Cardiothoracic Surgery*, vol. 1, no. 1, pp. 47–50, 2012.

[29] W. Wang, W. Yin, W. Shao et al., "Comparative study of systematic thoracoscopic lymphadenectomy and conventional thoracotomy in resectable non-small cell lung cancer," *Journal of Thoracic Disease*, vol. 6, no. 1, pp. 45–51, 2014.

[30] D. Gonzalez-Rivas, E. Fieira, M. Delgado, L. Mendez, R. Fernandez, and M. de la Torre, "Is uniportal thoracoscopic surgery a feasible approach for advanced stages of non-small cell lung cancer?" *Journal of Thoracic Disease*, vol. 6, no. 6, pp. 641–648, 2014.

[31] G. Veronesi, D. Galetta, P. Maisonneuve et al., "Four-arm robotic lobectomy for the treatment of early-stage lung cancer," *Journal of Thoracic and Cardiovascular Surgery*, vol. 140, no. 1, pp. 19–25, 2010.

Comparison of Diaphragmatic Breathing Exercise, Volume and Flow Incentive Spirometry, on Diaphragm Excursion and Pulmonary Function in Patients Undergoing Laparoscopic Surgery

Gopala Krishna Alaparthi,[1] Alfred Joseph Augustine,[2] R. Anand,[3] and Ajith Mahale[4]

[1]*Department of Physiotherapy, Kasturba Medical College, Manipal University, Bejai, Mangalore 575004, India*
[2]*Department of Surgery, Kasturba Medical College, Manipal University, Mangalore 575004, India*
[3]*Department of Pulmonary Medicine, Kasturba Medical College, Manipal University, Mangalore 575004, India*
[4]*Department of Radiodiagnosis, Kasturba Medical College, Manipal University, Mangalore 575004, India*

Correspondence should be addressed to Alfred Joseph Augustine; alfred.augustine@manipal.edu

Academic Editor: Casey M. Calkins

Objective. To evaluate the effects of diaphragmatic breathing exercises and flow and volume-oriented incentive spirometry on pulmonary function and diaphragm excursion in patients undergoing laparoscopic abdominal surgery. *Methodology.* We selected 260 patients posted for laparoscopic abdominal surgery and they were block randomization as follows: 65 patients performed diaphragmatic breathing exercises, 65 patients performed flow incentive spirometry, 65 patients performed volume incentive spirometry, and 65 patients participated as a control group. All of them underwent evaluation of pulmonary function with measurement of Forced Vital Capacity (FVC), Forced Expiratory Volume in the first second (FEV_1), Peak Expiratory Flow Rate (PEFR), and diaphragm excursion measurement by ultrasonography before the operation and on the first and second postoperative days. With the level of significance set at $p < 0.05$. *Results.* Pulmonary function and diaphragm excursion showed a significant decrease on the first postoperative day in all four groups ($p < 0.001$) but was evident more in the control group than in the experimental groups. On the second postoperative day pulmonary function (Forced Vital Capacity) and diaphragm excursion were found to be better preserved in volume incentive spirometry and diaphragmatic breathing exercise group than in the flow incentive spirometry group and the control group. Pulmonary function (Forced Vital Capacity) and diaphragm excursion showed statistically significant differences between volume incentive spirometry and diaphragmatic breathing exercise group ($p < 0.05$) as compared to that flow incentive spirometry group and the control group. *Conclusion.* Volume incentive spirometry and diaphragmatic breathing exercise can be recommended as an intervention for all patients pre- and postoperatively, over flow-oriented incentive spirometry for the generation and sustenance of pulmonary function and diaphragm excursion in the management of laparoscopic abdominal surgery.

1. Introduction

Chest physiotherapy is a common practice in patients undergoing cardiothoracic and abdominal surgery [1]. Abdominal surgery that was previously performed via a large incision is now more commonly performed laparoscopically [2]. The laparoscopic surgeries involve structures such as the gall bladder, colon, small intestine, stomach, liver, and pancreas [1].

In laparoscopy, intraoperative pulmonary changes are due to decreased pulmonary compliance secondary to upward movement of the diaphragm during insufflation and to changes in carbon dioxide (CO_2) homeostasis secondary to absorption of insufflated CO_2 from peritoneum [3]. General anesthesia and surgery related pain may lead to changes in the ventilation pattern resulting in the patient taking shallow breaths which reduce the ability to clear sputum from the chest [4–6].

Studies have reported altered pulmonary function after both conventional and laparoscopic abdominal surgeries [7–12]. Postoperative pulmonary dysfunction in laparoscopic surgery is approximately 20% to 25% depending upon the type of surgery [7–9]. Pulmonary dysfunction leads to pulmonary complications which includes atelectasis, pneumonia, tracheobronchial infection, and respiratory failure. These may have an adverse effect on the length of hospital stay [4].

Reduction of pulmonary function, Forced Vital Capacity (FVC), and Forced Expiratory Vital Capacity (FEV_1) have been reported on the basis of functional alterations [13]. Pathogenesis of postoperative pulmonary dysfunction has been attributed to diaphragmatic function impairment [14].

Chest physiotherapy has been employed as an alternative intervention to reduce occurrence of pulmonary function loss and its complications. Postoperative chest physiotherapy started being implemented in the beginning of the 20th century. It includes breathing exercises, percussion, vibration, splinted huffing/coughing, positioning, and mobilization [15].

Diaphragmatic breathing exercises are used in order to augment diaphragmatic descent while inhalation and diaphragmatic ascent while expiration. The beneficial effects of diaphragmatic breathing are as follows: inflation of the alveoli, reversing postoperative hypoxemia, improvement of ventilation and oxygenation, decreasing the work of breathing, and increasing the degree of excursion of the diaphragm [16, 17].

Mechanical breathing device such as the incentive spirometry (IS) has been introduced into clinical practice [13]. Incentive spirometry encourages the patient to take long, slow deep breath mimicking natural sighing and also provides a visual positive feedback. Incentive spirometers are available either by volume of inspiration (volume-oriented) or flow rate (flow-oriented) [4–6, 18–20].

The flow-oriented incentive spirometer (Triflow device) consists of three chambers in series, each of which contains a ball. When the patient's effort generates a subatmosphere pressure above the ball, it rises in the chamber. An inspiratory flow of 600 mL/s is required to raise the first ball, an inspiratory flow of 900 mL/s is required to elevate the first and second balls, and a flow of 1200 mL/s is required to elevate all three balls. The volume-oriented incentive spirometer is a compact device of 4000 mL capacity and has a one-way valve to prevent exhalation into the unit. A sliding pointer indicates the prescribed inspiratory volume and an inspiratory flow guide coaches the subject to inhale slowly [18–20].

Studies suggest a physiologically significant difference in the effect of the flow- and volume-oriented incentive spirometer. Flow-oriented devices (Triflow device) enforce more work of breathing and increase muscular activity of the upper chest. Volume-oriented devices (Coach 2 device) enforce less work of breathing and improve diaphragmatic activity [6, 18–21].

Earlier studies show that the volumetric incentive spirometer is better in case of cardiac and thoracic surgeries because it provides the appropriate feedback for a slow sustained inspiration and volume [18]. Studies show that slow sustained inspirations are much more effective to promote lung expansion rather than fast inspirations [18]. Studies also show that diaphragmatic breathing exercise encourages more diaphragmatic movement [17, 18].

Gastaldi et al. studied thirty-six subjects, in order to assess the effect of respiratory kinesiotherapy on respiratory muscle strength and pulmonary function following laparoscopic cholecystectomy. Subjects were randomly sorted into two groups: the exercise and the control. Three breathing exercises were performed by seventeen subjects while other nineteen served as a control group. All the subjects were assessed for Maximal Inspiratory Pressure (MIP) and Maximal Expiratory Pressure (MEP), PEF, and spirometry (FVC, FEV_1, and FEV_1/FVC). Both groups registered a decrease in all variables on the first day after surgery. On the second postoperative day, the exercise group showed decreased values for all variables. The values then normalized. However, values of all variables for the control group begin to normalize only on the fifth postoperative day [22].

El-Marakby et al. carried out a study on two experimental groups of patients in order to evaluate the effects of aerobic exercise training and incentive spirometry in controlling pulmonary complications following laparoscopic cholecystectomy. One group was given aerobic walking raining and incentive spirometry as well as traditional physical therapy (Group A); the other (Group B) was given traditional physical therapy. Results indicated a significant reduction in heart rate, SaO_2, and inspiratory capacity for both groups. The researchers concluded that aerobic exercise and incentive spirometry were beneficial in reducing the postoperative pulmonary complications after laparoscopic cholecystectomy [23].

Kundra et al. carried out a comparative study on the effect of preoperative and postoperative incentive spirometry on the pulmonary function of fifty patients who had undergone laparoscopic cholecystectomy. The study group had to carry out incentive spirometry fifteen times before surgery, every four hours, for one week. However, the control group underwent incentive spirometry only during the postoperative period. Pulmonary function was recorded before surgery and 6, 24, and 48 hours postoperatively and at the time of discharge. Result showed that pulmonary function improvement was seen after preoperative incentive Spirometry. The authors concluded that pulmonary function is well-preserved with preoperative than postoperative incentive spirometry [24].

Fagevik Olsén et al. reviewed forty-four studies in order to evaluate the effects of chest physiotherapy interventions in laparoscopic and open abdominal surgery. But the results showed that breathing exercises were efficacious in preventing postoperative pulmonary complications in patients undergoing open surgery. The review also showed that laparoscopic procedures impair respiratory function to a considerably lower degree than open surgery. One study in the review showed that routine treatment is not called for in upper gastrointestinal features such as, for instance, fundoplication and vertical banded gastroplasty [1].

Cattano et al. studied forty-one morbidly obese to assess use of incentive spirometry preoperatively which could help patients to preserve their pulmonary function (inspiratory capacity) better in the postoperative period following laparoscopic bariatric surgery. Subjects were randomly sorted into two groups (the exercise and the control group). The exercise group used the incentive spirometer for ten breaths, five times per day. The control group used incentive spirometer three breaths, once per day. Pulmonary function (inspiratory capacity) was recorded at the day of surgery and postoperative day 1. The author concluded that preoperative use of the incentive spirometer does not lead to significant improvement of pulmonary function (inspiratory capacity) [25].

Various chest physiotherapy techniques are used clinically as part of the routine prophylactic and therapeutic regimen in postoperative respiratory care. However, the efficacy of flow and volume incentive spirometry and diaphragmatic breathing exercise is still controversial [6, 17].

There are no retrievable studies that have been done on the clinical efficacy of diaphragmatic breathing exercise and flow and volume incentive spirometry after laparoscopic abdominal surgery. With this background the present study aim is to compare the effect of diaphragmatic breathing exercise, flow and volume incentive spirometry, on pulmonary function and diaphragm excursion, following laparoscopic surgery.

2. Material and Method

2.1. Inclusion Criteria. Inclusion criteria involved subjects of either gender in the age group of 18 to 80 years who were posted for laparoscopic abdominal surgery.

2.2. Exclusion Criteria. Exclusion criteria were as follows:

(i) Patients who had undergone open abdominal surgery and laparoscopic obstetrics and gynecological surgery.

(ii) Patients with unstable hemodynamic parameters (arterial pressure <100 mmHg systolic and <60 mmHg for diastolic and mean arterial pressure (MAP) <80 mmHg).

(iii) Patients with postoperative complications requiring mechanical ventilation.

(iv) Uncooperative patients or patients unable to understand or to use the device properly.

(v) Patients with inadequate inspiration characterized by vital capacity <10 mL/kg.

2.3. Equipment Used. Equipment used was as follows:

(i) Ultrasonography machine (Voluson730).

(ii) Pulmonary function test machine (EasyOne Plus Portable Diagnostic Spirometer Machine, ndd Medical Technologies, Inc. Massachusetts, USA).

(iii) Flow-oriented incentive spirometry machine (Triflow device, IGNA Medical Devices, Mumbai).

(iv) Volume-oriented incentive spirometry machine (Coach 2 device, Smiths Medical International Ltd., USA).

2.4. Procedure. The study was carried out in Kasturba Medical College Hospitals Mangalore over a period of four years starting from January 2011 to December 2014. The study was approved by the Institutional Ethics Committee of Kasturba Medical College Mangalore. Eligible patients were selected based on the inclusion and exclusion criteria. The purpose of study was made clear to each patient and a written informed consent was obtained prior to involving them in the study.

The patients were divided into four groups:

Flow-oriented incentive spirometry group (Triflow device).

Volume-oriented incentive spirometry group (Coach 2 device).

Diaphragmatic breathing exercise group.

Control group.

The patients were allocated to groups by block randomization done by primary investigator. The entire sample was divided into 13 blocks with 20 patients in each, 5 belonging to each group. Group information was concealed in a sealed opaque envelope and revealed to the patients only after they were recruited into the treatment group or the control group done by primary investigator.

Following the allocation to groups, the patients in the treatment group were visited one day prior to the surgery; preoperative information was offered and, based upon his/her group, flow-oriented incentive spirometry, volume-oriented incentive spirometry, or diaphragmatic breathing exercise was taught to each patient. Other therapies like airway clearance techniques, thoracic expansion exercise, and mobilization were also taught to every patient in all treatment groups (see Steps 1–5). Patients in the control group were not given any treatment or taught any exercises. The treatment protocol for postoperative laparoscopic abdominal surgery is as follows.

Step 1. The first step is diaphragmatic breathing exercise, flow or volume incentive spirometry (3 sets, 5 repetitions of deep breaths).

Step 2. The second step is airway clearance techniques (huffing or coughing).

Step 3. The third step is circulation (foot and ankle pumping, hip and knee bending 10 times each hour).

Step 4. The fourth step is thoracic expansion exercise (position patient in long sitting in bed/high sitting over the side of the bed).

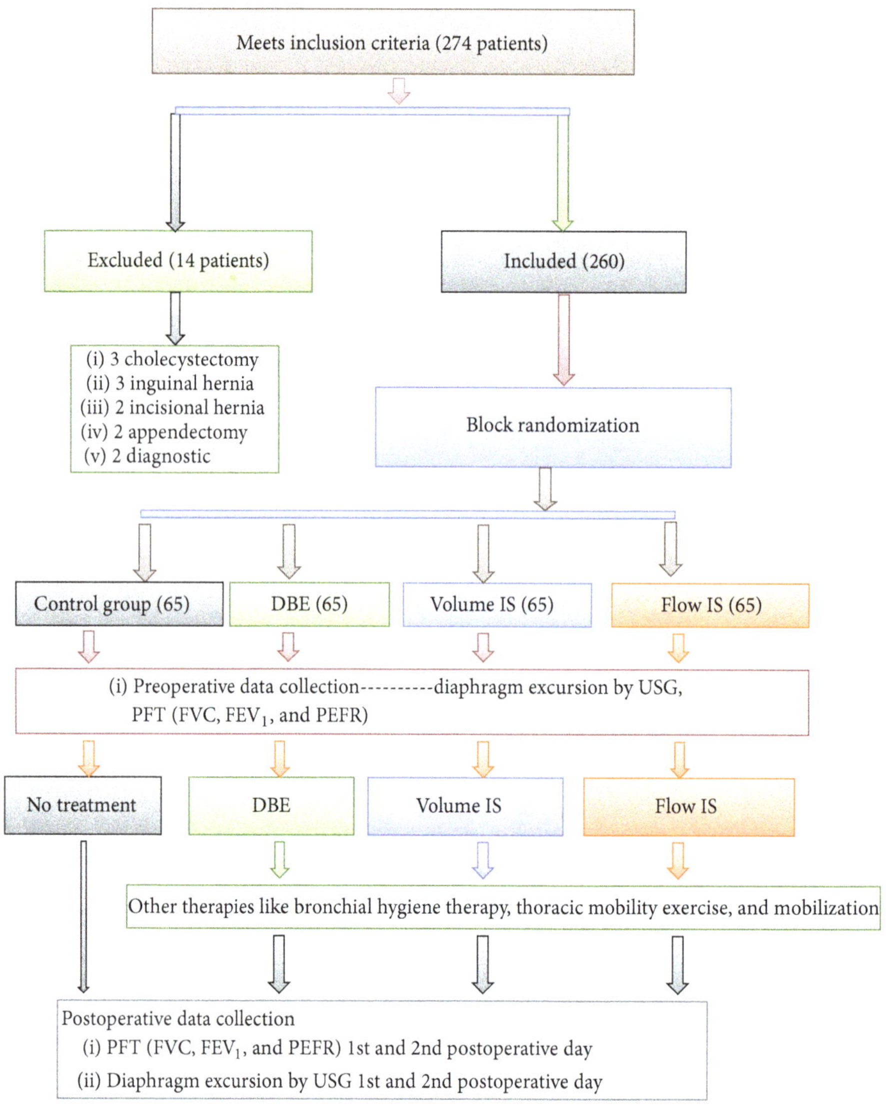

FIGURE 1: Consort flow diagram of the study.

Step 5. The fifth step is mobilization:

(a) Sitting out of the bed in a chair (one hour twice daily).

(b) Walking (three times per day).

(c) Stair climbing done before the patient was discharged from the hospital.

An experienced radiologist carried out ultrasonography for diaphragm excursion on the preoperative as well as the 1st and 2nd postoperative day, for all groups.

Pulmonary function tests (PFT) measured the following variables: Forced Vital Capacity (FVC), Forced Expiratory Volume in the first second (FEV_1), Peak Expiratory Flow Rate (PEFR). These were taken on the preoperative day and 1st and the 2nd postoperative day, for all groups. These measurements were taken by the primary investigator (Figure 1, flowchart).

3. Description of Outcome Measures

3.1. Diaphragm Excursion. The patient lays in the supine position and diaphragm movements were recorded in the B-Mode. The probe was positioned between the midclavicular and anterior axillary lines, in the subcostal area, so that the ultrasound beam entered the posterior third of the right hemidiaphragm perpendicularly. The procedure began at the end of normal expiration with the subjects being instructed to inhale as deeply as possible. A fixed point at the edge of the image on the screen and the diaphragm margin at maximal inspiration and again at maximal expiration served as reference points between which measurements were made, with the average of three values being taken for both maximal inspiration and maximal expiration [26, 27].

3.2. Pulmonary Function Test. Pulmonary function test procedures (EasyOne Plus Portable Diagnostic Spirometer

Machine) were carried out according to the American Thoracic Society/European Respiratory Society guidelines [28]. The following variables have been recorded: Forced Vital Capacity (FVC), Forced Expiratory Volume in the first second (FEV_1), and Peak Expiratory Flow Rate (PEFR) the best value of 3 acceptable tests [29].

3.3. Treatment Procedures

3.3.1. Methods to Perform Flow-Oriented and Volume-Oriented Incentive Spirometry. The patient was placed in a semirecumbent position (45°), with a pillow under the knees. The patient was instructed to inhale with a slow and deep sustained breath, holding it for a minimum of 5 seconds and then to exhale passively in order to avoid any forceful expiration. First, the patient was given demonstration and then asked to perform in order to ensure that she/he understood the process [15, 17]. The patient was instructed to hold the spirometer upright and to perform flow-oriented incentive spirometry by inhaling slowly and thereby raising the ball, followed by volume incentive spirometry in order to raise the piston or plate in the chamber to the set target [19, 20].

The patient was instructed to perform 3 sets of 5 repeated deep breaths. This had to be performed by the patient every waking hour. The therapist administered the exercise four times a day and the patient was instructed to perform the same for the rest of the day [19]. The patient was asked to keep a record of the exercise performed by entering in a log book which was provided beforehand.

3.3.2. Method to Perform Diaphragmatic Breathing Exercise. The patient assumed a semi-Fowler's position (back and head are fully supported and abdominal wall is relaxed) and performed diaphragmatic breathing. The therapist placed his hands just below the anterior costal margin, on the rectus abdominis, while the patient was instructed to inhale slowly and deeply through the nose, from functional residual capacity to total lung capacity with a three-second inspiratory hold. The patient was then instructed to relax the shoulders, keep the upper chest quiet in order that the abdomen be raised a little. The Patient was then instructed to exhale slowly through the mouth [16, 28].

The Patient was made to experience a slight rise and subsequent fall of the abdomen during inspiration and expiration, by placing his or her own hand below the anterior costal margin. The Patient was instructed to perform 3 sets of 5 deep breaths with the therapist administering them four times a day and the patient being instructed to perform the same once every waking hour for the rest of the day. In between the repetitions of the diaphragmatic breathing exercise, the patient was told to breathe normally [16, 28]. The patient was asked to keep a record of the exercise performed by entering in a log book which was provided beforehand.

3.4. Data Analysis

3.4.1. Sample Size. The sample size was calculated based on the values obtained from pulmonary function test in a pilot study (20 subjects, 5 in each group) [30, 31]. The following formula was used for calculating the same:

$$n = 2\left(\frac{Z\alpha + Z\beta}{D/S}\right)^2, \qquad (1)$$

where n is the number of subjects in each group and $Z\alpha$ and $Z\beta$ are constants and they are substituted. Selected power for the study was 90% and D is effect size which is the absolute value of the difference in means and represents what is considered a clinically meaningful or practically important difference in means.

D is taken from the pilot study which used the same variable, which compared pulmonary function test in subjects, and S is the standard deviation of the means. The sample size is 65 in each group (total 260 subjects).

Data was analyzed using SPSS package version 21. ANOVA and post hoc analysis (Bonferroni's t-test) were carried out to verify the within-groups differences. Between-groups differences were compared using two-factor ANOVA.

4. Results

We selected 274 patients posted for laparoscopic abdominal surgery, of which 260 were included in the study. Fourteen patients were excluded because they were converted to an open surgical procedure. There were 195 patients in the intervention groups and 65 in the control group.

Baseline demographic characteristics of the participants such as age, height, weight, BMI, risk factors, and duration of surgery are presented in Table 1. There were no statistically significant differences between the groups. Data about Patients who underwent different types of laparoscopic abdominal surgery are summarized in Table 1. Of the 260 patients included, 140 patients underwent cholecystectomy, 53 hernioplasty, 43 appendectomy, 11 umbilical hernia repair, 8 laparoscopic diagnostic, 3 bariatric surgery, and 2 hemicolectomy.

Forced Vital Capacity (FVC) was compared within the intervention groups and the control group before and after operation, and the same is summarized in Table 2. There was a statistically significant decrease in Forced Vital Capacity (FVC) in the 1st and 2nd post-op day when compared with the preoperative period in all groups.

Forced Expiratory Volume in one second (FEV_1) was compared within the intervention groups and the control group before and after the operation and is summarized in Table 3. There was a statistically significant decrease in Forced Expiratory Volume at the end of the first second (FEV_1) on the 1st and 2nd postoperative day when compared with the preoperative period in all groups.

Peak Expiratory Flow Rates (PEFR) were compared with the intervention groups and control group before and after operation and are summarized in Table 4. In all groups there was a statistically significant decrease in Peak Expiratory Flow Rate (PEFR) on the 1st and 2nd postoperative day compared to the preoperative period.

Diaphragm excursions were compared within intervention groups and the control group before and after operation

Table 1: Demographic characteristics of subjects undergoing laparoscopic abdominal surgery.

Variables	Intervention groups: Diaphragmatic breathing exercise ($N = 65$)	Flow incentive spirometry ($N = 65$)	Volume incentive spirometry ($N = 65$)	Control group ($N = 65$)	p value (<0.05)
Age (years) (mean ± SD)	41.8 ± 13.6	49.5 ± 16.1	45.5 ± 15.3	46.2 ± 16.4	0.055 NS
Gender (n) M : F	47 : 18	37 : 28	33 : 32	40 : 25	
Height (cm) (mean ± SD)	166.8 ± 11.6	165.0 ± 11.1	163.7 ± 10.0	163.5 ± 9.9	0.268 NS
Weight (kg) (mean ± SD)	65.2 ± 12.5	63.8 ± 12.6	62.7 ± 19.7	60.2 ± 12.3	0.266 NS
BMI (mean ± SD)	23.3 ± 3.3	23.0 ± 4.9	23.4 ± 6.1	22.5 ± 3.5	0.660 NS
H/o of smoking	3	2	3	1	
H/o of cardiac disease	1	2	2	2	
H/o of hypertension	6	9	6	3	
H/o of diabetes	2	3	5	7	
H/o of asthma	1	Nil	1	3	
Duration of surgery (Hrs)	1.78 ± 0.67	1.89 ± 0.59	1.76 ± 0.66	1.80 ± 0.53	0.63 NS
	Type of laparoscopic abdominal surgery				Total number
Cholecystectomy	28	39	44	29	140
Hernioplasty	14	15	11	13	53
Umbilical hernia repair	5	1	2	3	11
Appendectomy	16	6	6	15	43
Laparoscopic diagnostic	2	1	Nil	5	8
Bariatric surgery	Nil	1	2	Nil	3
Hemicolectomy	Nil	2	Nil	Nil	2

Table 2: Comparison of Forced Vital Capacity (FVC) before and after the laparoscopic abdominal surgery in the intervention groups and control group.

Forced Vital Capacity (FVC) (liters (L))	Preoperative (mean ± SD)	Postoperative 1st day (mean ± SD)	Postoperative 2nd day (mean ± SD)	Preoperative versus postoperative 1st day (mean difference)	Postoperative 1st day versus postoperative 2nd day (mean difference)	Preoperative versus postoperative 2nd day (mean difference)
Diaphragmatic breathing exercise ($n = 65$)	2.83 ± .79	2.19 ± .84	2.55 ± .79	0.63 (22.4%) $p < 0.001^{**}$	−0.35 (−16.2%) $p < 0.001^{**}$	0.28 (9.8%) $p < 0.001^{**}$
Flow incentive spirometry ($n = 65$)	2.50 ± .76	1.72 ± .70	2.13 ± .71	0.77 (31.0%) $p < 0.001^{**}$	−0.40 (−23.6%) $p < 0.001^{**}$	0.37 (14.7%) $p < 0.001^{**}$
Volume incentive spirometry ($n = 65$)	2.50 ± .73	1.86 ± .64	2.22 ± .70	0.64 (25.6%) $p < 0.001^{**}$	−0.36 (−19.4%) $p < 0.001^{**}$	0.28 (11.1%) $p < 0.001^{**}$
Control group ($n = 65$)	2.51 ± .80	1.78 ± .65	2.02 ± .67	0.73 (29.2%) $p < 0.001^{**}$	−0.24 (−13.7%) $p < 0.001^{**}$	0.49 (19.5%) $p < 0.001^{**}$

% change. **Highly significant at $p < 0.001$ level.

TABLE 3: Comparison of Forced Expiratory Volume in one second (FEV_1) before and after the laparoscopic abdominal surgery in the intervention groups and control group.

Forced Expiratory Volume in one second (FEV_1) (liters (L))	Preoperative (mean ± SD)	Postoperative 1st day (mean ± SD)	Postoperative 2nd day (mean ± SD)	Preoperative versus postoperative 1st day (mean difference)	Postoperative 1st day versus postoperative 2nd day (mean difference)	Preoperative versus postoperative 2nd day (mean difference)
Diaphragmatic breathing exercise ($n = 65$)	2.34 ± .70	1.76 ± .72	2.02 ± .69	0.57 (24.5%) $p < 0.001^{**}$	−0.25 (−14.3%) $p < 0.001^{**}$	0.32 (13.7%) $p < 0.001^{**}$
Flow incentive spirometry ($n = 65$)	2.06 ± .68	1.42 ± .64	1.74 ± .64	0.63 (30.9%) $p < 0.001^{**}$	−0.32 (−22.5%) $p < 0.001^{**}$	0.31 (15.3%) $p < 0.001^{**}$
Volume incentive spirometry ($n = 65$)	2.08 ± .64	1.53 ± .55	1.82 ± .64	0.55 (26.3%) $p < 0.001^{**}$	−0.29 (−19.1%) $p < 0.001^{**}$	0.25 (12.2%) $p < 0.001^{**}$
Control group ($n = 65$)	2.06 ± .67	1.42 ± .55	1.62 ± .59	0.64 (31.0%) $p < 0.001^{**}$	−0.20 (−14.3%) $p < 0.001^{**}$	0.43 (21.1%) $p < 0.001^{**}$

% change. **Highly significant at $p < 0.001$ level.

TABLE 4: Comparison of Peak Expiratory Flow Rate (PEFR) before and after the laparoscopic abdominal surgery in the intervention groups and the control group.

Peak Expiratory Flow Rate (PEFR) L/s	Preoperative (mean ± SD)	Postoperative 1st day (mean ± SD)	Postoperative 2nd day (mean ± SD)	Preoperative versus postoperative 1st day (mean difference)	Postoperative 1st day versus postoperative 2nd day (mean difference)	Preoperative versus postoperative 2nd day (mean difference)
Diaphragmatic breathing exercise ($n = 65$)	5.83 ± 2.1	3.74 ± 1.8	4.78 ± 2.0	2.09 (35.8%) $p < 0.001^{**}$	−1.04 (−27.8%) $p < 0.001^{**}$	1.04 (17.9%) $p < 0.001^{**}$
Flow incentive spirometry ($n = 65$)	5.21 ± 2.0	2.95 ± 1.3	4.04 ± 1.5	2.25 (43.2%) $p < 0.001^{**}$	−1.08 (−36.6%) $p < 0.001^{**}$	1.17 (22.4%) $p < 0.001^{**}$
Volume incentive spirometry ($n = 65$)	5.52 ± 1.8	3.52 ± 1.3	4.50 ± 1.7	2.00 (36.1%) $p < 0.001^{**}$	−0.97 (−27.6%) $p < 0.001^{**}$	1.02 (18.5%) $p < 0.001^{**}$
Control group ($n = 65$)	5.15 ± 1.8	3.26 ± 1.3	3.89 ± 1.5	1.88 (36.6%) $p < 0.001^{**}$	−0.62 (−19.2%) $p < 0.001^{**}$	1.25 (24.4%) $p < 0.001^{**}$

% change. **Highly significant at $p < 0.001$ level.

and are summarized in Table 5. There was a statistically significant decrease in diaphragm excursion in the 1st and 2nd postoperative period when compared with the preoperative period in all groups except in diaphragmatic breathing exercise group and volume incentive spirometry group which almost came back to normal.

Forced Vital Capacity (FVC), Forced Expiratory Volume in one second (FEV_1), Peak Expiratory Flow Rate, and diaphragm excursion were compared between the intervention groups and the control group during the preoperative and 2nd postoperative day and are summarized in Table 6.

There was a statistically significant difference between intervention groups (diaphragmatic breathing exercise group and volume incentive spirometry group) and control group in terms of Forced Vital Capacity (FVC) and diaphragm excursion ($p < 0.001$), the said variables being significantly lower in the control group than in the diaphragmatic breathing exercise group and volume incentive spirometry group.

5. Discussion

The main purpose of this study was to compare diaphragmatic breathing exercise, flow- and volume incentive spirometry, on pulmonary function and diaphragmatic excursion in patients undergoing laparoscopic abdominal surgery. To the best of our knowledge, this study is the first to compare the effects of diaphragmatic breathing exercise with two different kinds of incentive spirometry and also against a control group. There were 65 patients included in each group and the four groups were homogenous in terms of all demographic parameters. In our study we found that diaphragmatic breathing exercise and volume incentive spirometry improve lung function and diaphragm excursion in patients undergoing laparoscopic abdominal surgery.

In our study pulmonary function (FVC, FEV_1, and PEFR) and diaphragm excursion showed a decrease on the 1st postoperative day when compared to the preoperative values

Table 5: Comparison of diaphragm excursion before and after the laparoscopic abdominal surgery in the intervention groups and the control group.

Diaphragm excursion (cm)	Preoperative (mean ± SD)	Postoperative 1st day (mean ± SD)	Postoperative 2nd day (mean ± SD)	Preoperative versus postoperative 1st day (mean difference)	Postoperative 1st day versus postoperative 2nd day (mean difference)	Preoperative versus postoperative 2nd day (mean difference)
Diaphragmatic breathing exercise ($n = 65$)	4.2 ± .90	3.3 ± .91	4.1 ± .99	0.8 (20.6%) $p < 0.001$**	−0.7 (−22.2%) $p < 0.001$**	0.1 (2.9%) $p > 0.20$#
Flow incentive spirometry ($n = 65$)	4.0 ± 1.0	2.9 ± 1.0	3.7 ± 1.0	1.1 (27.0%) $p < 0.001$**	−0.7 (−24.7%) $p < 0.001$**	0.3 (8.9%) $p < 0.001$**
Volume incentive spirometry ($n = 65$)	4.0 ± 0.8	3.1 ± 0.8	3.9 ± 0.9	0.9 (23.7%) $p < 0.001$**	−0.8 (−26.4%) $p < 0.001$**	0.1 (3.5%) $p > 0.39$#
Control group ($n = 65$)	4.0 ± 1.0	2.8 ± 0.8	3.4 ± 0.9	1.1 (28.4%) $p < 0.001$**	−0.5 (−19.0%) $p < 0.001$**	0.5 (14.8%) $p < 0.001$**

% change. #Not significant at $p > 0.05$. **Highly significant at $p < 0.001$ level.

Table 6: Showing difference between preoperative and postoperative 2nd day between intervention groups and control group of Forced Vital Capacity, Forced Expiratory Volume in one second, Peak Expiratory Flow Rate, and diaphragm excursion.

Preoperative minus postoperative 2nd day (mean difference)	Forced Vital Capacity (FVC) (liters (L))	Forced Expiratory Volume in one second (FEV_1) (liters (L))	Peak Expiratory Flow Rate (PEFR) L/s	Diaphragm excursion (cm)
Diaphragmatic breathing exercise group versus flow incentive spirometry group	−0.09 p value 1.00#	0.00 p value 1.00#	−0.12 p value 1.00#	−0.23 p value 0.16#
Diaphragmatic breathing exercise group versus volume incentive spirometry group	−0.00 p value 1.00#	0.06 p value 1.00#	0.02 p value 1.00#	−0.15 p value 1.00#
Diaphragmatic breathing exercise group versus control group	−0.21 p value 0.03*	−0.11 p value 0.85#	−0.21 p value 1.00#	−0.46 p value < 0.001**
Flow incentive spirometry group versus volume incentive spirometry group	0.88 p value 1.00#	0.06 p value 1.00#	0.14 p value 1.00#	0.22 p value 0.23#
Flow incentive spirometry group versus control group	−0.12 p value 0.66#	−0.11 p value 0.75#	−0.08 p value 1.00#	−0.23 p value 0.20#
Volume incentive spirometry group versus control group	−0.21 p value 0.03*	−0.17 p value 0.12#	−0.23 p value 1.00#	−0.45 p value < 0.001**

#Not significant at $p > 0.05$. *Significant at $p < 0.05$ level. **Highly significant at $p < 0.001$ level.

in all four groups with an average decrease of 27% in Forced Vital Capacity, 28% in Forced Expiratory Volume in one second, 37% in Peak Expiratory Flow Rate, and 28% in diaphragm excursion. The present study finding of reduction in pulmonary function during postoperative day is similar to those reported in a previous study [3, 21–24].

Our results are in accordance with Schauer et al. who found 30% to 38% reduction in postoperative pulmonary function (FVC, FEV_1, and FEF25%–75%) in laparoscopic cholecystectomy [9]. Karayiannakis et al. found 22% of FVC and 19% of FEV_1 reduction after laparoscopic cholecystectomy [32]. Ramos et al. found 20% to 30% reduction in postoperative pulmonary function (FVC and FEV_1) in laparoscopic cholecystectomy [33]. Ravimohan et al. found 21% to 31% reduction in postoperative day pulmonary function variables (FVC, FEV_1, and FEF25%–75%) in laparoscopic cholecystectomy [7].

Possible reasons for decrease in pulmonary function and diaphragm excursion during the postoperative period in laparoscopic abdominal surgery are as follows. During the postoperative period, patients exhibit shallow breathing without the intermittent sigh or breaths which are inspired approximately ten times an hour. Patients will breathe shallowly which leads to a decrease in ventilation to dependent lung regions [7, 32, 33]. In the present study, reduced pulmonary function (FVC, FEV_1, and PEFR) and diaphragm excursion in postoperative laparoscopic abdominal surgery subjects might be due to postoperative pain, location of surgical ports, along with anaesthetic, analgesic usage [7, 34].

The effects of general anaesthesia on distribution of ventilation and chest wall and lung mechanics lead to ventilation-perfusion mismatch, increased dead space, shunt, and hypoxemia [9, 35, 36]. Narcotic/opioid analgesics and other drugs affect the central regulation of breathing, changing the neural drive of the upper airway and chest wall muscles, which lead to hypoventilation, a diminished sensitivity of the respiratory center to carbon dioxide stimulation, an increase of obstructive breathlessness, the suppression of the cough reflex, and irregular mucus production [37].

The location of surgical ports involves trauma near the diaphragm and chest wall/ribs, leading to postoperative incisional pain and reflex inhibition of the phrenic nerve and diaphragmatic reflex paresis resulting in functional disruption of respiratory muscle movement. In addition, when patients remain lying down for long periods during the postoperative period their abdominal content limits diaphragmatic movement [34].

Several studies found that diaphragmatic dysfunction is due to gas insufflation in the abdominal cavity which might also be responsible for the increase of resistance and reduced diaphragmatic excursion, leading to reduced lung volume [38]. All these factors lead to a change in postoperative lung function usually resulting in development of a restrictive pattern and decreased diaphragm excursion in laparoscopic abdominal surgery.

Our results are in accordance with Ford et al., who showed that reduction in inspiratory muscle activity, mainly the diaphragm, was the main determinant of impaired pulmonary function. Diaphragm dysfunction may be due to reflex inhibition of efferent phrenic activity [39]. Several studies suggested that laparoscopic abdominal surgery causes reflex inhibition of the phrenic nerve which might lead to shallow breaths and reduced pulmonary ventilation [34]. Erice et al. explained reduced pulmonary ventilation mainly due to decreased inspiratory muscle activity [40]. Lunardi et al. showed a decrease of 27% in the respiratory muscular activity of patients who underwent laparoscopy abdominal surgery [41].

Possible reasons for improved pulmonary function and diaphragm excursion in the diaphragmatic breathing exercise group are as follows. The present study showed that the diaphragmatic breathing exercise group was able to improve pulmonary mechanics thus leading to a beneficial effect on pulmonary function (FVC) and diaphragm excursion. Diaphragmatic breathing exercise improves diaphragmatic descent and diaphragmatic ascent during inspiration and expiration, respectively. Slower deep inspiration ensures more even distribution of air throughout the lung, particularly to the dependent lung [16]. The physiological effects of diaphragmatic breathing exercise are that breathing through full vital capacity and holding for 3–5 seconds ensure full inflation of the lungs thus opening up alveoli which have low volume and stimulating the production of surfactant. Diaphragmatic breathing exercise will also decrease activity of accessory muscles, ensure that breathing patterns are as close to normal as possible, and also reduce the work of breathing [16, 31].

Our results are in accordance with the findings of Tahir et al. who showed that diaphragmatic breathing exercise will improve basal ventilation [42]. Weber and Prayar and Menkes and Britt found that diaphragmatic breathing exercise will improve tidal volume and also facilitate secretion removal [43, 44]. Blaney and Sawyer observed that tactile stimulation over the subject's lower costal margin as well as verbal instruction served to significantly increase diaphragmatic movement during diaphragmatic breathing exercises [45]. Manzano et al. found that diaphragmatic breathing exercise was able to improve pulmonary mechanics and lead to beneficial effect on Forced Vital Capacity (FVC) [46]. Grams et al. evaluated the efficacy of diaphragmatic breathing exercise for the prevention of postoperative pulmonary complications and for the recovery of pulmonary mechanics and found that diaphragmatic breathing exercise appeared to be more effective [17].

Possible reasons for improved pulmonary function and diaphragmatic excursion in the volume incentive spirometry group are as follows. The present study showed that the volume incentive spirometry group also had improved pulmonary mechanics that led to a beneficial effect on pulmonary function (FVC) and diaphragm excursion. After laparoscopic abdominal surgery, it may be hard to take a deep breath and if patients do not breathe deeply it may lead to postoperative pulmonary complications. The volume incentive spirometer is a mechanical device used to take slow, deep long breaths that encourage patients to breathe to total lung capacity, to sustain that inflation and open up collapsed alveoli [18].

The volume incentive spirometer will be more "physiological" because the training volume is constant until it reaches the maximum inspiratory capacity (level preset by physiotherapist). It provides a low level of resistance training while minimizing the potential fatigue to the diaphragm [19]. Our study results are in accordance with Paisani et al. who showed that when volume incentive spirometry was performed with low inspiratory flow it promoted diaphragmatic excursion and improved the expansion of the basal area of chest wall [21]. Minschaert et al. observed that patients treated with incentive spirometry would have early recovery of the pulmonary volume [47]. Kundra et al. found that the use of incentive spirometry in the preoperative period leads to greater improvement in the lung functions than if given in the postoperative period. So use of the volume incentive spirometer will result in active recruitment of the diaphragm and other inspiration muscles which may lead to improved pulmonary function and diaphragm excursion [24].

Limitation of the Study. There was no blinding in the study procedure; the same investigator who randomized the patients into the experimental groups and the control group measured the outcome variables (pulmonary function test) and the same investigator taught the exercises to all experimental groups. Diaphragm excursion measurement was not done by the same radiologist throughout the study and the finding would have been confounded by the expertise of professional. Type of anaesthesia, analgesia, and postoperative pain was not recorded which could affect the findings.

There was no follow-up in the study as all patients were discharged on the 2nd postoperative day. As a result we are unaware which group values returned to normal. Patient adherence to the intervention programs was recorded by providing a log book to each subject, in which they had to make an entry the very time they did the prescribed technique but there is no way to verify the authenticity of these entries.

6. Suggestions for the Future Research

Future research could be directed at long-term follow-up to see which group sustains improvement for a long duration and the functional aspect of recovery. Future studies can be carried out to compare the effect of the techniques on patients who have undergone upper and lower abdominal laparoscopic surgeries, using a larger sample size. Effect of combining therapy like incentive spirometer and diaphragmatic breathing exercise can be studied on laparoscopic abdominal surgery patients. Future research can be done by assessing and using respiratory muscle strength and patient comfort with different technique as an outcome in laparoscopic abdominal surgery. Similar studies can be conducted on patients following open abdominal surgeries and cardiac and thoracic surgeries.

7. Clinical Implication

Based on the results of the study we strongly recommend the following:

> Volume-oriented incentive spirometry and diaphragmatic breathing exercise can be recommended for all patients preoperatively and postoperatively over flow-oriented incentive spirometry as an intervention for the generation and sustenance of pulmonary function and diaphragm excursion in the management of laparoscopic abdominal surgery.

8. Conclusion

(i) From our study we conclude that in laparoscopic abdominal surgery patients there is a significant decrease in pulmonary function (FVC, FEV_1, and PEFR) and diaphragm excursion in all four groups on the 1st postoperative day when compared with the preoperative day.

(ii) A greater improvement in pulmonary function and diaphragm excursion between the first and second postoperative day was seen in all experimental groups when compared to the control group.

(iii) From our study we conclude that pulmonary function and diaphragm excursion was better preserved in the diaphragmatic breathing exercise group and volume incentive spirometry group when compared with the flow incentive spirometry group and the control group.

Competing Interests

The authors declare that there are no competing interests.

Acknowledgments

The authors are extremely grateful to Dr. Anil Sharma, Senior Consultant Surgeon, Max Super Specialty Hospital, New Delhi, for all timely help, for valuable expert advice and suggestion, and for being the source of inspiration.

References

[1] M. Fagevik Olsén, K. Josefson, and H. Lönroth, "Chest physiotherapy does not improve the outcome in laparoscopic fundoplication and vertical-banded gastroplasty," *Surgical Endoscopy*, vol. 13, no. 3, pp. 260–263, 1999.

[2] L. Denehy and L. Browing, "Abdominal surgery: the evidence for physiotherapy intervention," in *Recent Advances in Physiotherapy*, C. Partridge, Ed., pp. 43–73, John Wiley & Sons, 1st edition, 2007.

[3] R. W. M. Wahba, F. Béïque, and S. J. Kleiman, "Cardiopulmonary function and laparoscopic cholecystectomy," *Canadian Journal of Anaesthesia*, vol. 42, no. 1, pp. 51–63, 1995.

[4] M. M. Guimarães, R. El Dib, A. F. Smith, and D. Matos, "Incentive spirometry for prevention of postoperative pulmonary complications in upper abdominal surgery," *Cochrane Database of Systematic Reviews*, vol. 8, no. 2, Article ID CD006058, 2009.

[5] C. R. F. Carvalho, D. M. Paisani, and A. C. Lunardi, "Incentive spirometry in major surgeries: a systematic review," *Brazilian Journal of Physical Therapy*, vol. 15, no. 5, pp. 343–350, 2011.

[6] P. do Nascimento Junior, N. S. P. Módolo, S. Andrade, M. M. F. Guimarães, L. G. Braz, and R. El Dib, "Incentive spirometry for prevention of postoperative pulmonary complications in upper abdominal surgery," *The Cochrane Database of Systematic Reviews*, vol. 2, Article ID CD006058, 2014.

[7] S. M. Ravimohan, L. Kaman, R. Jindal, R. Singh, and S. K. Jindal, "Postoperative pulmonary function in laparoscopic versus open cholecystectomy: a prospective, comparative study," *Indian Journal of Gastroenterology*, vol. 24, no. 1, pp. 6–8, 2005.

[8] R. C. Frazee, J. W. Roberts, G. C. Okeson et al., "Open versus laparoscopic cholecystectomy. A comparison of postoperative pulmonary function," *Annals of Surgery*, vol. 213, no. 6, pp. 651–654, 1991.

[9] P. R. Schauer, J. Luna, A. A. Ghiatas et al., "Pulmonary function after laparoscopic cholecystectomy," *Surgery*, vol. 114, no. 2, pp. 389–399, 1993.

[10] G. Putensen-Himmer, C. Putensen, H. Lammer, W. Lingnau, F. Aigner, and H. Benzer, "Comparison of postoperative respiratory function after laparoscopy or open laparotomy for cholecystectomy," *Anesthesiology*, vol. 77, no. 4, pp. 675–680, 1992.

[11] S. Hasukić, D. Mesić, E. Dizdarević, D. Keser, S. Hadziselimović, and M. Bazardzanović, "Pulmonary function after laparoscopic and open cholecystectomy," *Surgical Endoscopy*, vol. 16, no. 1, pp. 163–165, 2002.

[12] Y. Osman, A. Fusun, A. Serpil et al., "The comparison of pulmonary functions in open versus laparoscopic cholecystectomy," *Journal of the Pakistan Medical Association*, vol. 59, no. 4, pp. 201–204, 2009.

[13] G. Simonneau, A. Vivien, R. Sartene et al., "Diaphragm dysfunction induced by upper abdominal surgery. Role of postoperative pain," *American Review of Respiratory Disease*, vol. 128, no. 5, pp. 899–903, 1983.

[14] T. A. M. Chuter, C. Weissman, D. M. Mathews, and P. M. Starker, "Diaphragmatic breathing maneuvers and movement of the diaphragm after cholecystectomy," *Chest*, vol. 97, no. 5, pp. 1110–1114, 1990.

[15] P. Pasquina, M. R. Tramèr, J.-M. Granier, and B. Walder, "Respiratory physiotherapy to prevent pulmonary complications after abdominal surgery: a systematic review," *Chest*, vol. 130, no. 6, pp. 1887–1899, 2006.

[16] H. Nancy and J. S. Tecklin, "Respiratory treatment," in *Cardiopulmonary Physical Therapy; A Guide to Practice*, S. Irwin and J. S. Tecklin, Eds., pp. 356–374, Mosby, 1995.

[17] S. T. Grams, L. M. Ono, M. A. Noronha, C. I. S. Schivinski, and E. Paulin, "Breathing exercises in upper abdominal surgery: a systematic review and meta-analysis," *Brazilian Journal of Physical Therapy*, vol. 16, no. 5, pp. 345–353, 2012.

[18] P. Agostini and S. Singh, "Incentive spirometry following thoracic surgery: what should we be doing?" *Physiotherapy*, vol. 95, no. 2, pp. 76–82, 2009.

[19] R. D. Restrepo, R. Wettstein, L. Wittnebel, and M. Tracy, "AARC Clinical Practice Guidelines. Incentive spirometry: 2011," *Respiratory Care*, vol. 56, no. 10, pp. 1600–1604, 2011.

[20] R. H. Dean and D. B. Richard, "Devices for chest physiotherapy, incentive spirometry and intermittent positive-pressure breathing," in *Respiratory Care Equipment*, D. B. Richard, R. H. Dean, and L. C. Robert, Eds., pp. 245–263, J. B. Lippincott, Philadelphia, Pa, USA, 1995.

[21] D. D. M. Paisani, A. C. Lunardi, C. C. B. M. da Silva, D. Cano Porras, C. Tanaka, and C. R. Fernandes Carvalho, "Volume rather than flow incentive spirometry is effective in improving chest wall expansion and abdominal displacement using optoelectronic plethysmography," *Respiratory Care*, vol. 58, no. 8, pp. 1360–1366, 2013.

[22] A. C. Gastaldi, C. M. B. Magalhães, M. A. Baraúna, E. M. C. Silva, and H. C. D. Souza, "Benefits of postoperative respiratory kinesiotherapy following laparoscopic cholecystectomy," *Revista Brasileira de Fisioterapia*, vol. 12, no. 2, pp. 100–106, 2008.

[23] A. A. El-Marakby, A. Darwiesh, E. Anwar, A. Mostafa, and A. Jad, "Aerobic exercise training and incentive spirometry can control postoperative pulmonary complications after laparoscopic cholecystectomy," *Middle East Journal of Scientific Research*, vol. 13, no. 4, pp. 459–463, 2013.

[24] P. Kundra, M. Vitheeswaran, M. Nagappa, and S. Sistla, "Effect of preoperative and postoperative incentive spirometry on lung functions after laparoscopic cholecystectomy," *Surgical Laparoscopy, Endoscopy and Percutaneous Techniques*, vol. 20, no. 3, pp. 170–172, 2010.

[25] D. Cattano, A. Altamirano, A. Vannucci, V. Melnikov, C. Cone, and C. A. Hagberg, "Preoperative use of incentive spirometry does not affect postoperative lung function in bariatric surgery," *Translational Research*, vol. 156, no. 5, pp. 265–272, 2010.

[26] J. Ayoub, R. Cohendy, J. Prioux et al., "Diaphragm movement before and after cholecystectomy: a sonographic study," *Anesthesia and Analgesia*, vol. 92, no. 3, pp. 755–761, 2001.

[27] A. Boussuges, Y. Gole, and P. Blanc, "Diaphragmatic motion studied by M-mode ultrasonography: methods, reproducibility, and normal values," *Chest*, vol. 135, no. 2, pp. 391–400, 2009.

[28] Y. R. Silva, S. K. Li, and M. J. F. X. Rickard, "Does the addition of deep breathing exercises to physiotherapy-directed early mobilisation alter patient outcomes following high-risk open upper abdominal surgery? Cluster randomised controlled trial," *Physiotherapy (United Kingdom)*, vol. 99, no. 3, pp. 187–193, 2013.

[29] M. R. Miller, J. Hankinson, V. Brusasco et al., "Standardisation of spirometry," *European Respiratory Journal*, vol. 26, no. 2, pp. 319–338, 2005.

[30] G. K. Alaparthi, A. J. Augustine, R. Anand, and A. Mahale, "Chest physiotherapy during immediate postoperative period among patients undergoing laparoscopic surgery-a Randomized Controlled Pilot Trail," *International Journal of Biomedical and Advance Research*, vol. 4, no. 2, pp. 118–122, 2013.

[31] G. K. Alaparthi, A. J. Augustine, R. Anand, and A. Mahale, "Comparison of flow and volume oriented incentive spirometry on lung function and diaphragm movement after laparoscopic abdominal surgery: a randomized clinical pilot trial," *International Journal of Physiotherapy*, vol. 1, no. 5, pp. 274–278, 2013.

[32] A. J. Karayiannakis, G. G. Makri, A. Mantzioka, D. Karousos, and G. Karatzas, "Postoperative pulmonary function after laparoscopic and open cholecystectomy," *British Journal of Anaesthesia*, vol. 77, no. 4, pp. 448–452, 1996.

[33] G. C. Ramos, E. Pereira, S. Gabriel Neto, and E. C. de Oliveira, "Pulmonary function after laparoscopic cholecystectomy and abbreviated anesthetic-surgical time," *Revista do Colegio Brasileiro de Cirurgioes*, vol. 36, no. 4, pp. 307–311, 2009.

[34] S. Bhat, A. Katoch, L. Kalsotra, and R. K. Chrungoo, "A prospective comparative trial of post-operative pulmonary function: laparascopic versus open cholecystectomy," *JK Science*, vol. 9, no. 2, pp. 83–86, 2007.

[35] J. Ali, R. D. Weisel, A. B. Layug, B. J. Kripke, and H. B. Hechtman, "Consequences of postoperative alterations in respiratory mechanics," *The American Journal of Surgery*, vol. 128, no. 3, pp. 376–382, 1974.

[36] R. W. M. Wahba, "Perioperative functional residual capacity," *Canadian Journal of Anaesthesia*, vol. 38, no. 3, pp. 384–400, 1991.

[37] G. Gamsu, M. M. Singer, H. H. Vincent, S. Berry, and J. A. Nadel, "Postoperative impairment of mucous transport in the lung," *American Review of Respiratory Disease*, vol. 114, no. 4, pp. 673–679, 1976.

[38] J. Joris, A. Kaba, and M. Lamy, "Postoperative spirometry after laparoscopy for lower abdominal or upper abdominal surgical procedures," *British Journal of Anaesthesia*, vol. 79, no. 4, pp. 422–426, 1997.

[39] G. T. Ford, W. A. Whitelaw, T. W. Rosenal, P. J. Cruse, and C. A. Guenter, "Diaphragm function after upper abdominal surgery in humans," *American Review of Respiratory Disease*, vol. 127, no. 4, pp. 431–436, 1983.

[40] F. Erice, G. S. Fox, Y. M. Salib, E. Romano, J. L. Meakins, and S. A. Magder, "Diaphragmatic function before and after laparoscopic cholecystectomy," *Anesthesiology*, vol. 79, no. 5, pp. 966–975, 1993.

[41] A. C. Lunardi, D. D. M. Paisani, C. Tanaka, and C. R. F. Carvalho, "Impact of laparoscopic surgery on thoracoabdominal mechanics and inspiratory muscular activity," *Respiratory Physiology & Neurobiology*, vol. 186, no. 1, pp. 40–44, 2013.

[42] A. H. Tahir, R. B. George, H. Weill, and J. Adriani, "Effects of abdominal surgery upon diaphragmatic function and regional ventilation," *International Surgery*, vol. 58, no. 5, pp. 337–340, 1973.

[43] B. A. Weber and J. Prayar, “Physiotherapy skills: techniques and adjuncts,” in *Physiotherapy for Respiratory and Cardiac Problems*, B. A. Webber and J. Prayar, Eds., pp. 113–171, Churchill Levingstone, Edinburgh, UK, 1993.

[44] H. A. Menkes and J. Britt, “Rationale for physical therapy,” *American Review of Respiratory Disease*, vol. 122, no. 5, pp. 127–131, 1980.

[45] F. Blaney and T. Sawyer, “Sonographic measurement of diaphragmatic motion after upper abdominal surgery: a comparison of three breathing manoeuvres,” *Physiotherapy Theory and Practice*, vol. 13, no. 3, pp. 207–215, 1997.

[46] R. M. Manzano, C. R. F. De Carvalho, B. M. Saraiva-Romanholo, and J. E. Vieira, “Chest physiotherapy during immediate postoperative period among patients undergoing upper abdominal surgery: Randomized clinical trial,” *Sao Paulo Medical Journal*, vol. 126, no. 5, pp. 269–273, 2008.

[47] M. Minschaert, J. L. Vincent, A. M. Ros, and R. J. Kahn, “Influence of incentive spirometry on pulmonary volumes after laparotomy,” *Acta Anaesthesiologica Belgica*, vol. 33, no. 3, pp. 203–209, 1982.

21

The Role of Minimally Invasive Techniques in Scoliosis Correction Surgery

Michael B. Cloney,[1] Jack A. Goergen,[2] Angela M. Bohnen,[1] Zachary A. Smith,[1] Tyler Koski,[1] and Nader Dahdaleh[1]

[1] *Department of Neurological Surgery, Feinberg School of Medicine, Chicago, IL, USA*
[2] *Feinberg School of Medicine, Chicago, IL, USA*

Correspondence should be addressed to Michael B. Cloney; michael.cloney@yahoo.com

Academic Editor: Stephen Kavic

Objective. Recently, minimally invasive surgery (MIS) has been included among the treatment modalities for scoliosis. However, literature comparing MIS to open surgery for scoliosis correction is limited. The objective of this study was to compare outcomes for scoliosis correction patients undergoing MIS versus open approach. *Methods.* We retrospectively collected data on demographics, procedure characteristics, and outcomes for 207 consecutive scoliosis correction surgeries at our institution between 2009 and 2015. *Results.* MIS patients had lower number of levels fused ($p < 0.0001$), shorter surgeries ($p = 0.0023$), and shorter overall lengths of stay ($p < 0.0001$), were less likely to be admitted to the ICU ($p < 0.0001$), and had shorter ICU stays ($p = 0.0015$). On multivariable regression, number of levels fused predicted selection for MIS procedure ($p = 0.004$), and multiple other variables showed trends toward significance. Age predicted ICU admission and VTE. BMI predicted any VTE, and DVT specifically. Comorbid disease burden predicted readmission, need for transfusion, and ICU admission. Number of levels fused predicted prolonged surgery, need for transfusion, and ICU admission. *Conclusions.* Patients undergoing MIS correction had shorter surgeries, shorter lengths of stay, and shorter and fewer ICU stays, but there was a significant selection effect. Accounting for other variables, MIS did not independently predict any of the outcomes.

1. Introduction

Adult scoliosis is a spinal deformity typically caused by asymmetrical disc degeneration, osteoporosis, and vertebral body compression fractures [1]. When nonsurgical treatment fails, there are multiple surgical techniques that can be used [2]. The goals of surgery are to improve functionality, relieve pain, improve cosmesis, and prevent curve progression [3]. Whether performed posteriorly or anteriorly, open techniques are associated with large blood loss, muscle injury and denervation, significant postoperative pain, and other complications [4, 5].

Minimally invasive surgery (MIS) potentially avoids or lessens these complications due to its ability to reduce intraoperative blood loss, soft tissue damage, infection, postoperative pain, and recovery time [6]. The safety and feasibility of MIS for adult degenerative scoliosis have already been established [7]. Also, results have previously been reported that showed similar clinical improvement for patients who underwent open surgery versus MIS [8]. Furthermore, the patients who underwent MIS had lower morbidity and complication rates and significantly shorter hospital stays [8].

While these initial results are promising, these studies were on small subsets of patients with many confounding variables. The literature comparing open surgery versus MIS for scoliosis correction is limited; therefore, the need exists for further investigation to determine the efficacy of MIS. Here, we compared MIS and open scoliosis surgery with respect to selection for surgical technique and outcomes, including readmission rates, reoperation rates, bleeding, and clotting complications.

Table 1: Approaches and techniques used in minimally invasive operations.

	Number of operations using technique
Anterior approach	2
Posterior approach	11
Lateral approach	1
Percutaneous screws	9
Interbody fusion	10

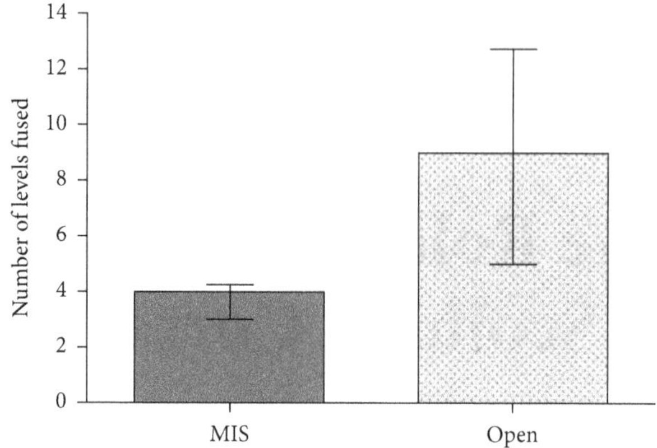

Figure 1: Number of levels fused for patients undergoing MIS approach versus open approach.

2. Methods

2.1. Patient Population. Patients were identified using the Northwestern University Electronic Data Warehouse (EDW). The EDW is an institution-specific registry clinical data repository jointly funded by Northwestern Memorial Hospital (NMH), Northwestern Medical Faculty Foundation (NMFF), and Northwestern University Feinberg School of Medicine. We identified all patients who underwent surgery for scoliosis in the Departments of Neurological Surgery or Orthopedic Surgery at Northwestern University between January 1, 2009, and May 31, 2015, as determined by the preoperative indication for surgery provided by the surgeon.

2.2. Clinical and Demographic Data. Data on patients' age, sex, race, BMI, smoking status (ever smoker versus never smoker), number of comorbid diagnoses, and insurance type (private versus other, including Medicare, Medicaid, and disability insurance) at the time of presentation were retrospectively collected for analysis. Data were also collected on the number of levels fused and length of surgery, as well as whether the patients' scoliosis correction involved a staged procedure, interbody fusion, laminectomy, or osteotomy. Data on surgical techniques and approaches used were also collected. The approaches used included lateral, posterior, and anterior. Of the 14 minimally invasive operations, most utilized an interbody fusion with percutaneous screws; see Table 1 for details.

2.3. Outcome Measures. Information about complications within 30 days after the surgery included the cumulative 30-day incidence and timing of VTEs (defined as either DVT or PE), all-cause readmissions, reoperations, ICU admission, length of ICU stay, length of hospital stay, and incidence of death.

2.4. Statistical Methods. Microsoft Excel 2011 (Microsoft, Redmond, WA, USA) was used to manage data. Statistical analysis was performed using Stata 12.0 (StataCorp, College Station, TX, USA) and Prism 6.0b (GraphPad Software, Inc., La Jolla, CA, USA). Parametric data was given as mean ± standard deviation and compared using a t-test. Nonparametric data was compared using Mann–Whitney U test or Chi-square test, as appropriate. Regression analysis was performed using stepwise logistic regression, with an inclusion threshold for the multivariable model of $p < 0.10$ for candidate variables on single-variable logistic regression. A value of $p < 0.05$ was considered statistically significant.

3. Results

3.1. Demographic Characteristics. There was no difference in age (64.5 ± 1.4 versus 58.1 ± 1.2, Δ−6.44 [−15.11, 2.22], p = 0.1442), gender (35.7% male versus 25.9% male, 1.588889 [0.5081890, 4.967774], p = 0.5304), race (p = 0.3243), insurance type (p = 0.6694), smoking status (p = 0.4284), BMI (26.1 ± 0.6 versus 26.8 ± 0.4, Δ0.72 ± 1.47 [−2.17, 3.61], p = 0.6242), or comorbid disease burden (p = 0.4499). On multivariable regression, age (OR 1.076323 [0.9977851, 1.161042], p = 0.057) and having private insurance (OR 3.735077 [0.9058839, 15.40021], p = 0.068) showed trends toward selection for MIS surgery (see Table 2).

3.2. Procedure Data. MIS patients were equally likely to have staged surgery (OR 0.6507177 [0.1749019, 2.420978], p = 0.5186), decompression (OR 0.3597285 [0.04548798, 2.844809], p = 0.3127), osteotomy (OR 0.2604895 [0.03313165, 2.048035], p = 0.1703), and allograft (OR 0.6491885 [0.2098068, 2.008732], p = 0.4505). There was a trend toward significance in surgical approach (p = 0.0857) and surgery involving the thoracic spine (OR 0.1539582 [0.008965574, 2.643795], p = 0.0805). MIS patients were less likely to have autograft (OR 0.1382386 [0.01769585, 1.079909], p = 0.0289) and had a lower number of levels fused (4.0 versus 9.0, Δ5.0 [2.0, 7.0], $p < 0.0001$, Figure 1). There was significantly more variance in the number of levels fused among patients undergoing open surgery ($p <$ 0.0001). On multivariable regression, the number of levels fused predicted selection for MIS procedure (OR 0.6079009 [0.4340611, 0.8513629], p = 0.004), and there was a trend toward significance for selection for MIS among patients undergoing a posterior approach (OR 3.43426 [0.8365153, 14.09913], p = 0.087) and not requiring surgical decompression (OR 0.1319887 [0.0147237, 1.183196], p = 0.070) (see Table 3).

TABLE 2: Patient demographic data for MIS approach versus open approach.

	MIS patients	Open patients	p value
Age	64.5 years (mean)	58.1 years (mean)	0.1442
Gender	35.7% male	25.9% male	0.5304
Race	100% Caucasian	86.01% Caucasian, 4.15% African American, 9.84% other	0.3243
Insurance type	10 private, 4 Medicare	108 private, 77 Medicare, 7 Medicaid, 1 other	0.6694
Smoking status	11 never smoked, 3 quit more than 12 months ago	119 never smoked, 53 quit more than 12 months ago, 21 current smokers or smoked within last 12 months	0.4284
BMI	26.1 (mean)	26.8 (mean)	0.6242
Comorbidities	2.43 comorbidities per patient (cardiac, renal, pulmonary, endocrine, or hypertension)	2.8 comorbidities per patient (cardiac, renal, pulmonary, endocrine, or hypertension)	0.4499

TABLE 3: Surgical procedure data for MIS approach versus open approach.

	Odds ratio for MIS patients/open approach patients	Confidence interval	p value
Posterior approach	3.43426	[0.8365153, 14.09913]	0.087
Number of levels fused	0.6079009	[0.4340611, 0.8513629]	0.004
Staged procedure	0.6507177	[0.1749019, 2.420978]	0.5186
Osteotomy	0.2604895	[0.03313165, 2.048035]	0.1703
Decompression	0.3597285	[0.04548798, 2.844809]	0.3127
Allograft	0.6491885	[0.2098068, 2.008732]	0.4505
Autograft	0.1382386	[0.01769585, 1.079909]	0.0289
Operation involving Thoracic spine	0.1539582	[0.008965574, 2.643795]	0.0805

3.3. Outcomes for MIS versus Open Scoliosis Correction. MIS surgery was significantly shorter (287.0 minutes versus 433.0 minutes, HR 2.319 [1.604, 8.342], $p = 0.0023$, Figure 2) and was less likely to last ≥6 hours (OR 0.2280405 [0.0751441, 0.6920369], $p = 0.0051$). MIS patients had shorter overall lengths of stay (4.5 days versus 8.0 days, HR 3.032 [3.725, 22.61], $p < 0.0001$, Figure 3), were less likely to be admitted to the ICU (OR 0.08779576 [0.02348702, 0.3281854], $p < 0.0001$), and had shorter ICU stays (19.0 hours versus 48.5 hours, HR 5.174 [5.200, 866.7], $p = 0.0015$).

On single-variable analysis, MIS patients were equally likely to experience the following within 30 days of surgery: readmission (OR 0.3271202 [0.01872778, 5.713847], $p = 0.2318$), reoperation (OR 1.181818 [0.06218783, 22.45929], $p = 1.0000$), DVT (OR 0.3477832 [0.01986991, 6.087253], $p = 0.2464$), PE (OR 3.634615 [0.3782204, 34.92786], $p = 0.2328$), any VTE (OR 0.8509616 [0.1044311, 6.934095], $p = 0.8800$), and postoperative death (OR 2.668966 [0.1222150, 58.28564], $p = 0.7034$). MIS patients were less likely to require transfusion (OR 0.1231231 [0.02681325, 0.5653661], $p = 0.0017$).

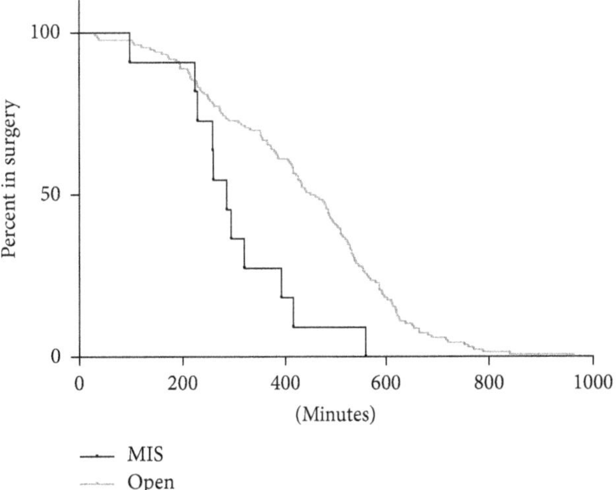

FIGURE 2: Comparison in surgery length between MIS and open approach patients.

3.4. Predictors of Outcomes after Scoliosis Correction. On multivariable regression, BMI predicted DVT within 30 days postoperatively (OR 1.130749 [1.021063, 1.252219], $p = 0.018$), and age (OR 1.048752 [0.9975131, 1.102623], $p = 0.063$) showed a trend toward significance. Number of levels fused showed a trend toward significance in predicting PE 30 days postop (OR 1.251054 [0.9814253, 1.594758], $p = 0.071$). Age (OR 1.053943 [1.000293, 1.11047], $p = 0.049$) and BMI (OR 1.143371 [1.037006, 1.260645], $p = 0.007$) predicted VTE within 30 days postop. Comorbid disease burden predicted readmission within 30 days postop (OR

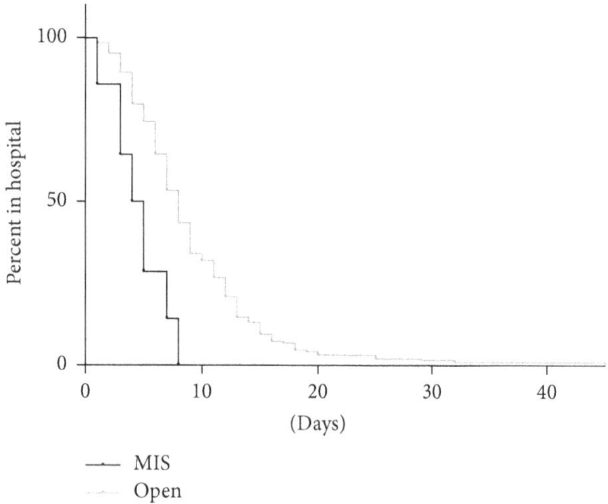

Figure 3: Comparison in LOS between MIS and open approach patients.

2.543268 [1.376737, 4.698219], $p = 0.003$), and involvement of the thoracic spine showed a trend toward significance (OR 0.1084136 [0.0109545, 1.072934], $p = 0.057$). Number of levels fused predicted prolonged surgery (surgery > 6 h) (OR 1.452142 [1.233844, 1.709062], $p < 0.001$), and a history of smoking showed a trend toward significance (OR 0.0040854 [$7.33e - 06$, 2.275654], $p = 0.088$). Number of levels fused (OR 1.297174 [1.182993, 1.422377], $p < 0.001$) and comorbid disease burden (OR 1.297174 [1.182993, 1.422377], $p < 0.001$) predicted the need for transfusion, and osteotomy showed a trend toward significance (OR 2.359625 [0.9492208, 5.865686], $p = 0.065$). Age (OR 0.9512098 [0.9089738, 0.9954083], $p = 0.031$), gender (OR 3.299076 [1.06138, 10.25448], $p = 0.039$), comorbid disease burden (OR 1.686387 [1.123766, 2.530687], $p = 0.012$), number of levels fused (OR 2.089387 [1.615015, 2.703095], $p < 0.001$), and undergoing a staged procedure (OR 5.321398 [1.470397, 19.25826], $p = 0.011$) all predicted ICU admission.

4. Discussion

Minimally invasive surgical techniques could potentially reduce the morbidity associated with traditional open surgical techniques in scoliosis correction [9–11]. Currently, the literature on MIS for scoliosis correction is limited. Many of the studies performed to date observed relatively few patients, and multiple systematic reviews have concluded that more research is needed [9, 12]. Our study examined 207 scoliosis correction surgeries and identified selection factors for MIS, how MIS outcomes compare to open surgery outcomes, and predictors of outcomes for each technique.

Importantly, the median number of levels fused predicted selection for MIS technique with MIS patients having fewer levels fused (4 versus 9, $p < 0.0001$). Many previous studies did not search for a selection effect for MIS versus open surgery selection. One meta-analysis on scoliosis correction, by Dangelmajer et al., did examine selection bias and found that both older patients and patients with less severe deformities were more likely to be selected for an MIS technique [13]. Our analysis agrees with this finding.

Furthermore, having private insurance ($p = 0.068$), undergoing a posterior approach ($p = 0.087$), and not requiring surgical decompression ($p = 0.070$) each showed a trend toward selection for MIS. Similarly to our finding that private insurance was an important determinant of surgery choice, a study by Park and Ha revealed that the cost of the MIS technique determined which patients underwent MIS versus open technique [6]. Another group separated the patients by allocating the private hospital patients to receive MIS and the public hospital patients in their study to receive the open technique [14]. This trend of selection biases between the two groups was consistent across most of the studies that reported patient selection information, limiting the ability to conclude a true difference in outcomes between the MIS and open techniques.

In our study, there was significantly more variance in the number of levels fused among patients undergoing open surgery ($p < 0.0001$). Dangelmajer et al. came to the same conclusion in their systematic review and attributed it to the fact that patients undergoing open procedure had a larger preoperative scoliosis [13]. This result shows that an open technique can be used for a broader range of spinal levels than MIS.

MIS surgery was significantly shorter (287.0 minutes versus 433.0 minutes, $p = 0.0023$, Figure 2) and patients undergoing MIS were less likely to have surgery last >6 hours ($p = 0.0051$) based on single-variable analysis. Anand et al. noted that their surgical outcomes data for MIS scoliosis correction was similar to open correction outcomes data when compared to the literature [8]. However, a meta-analysis on MIS versus open approach in degenerative lumbar disease revealed significant variability in operating times [15]. For example, one study found an average operating time of 161 minutes for the MIS approach compared to 375 minutes for the open approach [16]. In contrast, a study in the same meta-analysis found an average operating time of 159.2 minutes for the MIS approach versus 113.06 minutes for the open approach [17]. We suspect that confounding variables have an important impact on operating time, which would explain the significant variability between studies.

MIS patients also had shorter overall lengths of stay based on single-variable analysis (4.5 days versus 8.0 days, $p < 0.0001$, Figure 3). While it seems promising that MIS patients typically had a shorter length of stay, the results from other studies are variable, potentially indicating a selection effect [6, 14, 18]. Our length of stay results were consistent with a meta-analysis by Phan et al. that found a median length of stay of 4.7 days for the MIS approach and 8 days for the open approach [15]. Although our results are consistent with the meta-analysis, the presence of confounding variables makes it uncertain if MIS versus open surgery is the etiology of the variability in length of stay.

Compared to patients undergoing open surgery, MIS patients were less likely to be admitted to the ICU ($p < 0.0001$) but did have shorter ICU stays when it was required

(19.0 hours versus 48.5 hours, $p = 0.0015$). These results are consistent with previous groups who found that open surgery patients typically had more complications following surgical treatment [13, 19]. However, similarly to our study, these groups also noted the presence of confounding variables such as age and preoperation severity of deformity that could have attributed to these results. In fact, in our analysis, open surgery did not predict ICU admission on multivariable regression.

While MIS or open correction was not independently associated with ICU admission, the number of levels fused did independently predict ICU admission ($p < 0.001$). As the number of levels fused was also independently associated with the selection of technique, it may be a confounding factor that accounts for the significant difference in likelihood of ICU admission on single-variable analysis. Similarly, age was likely a confounding factor, as age showed a trend toward significance in predicting technique, and was a significant predictor of ICU admission ($p = 0.031$).

Our finding that comorbid disease burden independently predicted ICU admission ($p = 0.012$) and readmission within 30 days ($p = 0.003$) is consistent with the existing spine surgery literature [20, 21]. Cardiac, GI, and respiratory issues that were present before the operation are frequent causes of ICU admission and readmission and appear to be an important factor when comparing MIS versus open technique for scoliosis correction as well.

On multivariable regression analysis, age ($p = 0.049$) and BMI ($p = 0.007$) predicted VTE within 30 days postop. These variables are typically found to be strongly associated with such outcomes in spinal surgery, as evidenced in numerous previous studies [22–24]. Importantly, MIS surgery was not found to be an independent predictor of any outcome analyzed during multivariable regression. So, although we found that the typical outcome predictors (age, BMI, and comorbid disease burden) were significant in this study, we did not find any significant difference in patient outcome based on MIS versus open technique alone.

Our study has a number of important limitations. The study was conducted retrospectively and is subject to the biases inherent to this study design. A prospective study would enable us to further understand if the trends we discovered (private insurance, number of levels fused showing selection for MIS) were actively affecting the surgeon's decision whether to use an MIS or open approach. The operations we collected data on varied in the minimally invasive technique and approach used, which made it a less homogenous population to draw conclusions from. As a single-institution study, it only reflects the clinical decision-making of our spine surgeons with respect to patient selection and management. Our series is limited by its size, and a larger series would allow for a more thorough comparison between MIS and open surgery. Our study does not provide radiographic comparisons of corrections, as is common in the scoliosis literature. However, multiple prior studies have compared radiographic outcome for MIS and open scoliosis correction, the results of which have been meta-analyzed [2, 5, 7, 13, 25–27]. Despite its limitations, our study contributes to the existing literature on scoliosis correction by examining selection factors for MIS versus open surgery, as well as a variety of perioperative outcomes.

5. Conclusion

Patients undergoing MIS scoliosis correction had shorter surgeries, shorter lengths of stay, and shorter and fewer ICU stays, but there was a significant selection effect. Accounting for other clinical variables, undergoing MIS surgery did not independently predict any of the outcomes analyzed.

References

[1] M. Aebi, "The adult scoliosis," *European Spine Journal*, vol. 14, no. 10, pp. 925–948, 2005.

[2] S. Yadla, M. G. Maltenfort, J. K. Ratliff, and J. S. Harrop, "Adult scoliosis surgery outcomes: a systematic review," *Neurosurg Focus*, vol. 28, no. E3, 2010.

[3] N. Anand, E. M. Baron, and B. Khandehroo, "Is circumferential minimally invasive surgery effective in the treatment of moderate adult idiopathic scoliosis?" *Clinical Orthopaedics and Related Research*, vol. 472, pp. 1762–1768, 2014.

[4] J. J. Regan, H. Yuan, and P. C. McAfee, "Laparoscopic fusion of the lumbar spine: Minimally invasive spine surgery: A prospective multicenter study evaluating open and laparoscopic lumbar fusion," *The Spine Journal*, vol. 24, no. 4, pp. 402–411, 1999.

[5] M. Y. Wang and P. V. Mummaneni, "Minimally invasive surgery for thoracolumbar spinal deformity: initial clinical experience with clinical and radiographic outcomes," *Neurosurg Focus*, vol. 28, p. E9, 2010.

[6] Y. Park and J. W. Ha, "Comparison of one-level posterior lumbar interbody fusion performed with a minimally invasive approach or a traditional open approach," *The Spine Journal*, vol. 32, no. 5, pp. 537–543, 2007.

[7] E. Dakwar, R. F. Cardona, D. A. Smith, and J. S. Uribe, "Early outcomes and safety of the minimally invasive, lateral retroperitoneal transpsoas approach for adult degenerative scoliosis," *Neurosurg Focus*, vol. 28, no. 3, p. E8, 2010.

[8] N. Anand, R. Rosemann, B. Khalsa, and E. M. Baron, "Mid-term to long-term clinical and functional outcomes of minimally invasive correction and fusion for adults with scoliosis," *Neurosurg Focus*, vol. 28, E6, 2010.

[9] K. Bach, A. Ahmadian, A. Deukmedjian, and J. S. Uribe, "Minimally invasive surgical techniques in adult degenerative spinal deformity: a systematic review," *Clinical Orthopaedics and Related Research*, vol. 472, pp. 1749–1761, 2014.

[10] E. M. Baron and T. J. Albert, "Medical complications of surgical treatment of adult spinal deformity and how to avoid them," *Spine (Phila Pa 1976)*, vol. 31, pp. S106–118, 2006.

[11] S. S. Hu, "Blood loss in adult spinal surgery," *European Spine Journal*, vol. 13, no. S01, pp. S3–S5, 2004.

[12] N. Anand, E. M. Baron, and S. Kahwaty, "Evidence basis/ outcomes in minimally invasive spinal scoliosis surgery," *Neurosurgery Clinics of North America*, vol. 25, pp. 361–375, 2014.

[13] S. Dangelmajer, P. L. Zadnik, S. T. Rodriguez, Z. L. Gokaslan, and D. M. Sciubba, "Minimally invasive spine surgery for adult degenerative lumbar scoliosis," *Neurosurgical Focus*, vol. 36, no. 5, p. E7, 2014.

[14] R. J. Mobbs, P. Sivabalan, and J. Li, "Minimally invasive surgery compared to open spinal fusion for the treatment of degenerative lumbar spine pathologies," *Journal of Clinical Neuroscience*, vol. 19, pp. 829–835, 2012.

[15] K. Phan, P. J. Rao, A. C. Kam, and R. J. Mobbs, "Minimally invasive versus open transforaminal lumbar interbody fusion for treatment of degenerative lumbar disease: systematic review and meta-analysis," *European Spine Journal*, vol. 24, pp. 1017–1030, 2015.

[16] W. A. R. Sulaiman and M. Singh, "Minimally invasive versus open transforaminal lumbar interbody fusion for degenerative spondylolisthesis grades 1-2: patient-reported clinical outcomes and cost-utility analysis," *The Ochsner Journal*, vol. 14, no. 1, pp. 32–37, 2014.

[17] N.-F. Tian and F.-M. Mao, "Minimally invasive versus open transforaminal lumbar interbody fusion: a meta-analysis based on the current evidence," *European Spine Journal*, vol. 23, no. 4, pp. 929-930, 2014.

[18] F. Shunwu, Z. Xing, Z. Fengdong, and F. Xiangqian, "Minimally invasive transforaminal lumbar interbody fusion for the treatment of degenerative lumbar diseases," *The Spine Journal*, vol. 35, no. 17, pp. 1615–1620, 2010.

[19] R. E. Isaacs, J. Hyde, J. A. Goodrich, W. B. Rodgers, and F. M. Phillips, "A prospective, nonrandomized, multicenter evaluation of extreme lateral interbody fusion for the treatment of adult degenerative scoliosis: perioperative outcomes and complications," *The Spine Journal*, vol. 35, pp. S322–330, 2010.

[20] H. F. Kay, S. Chotai, J. B. Wick, D. P. Stonko, M. J. McGirt, and C. J. Devin, "Preoperative and surgical factors associated with postoperative intensive care unit admission following operative treatment for degenerative lumbar spine disease," *European Spine Journal*, vol. 25, no. 3, pp. 843–849, 2016.

[21] R. A. McCormack, T. Hunter, N. Ramos, R. Michels, L. Hutzler, and J. A. Bosco, "An Analysis of Causes of Readmission After Spine Surgery," *The Spine Journal*, vol. 37, no. 14, pp. 1260–1266, 2012.

[22] M. P. Glotzbecker, C. M. Bono, K. B. Wood, and M. B. Harris, "Thromboembolic disease in spinal surgery: a systematic review," *Spine (Phila Pa 1976)*, vol. 34, pp. 291–303, 2009.

[23] S. Z. Goldhaber and H. Bounameaux, "Pulmonary embolism and deep vein thrombosis," *Lancet*, vol. 379, pp. 1835–1846, 2012.

[24] K. Papadimitriou, A. G. Amin, R. M. Kretzer et al., "Thromboembolic events and spinal surgery," *Journal of Clinical Neuroscience*, vol. 19, no. 12, pp. 1617–1621, 2012.

[25] S. H. Berven, V. Deviren, J. A. Smith, S. H. Hu, and D. S. Bradford, "Management of fixed sagittal plane deformity: outcome of combined anterior and posterior surgery," *Spine (Phila Pa 1976)*, vol. 28, no. 15, pp. 1710–1715, 2003.

[26] M. O. Kelleher, M. Timlin, O. Persaud, and Y. R. Rampersaud, "Success and failure of minimally invasive decompression for focal lumbar spinal stenosis in patients with and without deformity," *The Spine Journal*, vol. 35, no. 19, pp. E981–E987, 2010.

[27] W. Liu, X. S. Chen, L. S. Jia, and D. W. Song, "The clinical features and surgical treatment of degenerative lumbar scoliosis: a review of 112 patients," *Orthopaedic Surgery*, vol. 1, pp. 176–183, 2009.

22

Tactile Electrosurgical Ablation: A Technique for the Treatment of Intractable Heavy and Prolonged Menstrual Bleeding

Ali M. El Saman,[1] Faten F. AbdelHafez,[1] Kamal M. Zahran,[1] Hazem Saad,[1] Mohamed Khalaf,[1] Mostafa Hussein,[1] Ibrahim M. A. Hassanin,[2] and Saba M. Shugaa Al Deen[3]

[1] *Women's Health Center, Department of Obstetrics & Gynecology, Faculty of Medicine, Assiut University, Assiut, Egypt*
[2] *Department of Obstetrics & Gynecology, Faculty of Medicine, Sohag University, Sohag, Egypt*
[3] *Department of Obstetrics & Gynecology, University Hospital of Sana'a, Yemen*

Correspondence should be addressed to Ali M. El Saman; ali_elsaman@yahoo.com

Academic Editor: Stephen Kavic

Objective. To study the efficacy and safety of tactile electrosurgical ablation (TEA) in stopping a persistent attack of abnormal uterine bleeding not responding to medical and hormonal therapy. *Methods.* This is a case series of 19 cases with intractable abnormal uterine bleeding, who underwent TEA at the Women's Health Center of Assiut University. The outcomes measured were; patient's acceptability, operative time, complications, menstrual outcomes, and reintervention. *Results.* None of the 19 counseled cases refused the TEA procedure which took 6–10 minutes without intraoperative complications. The procedure was successful in the immediate cessation of bleeding in 18 out of 19 cases. During the 24-month follow-up period, 9 cases developed amenorrhea, 5 had scanty menstrual bleeding, 3 were regularly menstruating, 1 case underwent repeat TEA ablation, and one underwent a hysterectomy. *Conclusions.* TEA represents a safe, inexpensive, and successful method for management of uterine bleeding emergencies with additional long-term beneficial effects. However, more studies with more cases and longer follow-up periods are warranted.

1. Introduction

Heavy and/or prolonged menstrual bleeding (HMB) stands among the most common presentations in the acute gynecology units and accounts for up to 70% of all gynecological consultations in the peri- and postmenopausal years [1]. Hysterectomy represents the ultimate treatment for HMB; however, it might have its potential psychosexual and depressing effects [2, 3]. In addition, hysterectomy is not an ideal option for medically unfit patients and/or those with deteriorated hemodynamics.

Several reports have proposed first generation endometrial ablation techniques [4–6]; however active bleeding may interfere with the appropriate visualization of the uterine cavity and increase the risk of complications. On the other hand, the second generation ablation devices [7, 8] require less skill but the high cost of their disposables limits their affordability in low income settings.

The authors are working in a setting of limited resources where offering expensive disposables for hysteroscopic ablators is not feasible all the time. They have experience in treating challenging cases of endometrial ablation using a specially designed monopolar electrosurgical coagulation probe able to perform electrosurgical ablation without hysteroscopy [9]. In a series of previous studies, the safety and the feasibility of TEA were investigated using an in vitro model of hysterectomy specimens [9] and a pilot clinical study under laparoscopic monitoring [10]. The experimental results showed complete coagulation of the endometrium along with 2–4 mm of the adjacent myometrium. No full thickness damage was observed, with the maximum depth involving only 16% of myometrial thickness [9]. Laparoscopic monitoring was performed in the initial clinical series to confirm that full thickness damage did not occur [10]. The aim of the present work was to investigate the role of tactile ablation in cases presenting with active uterine bleeding as an emergency minimally invasive procedure under ultrasonographic monitoring.

2. Materials and Methods

This study was approved by the ethics committee of Assiut University Hospitals. An institutional review board approval was obtained for using TEA in the management of heavy and/or prolonged menstrual bleeding that failed to respond to medical/hormonal treatment. A thorough history taking and clinical examination were completed for all patients. In addition, a routine ultrasonographic examination, followed by a dilatation and curettage biopsy were performed. Cases who desired further fertility, had a lower segment caesarean scars, with uterine size >10-week pregnancy, and presented with a coexisting gynecological pathology and/or their pathological examination showed atypical hyperplasia were excluded. Eligible cases were counseled regarding the risks, benefits, and available alternatives of the procedure. A written informed consent was then taken.

Under general anesthesia and in lithotomy position, the TEA procedure was preceded by cervical dilatation and uterine curettage to minimize the thickness of the endometrium and enhance the ablation efficacy. The procedure was performed under transabdominal ultrasonographic monitoring. When the uterus was well-visualized in a clear longitudinal scan, the uterine length was measured and the TEA probe was calibrated by sliding the flange depth gauge according to the measured uterine length (Figure 1). The power setting of electrosurgical coagulation unit was adjusted at 60 Watts at the coagulation mode; then the TEA probe was connected to its active monopolar socket.

The active end of TEA probe was introduced through the cervix until it touched the uterine fundus. The TEA probe was then directed to press gently on the anterior wall and the electrosurgical coagulation was activated while the TEA probe was slowly withdrawn down to the internal os. The electrosurgical coagulation was then switched off; the probe was reintroduced until the fundus and the procedure was repeated working from the right to the left side until complete coagulation of the anterior wall. Thereafter, the posterior uterine wall was coagulated in the same manner. Lastly the TEA probe was passed across the fundus slowly working from the right to the left uterine cornual ends to ensure the complete coagulation of the whole endometrium. The US transducer was tilted from side to side to better visualize the TEA probe inside the uterine cavity.

Coagulation was judged complete (first endpoint) when the activated TEA probe was passed over the whole uterine cavity. By the end of uterine cavity coagulation, tissue elasticity was lost and the uterine cavity underwent some shrinkage that impeded the easiness of moving the TEA probe up and down as if the uterine wall was clenching or holding it. This interesting sign was given the name "the grip sign" and it confirmed the fulfillment of the procedure. We theoretically evaluated other endpoints in the form of impending perforation (the occurrence of any penetration of the TEA probe through the myometrium in the ultrasonic scan), suspected or actual perforation, excessive vaginal bleeding, and/or unsatisfactory sonographic monitoring (inability to visualize the uterus in a clear longitudinal scan view with hyperechoic probe inside the uterine cavity between the two uterine walls and its tip below the fundus).

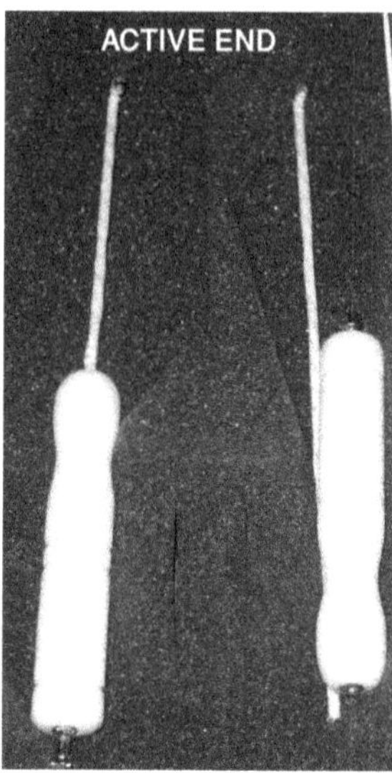

Figure 1: The tactile electrosurgical ablation (TEA) probe.

At the end of the procedure and after cessation of uterine bleeding, we performed a diagnostic hysteroscopy, for detection of missed foci of untreated endometrium. All cases were followed up every three months for one year. Longer-term follow-up for another one year was obtained by phone calls.

3. Results

Nineteen women presenting with heavy/prolonged menstrual bleeding were included in the current study. Their ages ranged from 40 to 47. The bleeding was heavy and prolonged in 15 cases and was on and off for three months in 2 cases, and continuous mild spotting was observed in the other 2 cases. Preoperative hemoglobin concentration ranged from 7 to 10 gm%. Two cases received preoperative blood transfusion, one received total dose iron infusion, and three cases were on oral iron.

Operative time ranged from 6 to 10 minutes depending on the size of the uterine cavity and proposed end points. No intraoperative difficulties, complications, or full thickness damage was reported. The grip sign was elicited very well in 17 cases and was not so obvious in the remaining 2 cases. Immediate diagnostic hysteroscopy was possible in 15 cases and showed complete coagulation (faint yellowish to dark brown color) apart from diminutive foci of uncoagulated endometrium (pinkish color) near the uterine cornua.

The TEA procedure was successful in the immediate cessation of the bleeding attack in 18 out of the 19 cases. During six- to 24-month follow-up period, 9 cases developed amenorrhea, 5 had light menstrual bleeding, 3 had regular menstruation, one case underwent a repeat ablation 6 months later (on request), and the last one had undergone a hysterectomy for recurrence of HMB.

4. Discussion

Tactile electrosurgical ablation (TEA) was successfully performed with satisfactory outcomes for 19 cases with heavy and/or prolonged uterine bleeding during an active, relentless bleeding attack. The TEA procedure was effective in the immediate cessation of the bleeding attack in 18 of the 19 cases. Although hysterectomy remains the definitive treatment for HMB, the associated morbidities are significant especially in medically unfit patients and/or in deteriorated hemodynamic states [9, 10]. The results of an applied patient's questionnaire in a hospital in Netherlands showed that approximately one-third of women undergoing hysterectomy due to abnormal uterine bleeding would have opted for endometrial ablation and 45% would have opted for a levonorgestrel-releasing IUD, despite a risk of 50% possibility of treatment failure [11].

However, for all types of hysteroscopic ablation, satisfactory proper visualization of the uterine cavity is vital for successful and safe performance. In addition, the number of well-trained personnel in hysteroscopic surgeries is still limited. Other challenges and financial constraints in developing countries result in difficulties in maintaining perfectly working hysteroscopic equipment [10].

In the present series, active heavy uterine bleeding was anticipated to result in failure to perform hysteroscopic endometrial ablation safely as it interferes with proper visualization. Other investigators reported such difficulties in hysteroscopic surgery [12]. Thermal balloons and other second generation ablators could play a backup role in such cases. However, financial constraints and scarce health resources limit the availability and affordability of expensive disposables [13, 14].

Hysteroscopic electrosurgeries are performed using appropriate distension media which should be electrolyte-free with monopolar electrosurgical coagulation. Nevertheless, electrolyte-free distension media has its own problems [15–17]. The most vulnerable subjects are those with unclear hysteroscopic view due to excessive bleeding. This requires too much washing at higher pressures, which pushes extra volumes of fluids into the open-mouthed bleeding vessels for a more prolonged duration. The use of TEA has the advantage of avoiding fluid overload especially in this vulnerable group of patients.

The technique of tactile electrosurgical ablation (TEA) is largely similar to the dilatation and curettage procedure. Hence, the procedure requires awareness of electrosurgical principles, satisfactory experience in ultrasonic monitoring, high resolution ultrasonic machine, and adequate experience in performing dilatation and curettage. Even if it seems that TEA is a blind technique, it is not underprivileged of direct external visual monitoring by ultrasonography. In addition, TEA is carried out under the great tactile sense of the experienced gynecologist, promoting the survival of that clinical sense before being a state-of-a-lost art [18].

The main weakness point of the present study is the limited number of cases that makes statistical and power analysis impractical. However, it opens a new perspective for a novel inexpensive backup approach for electrosurgical ablation without distension media, hysteroscopy, or expensive disposables especially in limited resources' settings. Moreover, TEA has the potential to be the procedure of choice in cases with heavy uterine bleeding as it depends on tactile rather than visual ablation and is found to be effective in stopping the active bleeding in 90% of cases.

5. Conclusions

Tactile endometrial ablation is a promising inexpensive management procedure of heavy uterine bleeding in low sources' setting. However larger studies are recommended to confirm its safety and cost effectiveness.

References

[1] R. C. Dicker, J. R. Greenspan, L. T. Strauss et al., "Complications of abdominal and vaginal hysterectomy among women of reproductive age in the United States: the collaborative review of sterilization," *The American Journal of Obstetrics and Gynecology*, vol. 144, no. 7, pp. 841–848, 1982.

[2] J. M. Y. Tsoh, H. C. M. Leung, G. S. Ungvari, and D. T. S. Lee, "Brief acute psychosis following hysterectomy in ethnopsychiatric context," *Singapore Medical Journal*, vol. 41, no. 7, pp. 359–362, 2000.

[3] Y. A. Helmy, I. M. A. Hassanin, T. A. Elraheem, A. A. Bedaiwy, R. S. Peterson, and M. A. Bedaiwy, "Psychiatric morbidity following hysterectomy in Egypt," *International Journal of Gynecology and Obstetrics*, vol. 102, no. 1, pp. 60–64, 2008.

[4] M. H. Goldrath, T. A. Fuller, and S. Segal, "Laser photovaporization of endometrium for the treatment of menorrhagia," *American Journal of Obstetrics and Gynecology*, vol. 140, no. 1, pp. 14–19, 1981.

[5] A. DeCherney and M. L. Polan, "Hysteroscopic management of intrauterine lesions and intractable uterine bleeding," *Obstetrics and Gynecology*, vol. 61, no. 3, pp. 392–396, 1983.

[6] T. G. Vancaillie, "Electrocoagulation of the endometrium with the ball-end resectoscope," *Obstetrics and Gynecology*, vol. 74, no. 3 I, pp. 425–427, 1989.

[7] A. Lethaby and M. Hickey, *Endometrial Destruction Techniques for Heavy Menstrual Bleeding (Cochrane Review)*, vol. 4 of *Update Software*, The Cochrane Library, Oxford, UK, 2002.

[8] R. S. Neuwirth, A.-A. Duran, A. Singer, R. MacDonald, and L. Bolduc, "The endometrial ablator: a new instrument," *Obstetrics and Gynecology*, vol. 83, no. 5, pp. 792–796, 1994.

[9] A. M. El-Saman, H. S. Mohamad, M. S. Zakhera, K. M. Zahran, E. M. Ahmad, and A. O. Salem, "Tactile electrosurgical ablation: a new technique for endometrial ablation. A preliminary study,"

The Medical Journal of Cairo University, vol. 78, no. 1, pp. 241–246, 2010.

[10] G. H. Sayed, A. M. El Saman, M. H. Mohamed, and S. M. S. Al Deen, "Outcomes and problems of hysteroscopic endometrial ablation in a University Hospital," *Middle East Fertility Society Journal*, vol. 19, no. 3, pp. 212–214, 2014.

[11] P. Bourdrez, M. Y. Bongers, and B. W. J. Mol, "Treatment of dysfunctional uterine bleeding: patient preferences for endometrial ablation, a levonorgestrel-releasing intrauterine device, or hysterectomy," *Fertility and Sterility*, vol. 82, no. 1, pp. 160–166, 265, 2004.

[12] K. McPherson, M. A. Metcalfe, A. Herbert et al., "Severe complications of hysterectomy: the value study," *BJOG*, vol. 111, no. 7, pp. 688–694, 2004.

[13] P. M. Brown, C. M. Farquhar, A. Lethaby, L. C. Sadler, and N. P. Johnson, "Cost-effectiveness analysis of levonorgestrel intrauterine system and thermal balloon ablation for heavy menstrual bleeding," *BJOG: An International Journal of Obstetrics & Gynaecology*, vol. 113, no. 7, pp. 797–803, 2006.

[14] J. T. Jensen, P. Lefebvre, F. Laliberté et al., "Cost burden and treatment patterns associated with management of heavy menstrual bleeding," *Journal of Women's Health*, vol. 21, no. 5, pp. 539–547, 2012.

[15] S. Izetbegović, "Early and late complications in patients treated with hysteroscopic surgery," *Medicinski arhiv*, vol. 56, no. 4, pp. 217–219, 2002.

[16] H.-W. Huang, S.-C. Lee, W.-M. Ho, H.-C. Lai, and S.-E. Juang, "Complications of fluid overloading with differential distention media in hysteroscopy—a report of two cases," *Acta Anaesthesiologica Sinica*, vol. 41, no. 3, pp. 149–154, 2003.

[17] P. D. Indman, P. G. Brooks, J. M. Cooper, F. D. Loffer, R. F. Valle, and T. G. Vancaillie, "Complications of fluid overload from resectoscopic surgery," *Journal of the American Association of Gynecologic Laparoscopists*, vol. 5, no. 1, pp. 63–67, 1998.

[18] A. M. El Saman, A. M. Darwish, M. S. Zakherah, H. O. Hamed, M. A. Bedaiwy, and A. M. Nasr, "Tactile cold scissor metroplasty as a novel backup method for hysteroscopic metroplasty," *Fertility and Sterility*, vol. 94, no. 3, pp. 1086–1089, 2010.

23

Association between Obesity, Surgical Route, and Perioperative Outcomes in Patients with Uterine Cancer

Entidhar Al Sawah,[1] Jason L. Salemi,[2] Mitchel Hoffman,[3] Anthony N. Imudia,[1] and Emad Mikhail[1]

[1]*Department of Obstetrics and Gynecology, University of South Florida Morsani College of Medicine, Tampa, FL, USA*
[2]*Department of Family and Community Medicine, Baylor College of Medicine, Houston, TX, USA*
[3]*Division of Gynecologic Oncology, Moffitt Cancer Center, University of South Florida, Tampa, FL, USA*

Correspondence should be addressed to Emad Mikhail; emikhail@health.usf.edu

Academic Editor: Saad Amer

Objective. To study temporal trends of hysterectomy routes performed for uterine cancer and their associations with body mass index (BMI) and perioperative morbidity. *Methods*. A retrospective review of the American College of Surgeons-National Surgical Quality Improvement Program (ACS-NSQIP) 2005-2013 databases was conducted. All patients who were 18 years old and older with a diagnosis of uterine cancer and underwent hysterectomy were identified using ICD-9-CM and CPT codes. Surgical route was classified into four groups: total abdominal hysterectomy (TAH), total vaginal hysterectomy (TVH), laparoscopic assisted vaginal hysterectomy (LAVH), and total laparoscopic hysterectomy (TLH) including both conventional and robotically assisted. Patients were then stratified according to BMI. *Results*. 7199 records were included in the study. TLH was the most commonly performed route of hysterectomy regardless of BMI, with proportions of 50.9%, 48.9%, 50.4%, and 51.2% in ideal, overweight, obese, and morbidly obese patients, respectively. The median operative time for TAH was 2.2 hours compared to 2.7 hours for TLH ($p < 0.01$). The median length of stay for TAH was 3 days compared to 1 day for TLH ($p < 0.01$). The percentage of patients with an adverse outcome (composite indicator including transfusion, deep venous thrombosis, and infection) was 17.1 versus 3.7 for TAH and TLH, respectively ($p < 0.01$). *Conclusion*. During the last decade, TLH has been increasingly performed in women with uterine cancer. The increased adoption of TLH was seen in all BMI subgroups.

1. Introduction

Uterine cancer is the most common gynecologic cancer in USA [1], with the median age at presentation being 60 years [2]. Depending on the stage and grade, surgery is the mainstay of treatment of uterine tumors, with or without subsequent radiation. Early stage uterine cancer can be managed safely with conventional as well as robotically assisted laparoscopic approaches [3, 4].

Despite the evidence-based benefits associated with minimally invasive gynecologic surgical approaches, laparotomy remains the route of choice in more than 60% of the 600,000 hysterectomy procedures performed annually in USA [5]. The rate of abdominal hysterectomy in USA between 2003 and 2005 was still over 60% and only 12–14% of hysterectomies were being performed laparoscopically [6].

Greater degree of obesity is a well-known risk factor for the development of uterine cancer [7, 8]. Surgery for uterine cancer in obese patients can pose significant intra- and postoperative challenges to the surgeon. Obesity is associated with a higher rate of conversion of laparoscopic surgery to laparotomy and a lower completion rate of lymph node dissection [9].

Although obesity is associated with higher incidence of uterine cancer and recent studies have reported that the rate of abdominal hysterectomy performed for benign indications is increased in obese patients [10], the extent to which obesity plays a role in the surgical management of

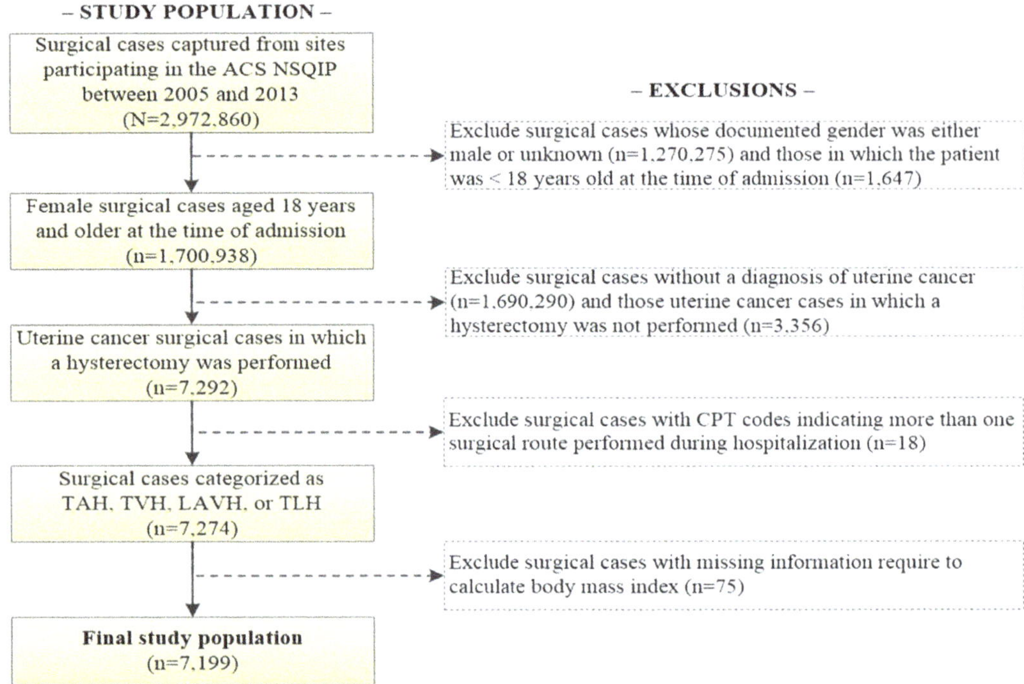

FIGURE 1: **Flow diagram representing the final determination of all patients in which a hysterectomy was performed among patients with a diagnosis of uterine cancer, ACS-NSQIP, 2005-2013**. ACS-NSQIP: American College of Surgeons-National Surgical Quality Improvement Program; TAH: total abdominal hysterectomy; TVH: total vaginal hysterectomy; LAVH: laparoscopic assisted vaginal hysterectomy; TLH: total laparoscopic hysterectomy.

uterine cancer is currently unknown. We hypothesize that, with increased obesity, the proportion of minimally invasive surgical approach might decrease. Therefore, in this study, we explore the association between obesity and surgical route for the treatment of uterine cancer, and we describe the extent to which the rate of perioperative complications differs by obesity status.

2. Materials and Methods

After obtaining exempt status from the University of South Florida's institutional review board, we used the American College of Surgeons-National Surgical Quality Improvement Program (ACS NSQIP) database from 2005 to 2013 to conduct a retrospective, cross-sectional analysis of female patients with uterine cancer who underwent hysterectomy. ACS-NSQIP is a publically available and deidentified database created as part of a quality improvement initiative originally developed by the Veterans' Health Administration in 1991 and adopted by the American College of Surgeons in 2001 [11, 12]. The database includes more than 450 participating community and academic hospitals nationwide. Data captured include but are not limited to demographics, comorbidities, laboratory values, and operative variables, as well as 30-day postoperative outcomes, complications, mortality, reoperation, and length of stay. Quality improvement and assurance protocols include routine auditing and the use of specially trained surgical nurses to record patient variables. A random 8-day sampling method is used to ensure that a diverse range of surgical procedures is captured.

In patients aged 18 years or above, we identified women with uterine cancer using the principal postoperative diagnosis (ICD-9-CM code 182.0, 182.1, or 182.8). We then used current procedural terminology (CPT) procedure codes to identify 7,292 surgical cases in which hysterectomy was performed and then specific codes were used to subclassify cases as (1) total abdominal hysterectomy (TAH, 58150 and 58200); (2) total vaginal hysterectomy (TVH, 58260, 58262, 58263, 58270, 58275, 58280, 58290, 58291, 58292, and 58294); (3) laparoscopic assisted vaginal hysterectomy (LAVH, 58550, 58552, 58553, and 58554); and (4) total laparoscopic hysterectomy (TLH, 58570, 58571, 58572, and 58573). We excluded 18 cases (0.2%) with CPT codes indicating more than one surgical route performed. Due to absence of specific CPT codes, we could not differentiate between robotically assisted laparoscopic hysterectomies from TLH; therefore, these groups are combined into a single group (TLH) (Figure 1).

Body mass index (BMI) was calculated as [(weight in pounds)/((height in inches)^2) $\times$ 703], and then patients were classified according to BMI as follows: normal and underweight (<25), overweight (25–29.9), obese (classes I and II; 30–39.9), and morbid obesity (class III; ≥40). We excluded 75 cases (1.0%) for which BMI could not be calculated due to missing information on presurgical weight and height. Data analyzed included patient age, race/ethnicity, operative time, length of hospital stay, blood transfusion,

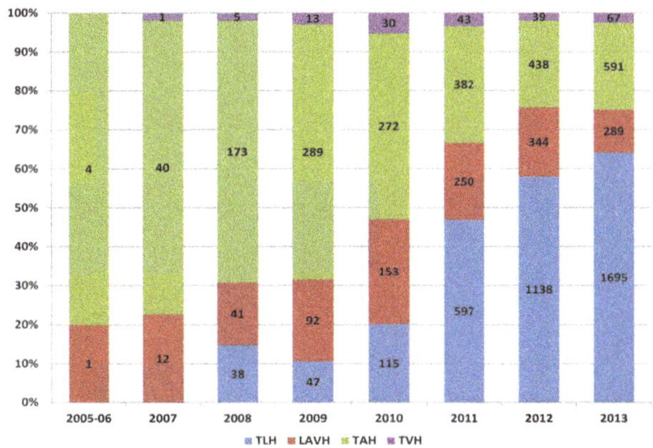

FIGURE 2: **Frequency and proportion of different types of hysterectomies performed among patients with a diagnosis of uterine cancer, ACS-NSQIP, 2005-2013.** TAH: total abdominal hysterectomy; TVH: total vaginal hysterectomy; LAVH: laparoscopic assisted vaginal hysterectomy; TLH: total laparoscopic hysterectomy.

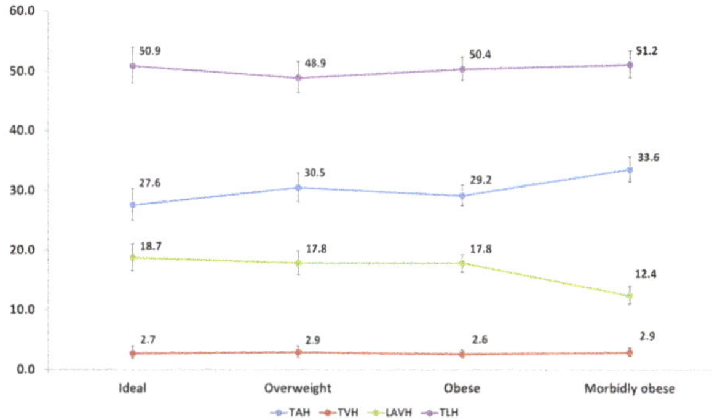

FIGURE 3: Rates of different types of hysterectomy performed among patients with a diagnosis of uterine cancer, by patient's body mass index, ACS-NSQIP, 2005-2013.

development of deep venous thrombosis, and development of surgical infection. Infection types included superficial surgical site (involving only skin or subcutaneous tissue) and deep incisional surgical site (involving deep soft tissues). When data were available (2011 or later), we also captured 30-day readmissions.

Descriptive statistics were used to describe the frequency and temporal trends in surgical approaches in the entire study population and stratified by patient's BMI level. Differences in the distribution of selected patient sociodemographic and hospital characteristics and in the rates of clinical outcomes by surgical approach were assessed using either a Wilcoxon-Mann–Whitney test (continuous variables) or chi-square test (categorical variables). For each hysterectomy route, we compared the rate of perioperative outcomes across levels of patient's BMI. All statistical analyses were conducted using SAS version 9.4 (SAS Institute, Inc., Cary, NC), using a 5% type I error rate and two-sided hypothesis tests. STrengthening the Reporting of OBservational studies in Epidemiology (STROBE) guidelines for reporting observational studies were followed for this study [13].

3. Results

Between 2005 and 2013, we identified a total of 7,199 uterine cancer surgical cases managed with hysterectomy and with documented presurgical weight and height (Figure 1). The most common route of hysterectomy was TLH (50.4%), followed by TAH (30.4%), LAVH (16.4%), and TVH (2.8%). During the study period, we observed a relative increase in the use of the TLH route (from 15% in 2008 to 64% in 2013) and a concomitant relative decrease in the use of TAH (from 67% in 2008 to 22% in 2013) (Figure 2). Until 2013, the proportion of hysterectomies using the LAVH route was relatively constant over time, as was the small proportion of surgical cases in which TVH was performed.

Total laparoscopic hysterectomy was the most performed procedure regardless of BMI, occurring in 50.9%, 48.9%, 50.4%, and 51.2% of patients with ideal, overweight, obese, and morbidly obese BMI, respectively (Figure 3). The overall rate of TAH was 30%; however, the rate tended to be slightly higher in patients who were morbidly obese (33.6%) relative to other patients. This increase in the rate of TAH in morbidly obese patients was at the expense of LAVH (12.4%); the LAVH rate among the morbidly obese was statistically significantly lower than the LAVH rate in each of the other BMI categories.

The median patient BMI differed significantly by surgical approach; patients who underwent TAH had overall higher BMI (34.0 kg/m^2) compared to those undergoing TVH (33.1 kg/m^2), LAVH (32.2 kg/m^2), and TLH (33.7 kg/m^2) (Table 1). Patients undergoing TAH and LAVH were more likely to be nonwhite than patients undergoing TVH and TLH ($p < 0.01$). The median operative room time was statistically significantly shorter for TAH (2.2 hours) compared to TLH (2.7 hours). However, the median length of hospital stay for TAH was three times longer than TLH, TVH, or LAVH ($p < 0.01$). Over 15% of patients who underwent TAH stayed in the hospital for 6 days or longer, compared to only 1.3% of patients undergoing TLH ($p < 0.01$). The rates of several perioperative complications were increased significantly in patients who underwent TAH compared to TLH; these complications include transfusion (10.3% versus 1.7%) ($p < 0.01$), surgical site infection (7.1% versus 1.7%) ($p < 0.01$), and readmission within 30 days (8.9% versus 3.8%) ($p < 0.01$).

Regardless of the route of hysterectomy, patients who were morbidly obese, obese, or overweight tended to have statistically significantly longer operation times than patients who had an ideal BMI ($p < 0.05$). Similarly, postoperative infections, including superficial or deep surgical site infections, were more common in higher BMI categories when compared with ideal BMI ($p < 0.05$), and patients who were morbidly obese experienced substantially higher rates of any surgical site or wound infection (6.4%) compared to patients who had an ideal BMI (1.6%). The 30-day readmission rates were similar across all BMI categories (Table 2).

The rate of readmission and the rate of a composite infection outcome (including superficial surgical site infection,

Table 1: Distribution of selected patient sociodemographic and hospital characteristics among patients with a diagnosis of uterine cancer and in which a hysterectomy was performed, by route of hysterectomy, ACS-NSQIP, 2005-2013.

	TAH (n=2,189)		TVH (n=198)		LAVH (n=1,182)		TLH (n=3,630)		P[a]
BMI (kg/m^2), med (Q1-Q3)	34.0	28.0-42.2	33.1	27.8-41.6	32.2	26.6-38.7	33.7	27.4-41.2	<.01
BMI (kg/m^2)									<.01
<25	313	14.3	31	15.7	212	17.9	577	15.9	
25-30	428	19.6	40	20.2	250	21.2	687	18.9	
30-40	776	35.4	70	35.4	472	39.9	1,341	36.9	
≥40	672	30.7	57	28.8	248	21.0	1,025	28.2	
Age at admission (years)									<.01
<50	260	11.9	23	11.6	138	11.7	358	9.9	
50-59	572	26.1	40	20.2	325	27.5	1,029	28.3	
60-69	741	33.9	68	34.3	411	34.8	1,354	37.3	
70-79	284	17.5	30	15.2	214	18.1	655	18.0	
≥80	232	10.6	37	18.7	94	8.0	234	6.4	
Race/ethnicity									<.01
Non-Hispanic white	1,426	65.1	162	81.8	790	66.8	2,939	81.0	
Non-Hispanic black	228	10.4	4	2.0	85	7.2	187	5.2	
Hispanic	140	6.4	9	4.5	95	8.0	157	4.3	
Other	82	3.7	12	6.1	49	4.1	190	5.2	
Missing	313	14.3	11	5.6	163	13.8	157	4.3	
Total operation time (hours), med (Q1-Q3)	2.2	1.6-3.0	1.6	1.1-2.8	2.6	1.9-3.6	2.7	2.0-3.5	<.01
Total operation time (hours)									<.01
<2	928	42.4	125	63.1	320	27.1	857	23.6	
2-3	700	32.0	29	14.6	394	33.3	1,374	37.9	
3-4	369	16.9	20	10.1	245	20.7	842	23.2	
4-5	115	5.3	14	7.1	144	12.2	371	10.2	
≥5	77	3.5	10	5.1	79	6.7	184	5.1	
Length of stay (days), med (Q1-Q3)	3.0	2.0-4.0	1.0	1.0-2.0	1.0	1.0-2.0	1.0	1.0-1.0	<.01
Length of stay (days)									<.01
0-1	97	4.4	140	70.7	833	70.5	2,920	80.4	
2	484	22.1	44	22.2	240	20.3	467	12.9	
3-5	1,271	58.1	11	5.6	90	7.6	193	5.3	
≥6	336	15.3	3	1.5	19	1.6	49	1.3	
Bleeding transfusion[b]	225	10.3	7	3.5	29	2.5	60	1.7	<.01
DVT/thrombophlebitis	20	0.9	3	1.5	6	0.5	17	0.5	0.07
Superficial surgical site infection[c]	107	4.9	2	1.0	3	0.3	33	0.9	<.01
Open wound/wound infection[d]	20	0.9	2	1.0	4	0.3	22	0.6	0.21
Deep incisional surgical site infection[e]	31	1.4	0	0.0	0	0.0	8	0.2	<.01
Any infection listed above	156	7.1	4	2.0	7	0.6	63	1.7	<.01
Any adverse outcome listed above	375	17.1	13	6.6	41	3.5	135	3.7	<.01
Readmission within 30 days[f]	125	8.9	8	5.4	30	3.4	129	3.8	<.01

ACS-NSQIP: American College of Surgeons-National Surgical Quality Improvement Program; BMI: body mass index; DVT: deep vein thrombosis.
Unless otherwise indicated, values listed are the frequency and percent.

[a]P value from either a Wilcoxon-Mann–Whitney test (continuous variables) or chi-square test (categorical variables).

[b]At least 1 unit of packed or whole red blood cells given from the surgical start time up to and including 72 hours postoperatively.

[c]Infection that occurs within 30 days after the operation and the infection involves only skin or subcutaneous tissue of the incision.

[d]Preoperative evidence of a documented open wound at the time of the principal operative procedure. An open wound is a breach in the integrity of the skin or separation of skin edges and includes open surgical wounds, with or without cellulitis or purulent exudate. This does not include osteomyelitis or localized abscesses.

[e]Infection that occurs within 30 days after the operation and the infection appears to be related to the operation and infection involved deep soft tissues (e.g., fascial and muscle layers) of the incision.

[f]Readmission within 30 days was only available beginning in 2011; therefore, the percent provided reflects only the proportion of 2011-13 cases who were readmitted.

TABLE 2: Perioperative outcomes stratified by patient's body mass index, ACS-NSQIP, 2005-2013.

Characteristic/outcome	BMI classification Ideal	Overweight	Obese	Morbidly obese
Patient age (years)[a]	63 (55-74)	65 (57-73)	63 (57-71)	60 (54-65)*
Operation time (min)[a]	137 (100-189)	143 (102-193)*	149 (110-200)*	164 (124-214)*
Length of hospital stay (days)[a]	1 (1-2)	1 (1-3)	1 (1-3)	1 (1-3)*
Bleeding transfusion[b]	79 (7.0)	70 (5.0)*	90 (3.4)*	82 (4.1)*
DVT/thrombophlebitis	3 (0.3)	11 (0.8)	18 (0.7)	14 (0.7)
Superficial surgical site infection[c]	11 (1.0)	10 (0.7)	53 (2.0)*	71 (3.5)*
Open wound/wound infection[d]	5 (0.4)	4 (0.3)	10 (0.4)	29 (1.4)*
Deep incisional surgical site infection[e]	2 (0.2)	2 (0.1)	7 (0.3)	28 (1.4)*
Any infection listed above	18 (1.6)	16 (1.1)	68 (2.6)	128 (6.4)*
Any adverse outcome listed above	96 (8.5)	91 (6.5)	167 (6.3)*	210 (10.5)
Readmission within 30 days[f]	46 (5.0)	47 (4.1)	101 (4.6)	98 (6.0)

ACS NSQIP = American College of Surgeons National Surgical Quality Improvement Program; BMI = body mass index; DVT = deep vein thrombosis.
*P-value<0.05 from either a Wilcoxon-Mann Whitney test (continuous variables) or chi-square test (categorical variables). For each outcome, three tests are performed: overweight vs. ideal BMI, obese vs. ideal BMI, morbidly obese vs. ideal BMI.
[a]Values presented as median (Q1-Q3); all others are presented as frequency (%).
[b]At least 1 unit of packed or whole red blood cells given from the surgical start time up to and including 72 hours postoperatively.
[c]Infection that occurs within 30 days after the operation and the infection involves only skin or subcutaneous tissue of the incision.
[d]Preoperative evidence of a documented open wound at the time of the principal operative procedure. An open wound is a breach in the integrity of the skin or separation of skin edges and includes open surgical wounds, with or without cellulitis or purulent exudate. This does not include osteomyelitis or localized abscesses.
[e]Infection that occurs within 30 days after the operation and the infection appears to be related to the operation and infection involved deep soft tissues (e.g., fascial and muscle layers) of the incision.
[f]Readmission within 30 days was only available beginning in 2011; therefore, the percent provided reflects only the proportion of 2011-13 cases who were readmitted.

open wound/wound infection, and deep incisional surgical site infection) within 30 days were significantly lower for TLH and LAVH compared to TAH in all BMI subgroups except for the overweight group (Supplemental Tables S1-S4).

In comparing perioperative outcomes of TLH stratified by patient's BMI category, it was noted that increasing degree of obesity was associated with longer operative time. The mean operation time in patients of ideal weight (145 min) was shorter compared to overweight, obese, and morbidly obese women (159, 158, and 171 minutes, resp., $p < 0.05$). Also, the rate of open surgical wound or wound infection was higher in the morbidly obese group (1.3%) compared to ideal weight patients (0.2%) ($p < 0.05$). All other perioperative outcomes were not statistically significantly different across BMI levels (Table 3).

4. Discussion

In this study, using the ACS-NSQIP database, TLH (including conventional or robotically assisted) was found to be the most frequently chosen route for hysterectomy for surgical management of patients with uterine cancer. Performance of TLH increased from 16.5% in 2008 to 64.1% in 2013. We also found that TLH is the most commonly chosen route regardless of the degree of obesity. Despite increased operative time compared to abdominal hysterectomy, the minimally invasive approach provided better perioperative outcomes manifesting in decreased length of hospital stay and decreased rates of transfusion, surgical site infection, and readmission within 30 days. The utilization of TLH was not negatively impacted by the degree of obesity, despite the increase in operative time and surgical infection.

The results from current study are consistent with data from the SEER database, which showed that performance of minimally invasive hysterectomy has increased from 9.3% in 2006 to 61.7% in 2011 [14]. Minimally invasive surgery improved outcomes including decreased hospital stay, increased patient quality of life, consistency with patient preference, and enhanced cosmesis [15]. These factors have been considered as important drivers of cost and efficiency in the era of the Affordable Care Act [16].

Compared to other routes, TAH rates among patients with uterine cancer were higher in morbidly obese women compared to women with lower BMI levels. This might be explained by the increased and persistent technical challenges encountered by surgeons during minimally invasive surgery in patients with higher degrees of obesity [17]. Excessive adiposity poses several challenges to the surgical team, including poor patient tolerance to Trendelenburg positioning and positive intra-abdominal pressure, surgeons' fatigue, and the inability to correctly expose and develop the anatomical spaces [18].

On the other hand, TAH was found to be associated with an increased risk for perioperative complications when compared with other surgical routes. This is reflected by longer hospital stay, higher rates of surgical sites infections, and higher 30-day readmission rates. Since higher perioperative complications can compromise overall survival and success of adjuvant therapy, it is critical to take active measures to avoid

TABLE 3: Perioperative outcomes among uterine cancer patients undergoing total laparoscopic hysterectomy, stratified by patient's body mass index, ACS-NSQIP, 2005-2013.

Characteristic/outcome	BMI classification			
	Ideal	Overweight	Obese	Morbidly obese
Patient age (years)[a]	63 (55-72)	65 (57-72)*	63 (57-70)	60 (54-66)*
Operation time (min)[a]	145 (113-194)	159 (119-205)*	158 (120-206)*	171 (134-218)*
Length of hospital stay (days)[a]	1 (1-1)	1 (1-1)	1 (1-1)	1 (1-1)*
Bleeding transfusion[b]	16 (2.8)	12 (1.7)	18 (1.3)*	14 (1.4)
DVT/thrombophlebitis	0 (0.0)	4 (0.6)	6 (0.4)	7 (0.7)
Superficial surgical site infection[c]	3 (0.5)	4 (0.6)	13 (1.0)	13 (1.3)
Open wound/wound infection[d]	1 (0.2)	1 (0.1)	7 (0.5)	13 (1.3)*
Deep incisional surgical site infection[e]	0 (0.0)	1 (0.1)	2 (0.1)	5 (0.5)
Any infection listed above	4 (0.7)	6 (0.9)	22 (1.6)	31 (3.0)*
Any adverse outcome listed above	20 (3.5)	20 (2.9)	44 (3.3)	51 (5.0)
Readmission within 30 days[f]	15 (2.8)	23 (3.6)	50 (3.9)	41 (4.2)

ACS NSQIP = American College of Surgeons National Surgical Quality Improvement Program; BMI = body mass index; DVT = deep vein thrombosis.
*P-value<0.05 from either a Wilcoxon-Mann Whitney test (continuous variables) or chi-square test (categorical variables). For each outcome, three tests are performed: overweight vs. ideal BMI, obese vs. ideal BMI, morbidly obese vs. ideal BMI.
[a]Values presented as median (Q1-Q3); all others are presented as frequency (%).
[b]At least 1 unit of packed or whole red blood cells given from the surgical start time up to and including 72 hours postoperatively.
[c]Infection that occurs within 30 days after the operation and the infection involves only skin or subcutaneous tissue of the incision.
[d]Preoperative evidence of a documented open wound at the time of the principal operative procedure. An open wound is a breach in the integrity of the skin or separation of skin edges and includes open surgical wounds, with or without cellulitis or purulent exudate. This does not include osteomyelitis or localized abscesses.
[e]Infection that occurs within 30 days after the operation and the infection appears to be related to the operation and infection involved deep soft tissues (e.g., fascial and muscle layers) of the incision.
[f]Readmission within 30 days was only available beginning in 2011; therefore, the percent provided reflects only the proportion of 2011-13 cases who were readmitted.

or reduce the incidence of such complications [19]. With accumulating experience and increased training in minimally invasive surgeries, including robotically assisted procedures, the adoption of such techniques is likely to increase in the future; we suspect a concomitant improvement in perioperative outcomes in patients with uterine cancer [5].

In cases where pelvic lymph node dissection is performed, the preferred route for hysterectomy is either abdominal or laparoscopic. The utilization of TVH for uterine cancer surgery is controversial and the utility of nodal dissection in uterine cancer patients lacks a consensus opinion [20]. The role of TVH in uterine cancer depends on the type of the tumor, the stage of tumor, BMI, and presence of comorbidities. For stage I grade I uterine cancer, TVH may be reasonable, especially if CA-125 level <20 U/mL because of the low likelihood of extrauterine tumor invasion [21]. TVH utilization is limited in more advanced uterine cancer due to the limited ability to complete cancer staging.

In comparison with higher degrees of obesity, ideal body weight was found to be associated with the most favorable perioperative outcomes. This is supported by other studies showing obesity to be associated with increased complication rates in elective hysterectomy procedures, independent of the surgical route. Morbid obesity was found to be associated with increased conversion of laparoscopic surgery to laparotomy and less complete lymph node dissection [19, 22, 23]. Obesity is now considered as a pandemic with increasing prevalence [24]. It has been shown that patients who are obese experience some of the greatest differential benefits from minimally invasive techniques [10]. Obesity increased the risk of unintended conversion to laparotomy, where patients with BMI >40 have 4-fold increase in the conversion rate [18].

The ACS-NSQIP database that was used in this study represents a major strength due to its multi-institutional nature and is widely considered to be accurate, reproducible, and reliable. Data are collected by specially trained surgical clinical nurse reviewers who collect more than 100 clinical variables, including preoperative risk factors, intraoperative variables, and 30-day postoperative mortality and morbidity outcomes for patients undergoing major surgical procedures [25].

A weakness of this study is its observational nature. Although clinical trials can be the best research path to delineate optimum surgical approach for uterine cancer in morbidly obese patients, observational studies can be invaluable tool for hypothesis generation and prediction of patients who are at higher risk of complication of a certain therapeutic approach. Another weakness of the study is the fact that it lacked data on patient survival and its association with BMI categories and the inability to differentiate between conventional laparoscopic and robotic procedures. The data in the ACS-NSQIP are only from participating hospitals and, despite being distributed throughout USA, they do not collectively represent a statistically selected nationally representative sample. This study also lacks data regarding lymph node dissection; traditionally obesity is thought to be associated with less complete lymph node dissection; interestingly, in a study by Uccella et al, it was found that the number of lymph nodes removed was not affected by BMI [18]. TLH is currently the most commonly performed route for hysterectomy for patients with uterine cancer, regardless of the degree of obesity. Other confounding variables including surgical experience, hospital to hospital variation, and ethnicity could not be controlled for in this analysis.

Obesity poses an important challenge for the surgeon in selecting the surgical modality that balances between the technical difficultly and obtaining the best perioperative surgical outcomes.

Abbreviations

BMI: Body mass index
ACS-NSQIP: American College of Surgeons-National Surgical Quality Improvement Program
CPT: Current procedural terminology
ICD-9-CM: International Classification of Disease, Ninth Revision, Clinical Modification
TAH: Total abdominal hysterectomy
TVH: Total vaginal hysterectomy
LAVH: Laparoscopic assisted vaginal hysterectomy
TLH: Total laparoscopic hysterectomy.

Disclosure

An earlier abstract of this paper was presented in the following link: http://www.jmig.org/article/S1553-4650(16)30281-3/fulltext, November-December, 2016, Volume 23, Issue 7. A preliminary version of this data was presented at Minimally Invasive Surgery Week 2016-SLS Annual Meeting, September 2016, Boston, Massachusetts; the AAGL-Global Congress on Minimally Invasive Gynecology, November 2016, Orlando, FL; and ACOG Annual Meeting, May 2017, San Diego, California.

Supplementary Materials

Table S1: perioperative outcomes among uterine cancer patients with ideal BMI, stratified by route of hysterectomy, ACS-NSQIP, 2005-2013. Table S2: perioperative outcomes among uterine cancer patients with overweight BMI, stratified by route of hysterectomy, ACS-NSQIP, 2005-2013. Table S3: perioperative outcomes among uterine cancer patients with obese BMI, stratified by route of hysterectomy, ACS-NSQIP, 2005-2013. Table S4: perioperative outcomes among uterine cancer patients with morbidly obese BMI, stratified by route of hysterectomy, ACS-NSQIP, 2005-2013. *(Supplementary Materials)*

References

[1] J. Cardenas-Goicoechea, A. Shepherd, M. Momeni et al., "Survival analysis of robotic versus traditional laparoscopic surgical staging for endometrial cancer," *American Journal of Obstetrics & Gynecology*, vol. 210, no. 2, pp. 160.e1–160.e11, 2014.

[2] F.F. Ferri, "Ferri's clinical advisor," in *5 books in 1*, Ferri's clinical advisor 2014, 5 books in 1, 2014.

[3] G. H. Eltabbakh, M. I. Shamonki, J. M. Moody, and L. L. Garafano, "Hysterectomy for obese women with endometrial cancer: Laparoscopy or laparotomy?" *Gynecologic Oncology*, vol. 78, no. 3 I, pp. 329–335, 2000.

[4] M. Q. Bernardini, L. T. Gien, H. Tipping, J. Murphy, and B. P. Rosen, "Surgical outcome of robotic surgery in morbidly obese patient with endometrial cancer compared to laparotomy," *International Journal of Gynecological Cancer*, vol. 22, no. 1, pp. 76–81, 2012.

[5] T. N. Payne and M. C. Pitter, "Robotic-assisted surgery for the community gynecologist: Can it be adopted?" *Clinical Obstetrics and Gynecology*, vol. 54, no. 3, pp. 391–411, 2011.

[6] D. Sarlos and L. A. Kots, "Robotic versus laparoscopic hysterectomy: A review of recent comparative studies," *Current Opinion in Obstetrics and Gynecology*, vol. 23, no. 4, pp. 283–288, 2011.

[7] R. Ballard-Barbash and C. A. Swanson, "Body weight: estimation of risk for breast and endometrial cancers," *American Journal of Clinical Nutrition*, vol. 63, no. 3, pp. 437S–441S, 1996.

[8] D. Aune, D. A. Navarro Rosenblatt, D. S. M. Chan et al., "Anthropometric factors and endometrial cancer risk: A systematic review and dose-response meta-analysis of prospective studies," *Annals of Oncology*, vol. 26, no. 8, pp. 1635–1648, 2015.

[9] R. W. Holloway and S. Ahmad, "Robotic-assisted surgery in the management of endometrial cancer," *Journal of Obstetrics and Gynaecology Research*, vol. 38, no. 1, pp. 1–8, 2012.

[10] E. Mikhail, B. Miladinovic, V. Velanovich, M. A. Finan, S. Hart, and A. N. Imudia, "Association between obesity and the trends of routes of hysterectomy performed for benign indications," *Obstetrics & Gynecology*, vol. 125, no. 4, pp. 912–918, 2015.

[11] S. F. Khuri, J. Daley, W. Henderson et al., "The Department of Veterans Affairs' NSQIP: The first national, validated, outcome-based, risk-adjusted, and peer-controlled program for the measurement and enhancement of the quality of surgical care," *Annals of Surgery*, vol. 228, no. 4, pp. 491–507, 1998.

[12] W. G. Henderson and J. Daley, "Design and statistical methodology of the National Surgical Quality Improvement Program: why is it what it is?" *The American Journal of Surgery*, vol. 198, no. 5, pp. S19–S27, 2009.

[13] E. von Elm, D. G. Altman, M. Egger et al., "The strengthening the reporting of observational studies in epidemiology (STROBE) statement: guidelines for reporting observational studies," *PLoS Medicine*, vol. 4, no. 10, article e297, 2007.

[14] J. D. Wright, W. M. Burke, A. I. Tergas et al., "Comparative effectiveness of minimally invasive hysterectomy for endometrial cancer," *Journal of Clinical Oncology*, vol. 34, no. 10, pp. 1087–1096, 2016.

[15] M. Frumovitz, P. T. Ramirez, M. Greer et al., "Laparoscopic training and practice in gynecologic oncology among Society of Gynecologic Oncologists members and fellows-in-training," *Gynecologic Oncology*, vol. 94, no. 3, pp. 746–753, 2004.

[16] E. Litvak and M. Bisognano, "Analysis & commentary: More patients, less payment: Increasing hospital efficiency in the aftermath of health reform," *Health Affairs*, vol. 30, no. 1, pp. 76–80, 2011.

[17] G. S. Leiserowitz, G. Xing, A. Parikh-Patel et al., "Laparoscopic versus abdominal hysterectomy for endometrial cancer comparison of patient outcomes," *International Journal of Gynecological Cancer*, vol. 19, no. 8, pp. 1370–1376, 2009.

[18] S. Uccella, M. Bonzini, S. Palomba et al., "Impact of Obesity on Surgical Treatment for Endometrial Cancer: A Multicenter Study Comparing Laparoscopy vs Open Surgery, with Propensity-Matched Analysis," *Journal of Minimally Invasive Gynecology*, vol. 23, no. 1, pp. 53–61, 2016.

[19] F. Bouwman, A. Smits, A. Lopes et al., "The impact of BMI on surgical complications and outcomes in endometrial cancer surgery - An institutional study and systematic review of the literature," *Gynecologic Oncology*, vol. 139, no. 2, pp. 369–376, 2015.

[20] S. Uccella, K. C. Podratz, G. D. Aletti, and A. Mariani, "Lymphadenectomy in endometrial cancer," *The Lancet*, vol. 373, no. 9670, p. 1170, 2009.

[21] A. K. Sood, R. E. Buller, R. A. Burger, J. D. Dawson, J. I. Sorosky, and M. Berman, "Value of preoperative CA 125 level in the management of uterine cancer and prediction of clinical outcome," *Obstetrics & Gynecology*, vol. 90, no. 3, pp. 441–447, 1997.

[22] K. Matsuo, C. E. Jung, M. S. Hom et al., "Predictive Factor of Conversion to Laparotomy in Minimally Invasive Surgical Staging for Endometrial Cancer," *International Journal of Gynecological Cancer*, vol. 26, no. 2, pp. 290–300, 2016.

[23] T.-J. Kim, G. Yoon, Y.-Y. Lee et al., "Robotic high para-aortic lymph node dissection with high port placement using same port for pelvic surgery in gynecologic cancer patients," *Journal of Gynecologic Oncology*, vol. 26, no. 3, pp. 222–226, 2015.

[24] M. Korenkov and S. Sauerland, "Clinical update: bariatric surgery," *The Lancet*, vol. 370, no. 9604, pp. 1988–1990, 2007.

[25] P. R. Fuchshuber, W. Greif, C. R. Tidwell et al., "The power of the National Surgical Quality Improvement Program–achieving a zero pneumonia rate in general surgery patients.," *The Permanente Journal*, vol. 16, no. 1, pp. 39–45, 2012.

24

A Comparative Study in Learning Curves of Two Different Intracorporeal Knot Tying Techniques

Manuneethimaran Thiyagarajan and Chandru Ravindrakumar

General Surgery Department, Sri Ramachandra Medical University, Chennai, India

Correspondence should be addressed to Manuneethimaran Thiyagarajan; profmaran@gmail.com

Academic Editor: Isaac Kim

Objectives. In our study we are aiming to analyse the learning curves in our surgical trainees by using two standard methods of intracorporeal knot tying. *Material and Method*. Two randomized groups of trainees are trained with two different intracorporeal knot tying techniques (loop and winding) by single surgeon for eight sessions. In each session participants were allowed to make as many numbers of knots in thirty minutes. The duration for each set of knots and the number of knots for each session were calculated. At the end each session, participants were asked about their frustration level, difficulty in making knot, and dexterity. *Results*. In winding method the number of knots tied was increasing significantly in each session with less frustration and less difficulty level. *Discussion*. The suturing and knotting skill improved in every session in both groups. But group B (winding method) trainees made significantly higher number of knots and they took less time for each set of knots than group A (loop method). Although both knotting methods are standard methods, the learning curve is better in loop method. *Conclusion*. The winding method of knotting is simpler and easier to perform, especially for the surgeons who have limited laparoscopic experience.

1. Introduction

A surgeon needs to improve his laparoscopic skills to overcome the difficulties in laparoscopy, which can be achieved through multiple and repetitive sessions in an alternative training method rather than getting trained in the patients directly. All must master the difficulties such as loss of depth perception, fulcrum effect of abdominal wall, limited motion freedom, and manipulation of tissues. This can be made easy by practicing in any of the training materials such as surgical simulators, virtual simulating trainers, and box-trainers. But the haptic feedback is best learnt in a box-trainer [1], which is an essential thing for learning the skills.

One of the most difficult tasks in laparoscopic surgery is intracorporeal knot tying and suturing technique. The fundamental elements of knot tying are its safety, easiness, rapidity of execution and tightness, and maintaining the knot. It has been an obstacle to all learners as it requires a lot of technical movement in a limited space. The extracorporeal knot tying is one of the alternate methods to overcome this difficulty [2].

When angle between the working instruments is narrow, the ligation and suturing are very difficult to perform. A side winding intracorporeal suturing can overcome this difficulty [3]. Most importantly geometric factors of endoscopic reconstruction, such as optimal distances between the working trocars, length of instruments, and angles between the instruments and the object will make lot of difference in suturing. Optimal geometry for intracorporeal suturing can be achieved by creating an isosceles triangle between the instruments with an angle between 25° and 45° and an angle <55° between the instruments and the horizontal line. These data should be considered when planning reconstructive laparoscopic procedure [4]. To make secured intracorporeal knot, surgeons knot is the ideal knotting method which consists of 2 × 1 configuration. The main aim of intracorporeal knot tying is to control suture tension and to create square knot in secured method. For basic laparoscopic surgery like appendectomy, a pretied loop can be used [5]. For single instrument knotting *Dowais Tie* technique [6] can be used. In a conventional knotting method with two instruments, the *loop* is

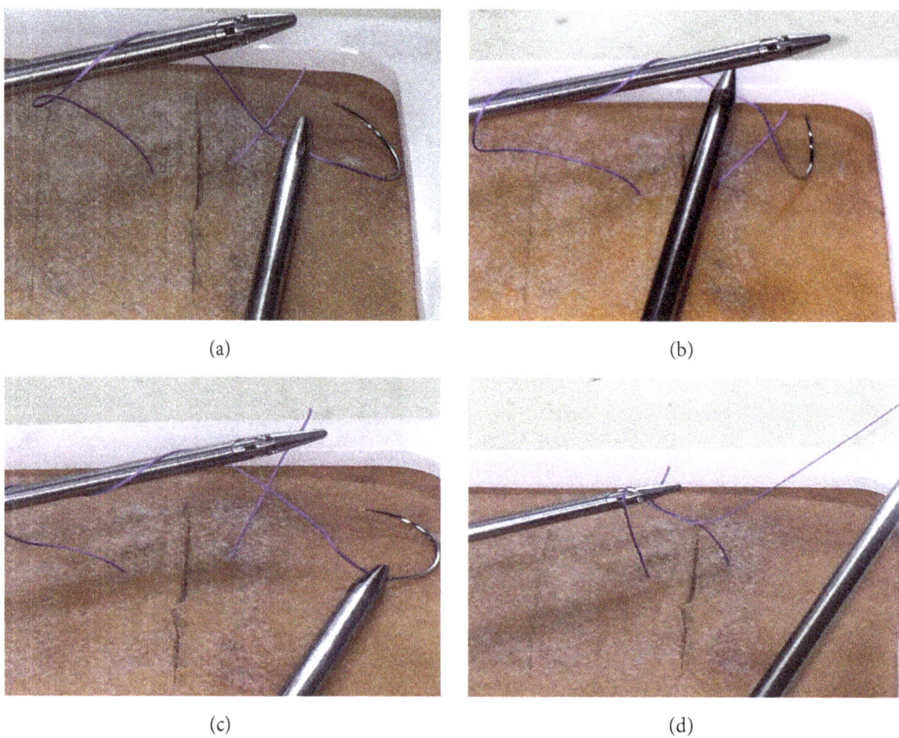

FIGURE 1: (a) (Step 1) Starting the loop of suture by right hand needle driver over the left hand needle driver. (b) (Step 2) Making two loops over the left hand needle driver. (c) (Step 3) The left hand needle driver catching the tail end of the suture through the loops. (d) (Step 4) First throw of knot completed by pulling the tail end of suture through the loop.

made with one hand instrument and other hand instrument enters into it to catch the tail end. An alternative method is by holing the suture half centimeter distal to the needle with one hand instrument and to rotate to make *winds* [7, 8] while the other hand instrument maintains the winds to apply the knot. There are many studies explaining about the different types of intracorporeal knot and its learning curves. But there is no information available about the best method of knot tying for teaching the surgical trainees in the box-trainer. In our study we are aiming to analyse the learning curves in our surgical trainees by using two different intracorporeal knot tying methods.

2. Materials and Methods

Twenty postgraduate students studying in the Department of General Surgery at Sri Ramachandra Medical College and Research Institute were included in this study. They participated on a voluntary basis. Students with prior experience in laparoscopic suturing, suturing in box-trainer, and suturing in simulators were excluded. All participants were right handed and between 24 to 35 years. Participants were divided into two groups: A and B. They were randomized by using the website http://www.randomization.com/. There were ten participants for each group. Group A was asked to follow loop method of knot tying and group B was asked to follow winding method of knot tying.

Laparoscopic box-trainer was used. Two needle drivers were used for each participant. A ten-centimeter vicryl suture 2-0 (V62H-Ethicon) material was given to each participant for every set of knots ($2 \times 1 \times 1$). Handling of instrument with manipulation of button and handling of needle driver were allowed five minutes before starting the task. Suturing pad was used to anchor the suture material while applying the knot.

Prior to start with training, each participant was given explanation about the surgical technique with a video and live demonstration by a single examiner. Same examiner coached all participants throughout the entire study. Proper bite has to be taken in the suture pad at the premarked area. After pulling the needle from the suture pad $2 \times 1 \times 1$ configuration knots were made during the training, the time taken for each set of knots was calculated, and the examiner corrected the participants whenever necessary to make the knot in a standardized manner.

2.1. Knot Tying Methods

2.1.1. Group A (Loop Method). After delivering needle from suture pad the right hand needle driver will make two loops (double forward) over the left hand needle driver and left hand needle driver will catch the tail of the suture and squaring of knot must be done. This will be followed with single reverse loop and one forward loop (Figure 1).

2.1.2. Group B (Wind Method). After delivering the needle, the driver will drop the needle and the left needle driver will hold the suture half centimeter distal to the needle. Then

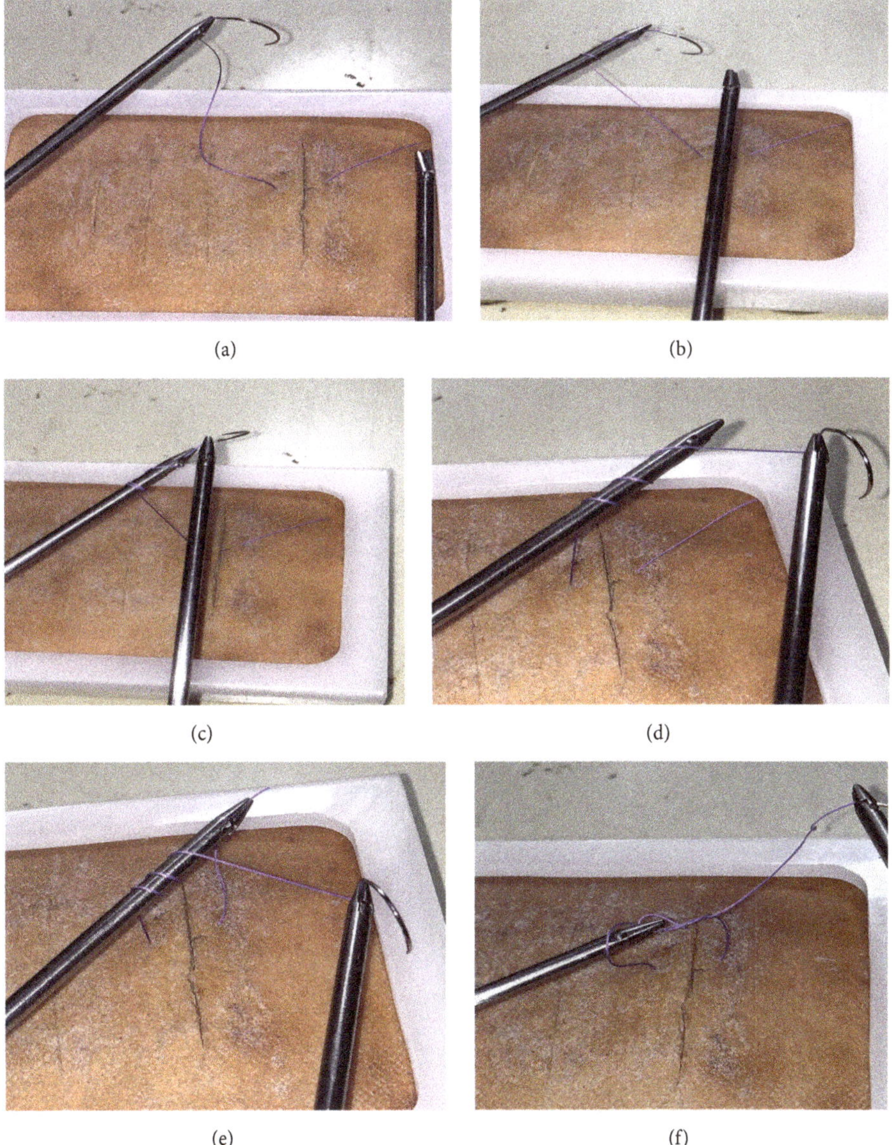

FIGURE 2: (a) (Step 1) Holding the suture material near the needle by left hand needle driver. (b) (Step 2) Winding of suture around the left hand needle driver. (c) (Step 3) Right hand needle driver receiving the needle from the left hand needle driver. (d) (Step 4) Right hand needle driver maintaining the wind on left needle driver. (e) (Step 5) Left hand needle driver catching the tail end of suture. (f) (Step 6) First throw of knot completed by pulling the tail end of suture.

the left needle driver has to rotate to wind the thread around its axis. The right needle driver has to then receive the needle once adequate winding was done followed by left needle driver to catch the tail end to make a square knot. The second throw will be done by reverse wind and last part will be done by forward wind (Figure 2).

Totally thirty-minute time was given for each participant for each session. Participants were allowed to make as many numbers of knots as possible for each session. Time calculation was done for each set of knots. The number of knots for each session was also calculated. At the end each session's participants were asked for information about frustration level (ranging from 1 to 5, 1 being the least and 5 being the maximum), difficulty in making knot (ranging from 1 to 5, 1 being the least and 5 being the maximum), and dexterity (ranging from 1 to 5, 1 being the least and 5 being the highest).

2.2. Statistical Methods. The collected data was analysed with SPSS 16.0 version software. To describe the data descriptive statistics, mean and standard deviation were used. To find the significant difference between the bivariate samples in paired groups (between sessions 1 to 8) Wilcoxon signed rank test was used and for independent groups (loop and wind) Mann-Whitney *U* test was used. For the repeated measures (from sessions 1 to 8) the Friedman test was used. In all the above statistical tools the probability value <0.05 is considered as significant level.

TABLE 1: Comparison of average number of knots was done between groups A and B (decimal number converted to whole number).

	Comparison of number of knots along the sessions between loop & winding method							
	S1	S2	S3	S4	S5	S6	S7	S8
Loop	3	4	5	5	6	7	7	7
Wind	3	6	8	9	11	12	14	15
Z-value	0.24	3.14	3.77	3.58	3.78	3.81	3.83	3.87
P value	0.853$^{\#}$	0.0001**	0.0001**	0.0001**	0.0001**	0.0001**	0.0001**	0.0001**

$^{\#}$Not sig. at $P \leq 0.05$ and **highly sig. at $P \leq 0.01$ level.

TABLE 2: Comparison of average time for one set of knots (2 × 1 × 1) in every session was done between groups A and B.

	Comparison of average time along the sessions between loop & winding method							
	S1	S2	S3	S4	S5	S6	S7	S8
Loop	615.7	525.0	395.9	378.3	330.4	272.8	254.2	253.2
Wind	658.1	336.5	237.6	198.2	171.5	147.0	133.5	122.3
Z-value	0.795	3.176	3.704	3.593	3.78	3.781	3.781	3.784
P value	0.436$^{\#}$	0.0001**	0.0001**	0.0001**	0.0001**	0.0001**	0.0001**	0.0001**

$^{\#}$Not sig. at $P \leq 0.05$ and **highly sig. at $P \leq 0.01$ level.

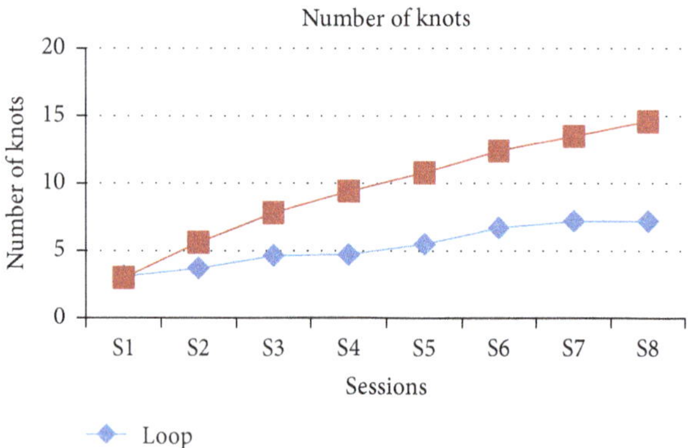

FIGURE 3: Graphical representation of both groups in view of number of knots in each session.

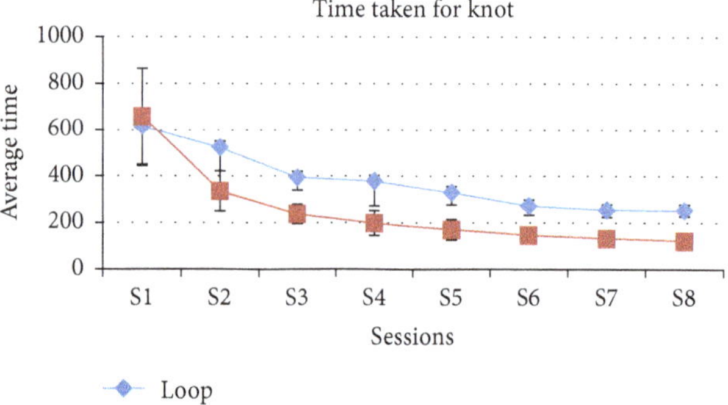

FIGURE 4: Graphical representation of both groups in view of average time in seconds for single set of knots in each session.

3. Results

3.1. Number of Knots. The comparison of number of knots along the sessions between the loop and winding methods showed that as the sessions were increasing the number of knots tied was increasing in the winding method compared with the loop method which is statistically significant except the first session, $P = 0.853 > 0.05$. The maximum number of knots made along the session in loop technique was seven and it shows a steady increase only from the sixth session, whereas in the winding technique there was a consistent increase in the number of knots from the first session to eighth session and it reached a maximum of fifteen knots at the end of the eighth session itself (Table 1, Figure 3).

3.2. Average Time Taken. The comparison of average time taken along the sessions between the loop and winding method shows that as the sessions were increasing the average time decreases in the winding method compared with the loop method which is statistically significant except the first session, $P = 0.436 > 0.05$ (Table 2, Figure 4).

3.3. Frustration Level. The comparison of frustration level along the sessions between the loop and winding method shows that as the sessions were increasing the frustration score is decreasing in the winding method and becomes steadily 1 from sixth session onwards compared with the loop method which is 2 till the end of the eighth session and which is statistically significant except the first three sessions (Table 3, Figure 5).

3.4. Difficulty Level. The comparison of difficulty level along the sessions between the loop and winding method shows that as the sessions were increasing the difficulty score is decreasing in the winding method and becomes steadily 1 from sixth session onwards compared with the loop method which is 2 till the end of the eighth session and which is statistically significant except the first three sessions (Table 4, Figure 6).

3.5. Dexterity. The comparison of dexterity along the sessions between the loop and winding method shows that as the sessions were increasing the dexterity score is increasing in

TABLE 3: Comparison of frustration level at the end of every session was done between groups A and B (from 1, least frustration, to 5, maximum frustration).

Comparison of frustration score along the sessions between loop & winding method								
	S1	S2	S3	S4	S5	S6	S7	S8
Loop	5	5	4	4	3	3	2	2
Wind	5	4	3	2	2	1	1	1
Z-value	1.129	1.258	1.802	3.297	2.457	3.17	2.675	3.442
P value	$0.353^{\#}$	$0.28^{\#}$	$0.089^{\#}$	0.001^{**}	0.019^{**}	0.002^{**}	0.011^{**}	0.001^{**}

$^{\#}$Not sig. at $P \leq 0.05$ and **highly sig. at $P \leq 0.01$ level.

TABLE 4: Comparison of difficulty level at the end of every session was done between groups A and B (from 1, least difficult level, to 5, highest difficult level).

Comparison of difficulty score along the sessions between loop & winding method								
	S1	S2	S3	S4	S5	S6	S7	S8
Loop	4	4	4	3	3	3	2	2
Wind	5	4	3	2	2	1	1	1
Z-value	1.314	1.849	1.961	2.737	3.071	3.006	3.88	3.943
P value	$0.280^{\#}$	$0.089^{\#}$	$0.063^{\#}$	0.011^{**}	0.002^{**}	0.003^{**}	0.0001^{**}	0.0001^{**}

$^{\#}$Not sig. at $P < 0.05$ and **highly sig. at $P < 0.01$ level.

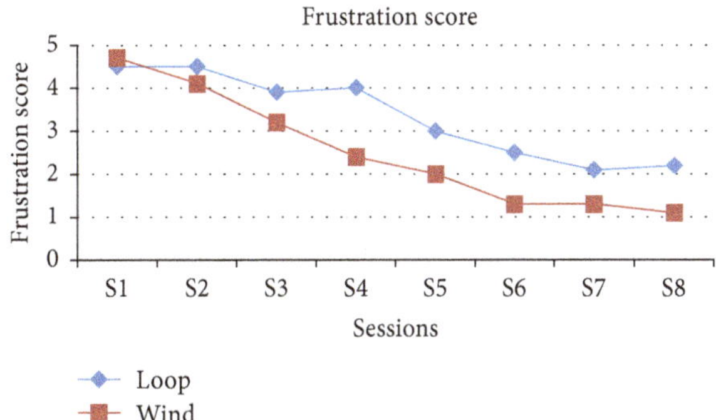

FIGURE 5: Graphical representation of both groups in view of frustration in the end of each session.

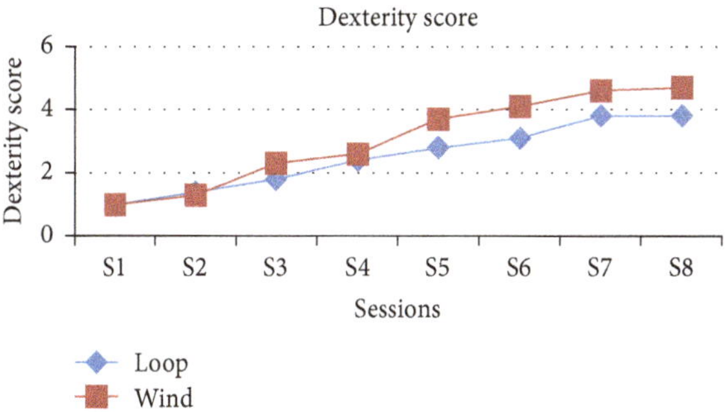

FIGURE 7: Graphical representation of both groups in view of dexterity of complete procedure in the end of each session.

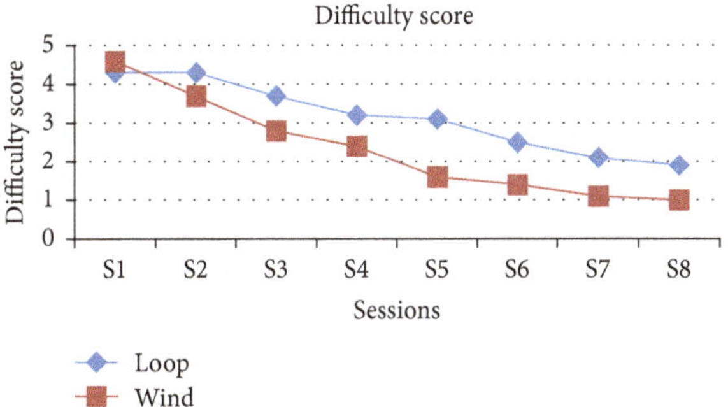

FIGURE 6: Graphical representation of both groups in view of difficulty in making knot in the end of each session.

the winding method and becomes steadily 5 on seventh session itself compared with the loop method which is 4 till the end of the eighth session and which is statistically significant except the first three sessions (Table 5, Figure 7).

3.6. Comparison of Session 8 with All Other Sessions in Both Loop Method and Winding Method. In winding method, while comparing the average time for suturing in S8 with other sessions, there is significant improvement in every session (P value < 0.01). It means average time taken for knot tying decreases significantly from S1 to S8 (Table 6).

In loop method, while doing the same type of comparison, there is significant improvement seen only up to S5. In S6 and S7 no significant improvement was seen. It means that there is no significant reduction in average time of knot tying from session 6 to session 8.

4. Discussion

It is well established that minimally invasive surgical skill must be acquired by proper training in box-trainers, rather than directly performing in a clinical setting to ensure patient safety. Training method has been changed currently like "see one, do one, and teach one." But in laparoscopy this may not be applicable since there is a long learning curve. The haptic

Table 5: Comparison of dexterity (1–5) in the end of session was done between groups A and B.

	Comparison of dexterity score along the sessions between loop & winding method							
	S1	S2	S3	S4	S5	S6	S7	S8
Loop	1	1	2	2	3	3	4	4
Wind	1	1	2	3	4	4	5	5
Z-value	0	0.457	1.832	0.602	2.669	2.523	2.437	2.466
P value	0.280#	0.089#	0.063#	0.011**	0.002**	0.003**	0.0001**	0.0001**

#Not sig. at $P < 0.05$ and **highly sig. at $P < 0.01$ level.

Table 6: Comparison of statistical significance for every session in both groups.

			P values						
	Session 1	Session 8	S1 versus S8	S2 versus S8	S3 versus S8	S4 versus S8	S5 versus S8	S6 versus S8	S7 versus S8
LOOP	615.7 ± 170	253.1 ± 25	0.005**	0.005**	0.005**	0.005**	0.005**	0.025*	0.159#
WIND	658.3 ± 207	122.3 ± 20	0.005**	0.005**	0.005**	0.005**	0.005**	0.005**	0.007**

#Not sig. at $P \le 0.05$, *sig. at $P < 0.05$ level, and **highly sig. at $P < 0.01$ level.

feedback in box-trainer will definitely improve the surgeon's skill. To avoid the injury to the abdominal organs during surgery the moving part of instrument must be in the optic field [9]. This training can be achieved in box-trainer. The working port placement must be either side of camera to make adequate triangulation, which will make knot tying easier. In box-trainer the port placement will be ideal for making triangulation. For suturing and knotting standard technique must be followed. After taking bite from tissue surgeon must pull the suture to make tail end shorter as 2 cm and he should position it before making knot. This will make grasping the tail end after making wind or loop easy [10]. To make knot in the tissue there are many knots tying methods available. For single port users extracorporeal knot tying method may be useful. To make knot tying as strong as open surgery at least two hands instruments (right and left) must be used [11, 12].

There is no study to compare the different suturing techniques in trainees. Zhou et al. work was a comparative study of suturing practice with haptic feedback and without haptic feedback. In this study result showed haptic feedback may not be warranted in laparoscopic surgical trainers at all stages of training [1]. In our study the training was given in the box-trainer. Haptic feedback of box-trainer definitely improved the suturing skills among our postgraduate students. From session 1 to session 8 there is lot of improvement in speed and dexterity in both groups. This shows the learning curve of both groups going up by our box-training. The suturing and knotting skill improved in every session in both groups. In comparison, group B (winding method) students made significantly higher number of knots and they took less time for each knot than group A (loop method) in all sessions except session 1. The feedback results of the candidates show no significant difference in view of frustration, difficulty, and dexterity from S1 to S3. On the other hand from S4 to S8, the difficulty and frustration significantly reduced and dexterity improved in group B (winding method) compared with group A (loop method).

While comparing each session with last session, in Group A (loop method) there is statistically significant improvement from S1 to S5, but from S6 to S8 there is no significant improvement in knot tying. In contrast there is significant improvement in winding method completely from S1 to S8.

All the above results show there is significant improvement in the learning curve in every session of training in both groups. Although both knotting methods are standard methods to apply in patients, the winding method of knotting will be simple and easy for the beginners to learn. In winding method of suturing the triangulation of working instrument is not completely required but in loop method of suturing the triangulation and adequate distance between instruments are required. Jagad explained the advantage of this winding method of suturing. It explains that winding method of suturing is more simple and easy to perform, especially for those who have limited experience in intracorporeal suturing and knot tying. It is easy to perform in narrow space. No special instrument is required to perform knot tying with this technique [8]. Even in our study frustration level and difficulty level in winding method are less comparing with loop method and reason could be the same as that mentioned by Jagad. The ergonomics of suturing is very important which will make surgery easier and faster. In winding method of suturing the ergonomic is improved and that is the reason why trainees can make more number of sutures with less difficulty. Rassweiler et al. explain that an ergonomic chair will improve the suturing in laparoscopic surgery [13]. In our study results show the winding method suturing is easier than loop method suturing. So This method of suturing can improve ergonomics and can make reconstructive laparoscopic surgeries easier. Murphy explained about advance modern surgical techniques of endoscopic knot tying, a new appreciation of knot tying theory, and application of these new techniques in many fields of minimally invasive surgery. In our study two standard methods of suturing techniques were compared which may give useful information to identify the best method of suturing technique in various types of minimally invasive surgeries.

5. Conclusion

Laparoscopic suturing and knotting are difficult skills to develop especially in new learners. Even though there are many methods of intracorporeal suturing available, two best methods of suturing techniques were compared in view of learning curves. While comparing with loop method of knotting, the winding method of knotting is simpler and easier to perform, especially for the surgeons who have limited experience in intracorporeal suturing and knot tying. The winding method essay for the learners probably does not require much triangulation while making knot.

Authors' Contribution

Manuneethimaran Thiyagarajan is responsible for acquisition of data, analysis and interpretation of data, critical revising of important intellectual content, and final approval of the version to be published. Chandru Ravindrakumar made substantial contribution to conception and design and revising the paper critically for important intellectual content.

References

[1] M. Zhou, S. Tse, A. Derevianko, D. B. Jones, S. D. Schwaitzberg, and C. G. L. Cao, "Effect of haptic feedback in laparoscopic surgery skill acquisition," *Surgical Endoscopy*, vol. 26, no. 4, pp. 1128–1134, 2012.

[2] Y. H. Lee, M. J. Kim, G. O. Chong, D. G. Hong, J. Lee, and Y. S. Lee, "YS knot: a new technique for a tension-controlled slip knot using a trocar," *Obstetrics & Gynecology Science*, vol. 58, no. 2, pp. 171–174, 2015.

[3] B. Ekçi, "A simple technique for knot tying in single incision laparoscopic surgery (SILS)," *Clinics*, vol. 65, no. 10, pp. 1055–1057, 2010.

[4] T. Frede, C. Stock, C. Renner, Z. Budair, Y. Abdel-Salam, and J. Rassweiler, "Geometry of laparoscopic suturing and knotting techniques," *Journal of Endourology*, vol. 13, no. 3, pp. 191–198, 1999.

[5] Y. Nouira and A. Horchani, "The pre-looped intracorporeal knot: a new technique for knot tying in laparoscopic surgery," *The Journal of Urology*, vol. 166, no. 1, pp. 195–197, 2001.

[6] A. Dowais and H. Samei, "Tying laparoscopic intracorporeal knots with one instrument: 'Dowais tie'," *The Internet Journal of Surgery*, vol. 21, no. 2, 2008.

[7] E. Croce and S. Olmi, "Intracorporeal knot-tying and suturing techniques in laparoscopic surgery: technical details," *Journal of the Society of Laparoendoscopic Surgeons*, vol. 4, no. 1, pp. 17–22, 2000.

[8] R. B. Jagad, "A new technique for intracorporeal knot tying in laparoscopic surgery," *Journal of Laparoendoscopic and Advanced Surgical Techniques*, vol. 18, no. 4, pp. 626–628, 2008.

[9] H. C. Topel, *Endoscopic Suturing and Knot Tying Manual*, Ethicon, 1991.

[10] J. L. Pennings, T. Kenyon, and L. Swanstrom, "The knit stitch—an improved method of laparoscopic knot tying," *Surgical Endoscopy*, vol. 9, no. 5, pp. 537–540, 1995.

[11] D. L. Murphy, "A new method of laparoscopic instrument knot tying," *Surgical Technology International*, vol. 4, pp. 199–202, 1995.

[12] D. L. Murphy, "Endoscopic knot tying made easier," *Australian and New Zealand Journal of Surgery*, vol. 65, no. 7, pp. 507–509, 1995.

[13] J. J. Rassweiler, A. S. Goezen, A. A. Jalal et al., "A new platform improving the ergonomics of laparoscopic surgery: initial clinical evaluation of the prototype," *European Urology*, vol. 61, no. 1, pp. 226–229, 2012.

25

The Frequency of Resurgery after Percutaneous Lumbar Surgery Using Dekompressor in a Ten-Year Period

Stephan Klessinger [1,2]

[1] *Department of Neurosurgery, Nova Clinic Biberach, Eichendorffweg 5, 88400 Biberach, Germany*
[2] *Department of Neurosurgery, University of Ulm, Albert-Einstein-Allee 23, 89081 Ulm, Germany*

Correspondence should be addressed to Stephan Klessinger; klessinger@nova-clinic.de

Academic Editor: Peng Hui Wang

To prevent open surgical procedures, minimally invasive techniques, like Dekompressor (PLDD), have been developed. The absence of reherniation is an important factor correlating with clinical success after lumbar surgery. In this retrospective, observational study, the frequency of additional open surgery after PLDD in a long time retrospective was examined. The correlation between clinical symptoms and outcome was assessed, and the time between PLDD and open surgery was analyzed. Consecutive patients after PLDD between 2005 and 2007 were included. MacNab's outcome criteria were used to evaluate patient satisfaction. The need for additional open surgery of the lumbar spine, the period between Dekompressor and resurgery, and the treated levels were analyzed. In total, 73 patients were included in this study. The patients were seen one month after PLDD. The majority of patients (76.7%) had additional radicular pain. The most common level treated was L4-5 (58.9%). The follow-up time was longer than 5 years in 30.1% of the patients and longer than 10 years in 6.82%. The short-term success rate was 67.1%. Additional surgery was performed in 26.0% of patients, with 78.9% of the reoperations undertaken during the first year after PLDD. These patients had a statistically significant worse outcome ($P = 0.025$). Radicular pain was present in all patients with an early subsequent surgery, but only in 50% of patients with late surgery ($P = 0.035$). Significantly more patients with poor pain relief had radicular pain ($P = 0.04$). The short-term success rate was worsened by a resurgery rate of 26.0%. Subsequent surgery, a short time after PLDD, suggests that PLDD is not a replacement for open discectomy. Because patients with radicular pain had a worse outcome and more frequent resurgeries, whether radicular pain is an ideal indication for PLDD should be discussed.

1. Introduction

Lumbar radicular pain caused by disc herniation is often treated with open discectomy [1]. Its effectiveness has been demonstrated in controlled trials [2–4] and in long-term follow-up studies [5]. Minimally invasive techniques have been developed to prevent open surgery. The paucity of evidence supporting these minimally invasive techniques highlights the need for more data. Only limited evidence exists for Nucleoplasty and Dekompressor [6, 7].

Percutaneous lumbar disc decompression with Dekompressor (PLDD) uses the Archimedes' pump principle to mechanically remove a predetermined amount of disc material, reducing the pressure in the disc. The placement of the 1.5 mm cannula is similar to that used in a standard discography.

PLDD has been shown to be superior to conservative treatment [6, 8, 9] and has been associated with a low rate of complications [8]. However, limited outcome data are available. While preliminary studies revealed a favorable outcome [9–13], only two assessed clinical outcomes beyond one year [6, 10], and only one study measured the open surgery rate after PLDD [6]. The absence of reherniation is an important factor for patient satisfaction after discectomy [14]. The expected outcomes after revision surgery are less well defined than for primary discectomy [14]. Therefore, the number of subsequent surgeries after PLDD is of great importance.

It is important to find an ideal indication for PLDD. Unsuccessful conservative treatment is a prerequisite of any spine surgery. Patients with a clear indication for open discectomy are also not ideal candidates for a percutaneous technique. It seems that outcomes after microdiscectomy for contained herniations are worse than for sequestered herniations [15]. As such, Dekompressor has been devised

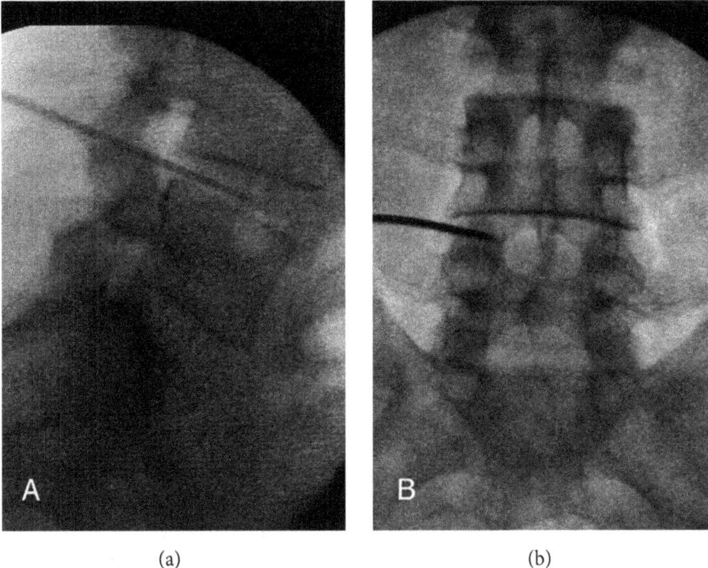

(a) (b)

FIGURE 1: AP and lateral fluoroscopy image of the position of the PLDD wand at L4-5.

for small contained disc herniations [1]. The idea is that the nucleus and annulus are in a closed system where the herniated part can move back towards the center after a decrease in volume. A contained disc is regarded as an important prerequisite to the success of PLDD [8].

Advantages of the Dekompressor system are the minimal damage to adjacent tissues [11]. Proponents of the system state that Dekompressor does not substitute disc degeneration [11]. Less pertinent scarring and less postoperative fibrosis may be expected [12].

The aim of this retrospective, observational study was to investigate the frequency of an additional open surgery after PLDD in a more than ten-year retrospective. The time between PLDD and open surgery was analyzed, and a correlation between the clinical symptoms and outcome was assessed.

2. Materials and Methods

In this retrospective observational study, the patient data were drawn from an electronic medical record system. PLDD was performed in a practice setting. Open disc surgery was performed in a general hospital.

Inclusion criteria were as follows: consecutive patients who underwent PLDD between January 2005 and December 2007. A history of pain for a minimum of 3 months was mandatory. Patients had either low back pain or radicular pain with or without a sensory loss. Patients with a lumbar spine surgery in their history were excluded.

For PLDD, the 17-gauge Dekompressor probe (Stryker, Kalamazoo, Michigan) was used. Prophylactic antibiotics were administered prior to the procedure. A standard approach was used to place the introducer cannula with the stylet under fluoroscopic view intradiscally. The correct cannula placement was confirmed with anterior-posterior and lateral fluoroscopic images (Figure 1). The Dekompressor probe was advanced into the cannula and switched on. Disc material was harvested by moving the cannula along several passes intradiscally.

Every patient was seen in the practice personally one month after the operation for follow-up and later according to the complaints of the patient. A physician interview and a clinical examination were performed. A long-term follow-up of more than ten years was possible.

The age and gender of the patients, the treated levels, the follow-up time, and the pain characteristics (only lumbago or radicular pain with or without sensory loss) were evaluated. MacNab's outcome criteria [14] (1 = Excellent, no pain, no restriction of activity; 2 = Good, occasional pain; 3 = Fair, improved but handicapped by intermittent pain; 4 = Poor, no improvement) were used to measure the success after PLDD. The evaluation of the necessity of an additional open lumbar spine surgery was the focus of this study. The period of time between the PLDD and the resurgery and the treated levels and the symptoms of the patients (back pain or radicular complaints) were analyzed.

The Exact-Fisher-test was used to compare values of patients with substantial pain relief and poor pain relief. Welch's t-test was used to test the hypothesis that two populations had equal means. $P < 0.05$ was set as the threshold for interpreting the results as significant.

3. Results

Between January 2005 and December 2007, 86 patients were treated with PLDD. Because of spine surgery in their history, eleven patients were excluded. Two patients were lost to follow-up. Therefore, 73 patients were included in this study. The data of these patients are shown in Table 1. In total, 33 patients (45.2%) were women and 40 were men. The age of the patients was between 17 and 85 years, with the mean age being 48.9 years.

Table 1: Patient characteristics.

	All Patients
n	73
Age (years)	
mean	48.9 ± 13.4
min-max	17–85
Female	33 (45.2%)
Level	
L2-3	2 (2.7%)
L3-4	4 (5.5%)
L3-4-5	3 (4.1%)
L4-5	43 (58.9%)
L4-5-S1	8 (11.0%)
L5-S1	13 (17.8%)
Side	
left	37 (50.7%)
right	31 (42.5%)
both	5 (6.8%)
Radicular Pain	56 (76.7%)
Sensory Loss	43 (58.9%)
Follow-up (months)	
mean	35.6 ± 40.2
min-max	1–132
Macnab's outcome criteria	
mean	2.2 ± 1.0
substantial pain relief (1+2)	49 (67.1%)
Additional surgery at index level	19 (26.0%)
Period until surgery (months)	
mean	10.1 ± 17.1
min-max	1–70

All patients had pain for more than three months (mean 6.6 months). Twenty-eight patients (38.4%) reported pain for more than one year before the treatment. Seventeen patients only had back pain. The majority of the patients (76.7%) had additional radicular pain. A sensory loss in the symptomatic leg was present in 43 patients (58.9%). No motor deficit was present.

The most common level treated was L4-5 (58.9%). Two levels (either L3-4-5 or L4-5-S1) were treated in 11 patients (15.1%). In 50.7% of patients the left side was symptomatic, while in 42.5 % of the patients, the right side was treated. Five patients (6.8%) were treated on both sides. No PLDD-related severe complications occurred.

The first follow-up examination one month after PLDD was mandatory for all patients. Further examinations were arranged according to the needs of the patients. This first follow-up was the only one in nine patients (12.3%). In 22 patients (30.1%), the follow-up was longer than 5 years, and in five patients (6.8%) it was longer than 10 years. The mean follow-up time was 35.6 months.

One month after the intervention, excellent results were achieved in 17 patients and good results, in 32 patients. Therefore, the short-term success rate was 67.1%. Subsequent surgery at the index level was necessary in 19 patients (26.0%). In these cases, the herniated disc fragment was removed, and a discectomy or a bony decompression of the spinal canal was performed.

Most reoperations (15 patients) had to be performed during the first year after PLDD (20.5% of all patients, 78.9% of all resurgeries). These patients (Table 2) had a statistically significant worse outcome (26.7% versus 75.0% satisfied patients, $|t|=2.467$, $(\alpha 1 = 0.025)t(7)=2.365$). Radicular pain was present in all patients with an early subsequent surgery, but only in 50% of patients with late surgery ($P = 0.035$). The mean time between PLDD and the additional surgery was at 10.8 ± 17.9 months (1–70 months).

Comparing the patients with excellent or good outcome (substantial pain relief) with the patients with poor pain relief (Table 3), significantly more patients with poor pain relief had radicular pain (91.7% versus 69.4 %, $P = 0.04$). As expected, the rate of resurgeries is higher if patients are not satisfied (50.0% versus 14.3%, $P = 0.002$).

4. Discussion

This retrospective observational study investigated the number of patients with a subsequent open surgery after PLDD. Patients with back pain only and patients with radicular pain were included. The short-term success rate was 67.1%; however, 26.0% of all patients had to undergo an additional surgery, most of them during the first year after PLDD. If resurgery was necessary, the primary outcome was worse compared to patients without surgery during follow-up. All patients with an early additional surgery had radicular pain. Patients with radicular pain had a worse outcome.

The short-term success rate is comparable with the few available studies from the literature. The recent study of McCormick et al. [6] found a 73% positive response after one year using a threshold of >50% improvement in NRS leg pain score and > 30% ODI improvement. This result builds on the other available studies with 6-to-24-month follow-up periods [9–13].

Also, the resurgery rate seems to be comparable with the only one study reporting these data. McCormick at al. [6] reported 36% additional surgery at the 8-year follow-up. All patients in his study had radicular pain. In the present study, the resurgery rate was 34% if only patients with radicular pain are taken into account. However, the patient selection in the McCormick study [6] and the present study is different. All patients in the McCormick study [6] were candidates for open discectomy. Therefore, it is concluded that PDLL had prevented spine surgery in 64% of cases. In the present study, no patient was a candidate for open surgery even though some of them had radicular pain or a sensory loss. However, no patient with a motor deficit or even bladder dysfunction was included. This means that the resurgery rate in the present study indicates additional surgery for a patient for whom conservative treatment was an alternative to PLDD. Recent studies found comparable resurgery rates for lumbar Nucleoplasty (18.7 %, [16]) and for cervical Nucleoplasty (19.5 % [17]).

TABLE 2: Patient characteristics dependent on the time of resurgery and significant differences between these two groups.

	All Patients with Resurgery	Resurgery during first year	Resurgery later	Significance
n	19	15 (78.9%)	4 (21.1%)	
Radicular pain	17 (89.5%)	15 (100.0%)	2 (50.0%)	**P = 0.035**
Macnab's outcome criteria				
mean	2.9 ± 0.8	3.1 ± 0.8	2.3 ± 0.5	**|t|=2.467, (α1 = 0.025)t(7)=2.365**
substantial pain relief (1+2)	7 (36.8%)	4 (26,7%)	3 (75.0%)	
Period until surgery (months)				
mean	10.8 ± 17.9	3.0 ± 2.3	40.3 ± 20.8	**|t|=3.588, (α1 = 0.025)t(3)=3.182**

TABLE 3: Patient characteristics dependent on the outcome and significant differences between these two groups.

	All Patients	Result substantial pain relief	Result poor pain relief	Significance
n	73	49 (67.1%)	24 (32.9%)	
Radicular pain	56 (76.7%)	34 (69.4%)	22 (91.7%)	**P = 0.04**
Additional surgery	19 (26.0%)	7 (14.3%)	12 (50.0%)	**P = 0.002**

Avoidance of surgery is an important goal in reducing morbidity and mortality [6]. From the data of this study it remains unclear whether PLDD can achieve this objective. It is also worth considering whether radicular pain is a good indication for PLDD. Generally, patient selection appears to be extremely important in the efficacy of PDD [8, 18]. The best results may be obtained when the disc herniation is contained [8, 18] and is limited to a single level [18]. For Ong et al. [8], the exact role of PLDD in the treatment of radicular pain is still up for debate, but PLDD should not be abandoned. Lee [19] concludes that, in spite of the lack of the evidence, the Dekompressor may be worth trying in patients with leg pain and contained disc herniations prior to open discectomy because the Dekompressor is easy to apply, is relatively safe, and causes less injurious to the disc. In contrast to the studies of Ong et al. [8] and Lee [19], the present study shows that radicular pain is an inferior indication compared to low back pain.

With an early resurgery, it was suspected that the indication for PLDD was too generous. Another explanation for early resurgery was the risk of acute herniation after the puncture of the disc with the 17-gauge needle. The risk of acute herniation is dependent on the needle diameter. The most vulnerable site is the inner annulus [20]. All patients with an early additional surgery had radicular pain. Patients with radicular pain had worse outcomes compared to patients with back pain only. As a consequence, a good indication might be a patient with low back pain without radicular symptoms with a contained disc. Trying Dekompressor in the first instance risks an additional surgery with lower success rates [1, 21]. This study suggests that Dekompressor is unable to replace open surgery.

There are limitations to this study. This audit is retrospective and observational and therefore does not represent a high level of evidence. However, the resurgery rate is an important factor for the outcome.

5. Conclusions

At first sight, a satisfied patient level of 67% seems to be a good result. However, this short-term result is significantly worsened due to a resurgery rate of 26.0%. Subsequent surgery a short time after PLDD suggests that PLDD is not a replacement for open discectomy. A contained disc herniation causing low back pain without radicular pain appears to be a good indication for Dekompressor. Because patients with radicular pain had a worse outcome and more frequent resurgeries, whether radicular pain is an ideal indication for PDLL should be discussed. Further studies are needed to compare the outcome and rate of subsequent surgery in patient populations with and without radicular symptoms to find the ideal indications for PLDD.

References

[1] Y. Vorobeychik, V. Gordin, D. Fuzaylov, and M. Kurowski, "Percutaneous Mechanical Disc Decompression Using Dekompressor Device: An Appraisal of the Current Literature," *Pain Medicine*, vol. 13, no. 5, pp. 640–646, 2012.

[2] H. Weber, "Lumbar disc herniation: a controlled, prospective study with ten years of observation," *The Spine Journal*, vol. 8, no. 2, pp. 131–140, 1983.

[3] J. N. Weinstein, T. D. Tosteson, J. D. Lurie et al., "Surgical vs nonoperative treatment for lumbar disk herniation. The Spine Patient Outcomes Research Trial (SPORT): A randomized trial," *Journal of the American Medical Association*, vol. 296, no. 20, pp. 2441–2450, 2006.

[4] J. N. Weinstein, J. D. Lurie, T. D. Tosteson et al., "Surgical versus nonoperative treatment for lumbar disc herniation: four-year results for the Spine Patient Outcomes Research Trial (SPORT)," *The Spine Journal*, vol. 33, no. 25, pp. 2789–2800, 2008.

[5] S. J. Atlas, R. B. Keller, Y. A. Wu, R. A. Deyo, and D. E. Singer, "Long-term outcomes of surgical and nonsurgical management

of sciatica secondary to a lumbar disc herniation: 10 year results from the Maine lumbar spine study," *The Spine Journal*, vol. 30, no. 8, pp. 927–935, 2005.

[6] Z. L. McCormick, C. Slipman, A. Kotcharian et al., "Percutaneous lumbar disc decompression using the dekompressor: A prospective long-term outcome study," *Pain Medicine*, vol. 17, no. 6, pp. 1023–1030, 2016.

[7] V. Singh, R. M. Benyamin, S. Datta, F. J. Falco, S. Helm II, and L. Manchikanti, "Systematic review of percutaneous lumbar mechanical disc decompression utilizing Dekompressor," *Pain Physician*, vol. 12, no. 3, pp. 589–599, 2009.

[8] D. Ong, N. H. L. Chua, and K. Vissers, "Percutaneous Disc Decompression for Lumbar Radicular Pain: A Review Article," *Pain Practice*, vol. 16, no. 1, pp. 111–126, 2016.

[9] D. Erginousakis, D. K. Filippiadis, A. Malagari et al., "Comparative prospective randomized study comparing conservative treatment and percutaneous disk decompression for treatment of intervertebral disk herniation," *Radiology*, vol. 260, no. 2, pp. 487–493, 2011.

[10] J. Aronsohn, K. Chapman, and M. Soliman, "Percutaneous microdiscectomy versus epidural injection for management of chronic spinal pain," *Proc West Pharmacol Soc*, pp. 16–19, 2010.

[11] K. M. Alò, R. E. Wright, J. Sutcliffe, and S. A. Brandt, "Percutaneous lumbar discectomy: One-year follow-up in an initial cohort of fifty consecutive patients with chronic radicular pain," *Pain Practice*, vol. 5, no. 2, pp. 116–124, 2005.

[12] P. Lierz, K. M. Alo, and P. Felleiter, "Percutaneous lumbar discectomy using the dekompressor® system under CT-control," *Pain Practice*, vol. 9, no. 3, pp. 216–220, 2009.

[13] J. Lemcke, F. Al-Zain, S. Mutze, and U. Meier, "Minimally invasive spinal surgery using nucleoplasty and the dekompressor tool: A comparison of two methods in a one year follow-up," *Minimally Invasive Neurosurgery*, vol. 53, no. 5-6, pp. 236–242, 2010.

[14] R. W. Abdu, W. A. Abdu, A. M. Pearson, W. Zhao, J. D. Lurie, and J. N. Weinstein, "Reoperation for Recurrent Intervertebral Disc Herniation in the Spine Patient Outcomes Research Trial," *The Spine Journal*, vol. 42, no. 14, pp. 1106–1114, 2017.

[15] C. B. Dewing, M. T. Provencher, R. H. Riffenburgh, S. Kerr, and R. E. Manos, "The outcomes of lumbar microdiscectomy in a young, active population: Correlation by herniation type and level," *The Spine Journal*, vol. 33, no. 1, pp. 33–38, 2008.

[16] S. Klessinger, "The frequency of re-surgery after lumbar disc Nucleoplasty in a ten-year period," *Clinical Neurology and Neurosurgery*, vol. 170, pp. 79–83, 2018.

[17] S. Klessinger, "The frequency of re-surgery after cervical disc nucleoplasty," *World Neurosurgery*, vol. 117, pp. e552–e556, 2018.

[18] L. Manchikanti, V. Singh, A. K. Calodney et al., "Percutaneous lumbar mechanical disc decompression utilizing Dekompressor®: an update of current evidence.," *Pain Physician*, vol. 16, no. 2, p. -24, 2013.

[19] S. C. Lee, "Percutaneous intradiscal treatments for discogenic pain," *Acta Anaesthesiologica Taiwanica*, vol. 50, no. 1, pp. 25–28, 2012.

[20] V. M. van Heeswijk, A. Thambyah, P. A. Robertson, and N. D. Broom, "Does an Annular Puncture Influence the Herniation Path?" *An In Vitro Mechanical and Structural Investigation*, 2017.

[21] A. Vik, J. A. Zwart, G. Hulleberg, and P. Nygaard, "Eight year outcome after surgery for lumbar disc herniation: A comparison of reoperated and not reoperated patients," *Acta Neurochirurgica*, vol. 143, no. 6, pp. 607–611, 2001.

26

Video-Assisted Thoracic Surgery for Tubercular Spondylitis

Roop Singh,[1] Paritosh Gogna,[1] Sanjeev Parshad,[2] Rajender Kumar Karwasra,[2] Parmod Kumar Karwasra,[1] and Kiranpreet Kaur[3]

[1] *Department of Orthopaedic Surgery, Paraplegia & Rehabilitation, Pt. B.D. Sharma PGIMS, 52 / 9-J, Medical Enclave, Rohtak, Haryana 124001, India*
[2] *Department of Surgery, Pt. B.D. Sharma PGIMS, Rohtak, Haryana 124001, India*
[3] *Department of Anaesthesia & Critical Care, Pt. B.D. Sharma PGIMS, Rohtak, Haryana 124001, India*

Correspondence should be addressed to Roop Singh; drroopsingh@rediffmail.com

Academic Editor: Othmar Schöb

The present study evaluated the outcome of video-assisted thoracic surgery (VATS) in 9 patients (males = 6, females = 3) with clinico-radiological diagnosis of tubercular spondylitis of the dorsal spine. The mean duration of surgery was 140.88 ± 20.09 minutes, mean blood was 417.77 ± 190.90 mL, and mean duration of postoperative hospital stay was 5.77 ± 0.97 days, Seven patients had a preoperative Grade A neurological involvement, while at the time of final followup the only deficit was Grade D power in 2 patients. In patients without bone graft placement ($n = 6$), average increase in Kyphosis angle was 16°, while in patients with bone graft placement ($n = 3$) the deformity remained stationary. At the time of final follow up, fusion was achieved in all patients, the VAS score for back pain improved from a pretreatment score of 8.3 to 2, and the function assessment yielded excellent ($n = 4$) to good ($n = 5$) results. In two patients minithoracotomy had to be resorted due to extensive pleural adhesions ($n = 1$) or difficulty in placement of graft ($n = 1$). Videoassisted thoracoscopic surgery provides a safe and effective approach in the management of spinal tuberculosis. It has the advantages of decreased blood loss and post operative morbidity with minimal complications.

1. Introduction

Tuberculous spondylitis, which is the most common form of skeletal TB (comprising 50% of all cases) and the most serious form of tuberculous lesions in various bones and joints, is reappearing as a problem [1–5]. In the developing world spinal TB is the main cause of kyphosis; 15% of patients treated conservatively have a considerable increase in kyphotic deformity, which in 3% to 5% is more than 60°. A severe kyphotic deformity is a major cosmetic and psychological disturbance in growing child and can result in secondary cardiorespiratory problems and late-onset paraplegia [6–9].

The standard surgical method of decompression of tubercular dorsal spine is either the anterolateral extrapleural or the open transthoracic transpleural approach. Both these approaches are sufficient for adequate decompression and graft placement but are associated with significant morbidity and require a prolonged hospital stay [10]. Video-assisted thoracic surgery (VATS) has developed very rapidly in the last two decades. The use of VATS retains the advantages of anterior spinal surgery and gives a comparable result of spinal deformity correction to that of the open approaches [11]. Although the advent of video-assisted thoracoscopic surgery (VATS) has given a valuable alternative to conventional thoracotomy with minimal morbidity there have been relatively few reports of VATS used for decompression and stabilization in active tuberculosis of thoracic spine [12, 13]. We report our preliminary experience of VATS in treating tubercular spondylitis of thoracic spine and report results and difficulties associated with the procedure.

2. Patients and Method

We performed video-assisted thoracoscopic surgery in 9 patients (males = 6, females = 7) with tubercular spondylitis of the dorsal spine at our centre from January 2009 to December 2011. The mean age was 37.11 ± 20.55 (range: 55–88 years) and the average final followup was 32 months (range: 24 to 41 months). The clinical diagnosis was made from patient's history and thorough general physical and neurological examination. It was then correlated with plain radiography and magnetic resonance imaging (MRI). Inclusion criteria were doubtful diagnosis, severe back pain and/or radicular pain persisting after conservative treatment, neurological deficit resulting from the presence of granulation tissue, abscess or sequestrated bone or a disc fragment compressing the dura, or a paravertebral abscess under tension. Exclusion criteria were multilevel disease, concomitant cervical or lumbar lesion, pleural adhesions, and intolerance to one-lung ventilation intraoperatively. Patients were given detailed information regarding surgical procedure. Prior written informed consent was taken from each patient explaining the procedure, risks, and benefits. They were also informed that VATS can be converted into open thoracotomy in conditions like inability to tolerate one-lung ventilation or severe pleural adhesions.

The surgery was performed under general anesthesia with a double-lumen endotracheal tube inserted for ipsilateral lung collapse and single lung ventilation. A close watch on all hemodynamic and respiratory parameters was maintained. The patients were placed in the right/left lateral decubitus position, depending on the radiologic findings (i.e., bulk of abscess and caseating tissue and destruction of body) and the relevant part was draped and prepared for a standard posterolateral thoracotomy (for conversion to standard thoracotomy in circumstance of intraoperative complication or the presence of severe pleural adhesion). With selective collapse of right/left lung, the initial trocar incision (2 cm) was made usually at the fifth or sixth intercostal space (ICS) or higher along the anterior axillary line depending upon the site of lesion. An 11-mm trocar was used to introduce the operating thoracoscope and an exploratory thoracoscopy was performed. The lesion site was identified and displayed on the video monitor. Two other stab incisions, the extended manipulating channels, usually 3-4 cm in length, were done 2-3 intercostal spaces above and below the first port, slightly posterior to the posterior axillary line. We encountered difficulty in making portals due to overcrowding of ribs in two patients.

Visualization of the spine was enhanced by tilting the patient forward so that the collapsed lung fell anteriorly and, if required, a fan retractor for further retraction of ipsilateral lung was inserted. The correct level of diseased vertebrae was determined by counting the ribs as seen through the endoscope. Putting a spinal needle from the marker site and visualizing the tip of needle through the thoracoscope further confirmed the correct level. With monopolar electrocautery accompanied by a suction tube the parietal pleura overlying the lesion was divided longitudinally. The larger intercostal arteries and veins were isolated, ligated, and divided if needed. The biopsy and decompression procedure was then performed with conventional disc roungeurs and elongated bone curettes and was carried out down to the epidural space. Additional procedures like placement of bone graft into the intervertebral space using a conventional bone impactor were done in 3 patients. In 2 patients, conversion to minithoracotomy was undertaken. A larger manipulating channel measuring 5 to 6 cm in length was created on the right/left lateral chest after introducing the thoracoscope and a short-segment rib of equal length was removed. The incision was made slightly behind the posterior axillary line at the level of right fifth rib. Then a rib spreader was used to open the intercostal space. Adhesionolysis by blunt dissection using finger was done. The following spinal procedures, including debridement, sequesterectomy, and interbody fusion with tricortical iliac crest bone grafting, could be manipulated with techniques used for standard open surgical procedures. The material was sent for histopathology, culture, and Ziehl-Neelsen staining. Hemostasis was carefully monitored and chest tube drain of appropriate size was inserted through one of the port sites in 7th or 8th intercostal space in midaxillary line and was connected to an underwater seal. The small wounds were closed. Figure 1 shows the various steps of VATS viz. placements of portal, fan retractor, chest tube drainage, opening abscess cavity and graft.

Patients were kept under close observation for 24 hours. A plain radiograph of the chest was obtained for adequate lung inflation. Chest tube was removed once collection in the chest tube bag was <50 mL in 24 hours. Postoperative X-rays were taken to assess the improvement. Stitches were removed after two weeks. Patient was advised bed rest for a minimal of 6 weeks. Mobilization was started after 6 weeks using a thoracolumbosacral orthosis (TLSO)/modified Taylor's brace with axillary support depending upon the clinical status of patient. ATT was given for 12 months. Patients were followed up at 2 weeks for 1 month, monthly for the next 6 months, and thereafter once in every 3 months. At each followup patient was examined clinicoradiologically and laboratory investigations (complete blood haemogram, serum glutamic oxaloacetic transaminase/serum glutamic pyruvic transaminase, serum bilirubin, serum protein, and albumin/globulin ratio) were done. At the time of final followup MRI and computed tomography (CT scan) of the dorsal spine were also performed.

The surgical outcome was assessed in terms of preoperative and postoperative neurologic status as per Frankel's grading, operative time, blood loss, average hospital stay, deformity correction and maintenance, fusion status, back pain using visual analogue scale, and complications. Fusion was assessed using both plain radiographs and CT scan and using Eck et al. criteria for fusion assessment [14]. Final functional outcome was assessed by modified Kirkaldy-Willis criteria [18].

3. Results

Patients were suffering from the symptomatology of the TB with a mean duration of 8.44 ± 3 months (range: 5–12 months). All the patients (n = 09) received antituberculous treatment (ATT) for a period of 3-4 weeks minimum before surgery and then postoperatively. The total duration of ATT was 12 months. The indication for surgery using VATS was failure to respond to chemotherapy (n = 01), neurological deficit not responding to chemotherapy (n = 07), and doubtful diagnosis (n = 01).

Using VATS, debridement, drainage of prevertebral and paravertebral abscess, and decompression of cord were done in six patients; debridement, drainage, decompression, and

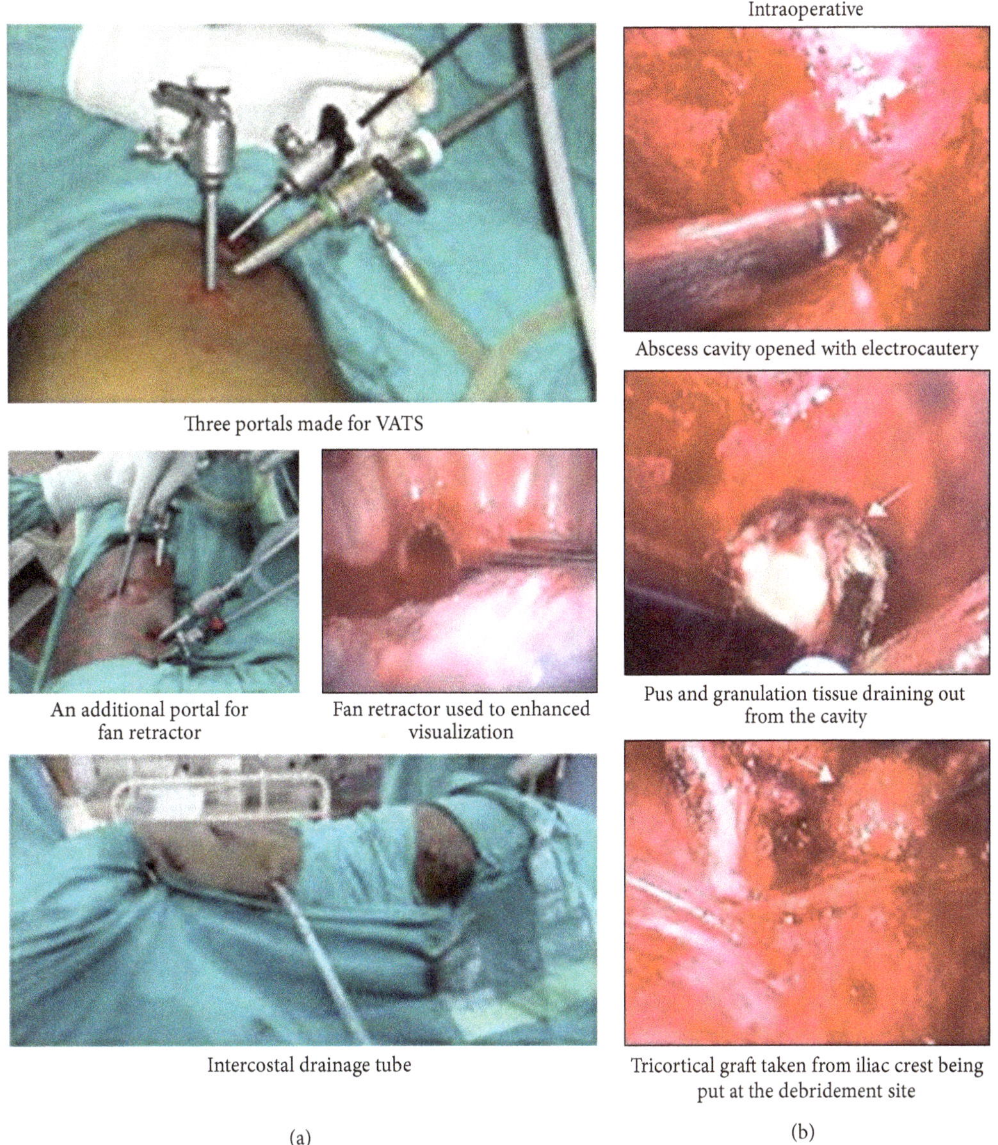

FIGURE 1: Peroperative and postoperative photographs of the VATS. (a) Portal placements and intraoperative and postoperative chest tube drainage. (b) Peroperative photographs showing opening of the lesion and debridement. Tricortical graft was put after debridement.

reconstruction with bone graft were done in one patient; and debridement, drainage, decompression, reconstruction with bone graft, and minithoracotomy were done in two patients. Sufficient tissue for histopathological examination was obtained and the clinical diagnosis of tuberculosis of spine was confirmed by pathologists in all the cases. The average operative time was 140.88 ± 20.09 minutes (range: 105–165 minutes), average blood loss was 417.77 ± 190.90 mL (range: 220–730 mL), and average hospital stay was 5.77±0.97 days (range: 4–7 days). As per Frankel's grading, 7 patients had Grade A neurological involvement preoperatively, which improved at subsequent followups (Table 1).

Radiographs of the spine revealed wedge collapse with contagious involvement in all patients. Average vertebral height loss, deformity angle, and kyphotic angle initially were 0.48, 11.8°, and 24.2°, respectively; the final values were 01, 22°, and 37°, respectively. As per CT the average percentage canal encroachment was 52.7% at initial presentation which improved to 10% at the time of final followup; it also revealed that fusion was present in 75% of the patients at their final followup. On MRI, all patients showed paradiscal and contiguous involvement of vertebrae; average vertebrae involvement per patient was 2.88 at presentation and 2.33 at the time of final followup. Paravertebral collection and subligamentous spread were seen in all patients at initial presentation, with an average vertebral extent of paravertebral soft tissue collection and subligamentous spread as 4.3 vertebrae each initially, which dropped to 2.7 and 1 vertebrae, respectively, at time of final followup.

The mean preoperative kyphosis angle in patient without ($n = 6$) and with ($n = 3$) bone graft was 25° and 23° and at time of final followup was 41° and 24°, respectively. Two

Table 1: Neurological improvement as per Frankel's grading.

Frankel's grades	Number of patients						
	Preop	Immediate postop	1 M	3 M	6 M	12 M	FFU
A	7	4	3	—	—	—	
B	—	1	2	2	—	—	
C	—	—	—	—	2	—	
D	—	2	2	3	3	3	2
E	2	2	2	4	4	6	7

M: months; FFU: final followup.

Table 2: Status of fusion in patients.

	Preop	6 months	12 months	Final followup
Fusion				
Without bone graft ($n = 06$)				
X-ray	—	04	06	06
CT		04	06	06
With bone graft (Eck et al. [14] grading) ($n = 03$)				
X-ray	—	03 (Grade II)	03 (Grade I)	03
CT	—	03 (Grade II)	03 (Grade I)	03

of the six patients without bone grafting achieved fusion at six months and another four at 12 months. Eck et al. criteria for fusion assessment were used to grade the fusion in 3 patients with bone grafting, according to which all 3 cases achieved Grade II fusion at six months and showed further improvement to Grade I at 12 months (Table 2).

Back pain as assessed using visual analogue scale improved from a pretreatment score of 8.3 to 2 at final followup. Functional outcome assessed as per the modified Kirkaldy-Willis criteria revealed 3 patients to have an excellent outcome, while good outcome was observed in 1 patient.

The most common complication was conversion to minithoracotomy in two patients. It was due to extensive pleural adhesions leading to difficulty in graft placement in one case and bleeding during placement of portals in another case. None of our cases had pneumothorax, pneumonitis, chylothorax, or Horner's syndrome. Postoperative histopathological examination showed caseation and/or granuloma formation suggestive of tuberculosis in all cases. Figures 2 and 3 are the photographs of X-rays, CT and MRI of the representative cases at presentation, six months, and 12 months.

4. Discussion

Evidence of tuberculous spondylitis, probably due to infection with mycobacterium bovis, was identified in mummies from the tomb of nebeveenenf, indicating that this process existed in dynastic Egypt as early as 3700 BC [19]. Skeletal tuberculosis still remains a major health concern as it accounts for at least 10% of cases of extrapulmonary infection, and spine is the most common site of bony involvement [10].

Absolute indications for surgery in patients with spinal tuberculosis under active treatment are approximately 6% in those without neurologic deficit and approximately 60% in those with neurologic deficit [20]. The standard surgical method of decompression of tubercular dorsal spine is either the anterolateral extrapleural or open transthoracic transpleural approach. Both these approaches are sufficient for adequate decompression and graft placement but are associated with significant morbidity and require a prolonged hospital stay [15]. Video-assisted thoracoscopic surgery (VATS) is a good surgical alternative to conventional thoracotomy with minimal morbidity [21], though surgically demanding. VATS has been used extensively in spinal deformities such as scoliosis with results comparable to open procedures, but there has been limited use of VATS for decompression in active tuberculosis of dorsal spine [16].

It is recommended to do bone grafting in tuberculous spine when significant bone loss has occurred. Once the adjacent vertebral bodies develop destructive lesions, vertebral collapse may follow, due to destruction of cancellous bone, producing anterior or lateral wedging. Bone graft provides the stability and prevents further collapse of spine [12]. In our study, bone grafting was done in three patients.

The operative time in our series ranged from 105 to 165 minutes, this variation was due to the different types of procedures performed, and, as expected, the operative time for each procedure was longer initially and decreased with experience. Our mean operative time was less as compared to other studies (Table 3) because we did not go for spinal instrumentation and bone grafting was done only in three patients in this short series. Average blood loss increases with the operative time and addition of an additional procedure.

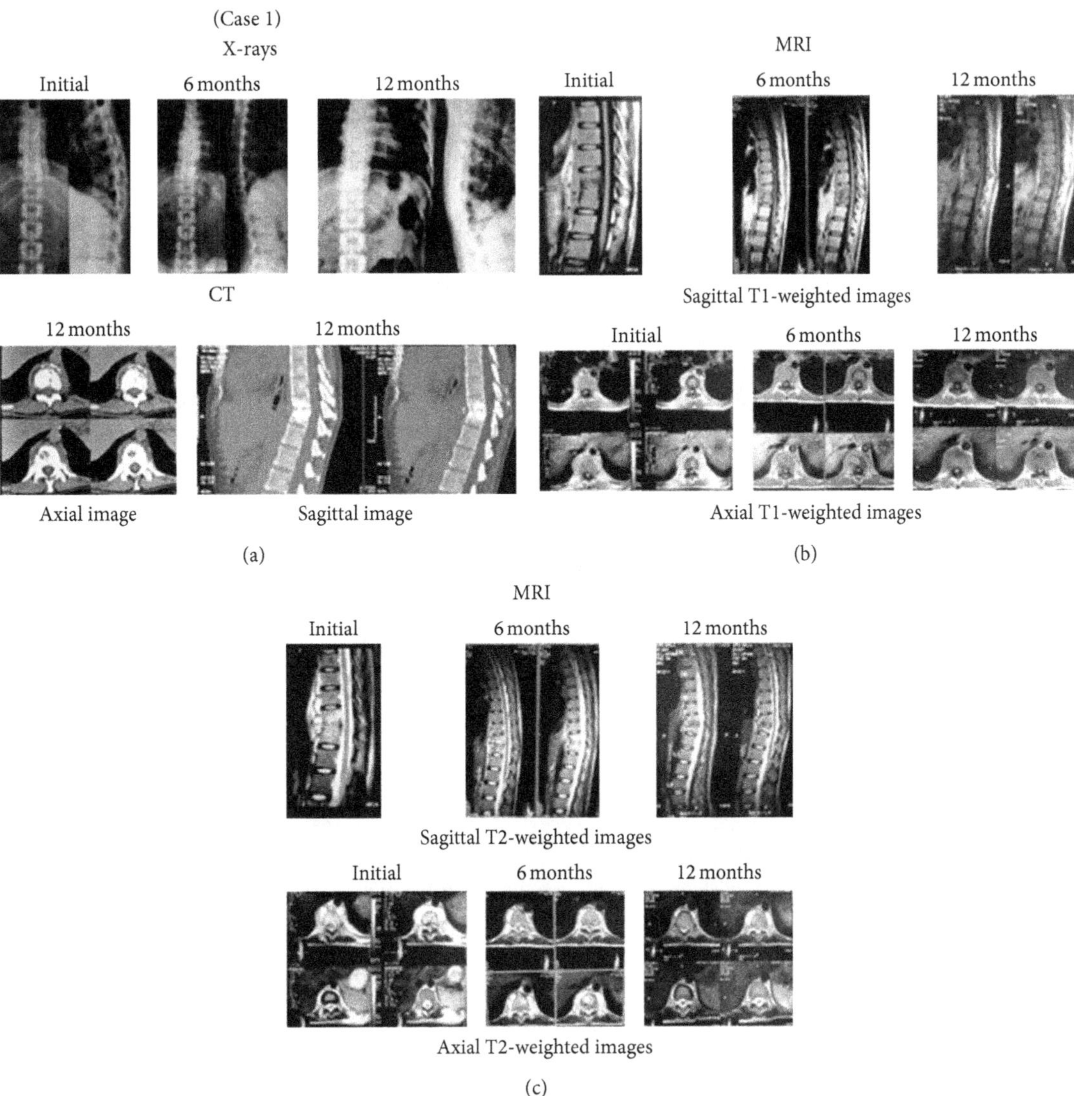

FIGURE 2: Tubercular spondylitis thoracic spine (D10-D11). Patient had a good subjective outcome and all changes in laboratory and radiological (MRI, CT, and X-rays) parameters showed improvement by the end of 12 months. Fusion was achieved at 12 months. No complications were seen and sinus which was present at initial presentation completely healed at her 18th month followup. (a) shows initial, 6-month, and 12-month X-rays and CT scan of the patient. (b) shows initial, 6-month, and 12-month sagittal and axial T1-weighted images. Disease completely healed at 12 months. (c) shows initial, 6-month, and 12-month sagittal and axial T2-weighted images. Disease completely healed at 12 months.

Better view provided by thoracoscopy and its preservation of wall structures (less extensive tissue dissection) probably are the explanations for less bleeding. Blood loss was comparative to other series of VATS in tuberculosis spine [13, 15, 16], except studies by Jayaswal et al. [12] and Kandwal et al. [17] where they used spinal instrumentation for stabilization in addition to the debridement. One of the major reported advantages of VATS was the reduction in postoperative hospital stay, and this was also observed in our series [22, 23]. Postoperative stay was less than reported by thoracotomy patients in other studies [23], which is a major consideration in developing countries with a high patient load in tertiary care hospitals.

One of the major goals of surgery was to achieve adequate neurological decompression through VATS in the present study. The decompression was adequate as indicated by the neurological recovery in all our cases. Our results are in accordance with available literature showing neurological recovery varying from 82 to 95% recovery of ambulatory status [12, 13, 15–17]. In a retrospective study done by Jayaswal et al. (2007), postoperatively 17 of the 18 patients with preoperative neurologic deficit attained ambulatory status and all patients showed improvement on the Frankel scale, with Grade C in one patient, Grade D in 10 patients, and Grade E in 12 patients [12]. In a series by Kapoor et al. (2005) of 16 patients, 14 (88%) had good neurologic recovery (improvement by 2-3 grades). In one patient, thoracoscopy was abandoned, and open thoracotomy was performed. Another patient did not recover and underwent anterolateral

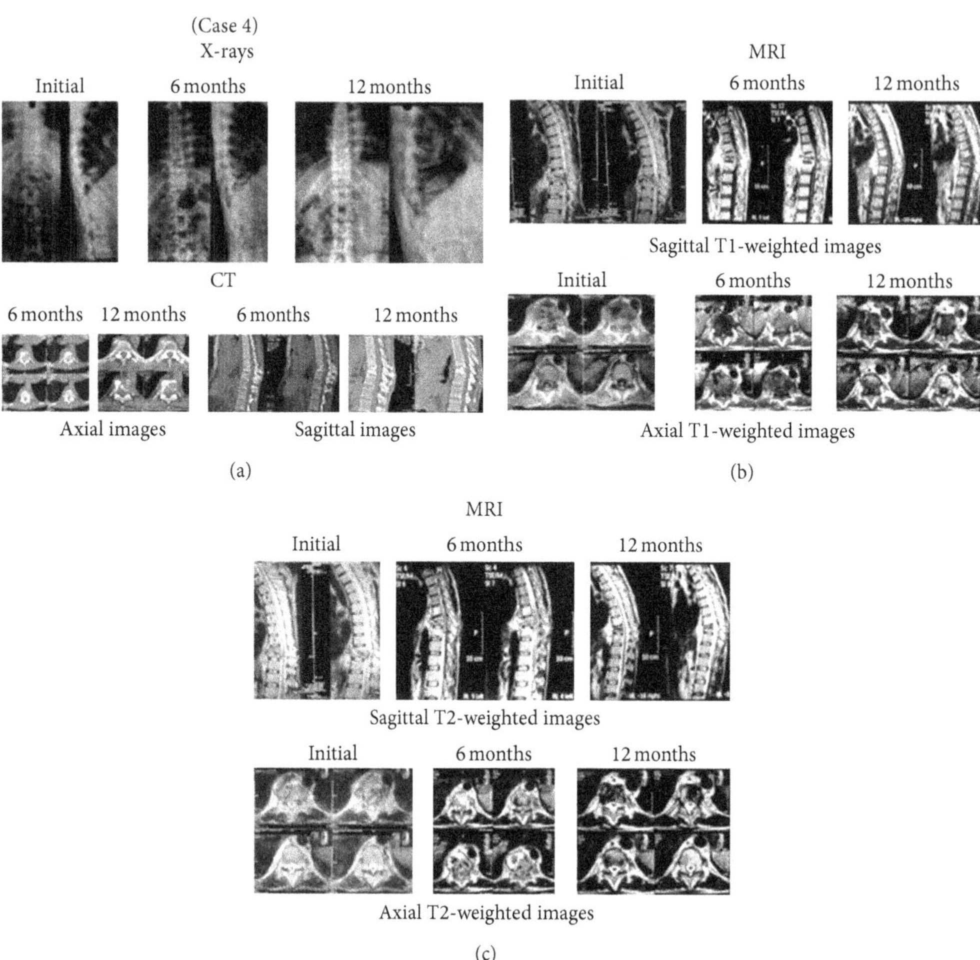

Figure 3: Tubercular spondylitisthoracic (D9-D10) with neurologic deficit. VATS along with minithoracotomy and placement of bone graft was done. Conversion to minithoracotomy was done because of dense pleural adhesions and difficulty in making portals was also encountered. Excellent subjective outcome and improvement in all laboratory and radiological (MRI, CT, and X-rays) parameters was seen by the end of 12 months. Patient attained ambulatory power (Grade A neurological deficit preoperatively) within 6 months of surgery. Grade I fusion was achieved at 12 months. (a) shows initial, 6-month, and 12-month X-rays and CT scan of the patient. (b) shows initial, 6-month, and 12-month sagittal and axial T1-weighted images. Disease completely healed at 12 months. (c) shows initial, 6-month, and 12-month sagittal and axial T2-weighted images. Disease completely healed at 12 months.

Table 3: Comparison of mean duration of surgery, average blood loss, and postoperative hospital stay with other studies.

Authors	Mean duration of surgery (minutes)	Average blood loss (mL)	Postoperative hospital stay (days)
Huang et al. (2000) [15]	172 (120–240)	485 (150–850)	21 (9–52)
Kapoor et al. (2005) [16]	223 (150–320)	497 (200–1200)	5.5 (4–9)
Jayaswal et al. (2007) [12]	228 (102–324)	780 (330–1180)	6 (3–12)
Kapoor et al. (2012) [13]	158.8	296.7	8.8
Kandwal et al. (2012) [17]	228 (102–330)	780 (330–1180)	—
Present study (2014)	141 (105–165)	418 (220–730)	5.7 (4–7)

decompression after 10 weeks [16]. In another series of 30 patients by Kapoor et al. (2012), all patients improved neurologically on a mean followup of 80 months. No patient had neurological deterioration and all of them regained ambulatory power with no cases of recurrence of tuberculosis [13]. In a series by Huang et al. (2000), after a followup of 24 months, the average neurologic recovery was 1.1 grades on Frankel's scale [15].

In our study, the mean preoperative, postoperative, 6-month, and 12-month kyphosis angle in patients without bone graft placement were 25°, 32°, and 41°, respectively. Therefore, final X-ray examination revealed an average increase in kyphosis angle by 16°. The mean preoperative, postoperative, 6-month, and 12-month kyphosis angle in patients with bone graft placement were 23°, 18°, and 24°, respectively. Therefore, there is an initial decrease in kyphosis angle with a subsequent slight increase at final followup, with deformity remaining stationary in the patients where bone grafting was done. Similar results were obtained by Jayaswal et al. (2007) with mean preoperative and 12-month follow-up kyphosis angles being 28° and 32° in patients without bone graft placement. The mean preoperative and 12-month follow-up kyphosis angles were 34° and 31° in patients in whom reconstruction with bone graft was done [12]. In a series by Huang et al. (2000), the mean preoperative, post-operative, and 2-year follow-up kyphosis angles were 26.8°, 16.8°, and 26°, respectively [15].

Adequate debridement and decompression also make room for healthy cancellous bone apposition resulting in high fusion rates [24, 25]. In a series of 23 patients who underwent VATS by Jayaswal et al. (2007), 22 achieved fusion with an average time for fusion of 16.5 weeks. Sixteen patients had Grade I fusion and six had Grade II fusion, and failure of fusion was seen in one patient [12]. In a series by Kandwal et al. (2012), 22 of 23 patients who underwent VATS had good fusion (Grade I and Grade II) and there was failure of fusion in one patient [17]. All our cases were able to attain fusion; this slight variation from that of literature can be attributable to small sample size of our study.

In our study, the VAS score for back pain improved from a pretreatment score of 8.3 to posttreatment 6-month and 12-month scores of 3.3 and 2, respectively. Kapoor et al. (2012) reported a statistically significant difference ($P < 0.001$ with Student's t-test) in VAS for back pain at three months compared to the preoperative period and at five-year followup compared to three months ($P < 0.001$) [13].

Functional outcome as assessed by modified Kirkaldy-Willis criteria at the time of final followup revealed result to be either excellent ($n = 5$) or good ($n = 4$). Huang et al. (2000) in their study of 10 patients followed for 24 months reported results as excellent ($n = 4$), good ($n = 5$), or fair ($n = 1$) [15]. In a series by Kapoor et al. (2012), out of 30 patients, excellent results were obtained in 24 patients, good in four, and fair in two, with 95% of patients having a good or excellent result [13].

As far as complications are concerned, all the complications of conventional thoracotomy are possible with the VATS procedure with a reported rate of 24.4–31.3% [16]. Dense pleural adhesion was encountered in two patients and to complete the procedure, we had to convert VATS into minithoracotomy. This has been reported as a complication of the procedure by others [12, 13, 15]. But we believe that this is not a complication of VATS per se, but a limitation of the procedure. None of the patients had intercostal neuralgia, which is a common complication in video-assisted thoracoscopic surgery (VATS). We did not encounter other complications of VATS reported in the literature like wound infection, dural tear, increase in neurologic deficit, chylothorax, Horner syndrome, encysted effusion, postoperative air leak, pneumothorax [26].

Our study has its own set of limitations. To name them, the study population was small and control group was lacking. Also, this series describes our early experiences with VATS. There is a steep learning curve before all the surgical goals of the open method can be attained through VATS. Adequate hand and eye coordination, which is necessary to perform remote bone and soft tissue dissection and to establish proper orientation under the angled endoscope, is required [12, 13, 15–17]. However, the strength of the study is that it is a single institutional study with cases operated by the same team of surgeons. The fact that this study comes from a centre in peripheral area of a developing country, where the prevalence of TB spondylitis is high, further adds to the relevance of this study.

To conclude, anterolateral decompression and transthoracic anterior decompression have been the two favoured approaches, but VATS can be considered as a valuable adjunct to the available options in the modern era of minimally invasive spine surgery. The findings of the present study suggest that video-assisted thoracoscopic surgery provides a safe and effective approach to the diagnosis and management of spinal tuberculosis.

It has inherent advantages of decreased blood loss and postoperative morbidity with good cosmetic acceptance but requires a learning curve and proper armamentarium. Proper selection of patients; competence of the anesthesiologist for monitoring single lung anesthesia; and surgical skills and experience of the surgeon comes handy in achieving ultimate good outcome. VATS leads to early recovery, cost effectivity, less morbidity, and shorter hospital stay. Our early experience of VATS in treating TB spondylitis is quiet encouraging and adds to the growing body in favour of minimally invasive surgery for the management of these lesions, though randomised studies with a larger followup are required to further support this observation.

References

[1] S. Rajasekaran, T. K. Shanmugasundaram, R. Prabhakar, J. Dheenadhayalan, A. P. Shetty, and D. K. Shetty, "Tuberculous lesions of the lumbosacral region: a 15-year follow-up of patients treated by ambulant chemotherapy," *Spine*, vol. 23, no. 10, pp. 1163–1167, 1998.

[2] M.-S. Moon, Y.-W. Moon, J.-L. Moon, S.-S. Kim, and D.-H. Sun, "Conservative treatment of tuberculosis of the lumbar and lumbosacral spine," *Clinical Orthopaedics and Related Research*, no. 398, pp. 40–49, 2002.

[3] S. M. Tuli, T. P. Srivastava, B. P. Varma, and G. P. Sinha, "Tuberculosis of spine," *Acta Orthopaedica Scandinavica*, vol. 38, no. 4, pp. 445–458, 1967.

[4] S. M. Tuli, Ed., *Tuberculosis of the Skeletal System*, Jaypee Brothers Medical, New Delhi, India, 3rd edition, 2004.

[5] L. B. Reichman, "Tuberculosis elimination. What's to stop us?" *International Journal of Tuberculosis and Lung Disease*, vol. 1, no. 1, pp. 3–11, 1997.

[6] M.-S. Moon, "Spine update tuberculosis of the spine: controversies and a new challenge," *Spine*, vol. 22, no. 15, pp. 1791–1797, 1997.

[7] S. M. Tuli, "Severe kyphotic deformity in tuberculosis of the spine," *International Orthopaedics*, vol. 19, no. 5, pp. 327–331, 1995.

[8] M.-S. Moon, I. Kim, Y.-K. Woo, and Y.-O. Park, "Conservative treatment of tuberculosis of the thoracic and lumbar spine in adults and children," *International Orthopaedics*, vol. 11, no. 4, pp. 315–322, 1987.

[9] A. C. M. C. Yau, L. C. S. Hsu, J. P. O'Brien, and A. R. Hodgson, "Tuberculous kyphosis. Correction with spinal osteotomy, halo pelvic distraction, and anterior and posterior fusion," *Journal of Bone and Joint Surgery. American*, vol. 56, no. 7, pp. 1419–1434, 1974.

[10] A. V. Slucky and F. Eismont, "Spinal infections," in *The Textbook of Spinal Surgery*, K. H. Bridwell and R. L. Dewald, Eds., pp. 2141–2183, Lippincott Raven, Philadelphia, Pa, USA, 1997.

[11] H.-K. Wong, H.-T. Hee, Z. Yu, and D. Wong, "Results of thoracoscopic instrumented fusion versus conventional posterior instrumented fusion in adolescent idiopathic scoliosis undergoing selective thoracic fusion," *Spine*, vol. 29, no. 18, pp. 2031–2038, 2004.

[12] A. Jayaswal, B. Upendra, A. Ahmed, B. Chowdhury, and A. Kumar, "Video-assisted thoracoscopic anterior surgery for tuberculous spondylitis," *Clinical Orthopaedics and Related Research*, no. 460, pp. 100–107, 2007.

[13] S. Kapoor, S. Kapoor, M. Agrawal, P. Aggarwal, and B. K. Jain Jr., "Thoracoscopic decompression in Pott's spine and its long-term follow-up," *International Orthopaedics*, vol. 36, no. 2, pp. 331–337, 2012.

[14] K. R. Eck, L. G. Lenke, K. H. Bridwell, L. A. Gilula, C. J. Lashgari, and K. D. Riew, "Radiographic assessment of anterior titanium mesh cages," *Journal of Spinal Disorders*, vol. 13, no. 6, pp. 501–509, 2000.

[15] T.-J. Huang, R. W.-W. Hsu, S.-H. Chen, and H.-P. Liu, "Video-assisted thoracoscopic surgery in managing tuberculous spondylitis," *Clinical Orthopaedics and Related Research*, no. 379, pp. 143–153, 2000.

[16] S. K. Kapoor, P. N. Agarwal, B. K. Jain Jr., and R. Kumar, "Video-assisted thoracoscopic decompression of tubercular spondylitis: clinical evaluation," *Spine*, vol. 30, no. 20, pp. E605–610, 2005.

[17] P. Kandwal, B. Garg, B. Upendra, B. Chowdhury, and A. Jayaswal, "Outcome of minimally invasive surgery in the management of tuberculous spondylitis," *Indian Journal of Orthopaedics*, vol. 46, no. 2, pp. 159–164, 2012.

[18] W. H. Kirkaldy-Willis and T. G. Thomas, "Anterior approaches in the diagnosis and treatment of infections of the vertebral bodies," *The Journal of Bone and Joint Surgery. American*, vol. 47, pp. 87–110, 1965.

[19] J. H. Bates and W. W. Stead, "The history of tuberculosis as a global epidemic," *Medical Clinics of North America*, vol. 77, no. 6, pp. 1205–1217, 1993.

[20] G. Bakalim, "Tuberculous spondylitis, a clinical study with special reference to the significance of spinal fusion and chemotherapy," *Acta Orthopaedica Scandinavica. Supplementum*, vol. 47, pp. 1–111, 1960.

[21] P. O. Newton, M. Marks, F. Faro et al., "Use of video-assisted thoracoscopic surgery to reduce perioperative morbidity in scoliosis surgery," *Spine*, vol. 28, no. 20, pp. S249–S254, 2003.

[22] P. Mangione, F. Vadier, and J. Sénégas, "Thoracoscopy versus thoracotomy for spinal surgery: comparison of two paired series," *Revue de Chirurgie Orthopedique et Reparatrice de l'Appareil Moteur*, vol. 85, no. 6, pp. 574–580, 1999.

[23] R. J. Landreneau, S. R. Hazelrigg, M. J. Mack et al., "Postoperative pain-related morbidity: video-assisted thoracic surgery versus thoracotomy," *Annals of Thoracic Surgery*, vol. 56, no. 6, pp. 1285–1289, 1993.

[24] V. J. Laheri, N. P. Badhe, and G. T. Dewnany, "Single stage decompression, anterior interbody fusion and posterior instrumentation for tuberculous kyphosis of the dorso-lumbar spine," *Spinal Cord*, vol. 39, no. 8, pp. 429–436, 2001.

[25] Medical Research Council, "A 10-year assessment of a controlled trial comparing debridement and anterior spinal fusion in the management of tuberculosis of the spine in patients on standard chemotherapy in Hong Kong. Eighth Report of the Medical Research Council Working Party on Tuberculosis of the Spine," *The Journal of Bone and Joint Surgery. British*, vol. 64, pp. 393–398, 1982.

[26] L. T. Khoo, R. Beisse, and M. Potulski, "Thoracoscopic-assisted treatment of thoracic and lumbar fractures: a series of 371 consecutive cases," *Neurosurgery*, vol. 51, no. 5, pp. 104–117, 2002.

27

Confocal Laser Endomicroscopy in Neurosurgery: A New Technique with Much Potential

David Breuskin,[1] Jana DiVincenzo,[1] Yoo-Jin Kim,[2] Steffi Urbschat,[1] and Joachim Oertel[1]

[1] *Department of Neurosurgery, Saarland University, 66421 Homburg, Germany*
[2] *Department of Pathology, Saarland University, 66421 Homburg, Germany*

Correspondence should be addressed to Joachim Oertel; joachim.oertel@uks.eu

Academic Editor: John Y. K. Lee

Technical innovations in brain tumour diagnostic and therapy have led to significant improvements of patient outcome and recurrence free interval. The use of technical devices such as surgical microscopes as well as neuronavigational systems have helped localising tumours as much as fluorescent agents, such as 5-aminolaevulinic acid, have helped visualizing pathologically altered tissue. Nonetheless, intraoperative instantaneous frozen sections and histological diagnosis remain the only method of gaining certainty of the nature of the resected tissue. This technique is time consuming and does not provide close-to-real-time information. In gastroenterology, confocal endoscopy closed the gap between tissue resection and histological examination, providing an almost real-time histological diagnosis. The potential of this technique using a confocal laser endoscope EndoMAG1 by Karl Storz Company was evaluated by our group on pig brains, tumour tissue cell cultures, and fresh human tumour specimen. Here, the authors report for the first time on the results of applying this new technique and provide first confocal endoscopic images of various brain and tumour structures. In all, the technique harbours a very promising potential to provide almost real-time intraoperative diagnosis, but further studies are needed to provide evidence for the technique's potential.

1. Introduction

Neurooncological diagnosis and treatment constitute a major part of neurosurgery. Obtaining histological diagnosis is frequently challenging. The resulting therapeutic options vary depending on the histological grade and the tumour type. The incidence of gliomas is expected to be around 5-6/100000 per year, with their survival rate depending heavily on their WHO grade. Even with today's high medical standards consisting of surgical removal and postoperative combined radiochemotherapy, median survival shows 18–21 months at its best for glioblastomas [1]. While it is frequently noted that malignant gliomas cannot be cured by surgical resection, recent studies show an improved life expectancy associated with a more extended tumour resection [1–3]. Thus, currently, research is focussing on increasing the extent of resection through various additional techniques such as neuronavigation [4] or 5-aminolaevulinic acid (5-ALA) fluorescent marking of tumour cells. While neuronavigation suggests precise imaging of the tumour, this can be misleading due to brain shift occurring during surgery and therefore tumour borders are not depicted according to reality [5]. For 5-ALA, randomized clinical trials showed a significant reduction of second resection in patients treated with 5-ALA compared to those who had surgery being performed solely under white light [6]. However, not all tumour cells show fluorescent activity; thus, neither the introduction of neuronavigation nor 5-ALA tumour imaging solved the problem of intraoperative precise separation of tumour tissue from adjacent intact brain parenchyma.

A new way of optical imaging is confocal laser endomicroscopy (CLE) which has recently been applied to other medical fields such as gastroenterology and pulmonology. As a patent dating back to 1957, confocal microscopy manages to reduce emitted light by molecules that are not in the desired focus plane. Opposed to conventional fluorescence microscopes where the tissue is widely lit upon, confocal laser microscopy only emits a punctual light beam from a laser source reducing the amount of scattered light that is then emitted by the sample. Because of an interposed pinhole blocking all remaining scattered light, only light emitted by the desired point is detected. The confocal light generates clear focused images without any out of focus signals. This technique has allowed visualizing the underlaying tissue on a microscopic scale with its features notably depending on the device in use. Through this method, however, it has been possible to achieve real-time imaging on a scale that has previously only been possible on histologic slices, making it a powerful diagnostic tool for tissue alterations. In gastroenterology as well as in pulmonology, the technique has been used in a combined method with standard endoscopy, giving the possibility of microscopic evaluation combined with targeted biopsies of altered tissue [7–9].

With these promising results, CLE was introduced to neurosurgery and is currently being evaluated in different settings. It is a common goal that this technique can be used in an easy intraoperative setting, allowing neurosurgeons to scan tumour borders, allowing for more precise resections to be made and improving the outcome of patients with brain tumours.

2. Materials and Methods

2.1. General Study Design. The application of a confocal endomicroscope (EndoMAG1) manufactured by KARL Storz company, Tuttlingen, Germany, on human tumour specimen and human tumour cell cultures in order to analyse the value of this device in neurooncology was investigated.

2.2. Confocal Endoscope. The imaging device comprises of a rigid endoscope with Hopkins-rod lenses mounted on a fixed frame connected to the imaging device and computer. The outer diameter is 5 mm, and the length amounts to 323 mm. The size of the circular scanning field covers 300 μm × 300 μm, and the highest achievable resolution is 2 μm. The wavelength of the laser signal is red, and scanning depth in 3D mode is approximately 80 μm. The detected signal consists of reflection and scattering. The frame rate (2D) is almost 40 frames per second allowing true real-time images to be evaluated. The setting of the CLE does not yet allow the investigation at location during surgery. Tissue samples had to be removed first and taken to the work station depicted in Figure 1 in order to be examined.

2.3. Tissue Investigation and Data Evaluation. In the first step, pig brain tissue was used to evaluate general handling aspects and to develop an algorithm to proceed with the tissue samples for optimal CLE results.

In the second step, samples of resected tumour tissue or primary cell cultures were covered in isotonic saline solution as a thin fluid layer improved image quality. The rigid endoscope was then placed on top of the sample, while a slight pressure to the tissue needed to be applied to ensure contact. All tissue samples were then investigated a second time after staining with methylene blue after incubation time of 20 minutes. Methylene blue is an in vivo as well as in vitro staining agent that is safe to use and of no toxic nature to the patient. In histology, it stains nuclei, making their examination favourable. Other than this histological use,

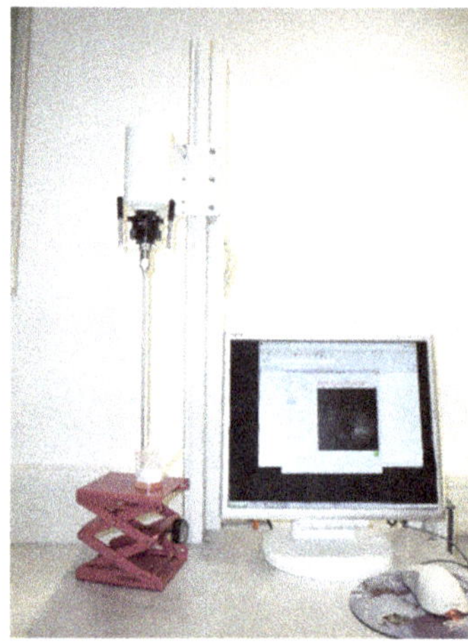

FIGURE 1: Confocal endomicroscope EndoMAG1.

MB serves as a spray dye in gastroenterologic endoscopic procedures in order to visualise altered tissue. After starting the software, images of the samples were viewed in real time. Samples were brought in focus by changing the height of the platform. When a clear image was achieved, the tissue was scanned by using the focus on the endoscope. These images were digitally saved and compared to their respective histological slices made by the neuropathologist. All three groups of images, tumour tissue samples, cell cultures, and histological slices were used to define similarities in respect to their original tumour entity, which focused mainly on cell shape and density, shape of the nuclei, and interstitial structures.

3. Results and Discussion

In this first trial using this specific device, images of unaltered pig brain tissue and of primary cell cultures were evaluated. It was possible to see structures on an endomicroscopic level detecting different cell structures on a highly focused plane. Additionally, different tissue structures, differences between grey and white substances, and arachnoid membranes could be visualized although the scanning field consisted only of 300 μm × 300 μm (Figures 2(a)–2(f)).

The preparation of the tissue before examination proved to be without difficulties. The samples needed no more than a small layer of liquid—in this series isotonic sodium chloride solution—to improve image quality. Compared to frozen sections done by the neuropathologist, this technique offers a quicker preparation and faster visualisation since staining does not necessarily need to be done.

Images of the grey substance, for example, showed a higher density in nuclei compared to white substance, giving impressions of the different structures and scale. The tissue structure was much denser compared to arachnoid mater with a more fibrous pattern including elongated cell bodies and fibrillar cytoplasm.

After this first examination, samples were partly stained with methylene blue (MB). For this, the tissue was simply put into MB solution. Depending on the size of the sample,

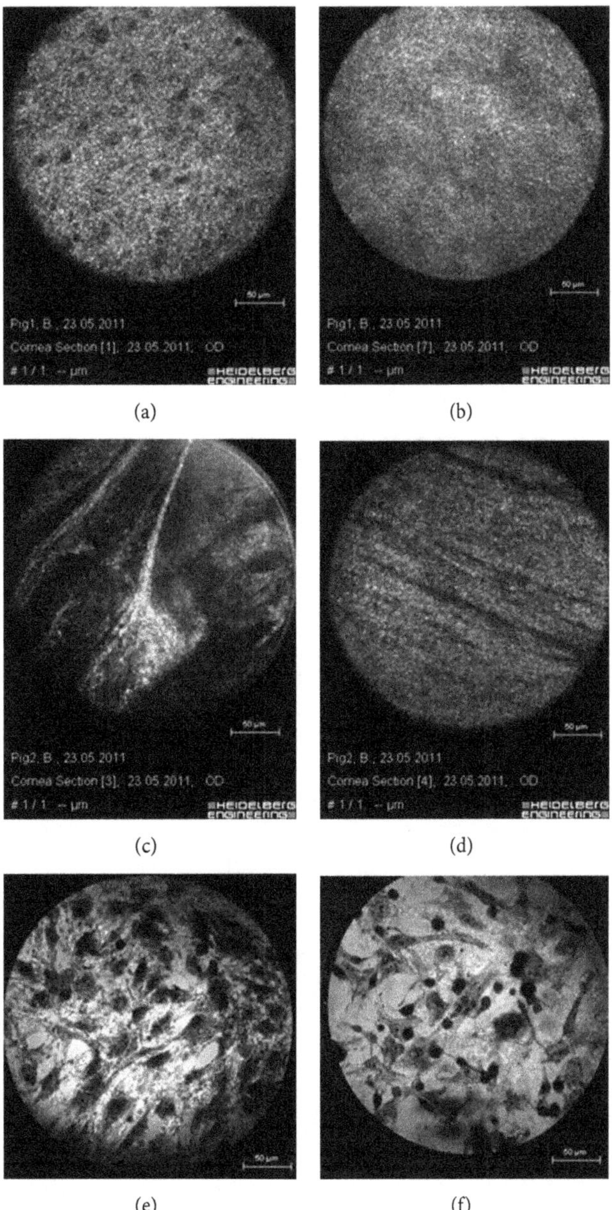

FIGURE 2: (a) Grey matter of the pig. (b) White matter of the pig. (c) Arachnoid membrane of the pig. (d) Ventricular wall of the pig. (e) Primary meningioma cell culture. (f) Primary glioblastoma cell culture.

it was best to divide the tissue in small pieces to create a larger contact surface for staining. After 20 minutes of incubation, analysis was performed likewise to the native examination. Results were mainly not very different from native samples. However, the application of MB helped in the evaluation of the nuclei in selected cases since the nuclei presented themselves darker with a more pronounced contrast depending on how well MB had been absorbed. For further investigation as well as intraoperative use, however, the need of MB staining seems to be questionable, as no significant benefit could be observed.

In the second step of analysis, more than 50 tumour specimens were evaluated. It was found that common histological paradigms could not entirely be applied for tumour tissue evaluation. Different endomicroscopic histological criteria were established which were found to be reoccurring amongst different tumour entities. These criteria mainly included the morphology of the nucleus and its location within the cell, the existence and the shape of the cytoplasm, the presence of psammoma bodies, the cell-to-cell contact, the cellular density within the specimen, the growth pattern (i.e., diffuse, well sorted), and the presence of blood vessels.

Confocal endomicroscopically, glioblastomas showed similarities to normal brain tissue although presenting a higher cellularity. Nuclei were mostly polymorphous and variable in shape, much of how they present themselves in histological findings. However, the most striking confocal diagnostic criterion was a very diffuse growth pattern with cell borders hardly being visible and fibrillar cytoplasm being less remarkable as in low grade gliomas or in normal tissue

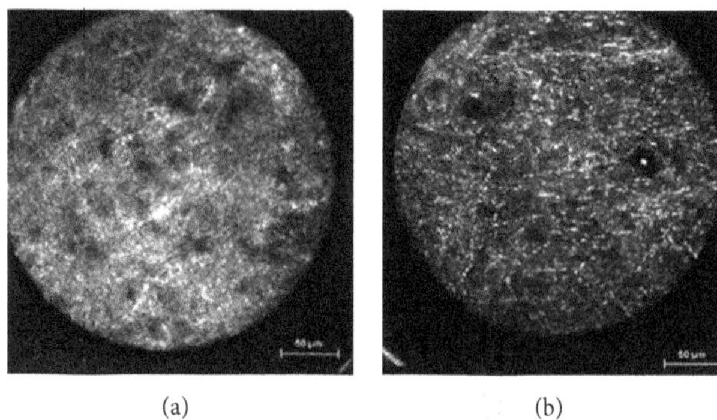

(a) (b)

FIGURE 3: (a) Glioblastoma. (b) Astrocytoma.

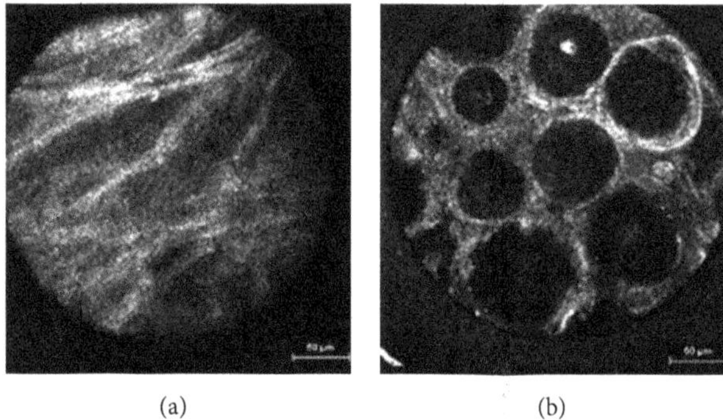

(a) (b)

FIGURE 4: (a) Meningioma. (b) Psammomatous meningioma.

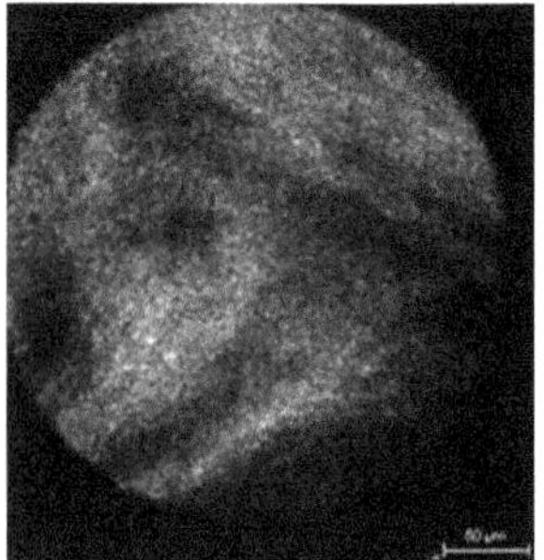

FIGURE 5: Schwannoma.

(Figure 3(a)). In low grade gliomas, cell borders showed a much sharper contrast and more definite glia-like structure (Figure 3(b)).

Meningiomas showed a very distinct image. Their origin being arachnoid cells, a very well distinguishable fibrous network with oval shaped nuclei and elongated spindle-like cytoplasm, was found (Figure 4(a)). This structure became even more apparent when scanning through the tissue using the focus. An even more precise diagnosis could be made in cases of psammomatous meningiomas when characteristic psammoma bodies were present and scattered throughout the samples (Figure 4(b)). Schwannomas resembled meningiomas in many ways but showed larger fibrous streaks (Figure 5).

As quintessence of this first evaluation of a new confocal laser endoscope, some peculiar aspects can be already summarised and have to be discussed.

Based on the results in the pig brain and on human tumour cell culture as well as based on the results of fresh human tumour specimen, brain cell and tissue as well as tumour specimen show a very characteristic appearance in confocal endoscopic imaging. Thus, at first sight, confocal endoscopy could provide almost real-time diagnosis of human brain tumours. But further studies are needed before any conclusions can be made.

These results reflect some of the aspects mentioned by other groups using confocal endomicroscopic techniques [10–12]. While the devices in use differ, examination of tumorous tissue provides images that allow a histological differentiation from healthy brain tissues. With the EndoMAG1, however, no fluorescent agents were needed in order to investigate the probes, which ultimately makes intraoperative use easier and, in cases of toxic agents, safer for patients.

Intraoperative detection of tumour margins as well as identification of altered cerebral tissue is one of the most demanding aspects of brain tumour surgery. Improving the quality of the surgical procedure through much technical advancement throughout the past recent years, operative visualisation still has many downsides. High grade gliomas infiltrate the tissue that seems unaltered under the surgical microscope, which is why many tumours cannot be radically removed yet. Confocal laser endomicroscopy is aiming to close this gap between molecular imaging and surgical microscopic imaging. Introduced and well established, the technique might very well have the potential to change the surgical strategy by its intraoperative application. The potential of gathering real-time histopathology will eventually help neurosurgeons to thoroughly scan borders of the resection area determining whether an extension of resection is needed. Surgical procedures could then be kept as minimally invasive as possible while removing as much as possible without causing neurologic damage because of excessive resection.

CLE is yet to be properly investigated in order to be fully integrated into standard neurosurgical procedures, but few groups are currently evaluating different devices as well as techniques, all of them benefiting from the knowledge of nonneurosurgical fields of application [10–12]. Further trials will see this device being used on different tumour entities to gather sufficient data for accurate intraoperative histological diagnosis. Whether ordinary histological paradigms are applicable is yet to be examined. It is possible that different criteria need to be found to evaluate the samples as it has been done in gastroenterology [13].

4. Conclusion

Confocal laser endoscopy with the EndoMAG1 provides reliable images applied at pig brain, cell tissue cultures, and fresh human brain tumour tissue. All structures seem to harbour a very characteristic endoscopic image. Thus, potentially, this technique could provide a real-time histological diagnosis. But before this even could be discussed, a further development of the endoscope and a detailed analysis of the correlation of confocal endoscopic imaging and histopathological diagnosis have to be done in further studies.

References

[1] W. Stummer, M. J. Van Den Bent, and M. Westphal, "Cytoreductive surgery of glioblastoma as the key to successful adjuvant therapies: new arguments in an old discussion," *Acta Neurochirurgica*, vol. 153, no. 6, pp. 1211–1218, 2011.

[2] M. Lacroix, D. Abi-Said, D. R. Fourney et al., "A multivariate analysis of 416 patients with glioblastoma multiforme: prognosis, extent of resection, and survival," *Journal of Neurosurgery*, vol. 95, no. 2, pp. 190–198, 2001.

[3] M. J. McGirt, K. L. Chaichana, M. Gathinji et al., "Independent association of extent of resection with survival in patients with malignant brain astrocytoma: clinical article," *Journal of Neurosurgery*, vol. 110, no. 1, pp. 156–162, 2009.

[4] Y. Tanaka, T. Nariai, T. Momose et al., "Glioma surgery using a multimodal navigation system with integrated metabolic images," *Journal of Neurosurgery*, vol. 110, no. 1, pp. 163–172, 2009.

[5] N. Sanai and M. S. Berger, "Operative techniques for gliomas and the value of extent of resection," *Neurotherapeutics*, vol. 6, no. 3, pp. 478–486, 2009.

[6] W. Stummer, J.-C. Tonn, H. M. Mehdorn et al., "Counterbalancing risks and gains from extended resections in malignant glioma surgery: a supplemental analysis from the randomized 5-aminolevulinic acid glioma resection study," *Journal of Neurosurgery*, vol. 114, no. 3, pp. 613–623, 2011.

[7] T. M. Yeung and N. J. Mortensen, "Advances in endoscopic visualization of colorectal polyps," *Colorectal Disease*, vol. 13, no. 4, pp. 352–359, 2011.

[8] L. Thiberville and M. Salaün, "Bronchoscopic advances: on the way to the cells," *Respiration*, vol. 79, no. 6, pp. 441–449, 2010.

[9] D. I. Gheonea, A. Saftoiu, T. Ciurea, C. Popescu, C. V. Georgescu, and A. Malos, "Confocal laser endomicroscopy of the colon," *Journal of Gastrointestinal and Liver Diseases*, vol. 19, no. 2, pp. 207–211, 2010.

[10] T. Sankar, P. M. Delaney, R. W. Ryan et al., "Miniaturized handheld confocal microscopy for neurosurgery: results in an experimental glioblastoma model," *Neurosurgery*, vol. 66, no. 2, pp. 410–417, 2010.

[11] S. Foersch, A. Heimann, A. Ayyad et al., "Confocal laser endomicroscopy for diagnosis and histomorphologic imaging of brain tumors *in vivo*," *PLoS One*, vol. 7, no. 7, Article ID e41760, 2012.

[12] H.-G. Schlosser, O. Suess, P. Vajkoczy, F. K. H. V. Landeghem, M. Zeitz, and C. Bojarski, "Confocal neurolasermicroscopy in human brain perspectives for neurosurgery on a cellular level (including additional Comments to this article)," *Zentralblatt für Neurochirurgie*, vol. 71, no. 1, pp. 13–16, 2010.

[13] T. Kuiper, F. J. C. Van Den Broek, S. Van Eeden et al., "New classification for probe-based confocal laser endomicroscopy in the colon," *Endoscopy*, vol. 43, no. 12, pp. 1076–1081, 2011.

28

Changes in Hysterectomy Route and Adnexal Removal for Benign Disease in Australia 2001–2015: A National Population-Based Study

Natalie De Cure[1] **and Stephen J. Robson**[2]

[1]Centenary Hospital for Women and Children, P.O. Box 11, Woden, ACT 2606, Australia
[2]Department of Obstetrics and Gynaecology, Australian National University Medical School, P.O. Box 5235, Garran, ACT 2605, Australia

Correspondence should be addressed to Stephen J. Robson; stephen.robson@anu.edu.au

Academic Editor: Saad Amer

Objective. Hysterectomy rates have fallen over recent years and there remains debate whether salpingectomy should be performed to reduce the lifetime risk of ovarian cancer. We examined trends in adnexal removal and route of hysterectomy in Australia between 2001 and 2015. *Methods.* Data were obtained from the national procedural dataset for hysterectomy approach (vaginal, VH; abdominal, AH; and, laparoscopic, LH) and rates of adnexal removal, as well as endometrial ablation. The total female population in two age groups ("younger age group," 35 to 54 years, and "older age group," 55 to 74 years) was obtained from the Australian Bureau of Statistics. *Results.* The rate of hysterectomy fell in both younger (61.7 versus 45.2/10000/year, $p < 0.005$) and older (38.8 versus 33.2/10000/year, $p < 0.005$) age groups. In both age groups there were significant decreases in the incidence rates for VH (by 53% in the younger age group and 29% in the older age group) and AH (by 53% and 55%, respectively). The rates of LH increased by 153% in the younger age group and 307% in the older age group. Overall, the proportion of hysterectomies involving adnexal removal increased (31% versus 65% in the younger age group, $p < 0.005$; 44% versus 58% in the older age group, $p < 0.005$). The increase occurred almost entirely after 2011. *Conclusion.* Hysterectomy is becoming less common, and both vaginal and abdominal hysterectomy are being replaced by laparoscopic hysterectomy. Removal of the adnexae is now more common in younger women.

1. Introduction

Hysterectomy for benign conditions remains a common procedure in Australia and internationally. Prior to 2000, the lifetime risk of hysterectomy in Australian women was estimated to be approximately 35% [1], similar to the rate in other developed countries [2, 3]. Since 2000—associated with the introduction of treatments such as the levonorgestrel-releasing intrauterine system (Mirena™) and second-generation endometrial ablation techniques—the rate of hysterectomy has fallen [4]. Over the same period nonsurgical treatments for fibroids such as uterine artery embolization and focussed ultrasound also might be expected to reduce further the rate of hysterectomy [5, 6].

A trend to decreased use of hysterectomy has been identified in some European countries and in North America [7, 8]. As treatments for heavy menstrual bleeding (HMB) have evolved so has the surgical approach to hysterectomy. Updating previous evidence [9, 10] a recent systematic review comparing total laparoscopic hysterectomy (TLH) with vaginal hysterectomy (VH) included 24 studies published to February 2016 and reported no difference between the two techniques in the rate of major or minor complications, risk of ureter and bladder injuries, intraoperative blood loss, and length of hospital stay [11]. VH was associated with a shorter operative time and lower rates of vaginal cuff dehiscence and conversion to laparotomy. However vaginal access and uterine size impose limitations on uptake of vaginal hysterectomy and there is a body of evidence supporting a laparoscopic approach as more appropriate where a vaginal approach is difficult [9, 10].

Further complicating the change in surgical paradigm is an evolving body of evidence that cells of the fallopian tube may be the origin of many high-grade serous ovarian tumours [12]. For this reason some professional societies now recommend discussion of opportunistic salpingectomy at the time of hysterectomy for benign conditions to reduce this risk [13, 14]. A systematic review of opportunistic salpingectomy identified ten comparative studies that cumulatively demonstrated a small to no increase in operative time and no additional blood loss, hospital stay, or complications attributable to salpingectomy at the time of hysterectomy for benign disease [15]. However, salpingectomy can be more challenging at VH and this has a potential to influence the choice of approach for hysterectomy [16]. We set out to determine how these factors might have influenced hysterectomy in Australia over the last 15 years. We wanted to determine if there had been a significant change in the incidence rate of hysterectomy; whether there had been changes in the approach to hysterectomy; and whether there has been an increasing trend to removal of the adnexae.

2. Materials and Methods

Data regarding hysterectomy and endometrial ablation were obtained from the Australian Institute of Health and Welfare (AIHW) national procedural database. The AIHW national procedural database holds information collected through the National Health Information Agreement as required by and specified in the National Minimum Data Set relating to hospitals. The data are supplied by all Australian state and territory health authorities. Procedures use an agreed national standard, the *Australian Classification of Health Interventions* (ACHI), which is based around the Australian National Medical Benefits Schedule (MBS). Validation studies of the AIHW dataset have reported 99.5% agreement with "true" morbidity in a female population (kappa 0.86) [17]. We selected data from 2001 to 2015 using procedures coded according to the ICD-10-AM/ACHI guidelines, as detailed in Box 1. Data were extracted only for benign disease: hysterectomy code numbers specific for malignant disease were identified but not extracted and were not included in the study dataset.

To provide a denominator, annual point estimates for the total female population in two age bands—35 to 54 years (the "younger age group") and 55 to 74 years (the "older age group")—were obtained from the Australian Bureau of Statistics (ABS). All extracted data were entered into Excel™ spreadsheets and statistical analysis was performed in GenStat (https://www.vsni.co.uk/software/genstat/). Polynomial linear regressions were performed to calculate the coefficient of determination (R^2 values) as measures of the closeness of fit and p values. The study received prospective approval from the Human Research Ethics Committee of the Australian National University (protocol 2015/347).

3. Results

The overall incidence rate of hysterectomy at a national level fell (from 54.7 to 40.7/10000/year, $p < 0.005$) and this change occurred in both the younger (from 61.7 to 45.2/10000/year, $p < 0.005$) and older (from 38.8 to 33.2/10000/year, $p < 0.005$) age groups over the study period (Figure 1). Over the same time period the rate of endometrial ablation in the younger age group increased from 11.0 to 22.4/10000/year ($p < 0.005$).

The total number of hysterectomies performed in Australia by each route is presented in Figure 2 (the younger age group) and Figure 3 (the older age group).

The incidence rates for the individual routes of hysterectomy (vaginal, abdominal, and laparoscopic) also changed in both age groups. In the younger age group (Figure 4) the rates fell for VH by 53% (from 18.9 to 8.9/10000/year, $p < 0.005$) and for AH also by 53% (from 35.1 to 16.5/10000/year, $p < 0.005$), while that of LH increased by 153% (from 7.8 to 19.7/10000/year, $p < 0.005$). In the older age group (Figure 5) the rate of VH fell by 29% (from 20.0 to 14.3/10000/year, $p < 0.005$) and for AH by 55% (from 15.9 to 7.1/10000/year, $p < 0.005$). The rate of LH increased by 307% (from 2.9 to 11.8/10000/year, $p < 0.005$).

The proportion of hysterectomies involving removal of adnexal structures increased significantly over the study period in the younger age group for each route of hysterectomy (Figure 6): by 623% in VH (from 2.2 to 15.9%, $p < 0.005$); by 44% in AH (from 46.6% to 66.9%, $p = 0.09$); and by 50% in LH (from 34.2% to 84.5%, $p = 0.012$). In the older age group (Figure 7) for AH the rate of adnexal removal was high and remained unchanged (from 91.5% to 91.9%, $p = 0.11$). The rate in LH increased from 76% to 95% ($p < 0.005$) and in VH the rate was low but increased from 2.6% to 10.6% ($p < 0.005$).

For hysterectomy by all approaches the proportion performed with associated adnexal removal has increased in both the younger (from 31% to 65%, $p < 0.005$) and older (from 44% to 58%, $p < 0.005$) (Figure 8). However, this increase has occurred almost entirely after 2011: there was no significant increase in the rate of adnexal removal from 2001 to 2011 in either the younger ($p = 0.41$) or older ($p = 0.32$) age groups.

4. Discussion

The findings of this study are consistent with published data from Europe and North America that have shown that hysterectomy is being undertaken less commonly in developed countries [2, 3]. Despite a weight of evidence supporting a vaginal approach [9, 10], the proportion of hysterectomies performed vaginally has fallen overall, with the greatest decrease has been seen in the younger age group. Importantly, the proportion of hysterectomies performed with associated adnexal removal has increased in the younger age group, but across both age groups there is a low rate with VH.

The findings of our study provide a comparison to other similar countries. A study from Denmark using data from

Descriptor XIII *"Gynaecological procedures"*
"Uterus" *Blocks 1259–1273*
Block 1263 Destructive procedures of uterus
15622-0 Endoscopic endometrial ablation
*Block 1268 Abdominal hysterectomy**
35653-00 Subtotal abdominal hysterectomy
35653-01 Total abdominal hysterectomy
35653-02 Abdominal hysterectomy with unilateral salpingo-oophorectomy
35653-03 Abdominal hysterectomy with bilateral salpingo-oophorectomy
35653-04 Abdominal hysterectomy with removal of adnexae
*Block 1269 Vaginal hysterectomy**
35657-00 Vaginal hysterectomy
35673-00 Vaginal hysterectomy with unilateral salpingo-oophorectomy
35673-02 Vaginal hysterectomy with removal of adnexae
35673-01 Vaginal hysterectomy with bilateral salpingo-oophorectomy
*Laparoscopic hysterectomy**
35750-00 Laparoscopically-assisted vaginal hysterectomy
35753-00 Laparoscopically-assisted vaginal hysterectomy with unilateral salpingo-oophorectomy
35753-01 Laparoscopically-assisted vaginal hysterectomy with bilateral salpingo-oophorectomy
35766-00 Laparoscopically-assisted vaginal hysterectomy proceeding to abdominal hysterectomy
35766-03 Laparoscopically-assisted vaginal hysterectomy proceeding to abdominal hysterectomy with removal of adnexae
From 2008:
90448-00 Subtotal laparoscopic abdominal hysterectomy
90448-01 Total laparoscopic abdominal hysterectomy
90448-02 Total laparoscopic abdominal hysterectomy with removal of adnexae.

Box 1: Search strategy. *Only descriptors for benign disease extracted.

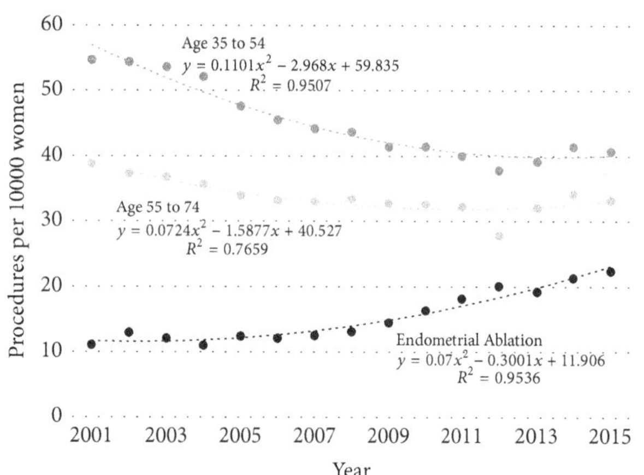

FIGURE 1: Age-stratified incidence rates of hysterectomy in Australia (procedures per 10000 women) for women aged 35–54 years and 55–74 years and incidence rate of endometrial ablation in women aged 35–54 years.

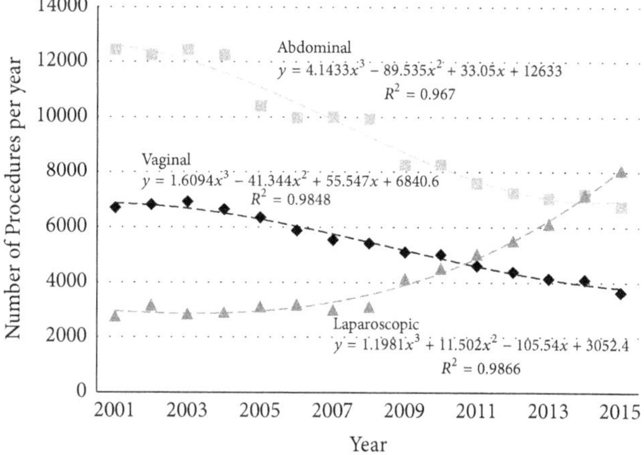

FIGURE 2: Absolute number of hysterectomies by different routes (◆ vaginal, ■ abdominal, and ▲ laparoscopic) in Australia in women aged 35–54 years.

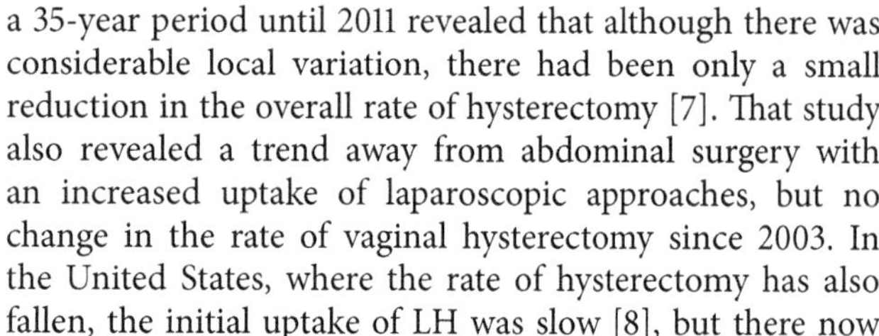
a 35-year period until 2011 revealed that although there was considerable local variation, there had been only a small reduction in the overall rate of hysterectomy [7]. That study also revealed a trend away from abdominal surgery with an increased uptake of laparoscopic approaches, but no change in the rate of vaginal hysterectomy since 2003. In the United States, where the rate of hysterectomy has also fallen, the initial uptake of LH was slow [8], but there now has been acceleration in the use of laparoscopic and robotic hysterectomy [18].

The increase in removal of adnexal structures noted in this study mirrors a similar trend noted in the United States. The change is likely to reflect the evolving literature describing a clear association between dysplastic changes occurring in the distal fallopian and their relationship to ovarian malignancy [12, 19]. Our study showed low rates of adnexal removal associated with VH in younger women. The technical challenges in performing adnexal surgery at the

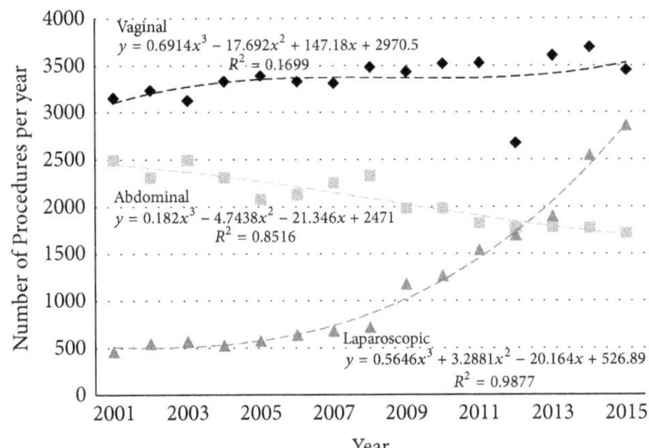

FIGURE 3: Absolute number of hysterectomies by different routes (◆ vaginal, ■ abdominal, and ▲ laparoscopic) in Australia in women aged 55–74 years.

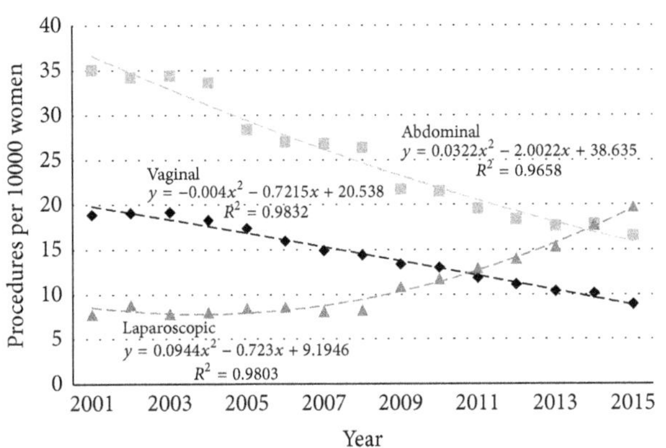

FIGURE 4: Age-stratified incidence rates for different routes of hysterectomy (◆ vaginal, ■ abdominal, and ▲ laparoscopic) in Australia (procedures per 10000 women) for women aged 35–54 years.

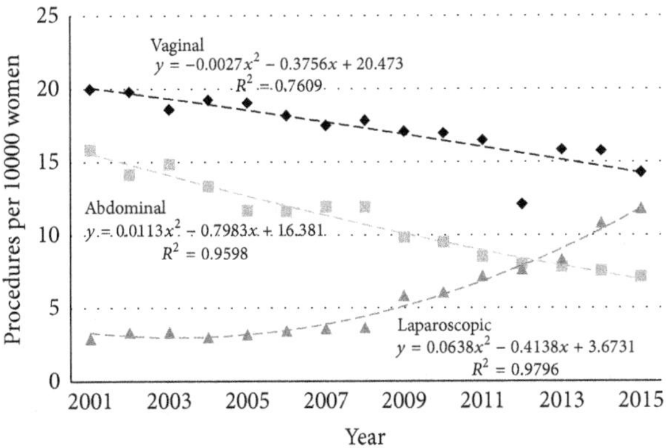

FIGURE 5: Age-stratified incidence rates for different routes of hysterectomy (◆ vaginal, ■ abdominal, and ▲ laparoscopic) in Australia (procedures per 10000 women) for women aged 55–74 years.

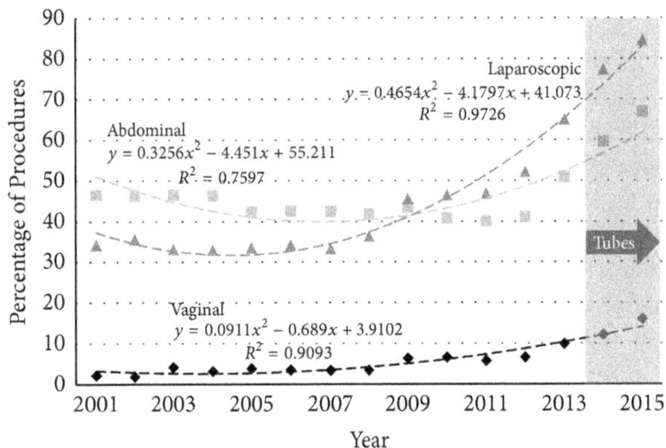

FIGURE 6: Percentage of procedures involving removal of the adnexae by route of hysterectomy (◆ vaginal, ■ abdominal, and ▲ laparoscopic) in Australia for women aged 35–54 years. The epoch in which guidance advised opportunistic salpingectomy is shaded.

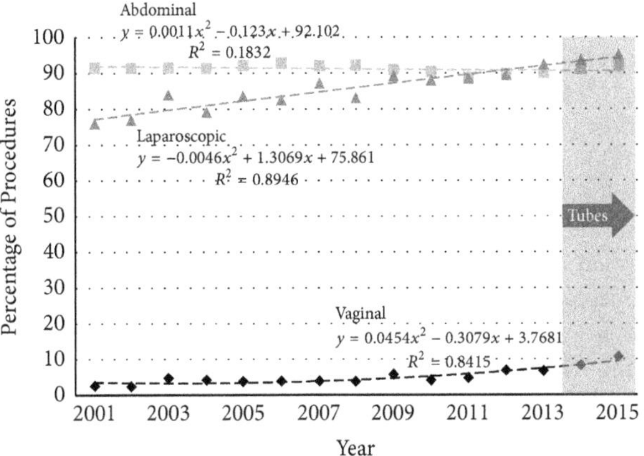

FIGURE 7: Percentage of procedures involving removal of the adnexae by route of hysterectomy (◆ vaginal, ■ abdominal, and ▲ laparoscopic) in Australia for women aged 55–74 years. The epoch in which guidance advised opportunistic salpingectomy is shaded.

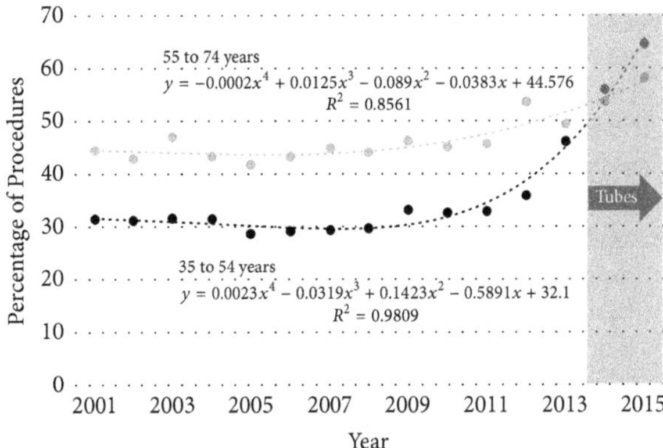

FIGURE 8: Percentage of all hysterectomies involving removal of the adnexae by age group (35 to 54 years, 55 to 74 years) for the period 2001 to 2015 in Australia. The epoch in which guidance advised possible opportunistic salpingectomy is shaded.

time of VH are well-recognised, with authors commenting that with "the decreasing rate of... [vaginal hysterectomy]... the vaginal approach and [the added] complexity of a salpingectomy may make this approach seem less appealing" [17]. A population-based study from Sweden reported that women who had undergone salpingectomy during hysterectomy for benign disease had a decrease in subsequent risk for ovarian cancer with a hazard ratio of 0.65 and that women undergoing bilateral salpingectomy had 50% lower risk than those undergoing unilateral salpingectomy [12]. Those authors concluded that removal of the fallopian tubes is an effective measure to reduce ovarian cancer risk in the general population.

While systematic reviews continue to report that the VH is preferable for hysterectomy in benign disease, the ideal route for women unsuitable for a vaginal approach remains to be determined [9]. Meta-analysis of published randomised controlled trials favours LH but with the trade-off of a longer operating time [20]. Despite evidence that VH is associated with the best outcome, the use of VH has fallen. The Cochrane review group concluded that VH should be performed where possible, but where VH is not considered possible, LH may have advantages over AH. However, the length of the surgery increases as the extent of the surgery performed laparoscopically increases.

The trend to an increasing prevalence of obesity in developed countries is likely to affect both the operating time and the rate of complications associated with LH. Women who are obese have an increased risk of developing gynaecological conditions such as endometrial hyperplasia and heavy menstrual bleeding, making them more likely to require hysterectomy [21]. Over the period of our study the proportion of women with a body mass index (BMI) of $30\,\mathrm{Kg/m^2}$ in Australia was estimated to have increased by more than 13%, up to a prevalence of 55.9% [22]. Women with a high body mass index (BMI) are likely to be overrepresented in the hysterectomy group, and their operations are likely to use more operative time. A high BMI increases the duration of abdominal hysterectomy [23], and even after adjustment for patient age, parity, history of open surgery, previous caesarean section, and menopausal status, a significantly longer operating time—as much as doubling—was noted in the case of obese patients [24]. Indeed, the operating time for LH increases almost linearly with increasing BMI [25].

There are two important limitations to this study. Firstly, it is not possible to determine background rates of preexisting hysterectomy, so the population incidence rates reported are for women irrespective of whether they have a uterus or not. The age-related likelihood that a woman has already undergone hysterectomy is obviously cumulative, so the incidence rates we have reported underestimate the true rate of hysterectomy in women eligible for the procedure, that is, women who still have a uterus. The second limitation is that coding in the national dataset reflects nonspecific data regarding whether "removal of adnexal structures" was undertaken, and we were not specifically able to determine whether either isolated salpingectomy or salpingo-oophorectomy was performed at the hysterectomy. However, it seems likely that this change in the younger age group reflects salpingectomy alone since Australian guidance is explicit in discouraging oophorectomy before women reach their 1960s [14].

5. Conclusion

This study has confirmed the findings of other international studies that hysterectomy is becoming less common [7, 8] and that both vaginal and abdominal hysterectomy are being replaced by laparoscopic hysterectomy. At the same time, removal of the adnexae at the time of hysterectomy is now becoming more common in younger women.

Acknowledgments

The authors wish to thank Dr. Steven Lyons for his careful review of the manuscript and very helpful advice.

References

[1] K. Spilsbury, J. B. Semmens, I. Hammond, and A. Bolck, "Persistent high rates of hysterectomy in Western Australia: a population-based study of 83 000 procedures over 23 years," *BJOG: An International Journal of Obstetrics & Gynaecology*, vol. 113, no. 7, pp. 804–809, 2006.

[2] R. M. Merrill, "Hysterectomy surveillance in the United States, 1997 through 2005," *Medical Science Monitor*, vol. 14, pp. CR24–CR31, 2008.

[3] C. Lundholm, C. Forsgren, A. L. V. Johansson, S. Cnattingius, and D. Altman, "Hysterectomy on benign indications in Sweden 1987-2003: a nationwide trend analysis," *Acta Obstetricia et Gynecologica Scandinavica*, vol. 88, no. 1, pp. 52–58, 2009.

[4] L. J. Middleton, R. Champaneria, J. P. Daniels et al., "Hysterectomy, endometrial destruction, and levonorgestrel releasing intrauterine system (Mirena) for heavy menstrual bleeding: Systematic review and meta-analysis of data from individual patients," *BMJ*, vol. 341, no. 7769, Article ID c3929, p. 379, 2010.

[5] E. Liang, B. Brown, R. Kirsop et al., "Efficacy of uterine artery embolization for treatment of symptomatic fibroids and adenomyosis - an interim report on an Australian experience," *Australian and New Zealand Journal of Obstetrics and Gynaecology*, vol. 52, pp. 106–112, 2012.

[6] G. A. Vilos, C. Allaire, P. Y. Laberge, N. Leyland et al., "The management of uterine leiomyomas," *Journal of Obstetrics and Gynaecology Canada*, vol. 37, pp. 157–181, 2015.

[7] R. Lykke, J. Blaakaer, B. Ottesen, and H. Gimbel, "Hysterectomy in Denmark 1977-2011: changes in rate, indications, and hospitalisation," *European Journal of Obstetrics and Gynecology and Reproductive*, vol. 171, pp. 333–338, 2013.

[8] J. M. Wu, M. E. Wechter, E. J. Geller, T. V. Nguyen, and A. G. Visco, "Hysterectomy rates in the United States, 2003," *Obstetrics & Gynecology*, vol. 110, no. 5, pp. 1091–1095, 2007.

[9] J. W. M. Aarts, T. E. Nieboer, N. Johnson et al., "Surgical approach to hysterectomy for benign gynaecological disease," *Cochrane Database of Systematic Reviews*, vol. 8, p. CD003677, 2015.

[10] N. Johnson, D. Barlow, A. Lethaby et al., "Methods of hysterectomy: systematic review and meta-analysis of randomised controlled trials," *BMJ*, vol. 330, pp. 1478–1485, 2005.

[11] E. M. Sandberg, A. R. H. Twijnstra, S. R. C. Driessen, and F. W. Jansen, "Total laparoscopic hysterectomy versus vaginal hysterectomy: a systematic review and meta-analysis," *Journal of Minimally Invasive Gynecology*, vol. 24, no. 2, pp. 206–217.e22, 2017.

[12] H. Falconer, L. Yin, H. Gronberg, and D. Altman, "Ovarian cancer risk after salpingectomy: a nationwide population-based study," *Journal of the National Cancer Institute*, p. 107, 2015.

[13] Committee on Gynecologic Practice, "Committee opinion no. 620: Salpingectomy for ovarian cancer prevention," *Obstetrics and Gynecology*, vol. 125, pp. 279–281, 2015.

[14] RANZCOG, "Managing the adnexae at the time of hysterectomy for benign gynaecological conditions," 2014, http://www.ranzcog.edu.au.

[15] R. M. Kho and M. E. Wechter, "Operative outcomes of opportunistic bilateral salpingectomy at the time of benign hysterectomy in low-risk premenopausal women: a systematic review," *Journal of Minimally Invasive Gynecology*, vol. 24, no. 2, pp. 218–229, 2017.

[16] M. Robert, D. Cenaiko, J. Sepandj, and S. Iwanicki, "Success and complications of salpingectomy at the time of vaginal hysterectomy," *Journal of Minimally Invasive Gynecology*, vol. 22, no. 5, pp. 864–869, 2015.

[17] C. L. Roberts, C. A. Cameron, J. C. Bell, C. S. Algert, and J. M. Morris, "Measuring maternal morbidity in routinely collected health data: development and validation of a maternal morbidity outcome indicator," *Medical Care*, vol. 46, no. 8, pp. 786–794, 2008.

[18] L. C. Turner, J. P. Shepherd, L. Wang, C. H. Bunker, and J. L. Lowder, "Hysterectomy surgery trends: a more accurate depiction of the last decade?" *American Journal of Obstetrics and Gynecology*, vol. 277, no. 2, pp. e1–e7, 2013.

[19] S. H. Yoon, S. N. Kim, S. H. Shim, S. B. Kang, and S. J. Lee, "Bilateral salpingectomy can reduce the risk of ovarian cancer in the general population: a meta-analysis," *European Journal of Cancer*, vol. 55, pp. 38–46, 2016.

[20] C. A. Walsh, S. R. Walsh, T. Y. Tang, and M. Slack, "Total abdominal hysterectomy versus total laparoscopic hysterectomy for benign disease: a meta-analysis," *European Journal of Obstetrics and Gynecology and Reproductive*, vol. 144, pp. 3–7, 2009.

[21] S. Pandey and S. Bhattacharya, "Impact of obesity on gynecology," *Women's Health*, vol. 6, pp. 107–177, 2010.

[22] Australian Bureau of Statistics, "4364.0.55.001 - National Health Survey: First Results, 2014-15. Overweight and obesity," http://www.abs.gov.au/ausstats/.

[23] O. Harmanli, V. Dandolu, J. Lidicker, R. Ayaz, U. R. Panganamamula, and E. F. Isik, "The effect of obesity on total abdominal hysterectomy," *Journal of Women's Health*, vol. 19, no. 10, pp. 1915–1918, 2010.

[24] N. Chopin, J. M. Malaret, M.-C. Lafay-Pillet, A. Fotso, H. Foulot, and C. Chapron, "Total laparoscopic hysterectomy for benign uterine pathologies: obesity does not increase the risk of complications," *Human Reproduction*, vol. 24, no. 12, pp. 3057–3062, 2009.

[25] D. Bardens, E. Sotomayer, S. Baum et al., "The impact of the body mass index (BMI) on laparoscopic hysterectomy for benign disease," *Archives of Gynecology and Obstetrics*, vol. 289, pp. 803–807, 2014.

The Role of the Single Incision Laparoscopic Approach in Liver and Pancreatic Resectional Surgery

Nikolaos A. Chatzizacharias,[1] Khaled Dajani,[1] Jun Kit Koong,[1,2] and Asif Jah[1]

[1]*Department of HPB and Transplant Surgery, Addenbrooke's Hospital, Cambridge University Hospitals NHS Foundation Trust, Cambridge, UK*
[2]*Department of Surgery, Faculty of Medicine, University of Malaya, Kuala Lumpur, Malaysia*

Correspondence should be addressed to Nikolaos A. Chatzizacharias; chatzizacharias@gmail.com

Academic Editor: Peng Hui Wang

Introduction. Single incision laparoscopic surgery (SILS) has gained increasing support over the last few years. The aim of this narrative review is to analyse the published evidence on the use and potential benefits of SILS in hepatic and pancreatic resectional surgery for benign and malignant pathology. *Methods.* Pubmed and Embase databases were searched using the search terms "single incision laparoscopic", "single port laparoscopic", "liver surgery", and "pancreas surgery". *Results.* Twenty relevant manuscripts for liver and 9 for pancreatic SILS resections were identified. With regard to liver surgery, despite the lack of comparative studies with other minimal invasive techniques, outcomes have been acceptable when certain limitations are taken into account. For pancreatic resections, when compared to the conventional laparoscopic approach, SILS produced comparable results with regard to intra- and postoperative parameters, including length of hospitalisation and complications. Similarly, the results were comparable to robotic pancreatectomies, with the exception of the longer operative time reported with the robotic approach. *Discussion.* Despite the limitations, the published evidence supports that SILS is safe and feasible for liver and pancreatic resections when performed by experienced teams in the tertiary setting. However, no substantial benefit has been identified yet, especially compared to other minimal invasive techniques.

1. Introduction

Single incision laparoscopic surgery (SILS), first described by Inoue et al. [1] more than two decades ago for an appendectomy procedure, has gained support for the benefit of improved cosmesis compared to the multiport laparoscopic approach, as well as the potential reduction in the risk of port-related complications, such as bleeding and visceral injury, less postoperative pain, shorter length of stay, and quicker return to work [2–6]. This innovative approach has been further applied to a broad range of operations, such as cholecystectomy, gastrectomy, colectomy, and splenectomy [7–11]. With regard to liver and pancreas surgery, data on the use of SILS are still limited to case reports and small series.

The purpose of this narrative review is to analyse the published evidence on the use and potential benefits of SILS in hepatic and pancreatic resectional surgery for benign and malignant pathology.

2. Methods

A literature search of the Pubmed and Embase databases was performed by two independent researchers (NAC and KD) using the search terms "single incision laparoscopic", "single port laparoscopic", "liver surgery", and "pancreas surgery". The search was confined to English manuscripts. As this is a narrative review, ethical approval was not required. Relevant references cited in the literature were reviewed and included where appropriate.

3. Results

Initial literature search identified 51 publications for liver and 21 for pancreatic surgery. Cases of liver cysts deroofing were excluded from the analysis. Due to the limited amount of data, case reports were included. After review of publications, 20 manuscripts for liver and 9 for pancreatic SILS resectional

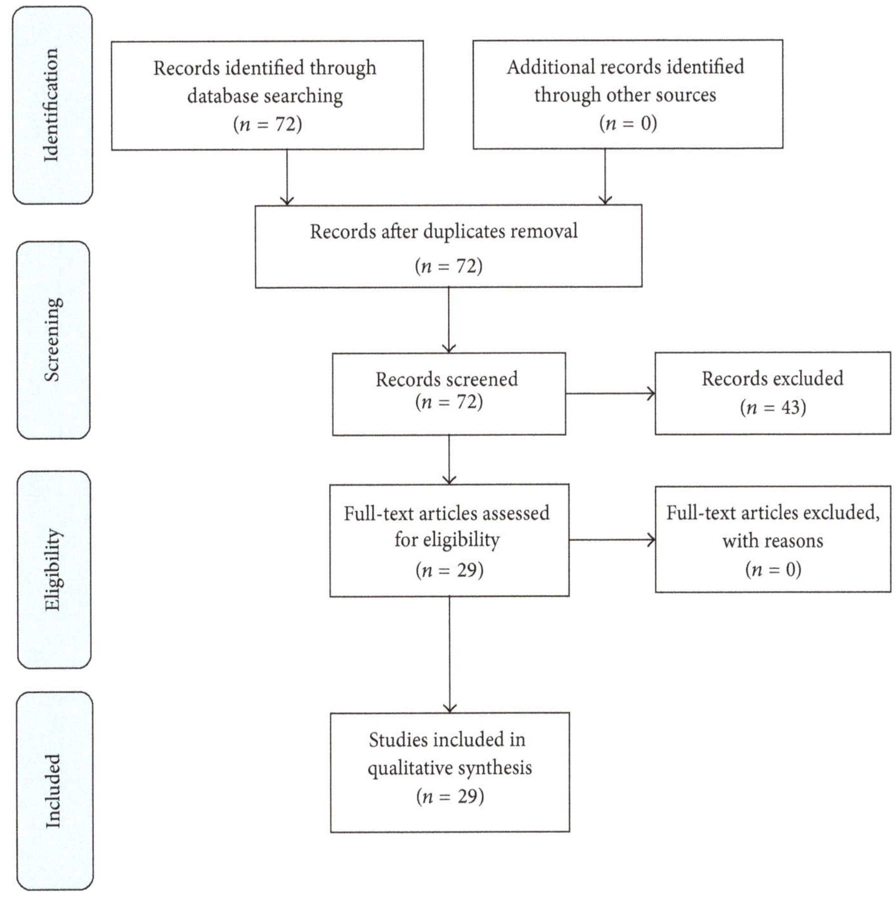

FIGURE 1

surgery were deemed relevant and included in the analysis (Figure 1).

3.1. Liver Resectional Surgery. Over the last couple of decades, significant progress has been made in the field of minimally invasive liver surgery. It is now well established that laparoscopic liver resections are feasible and safe and produce comparable oncological outcomes to open resections, while resulting in shorter hospital stay and blood loss [40–42]. SILS is the most recent development in the laparoscopic approaches to liver surgery with increasing amount of data presented in the literature. Nonetheless, no studies comparing SILS with open or conventional multiport laparoscopic or robotic liver resectional surgery are currently available in the literature.

Various limitations have been described with the SILS approach, mainly with regard to the size and location of the lesions and the body mass index (BMI) of the patient. Easily accessible, superficial lesions in segments II, III, IV, V, and VIII [20, 28] are preferable, even though bigger or more technically challenging resections for less favourably located tumours have been described with increased experience in the technique (Table 1). With regard to the size of the lesions, most groups adopted a cut-off of <2.5–5 cm in diameter for malignant and <10 cm for benign tumours [12, 14, 20–22, 27, 28, 31]. Resection of larger malignant lesions has also been described [15, 20, 22]; however the potential extension of the incision for extraction of large specimen defeats the purpose of SILS [27]. Other contraindications include vascular or extrahepatic involvement and morbid obesity [20, 27, 28]. Even though a history of upper abdominal surgery is a relative contraindication for some groups [28], SILS liver resections in patients with previous hepatectomies [22], as well as a synchronous liver and colonic resection [22], have been described.

A detailed description of the technique is beyond the remit of this review. Briefly, the patient is positioned supine in reverse Trendelenburg, with the legs apart to facilitate the position of the primary surgeon [15, 21, 22, 26–28]. Patient positioning in left lateral or semilateral positions has also been described [15]. Transumbilical incision with a 3-trocar technique has been used by most groups, while right upper quadrant incision has also been described [15, 24]. The latter may become useful in the setting of portal hypertension with umbilical varices or lesions in distant segments. Standard liver resection techniques were used with a combination of ultrasonic and other energy devices, clips, and staplers. Articulating instruments and scopes were also used in some cases.

Median operative time was between 70 and 227 minutes (Table 1). For larger resections (right or left hepatectomy) reported operative times varied between 110 and 545 minutes.

Table 1: Published evidence on the use of SILS in liver resectional surgery.

	Procedure (number)	Indication (number)	Location of lesion (number)	Size of lesion (mm) (median and range) or (mean ± SD)	Conversion rate (%)	Operative time (min) (median and range) or (mean ± SD)	Blood loss (mL) (median and range) or (mean ± SD)	LOS (days) (median and range) or (mean ± SD)	Complications (number)
Claude et al., 2014 [12]	NALR (7)	FNA (1) Adenoma (1) HCC (2) CRCLM (2) HM (1)	Segment III (2) Segment V (2) Segment VI (3)	20 (20–47)	0	110 (60–150)	50 (25–150)	5 (1–13)	0
Tzanis et al., 2014 [13]	LLR (1) NALR (2)	Adenoma (1) HCC (1) FNH (1)	Segment II/III (1) Segment VI (1) Segment VI/VII (1)	38 (12–90)	0	110 (100–120)	<50 (<50–150)	3 (1–3)	1 (allergic reaction)
Wu et al., 2014 [14]	Proximal left (1) LLR (8) NALR (9)	HM (8) FNH (1) CRCLM (2) HCC (2) Hepatolithiasis (2) Adenoma (2)	Segment II (3) Segment IV (1) Segment V/VI (3) Segment VIII (2)	49 (20–105)	0	117.9 (55–185)	256.5 (30–830)	7 (3–10)	Pleural effusion (2) Wound infection (1) Incisional hernia (1)
Shetty et al., 2012 [15]	NALR (6) SLR (11) LH (1) LLR (4) RH (1)	HCC (23)	Segment I/VI (2) Segment II (5) Segment II/III (1) Segment IV (2) Segment V (1) Segment VI (11) Segment VII (1) Segment VI/VII (1)	36 (10–90)	26	205 (95–545)	500 (100–2500)	8 (5–16)	Bile leak (1)
Røsok and Edwin, 2011 [16]	NALR(1)	CRCLM (1)	Segment V (1)	15	0	—	120	5	Pulmonary oedema (1)
Toyama et al., 2013 [17]	NALR (1)	HCC/CCA (1)	Segment VI (1)	30	0	180	Minimal	—	None
Kobayashi et al., 2010 [18]	NALR (1)	HCC (1)	Segment III (1)	20	0	70	Minimal	1	None
Belli et al., 2011 [19]	NALR (1)	HCC (1)	Segment III (1)	—	0	130	Minimal	2	None
Pan et al., 2012 [20]	LLR (3) NALR (5)	HCC (4) Multiple cysts (2) CRCLM (1) HM (1)	Segment II/III (4) Segment IV (2) Segment VI (2)	47 (35–110)	0	89 (67–123)	58 (50–100)	3 (2–6)	None

Table 1: Continued.

	Procedure (number)	Indication (number)	Location of lesion (number)	Size of lesion (mm) (median and range) or (mean ± SD)	Conversion rate (%)	Operative time (min) (median and range) or (mean ± SD)	Blood loss (mL) (median and range) or (mean ± SD)	LOS (days) (median and range) or (mean ± SD)	Complications (number)
Camps Lasa et al., 2014 [21]	LH (1) LLR (4)	CRCLM (4) Hydatid cyst (1)	Segment II (1) Segment III (2) Segment II/III (2)	24 (7–62)	0	135 (120–210)	—	3 (3-4)	None
Kim et al., 2014 [22]	LLR (1) NALR (2)	HCC (3)	Segment II (2) Segment III (1) Segment VI (1)	17 (10–36)	0	227 (142–228)	200 (200–250)	7 (3–8)	Pleural effusion (1)
Hu et al., 2011 [23]	LLR (1) NALR (1)	HM (2)	Segment II/III (1) Segment IV (1)	48 (15–80)	0	120	100	3	None
Gaujoux et al., 2011 [24]	LH (3) NALR (1)	HCC (1) Ovarian cancer metastasis (1) CRCLM (2)	Segment III (1) Segment IV (1) Segment III/IV (2)	14 (13–20)	0	115 (55–140)	38 (20–50)	2	None
Kim et al., 2013 [25]	LLR (1)	CRCLM (1)	Segments II/III (1)	80	0	315 (synchronous high anterior resection)	—	11	Atelectasis (1)
Machado et al., 2014 [26]	LLR (8)	Adenoma (6) FNH (1) CCA (1)	—	—	0	68 (45–100)	<100	1 (1-2)	None
Dapri et al., 2012 [27]	LLR (1) NALR (2)	Hydatid (2) CRCLM (1)	Segment II/III (1) Segment VII (1) Segment VIII (1)	—	0	158 (114–185)	350 (200–500)	5 (4-5)	None
Zhao et al., 2011 [28]	LLR (4) NALR (8)	HCC (2) Haemangioma (6) FNH (3) Adenoma (1)	Segment II/III (3) Segment III (5) Segment IV (1) Segment IV/V (1) Segment V (1) Segment V/VIII (1)	44 ± 26 (11–96)	17	80.4 ± 38.3 (35–160)	45 (20–800)	4 ± 1 (2–8)	Massive haemorrhage (1) Bile leak (1)
Cai et al., 2010 [29]	NALR (1)	HM (1)	Segment II/III (1)	38	0	75	80	2	None
Aldrighetti et al., 2011 [30]	LLR (1)	CRCLM (1)	Segment II/III (1)	35	0	145	50	4	None
Aikawa et al., 2012 [31]	NALR (8)	HCC (5) HM (1) Metastasis (1) NET (1)	Segment II (1) Segment III (2) Segment IV (2) Segment V (1) Segment VIII (2)	15 (9–30)	0	148 (141–235)	2 (0–10)	6 (3–11)	None

NALR: nonanatomical liver resection, LLR: left lateral resection, LH: left hepatectomy, RH: right hepatectomy, SLR: segmental liver resection, CRCLM: colorectal cancer liver metastasis, HCC: hepatocellular carcinoma, FNH: focal nodular hyperplasia, HM: haemangioma, CCA: cholangiocarcinoma.

A 0–26% conversion rate to multiport laparoscopic or open procedure and acceptable blood loss for liver resectional surgery were reported (Table 1). Median length of stay was reported between 1 and 11 days (between 2 and 10 days for large resections), with longer length of stay being attributed to postoperative complications.

3.2. Pancreatic Resectional Surgery. As with liver surgery, minimally invasive approaches have been gaining support in the field of pancreatic surgery. Published evidence suggest that laparoscopic pancreatic resections have comparable oncological outcomes to open surgery and additional benefits with regard to postoperative pain and morbidity [43–45]. The SILS approach is less well established, with only a few cases and small series reported in the literature. Indications for SILS pancreatic resections included a variety of pathologies, benign and malignant (Table 2). Due to the technical challenge, strict selection criteria are usually used. Smaller lesions (<3.5 cm) are preferable, even though resections of larger ones have been described. Ideally, patients should have a low BMI, no history of previous abdominal surgery, and strong preference for cosmesis [38]. All published cases have been performed for favourably located lesions in the body and/or tail of the pancreas and include distal pancreatectomies, with or without splenic preservation. Exceptions are two local excisions of lesions in infants, with one of them being a case of enucleation of pancreatoblastoma from the head of the pancreas [39].

As with every laparoscopic procedure, patient positioning is of high importance. Supine [2, 32, 34, 36, 38, 39], right lateral [35], and semilateral [33, 37] positions with [2, 32, 34, 38, 39] or without legs apart have been described, while reverse Trendelenburg after establishing the pneumoperitoneum was used by all groups. The surgical technique described is similar among the reports with minor modifications. Umbilical incision was used mainly, with one group describing left pararectal incision for very distal lesions [33]. Most commonly a 3-trocar technique [32, 34, 35, 37–39] was used, while the use of scope and instruments varied (angulating and straight both reported). Subsequent dissection followed the standard laparoscopic steps with the use of an energy device for the sealing of smaller vessels, while the main splenic vessels were secured generally with the use of staplers or clips. Staplers were used for the pancreatic parenchymal transection. Gastric traction sutures have been described by some groups to facilitate better exposure of the pancreas [2, 32, 34, 35, 37]. Median operative time has been reported between 145 and 330 minutes with a 0–19% conversion rate and acceptable levels of blood loss (Table 2). Median length of stay varied between 2 and 7 days, while the most commonly reported complication was postoperative pancreatic fistula formation.

Despite the small number of cases, two single centre retrospective studies compared the results of the SILS approach to those of conventional laparoscopic distal pancreatectomy [33, 38]. Both reported no significant difference in the patients' characteristics between the two groups. More specifically, there was no significant difference with regard to patients' age [33, 38], ASA class [33], gender [38], and weight and BMI [33, 38]. Similarly, there was no significant difference in the size [33, 38] or type [38] of the lesions. Intraoperative parameters, such as operative time [33, 38], blood loss [33, 38], and conversion rate to open procedure [38], were also comparable, as well as postoperative parameters, such as pain [38], length of stay [33, 38], and complications [33, 38].

A comparison between SILS and robotic distal pancreatectomy and splenectomy has also been reported, based also on a retrospective analysis of a single centre cohort, which included cases performed for malignant disease [36]. With the exception of the longer operative time reported with the robotic approach (297 versus 254 minutes, $p = 0.03$), no significant differences were identified with regard to patients' age, BMI, blood loss, conversion rate, and size of the tumours. Of note, the group acknowledged the preference towards the SILS approach in patients with normal or low BMI, as the operating space in these patients may not be sufficient for the effective use of the robotic arms. Postoperative complication rate was also comparable between the two groups; nonetheless a case of mortality was reported in the robotic group.

4. Discussion

SILS is one of the latest evolutions in minimal invasive surgery and has been increasingly utilised in abdominal surgery. The evidence on its use in liver and pancreatic resectional surgery is scarce and limited to published case reports and small case series.

The main advantage of SILS is cosmesis, with the benefits of minimal or no-scar access advocated by various groups [14, 15, 27, 30, 34]. It also carries a lower risk for port site related complications, such as visceral injury and bleeding, as well as potentially less postoperative pain, reduced length of stay, and quicker return to work [2–6]. In liver and pancreatic resectional surgery, the benefits of SILS are still unclear. Due to the lack of prospective and randomised comparative studies between SILS and other minimally invasive approaches, such as the conventional multiport or robotic techniques, the evidence is currently based on retrospective analyses of small case series [33, 36, 38]. However, as SILS is a relatively new approach and the international experience is still small, the potential benefits might be more obvious in the future.

SILS is considered less invasive than standard multiport laparoscopy but has significant technical difficulties and limitations. The main one arises from difficult instrumentation due to the lack of space and triangulation. Therefore, SILS is mainly limited to low BMI patients with no history of previous abdominal surgery. Articulated laparoscopic telescopes and instruments have also been utilised in order to overcome this problem, but with significant increase in the cost of the operation [34]. In the context of major resectional surgery, such as liver and pancreatic surgery, the lack of space and triangulation might compromise the dissection and potentially the resection margins, while important manoeuvres, such as access to the hilum, Pringle's, or other emergency haemostatic manoeuvres, become very difficult to apply [27]. The length of the instruments also poses a potential problem for liver resections and also for small distal pancreatic lesions. With SILS through an umbilical incision,

Table 2: Published evidence on the use of SILS in pancreatic resectional surgery.

	Procedure (number)	Indication (number)	Size of lesion (mm) (median and range) or (mean ± SD)	Conversion rate (%)	Operative time (min) (median and range) or (mean ± SD)	Blood loss (mL) (median and range) or (mean ± SD)	LOS (days) (median and range) or (mean ± SD)	Complications (number)
Barbaros et al., 2010 [2]	DP+S (1)	RCC metastases (2)	23 (15–30)	0	330	100	7	POPF grade A (1)
Chang et al., 2012 [32]	DP (1)	SCN (1)	35	0	233	<100	3	None
Haugvik et al., 2013 [33]	DP (5) DP+S (3)	5 NET (5) SCN (1) IPMN (1) Fibrosis (1)	21 (10–45)	0	145 (98–223)	225 (30–400)	6 (3–15)	Port site infection (1) Port site bleeding (1) POPF grade B (2)
Machado et al., 2015 [34]	DP (18) DP+S (2)	NET (11) IPMN (6) MCN (3)	31 (9–70)	0	176 (110–340)	<50 (<50–250)	2 (1–5)	POPF grade A (4)
Misawa et al., 2012 [35]	DP (1) DP+S (1)	Cystadenoma (1) MCN (1)	50 (35–65)	0 0	240 225	0 100	7 5	None None
Ryan et al., 2015 [36]	DP+S (16)	PDA (3) NET (2) IPMN (2) SCN (2) MCN (1) Splenunculi (1) Splenic HM (1)	38 ± 30 (8–117)	19	190 (197 ± 40.7)	150 (246 ± 263.9)	4 (6 ± 3.8)	AF (1) Pneumonia (1) Colonic abscess (1)
Srikanth et al., 2013 [37]	DP+S (1)	NET (1)	35	0	—	—	5	Collection (1)
Yao et al., 2014 [38]	DP+S (7) DP (7)	MCN (6) SCN (3) Pancreatic cysts (3) Splenic artery aneurysm (2)	43 ± 22 (12–110)	7	166 ± 55	157 ± 162	7 ± 1 (5–10)	POPF grade A/B (1)
Zhang et al., 2015 [39]	Local excision (2) DP (1)	Pancreatoblastoma (1) Nesidioblastosis (2)	—	0	153 (120–200)	Minimal	6-7	None

DP: distal pancreatectomy, DP+S: distal pancreatectomy and splenectomy, NET: neuroendocrine tumour, IPMN: intraductal papillary mucinous neoplasm, SCN: serous cystic neoplasm, MCN, mucinous cystic neoplasm, PDA: pancreatic ductal adenocarcinoma, HM: haemangioma, AF: atrial fibrillation, POPF: postoperative pancreatic fistula.

sometimes instruments are not long enough to reach the entire dissection surface. Some groups have described the use of right or left upper quadrant ports to overcome this problem [15, 24, 33] and even the design of customised longer instruments [15]. Furthermore, the small number of ports and space limit retraction capabilities. This is particularly important in the setting of pancreatic resectional surgery, where stomach traction sutures have been used by some groups [2, 32, 34, 35, 37].

Many surgeons prefer to leave an abdominal drain in the setting of liver and more commonly pancreatic resections. Some groups reported the use of the umbilical port as a drain exit site [2, 35], while the use of an additional 5 mm port that can subsequently be converted into the drain exit site has also been reported [34]. Although a potential disadvantage of SILS could be the increased risk for the development of incisional herniae due to the longer incision for the insertion of the SILS port system, this was not supported by the published evidence (Tables 1 and 2).

With regard to its main potential benefit, improved cosmesis, many reports suggest good to excellent results [13, 21, 26, 30, 34, 35, 38], with less scarring [38] and improved cosmesis [15, 28] for both liver [13, 15, 21, 26, 28, 30] and pancreatic resections [34, 35, 38]. Despite the fact that many series reported high levels of patient satisfaction [13, 14, 21, 28], only one study measured this during the first postoperative follow-up visit after SILS liver resection [21]. When asked to categorise their aesthetic satisfaction to poor, fair, good, or very good, the majority of patients ($n = 4$) were very satisfied, with one patient reporting good aesthetic result.

The vast majority of the experience with SILS in liver surgery refers to smaller resections (nonanatomical, left lateral sectionectomy and segmentectomies), with only 7 major hepatectomies reported in the literature (Table 1). The high level of technical difficulty limits, at least in the beginning of the learning curve, the use of the SILS approach to small, superficial, and easily accessible lesions. It is generally accepted that, ideally, patients should have a low BMI and no previous upper abdominal surgery, even though exceptions to these have also been reported [22]. Even though liver resections in cirrhotics may pose a greater challenge, SILS has also been described in this group of patients. Nonetheless, most cases were limited to early Child's A stage patients [12, 20, 28, 31], with only 3 cases reported in Child's B [12, 31] and 1 case in a Child's C patient [31]. The small number of reported SILS liver resections in the literature precludes direct comparison with laparoscopic surgery. Nonetheless, the median operative time of 70–227 minutes is not substantially different than the time (99–331 minutes) reported for laparoscopic hepatectomies [42]. Similarly, the estimated blood loss (<50–500 mL for SILS and 50–659 mLs for laparoscopic [42]) is also comparable. The wide range of the 0–26% conversion rate reflects the technical difficulties and long learning curve of the SILS approach. With increasing experience this is expected to approach the 4% conversion rate [42] of the laparoscopic approach. No mortality has been reported after SILS hepatectomy, while low complication rates and only 3 cases of liver specific complications were reported (Table 1). These results resemble the low mortality (0.3%) and morbidity (10.5%) rates after laparoscopic liver resections [42]. Keeping in mind the technical limitations of the SILS approach and despite the lack of randomised control trials and prospective comparative studies between SILS and multiport laparoscopic surgery, the published evidence generally supports the view that SILS is safe and feasible for liver resections when performed by experienced teams in the tertiary setting.

With regard to pancreatic surgery, only a limited number of reports is available with regard to SILS distal pancreatectomy with or without splenectomy, supporting its safety and feasibility in the appropriate setting. The vast majority of the cases were for benign disease with only 4 cases performed for malignant lesions (3 pancreatic ductal adenocarcinomas and 1 renal cancer metastasis to the pancreas) (Table 2). Any conclusions on the benefits of SILS for pancreatic resectional surgery should be made with caution, due to the lack of randomised trials and prospective studies. Based on two retrospective comparative case series, the results between SILS and the conventional multiport laparoscopic approach were comparable, without any substantial benefit in operative time, blood loss, postoperative pain, length of stay, and complication rate [33, 38]. This highlights the question of any real value of SILS in the context of pancreatic surgery. On the contrary, supporters of this approach would argue that its real benefits might become more obvious with increasing experience and evolving technology, an argument which was also valid in the early stages of development of laparoscopic surgery. Furthermore, this issue becomes more complicated after one retrospective case series reported comparable results between SILS and robotic surgery of the pancreas [36]. Once again, and in the absence of any strong evidence (prospective randomised trials), the value of SILS becomes questionable, especially as robotic pancreatic surgery has already gained wide acceptance in both benign and malignant resections. On the other hand, although no cost comparison has been published between the two techniques, the robotic approach is likely to have a higher capital cost.

In conclusion, published evidence has not shown any substantial benefit of SILS in the context of liver and pancreatic resectional surgery, especially compared to other minimal invasive techniques, such as multiport laparoscopic and robotic surgery. Further studies in the form of prospective and randomised controlled trials would be required to draw safe conclusions about the value of this innovative approach.

Abbreviations

SILS: Single incision laparoscopic surgery
BMI: Body mass index.

Competing Interests

All authors declare no conflict of interests.

Authors' Contributions

All authors contributed to the writing of the manuscript. Dr. Nikolaos A. Chatzizacharias and Dr. Khaled Dajani conducted the systematic review.

References

[1] H. Inoue, K. Takeshita, and M. Endo, "Single-port laparoscopy assisted appendectomy under local pneumoperitoneum condition," *Surgical Endoscopy*, vol. 8, no. 6, pp. 714–716, 1994.

[2] U. Barbaros, A. Sümer, T. Demirel et al., "Single incision laparoscopic pancreas resection for pancreatic metastasis of renal cell carcinoma," *Journal of the Society of Laparoendoscopic Surgeons*, vol. 14, no. 4, pp. 566–570, 2010.

[3] S. J. Binenbaum, J. A. Teixeira, G. J. Forrester et al., "Single-incision laparoscopic cholecystectomy using a flexible endoscope," *Archives of Surgery*, vol. 144, no. 8, pp. 734–738, 2009.

[4] S. E. Hodgett, J. M. Hernandez, C. A. Morton, S. B. Ross, M. Albrink, and A. S. Rosemurgy, "Laparoendoscopic single site (LESS) cholecystectomy," *Journal of Gastrointestinal Surgery*, vol. 13, no. 2, pp. 188–192, 2009.

[5] T. H. Hong, H. L. Kim, Y. S. Lee et al., "Transumbilical single-port laparoscopic appendectomy (TUSPLA): scarless intracorporeal appendectomy," *Journal of Laparoendoscopic & Advanced Surgical Techniques A*, vol. 19, no. 1, pp. 75–78, 2009.

[6] M. M. Desai, A. K. Berger, R. Brandina et al., "Laparoendoscopic single-site surgery: initial hundred patients," *Urology*, vol. 74, no. 4, pp. 805–812, 2009.

[7] S. A. Antoniou, O. O. Koch, G. A. Antoniou et al., "Meta-analysis of randomized trials on single-incision laparoscopic versus conventional laparoscopic appendectomy," *The American Journal of Surgery*, vol. 207, no. 4, pp. 613–622, 2014.

[8] S. A. Antoniou, R. Pointner, and F. A. Granderath, "Single-incision laparoscopic cholecystectomy: a systematic review," *Surgical Endoscopy*, vol. 25, no. 2, pp. 367–377, 2011.

[9] U. Barbaros and A. Dinccag, "Single incision laparoscopic splenectomy: the first two cases," *Journal of Gastrointestinal Surgery*, vol. 13, no. 8, pp. 1520–1523, 2009.

[10] T. Takahashi, H. Takeuchi, H. Kawakubo, Y. Saikawa, N. Wada, and Y. Kitagawa, "Single-incision laparoscopic surgery for partial gastrectomy in patients with a gastric submucosal tumor," *American Surgeon*, vol. 78, no. 4, pp. 447–450, 2012.

[11] K. Maeda, E. Noda, H. Nagahara et al., "A comparative study of single-incision versus conventional multiport laparoscopic ileocecal resection for Crohn's disease with strictures," *Asian Journal of Endoscopic Surgery*, vol. 5, no. 3, pp. 118–122, 2012.

[12] T. Claude, S. Daren, S. Chady, M. Alexandre, L. Alexis, and A. Daniel, "Single incision laparoscopic hepatectomy: advances in laparoscopic liver surgery," *Journal of Minimal Access Surgery*, vol. 10, no. 1, pp. 14–17, 2014.

[13] D. Tzanis, P. Lainas, H. Tranchart et al., "Atypical as well as anatomical liver resections are feasible by laparoendoscopic single-site surgery," *International Journal of Surgery Case Reports*, vol. 5, no. 9, pp. 580–583, 2014.

[14] S. Wu, X. P. Yu, Y. Tian et al., "Transumbilical single-incision laparoscopic resection of focal hepatic lesions," *Journal of the Society of Laparoendoscopic Surgeons*, vol. 18, no. 3, 2014.

[15] G. S. Shetty, Y. K. You, H. J. Choi, G. H. Na, T. H. Hong, and D. G. Kim, "Extending the limitations of liver surgery: outcomes of initial human experience in a high-volume center performing single-port laparoscopic liver resection for hepatocellular carcinoma," *Surgical Endoscopy*, vol. 26, no. 6, pp. 1602–1608, 2012.

[16] B. I. Røsok and B. Edwin, "Single-incision laparoscopic liver resection for colorectal metastasis through stoma site at time of reversal of diversion ileostomy: a case report," *Minimally Invasive Surgery*, vol. 2011, Article ID 502176, 3 pages, 2011.

[17] Y. Toyama, S. Yoshida, N. Okui, H. Kitamura, S. Yanagisawa, and K. Yanaga, "Transumbilical single-incision laparoscopic hepatectomy using precoagulation and clipless technique in apatient with combined hepatocellular-cholangiocarcinoma: a case report," *Surgical Laparoscopy, Endoscopy & Percutaneous Techniques*, vol. 23, no. 5, pp. e194–e199, 2013.

[18] S. Kobayashi, H. Nagano, S. Marubashi et al., "A single-incision laparoscopic hepatectomy for hepatocellular carcinoma: initial experience in a Japanese patient," *Minimally Invasive Therapy & Allied Technologies*, vol. 19, no. 6, pp. 367–371, 2010.

[19] G. Belli, C. Fantini, A. D'Agostino et al., "Laparoendoscopic single site liver resection for recurrent hepatocellular carcinoma in cirrhosis: first technical note," *Surgical Laparoscopy, Endoscopy & Percutaneous Techniques*, vol. 21, no. 4, pp. e166–e168, 2011.

[20] M. Pan, Z. Jiang, Y. Cheng et al., "Single-incision laparoscopic hepatectomy for benign and malignant hepatopathy: initial experience in 8 Chinese patients," *Surgical Innovation*, vol. 19, no. 4, pp. 446–451, 2012.

[21] J. Camps Lasa, E. Cugat Andorrà, E. Herrero Fonollosa et al., "Single-port laparoscopic approach of the left liver: initial experience," *Cirugía Española*, vol. 92, no. 9, pp. 589–594, 2014.

[22] G. Kim, A. C. Lau, and S. K. Chang, "Single-incision laparoscopic hepatic resection in patients with previous hepatic resections: a mini case series," *Asian Journal of Endoscopic Surgery*, vol. 7, no. 1, pp. 63–66, 2014.

[23] M.-G. Hu, G.-D. Zhao, D.-B. Xu, and R. Liu, "Transumbilical single-incision laparoscopic hepatectomy: an initial report," *Chinese Medical Journal*, vol. 124, no. 5, pp. 787–789, 2011.

[24] S. Gaujoux, T. P. Kingham, W. R. Jarnagin, M. I. D'Angelica, P. J. Allen, and Y. Fong, "Single-incision laparoscopic liver resection," *Surgical Endoscopy*, vol. 25, no. 5, pp. 1489–1494, 2011.

[25] G. Kim, D. Lomanto, M. M. Lawenko et al., "Single-port endo-laparoscopic surgery in combined abdominal procedures," *Asian Journal of Endoscopic Surgery*, vol. 6, no. 3, pp. 209–213, 2013.

[26] M. A. C. Machado, R. C. Surjan, and F. F. Makdissi, "Intrahepatic glissonian approach for single-port laparoscopic liver resection," *Journal of Laparoendoscopic & Advanced Surgical Techniques*, vol. 24, no. 8, pp. 534–537, 2014.

[27] G. Dapri, L. Dimarco, G.-B. Cadière, and V. Donckier, "Initial experience in single-incision transumbilical laparoscopic liver resection: indications, potential benefits, and limitations," *HPB Surgery*, vol. 2012, Article ID 921973, 9 pages, 2012.

[28] G. Zhao, M. Hu, R. Liu et al., "Laparoendoscopic single-site liver resection: a preliminary report of 12 cases," *Surgical Endoscopy*, vol. 25, no. 10, pp. 3286–3293, 2011.

[29] X.-J. Cai, Z.-Y. Zhu, X. Liang et al., "Single incision laparoscopic liver resection: a case report," *Chinese Medical Journal*, vol. 123, no. 18, pp. 2619–2620, 2010.

[30] L. Aldrighetti, E. Guzzetti, and G. Ferla, "Laparoscopic hepatic left lateral sectionectomy using the LaparoEndoscopic Single Site approach: evolution of minimally invasive liver surgery," *Journal of Hepato-Biliary-Pancreatic Sciences*, vol. 18, no. 1, pp. 103–105, 2011.

[31] M. Aikawa, M. Miyazawa, K. Okamoto et al., "Single-port laparoscopic hepatectomy: technique, safety, and feasibility in a clinical case series," *Surgical Endoscopy and Other Interventional Techniques*, vol. 26, no. 6, pp. 1696–1701, 2012.

[32] S. K. Y. Chang, D. Lomanto, and M. Mayasari, "Single-port laparoscopic spleen preserving distal pancreatectomy," *Minimally Invasive Surgery*, vol. 2012, Article ID 197429, 4 pages, 2012.

[33] S.-P. Haugvik, B. I. Røsok, A. Waage, Ø. Mathisen, and B. Edwin, "Single-incision versus conventional laparoscopic distal pancreatectomy: a single-institution case-control study," *Langenbeck's Archives of Surgery*, vol. 398, no. 8, pp. 1091–1096, 2013.

[34] M. A. C. Machado, R. C. Surjan, and F. F. Makdissi, "Laparoscopic distal pancreatectomy using single-port platform: technique, safety, and feasibility in a clinical case series," *Journal of Laparoendoscopic & Advanced Surgical Techniques A*, vol. 25, no. 7, pp. 581–585, 2015.

[35] T. Misawa, R. Ito, Y. Futagawa et al., "Single-incision laparoscopic distal pancreatectomy with or without splenic preservation: how we do it," *Asian Journal of Endoscopic Surgery*, vol. 5, no. 4, pp. 195–199, 2012.

[36] C. E. Ryan, S. B. Ross, P. B. Sukharamwala, B. D. Sadowitz, T. W. Wood, and A. S. Rosemurgy, "Distal pancreatectomy and splenectomy: a robotic or LESS approach," *Journal of the Society of Laparoendoscopic Surgeons*, vol. 19, no. 1, Article ID e2014.00246, 2015.

[37] G. Srikanth, N. Shetty, and D. Dubey, "Single incision laparoscopic distal pancreatectomy with splenectomy for neuroendocrine tumor of the tail of pancreas," *Journal of Minimal Access Surgery*, vol. 9, no. 3, pp. 132–135, 2013.

[38] D. Yao, S. Wu, Y. Li, Y. Chen, X. Yu, and J. Han, "Transumbilical single-incision laparoscopic distal pancreatectomy: preliminary experience and comparison to conventional multi-port laparoscopic surgery," *BMC Surgery*, vol. 14, article 105, 2014.

[39] J.-S. Zhang, L. Li, M. Diao et al., "Single-incision laparoscopic excision of pancreatic tumor in children," *Journal of Pediatric Surgery*, vol. 50, no. 5, pp. 882–885, 2015.

[40] D. Tzanis, N. Shivathirthan, A. Laurent et al., "European experience of laparoscopic major hepatectomy," *Journal of Hepato-Biliary-Pancreatic Sciences*, vol. 20, no. 2, pp. 120–124, 2013.

[41] N. W. Pearce, F. Di Fabio, M. J. Teng, S. Syed, J. N. Primrose, and M. Abu Hilal, "Laparoscopic right hepatectomy: a challenging, but feasible, safe and efficient procedure," *The American Journal of Surgery*, vol. 202, no. 5, pp. e52–e58, 2011.

[42] K. T. Nguyen, T. C. Gamblin, and D. A. Geller, "World review of laparoscopic liver resection—2,804 patients," *Annals of Surgery*, vol. 250, no. 5, pp. 831–841, 2009.

[43] L. Bencini, M. Annecchiarico, M. Farsi et al., "Minimally invasive surgical approach to pancreatic malignancies," *World Journal of Gastrointestinal Oncology*, vol. 7, no. 12, pp. 411–421, 2015.

[44] T. Jin, K. Altaf, J. J. Xiong et al., "A systematic review and meta-analysis of studies comparing laparoscopic and open distal pancreatectomy," *HPB*, vol. 14, no. 11, pp. 711–724, 2012.

[45] M. Nakamura and H. Nakashima, "Laparoscopic distal pancreatectomy and pancreatoduodenectomy: is it worthwhile? A meta-analysis of laparoscopic pancreatectomy," *Journal of Hepato-Biliary-Pancreatic Sciences*, vol. 20, no. 4, pp. 421–428, 2013.

Neuroendoscopic Resection of Intraventricular Tumors: A Systematic Outcomes Analysis

Sean M. Barber, Leonardo Rangel-Castilla, and David Baskin

Houston Methodist Neurological Institute, Department of Neurological Surgery, Suite 944, 6560 Fannin Street, Houston, TX 77030, USA

Correspondence should be addressed to Sean M. Barber; smbarber@tmhs.org

Academic Editor: Joachim Oertel

Introduction. Though traditional microsurgical techniques are the gold standard for intraventricular tumor resection, the morbidity and invasiveness of microsurgical approaches to the ventricular system have galvanized interest in neuroendoscopic resection. We present a systematic review of the literature to provide a better understanding of the virtues and limitations of endoscopic tumor resection. *Materials and Methods.* 40 articles describing 668 endoscopic tumor resections were selected from the Pubmed database and reviewed. *Results.* Complete or near-complete resection was achieved in 75.0% of the patients. 9.9% of resected tumors recurred during the follow-up period, and procedure-related complications occurred in 20.8% of the procedures. Tumor size ≤ 2cm ($P = 0.00146$), the presence of a cystic tumor component ($P < 0.0001$), and the use of navigation or stereotactic tools during the procedure ($P = 0.0003$) were each independently associated with a greater likelihood of complete or near-complete tumor resection. Additionally, the complication rate was significantly higher for noncystic masses than for cystic ones ($P < 0.0001$). *Discussion.* Neuroendoscopic outcomes for intraventricular tumor resection are significantly better when performed on small, cystic tumors and when neural navigation or stereotaxy is used. *Conclusion.* Neuroendoscopic resection appears to be a safe and reliable treatment option for patients with intraventricular tumors of a particular morphology.

1. Introduction

Intraventricular tumors present a unique challenge for the neurosurgeon. Their deep location and proximity to eloquent neurovascular anatomy complicate surgical approach and resection [1]. Microsurgery remains the gold standard for the treatment of intraventricular tumors [1–4], but microsurgical approaches are not without limitations [5–12]. The desire for a less invasive but equally effective surgical approach to intraventricular pathology has directed the attention of many in the neurosurgical community towards neuroendoscopy.

Neuroendoscopy was introduced in the early 1900s, adopted initially by Dandy [13] and others [14, 15] as a novel means of treating hydrocephalus [16], but the technique was overshadowed midcentury by the advent of the valved ventriculoperitoneal (VP) shunt [17, 18]. Years later, neuroendoscopy regained popularity due to improvements in optical technology and the introduction of the rigid and flexible neuroendoscopes [16, 19, 20]. Today, neuroendoscopic techniques have further evolved, and the spectrum of intracranial pathologies treatable by modern neuro-endoscopic means continues to expand.

Early reports have demonstrated endoscopic resection of intraventricular masses to be effective and safe [21, 22]. The large majority of data in the neurosurgical literature, however, originate from studies of endoscopic colloid cyst resection [11, 23, 24]. Data regarding endoscopic resection of other intraventricular tumors exist primarily in case reports and small series with insufficient sample size to draw meaningful conclusions.

The goal of this report is to review the relevant literature describing the endoscopic resection of intraventricular masses as a whole, both cystic and solid, to provide a better understanding of this technique's virtues and limitations.

2. Materials and Methods

Pubmed literature searches were performed using search terms "(endoscop*) AND ventric*", "(endoscop*) AND tumor", "((neuro-endoscop*) OR neuroendoscop*) AND tumor", and "(tumor) AND ventric*". Additional articles were located via cross-referencing of articles discovered initially through Pubmed searches. Articles included in the study were required to originate from peer-reviewed, English language journals describing the attempted resection (e.g., biopsies and cyst fenestrations without attempted resection were excluded) of an intraventricular tumor (e.g., suprasellar neoplasms without intraventricular extension were excluded) by purely endoscopic means (e.g., "endoscope-assisted" microsurgical resections were excluded) through a single endoscope ("dual-port" resections were excluded). Care was taken to exclude any redundant patient data from the analysis, and five articles required exclusion from the study due to an inability to definitively distinguish study patients in these five articles from patients in other study articles by the same author. In these five cases, the earlier of the two conflicting publications was omitted. Selected articles were also required to report on one or more of the following variables: (1) estimated completeness of resection achieved, (2) radiographic recurrence rates, and/or (3) complications related to the procedure. Cases involving the use of stereotactic radiosurgery, chemotherapy, or other nonsurgical treatment adjuncts were included. Two hundred and twenty articles were reviewed, and 40 were selected based on the above criteria.

Data collected from these 40 studies included tumor type, location within the ventricular system, tumor size, the presence of hydrocephalus preoperatively, operative technique, success of endoscopic resection, rates of intraoperative hemorrhage, and other procedure-related complications, rates of tumor recurrence, and length of clinical and/or radiographic follow-up.

Estimates regarding the completeness of endoscopic resection were obtained most commonly by surgeon or observer recollection and self-report, but were also obtained through assessments of postoperative imaging studies and chart review in some cases. Complete endoscopic resection was defined as gross total resection of all visible tumor as confirmed by visual intraoperative assessment or by the absence of any visible tumor residual on postoperative contrast magnetic resonance imaging (MRI). Near-complete resection was defined as resection of all but a very small amount of tumor adherent to nearby tissues. Partial resection was defined by a considerable tumor remnant as assessed either intraoperatively or on postoperative contrast MRI.

Statistical analysis was performed using the Student t-test and chi-square analysis using Microsoft Excel and GraphPad Instat 3 software. If the sample size was insufficient for chi-square testing ($n < 5$), the Fisher exact text was used. A P value of 0.05 was considered statistically significant.

3. Results

3.1. Patients and Tumor Types. The entire patient population consisted of 668 patients with intraventricular tumors who underwent attempted endoscopic resection. The publication dates of the 40 articles ranged from 1994 to 2012, and the number of patients (n) in each article ranged from 1 to 90 patients (mean, 16 patients). Hydrocephalus was seen preoperatively in 296 of 352 patients (84.1%) for whom relevant data was reported.

Colloid cysts were the most frequently encountered tumor by far ($n = 569$, 85.2% of study patients) followed by hypothalamic hamartomas ($n = 30$, 4.5% of study patients), craniopharyngiomas ($n = 8$, 1.2% of study patients), and ependymomas ($n = 7$, 1.0% of study patients). In 14 patients (2.1% of study patients) from 3 articles, the histological tumor type was either unknown or not reported. Tumor diameter ranged from 0.5 to 4.5 cm in 274 tumors from series where tumor size was reported (mean diameter, 1.5 cm). The most common tumor location was the third ventricle ($n = 572$, 85.2% of reported locations). Patient information and tumor types are summarized in Tables 1 and 2, respectively.

3.2. Operative Technique. Various techniques for neuroendoscopic resection of intraventricular tumors have been described in detail elsewhere [2, 12, 16, 20, 25–35]. Individual techniques differed throughout the included studies between surgeons as well as variances in tumor morphology and patient anatomy.

All procedures were performed with the patient under general anesthesia in a supine position. The patient's head was most commonly placed on a soft headrest, except where neuronavigation or stereotaxy was used, in which case the patient's head was placed in a 3-point pin fixation device. Preoperative antibiotics were always administered, but prophylactic antiepileptics frequently were not. The average operative time was 107.5 minutes and the average hospital stay was 4.8 ± 2.9 days.

Ventricular access was most commonly attained through a right-sided approach (unless asymmetric left-sided ventriculomegaly was present, in which case a left-sided approach was preferred). In all cases of hypothalamic hamartoma resection, ventricular access was performed contralateral to the greatest extent of tumor mass. Incision was made over the intended ventricular access site and a standard burr hole was created. The burr hole was most commonly placed at some variant of Kocher's point, although slightly more lateral (5–7 cm lateral to midline) on occasion. [3, 11, 36] Several authors make note of the importance of beveling the burr hole into a conical shape to allow for a greater degree of scope manipulation and visualization during the procedure [11, 37]. In some cases, the burr hole was placed more anteriorly (e.g., 5 cm anterior to the coronal suture, $n = 183$ [25, 26, 30, 31, 38, 39]; or 1.5–3 cm above the orbital rim in cases where a supraorbital trajectory was used, ($n = 8$ [27, 40])) to allow for better visualization of more posteriorly located tumors. In two cases, ventricular access was obtained via a transcallosal approach [12], and in the case of two pineal masses [41], a subtorcular approach was used.

The dura is incised in cruciate fashion and coagulated, followed by ventricular puncture and the introduction of an endoscope. Often a small-diameter peel-away introducer sheath containing a navigation probe and/or small-diameter rigid endoscope is used for initial ventricular puncture, although some authors preferred to perform initial ventricular puncture with a ventricular needle or catheter, followed by the introduction of an endoscope into the needle or catheter tract [31, 33].

3.3. Instruments. After entry into the ventricle, the tumor is inspected and its relationship to the surrounding anatomy is assessed. In some cases, visualization required the use of a 30° rigid endoscope or flexible neuroendoscope. A larger diameter rigid endoscope with multiple working channels is then introduced, through which tumor manipulation, coagulation, and resection take place. In the case of 59 colloid cysts and a single ependymoma, flexible neuroendoscopes were used for the majority of the procedure [2, 42, 43].

Cystic tumors were frequently penetrated and gently aspirated, after which the cyst wall was coagulated and resected piecemeal or *en bloc* with forceps, scissors, and other tools. In several cases, an adjunctive endoscopic aspiration tool (CUSA (Tyco Healthcare Radionics, Burlington, MA, USA) (n = 2) [41], NICO Myriad aspirator (NICO Corporation, Indianapolis, IN, USA) (n = 9) [41, 44, 45], Micro ENP Ultrasonic Hand Piece (Scoring GmbH, Medizintechnik, Germany) (n = 1) [42], or the Suros device (Suros Surgical Systems, Inc., Indianapolis, IN) (n = 2) [46]) assisted with tumor debulking and removal.

3.4. Navigation/Stereotaxy. Navigation and/or stereotactic localization tools were used in 266 procedures (45.1% of 581 procedures reporting such data) [12, 25–29, 31, 33–35, 38, 39, 42, 46–49]. In some cases, navigation and/or stereotactic tools were used only in those patients lacking ventriculomegaly on preoperative imaging, due to the enhanced difficulty associated with endoscopic visualization and maneuverability in the absence of hydrocephalus. A single author describes the intraventricular insufflation of saline in cases where small ventricles are encountered in attempts to improve operative success in this setting [28]. Data regarding the use of navigation or stereotactic tools is summarized in Table 1.

3.5. Completeness of Resection. Complete or near-complete tumor resection was achieved in 487 of 649 patients (75.0%) for whom completeness of endoscopic resection was reported. Complete resections were seen after initial resection attempts in 80.2% of colloid cysts, compared with 45.5% of other tumors (P < 0.0001). Complete or near-complete resection was more commonly attained amongst tumors with a substantial cystic component (79%) when compared with noncystic tumors (38.2%) (P < 0.0001). Complete or near-complete resection was also significantly more likely for tumors ≤2 cm in diameter when compared with larger tumors (P = 0.0146), and for tumors resected with the aid of navigation/stereotaxy (P = 0.0003) compared with those where these tools were not used. Resection outcomes are displayed in Figure 1 and Tables 1 and 2.

3.6. Adjunctive Procedures. Procedures in addition to the tumor resection were attempted during the same operative session in 70 patients (12.0% of patients for whom such data was reported). These adjunctive procedures included endoscopic third ventriculostomy (n = 27) [12, 16, 19, 29, 30, 42, 49, 50], septum pellucidostomy (n = 28) [12, 36, 49, 51], stent placement within the foramen of Monro and/or aqueduct of Sylvius (n = 2) [12, 19], placement of a VP-shunt [44] (n = 2), and postresection fluorescent ventriculography (n = 11) [34].

3.7. Procedure-Related Complications. Perioperative complications were seen in 123 out of 592 patients (20.8%) for whom data regarding complications was reported. These complications included hemorrhage (intraventricular, n = 41; intraparenchymal or along the introducer tract, n = 2; or epidural, n = 2), meningitis and/or ventriculitis (n = 15), "memory disturbance" (n = 14), CSF leak (n = 6), infarct (n = 5), cranial nerve deficit (n = 4), and hormonal disturbance (n = 2). The presence of a cystic component was associated with a significantly lower complication rate when compared to noncystic tumors (P < 0.0001). No significant relationship was observed between tumor size (P = 0.355) or the use of navigation/stereotaxy (P = 0.196) and complication rate. Data regarding procedure-related complications are shown in Figure 1 and Tables 1 and 2.

3.8. Clinical Outcomes. In the large majority of study patients, clinical morbidity was either unchanged or improved at most latent follow-up. There were no deaths reported to have occurred as a result of any of the 668 procedures. Postoperative morbidity increases were seen in 54 patients (9.5% of 569 patients for whom the relevant data was supplied) due to a variety of complications, including post-operative infarct, intraventricular hemorrhage, and meningitis or ventriculitis. Clinical outcomes are summarized in Table 1.

3.9. Tumor Recurrence. Tumor recurrence was seen in 53 of the 533 patients (9.9%) for whom data regarding recurrence was reported throughout an average of 31 months of follow-up. Recurrence was discovered, on average, 39 months after the initial resection in these 53 patients (range, 6–79 months). Tumor recurrence was seen in 9.8% of colloid cysts (49/498 patients reporting) compared with 11.1% of other tumors (4/36 patients reporting) (P = 0.805). Recurrence was seen most frequently with epidermoid cysts (n = 1, 100% recurrence), craniopharyngiomas (n = 5, 40% recurrence), and ependymomas (n = 1, 14.3% recurrence). No significant relationship was observed between tumor size (P = 0.546) or the presence of a cystic component (P = 0.325) and recurrence rates. Data regarding tumor recurrence are seen in Figure 1 and Tables 1 and 2.

4. Discussion

4.1. Virtues of Neuroendoscopic Tumor Resection. Neuroendoscopy offers solutions to some of the challenges faced with intraventricular tumor surgery. Endoscopic approaches to intraventricular pathology provide improved illumination

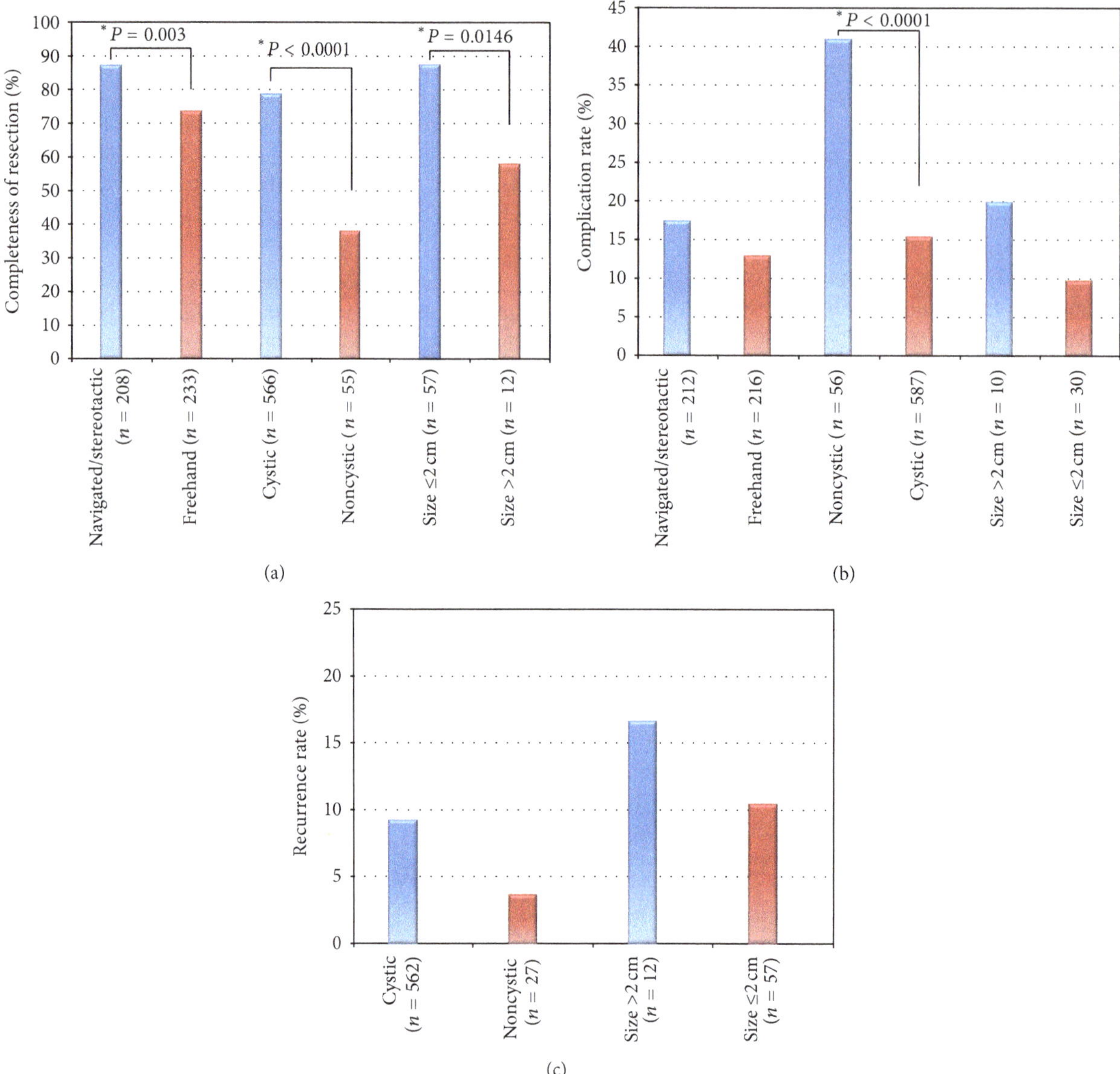

FIGURE 1: Column graphs displaying the variances in (a) resection success, (b) recurrence rate, and (c) complication rate seen with navigated endoscopic resection versus freehand, cystic tumors versus non-cystic, and large tumors (size > 2 cm) versus small (size ≤ 2 cm). * = statistically significant result.

and visualization of an anatomically remote and otherwise-difficult-to-reach location without the degree of tissue dissection and retraction often required with microsurgical techniques [24, 52]. Early results taken from colloid cyst resection demonstrate a reduction in complication rates, overall morbidity, operative time, and hospital stay [20–22, 25].

Neuroendoscopic approaches to intraventricular pathology also afford the surgeon an opportunity to treat associated hydrocephalus concomitantly, although tumor resection alone may be sufficient to restore cerebrospinal fluid (CSF) flow in some cases [12, 24, 53, 54]. In our study, hydrocephalus was seen on presentation in 84.1% of intraventricular tumors undergoing endoscopic resection, yet adjunctive cerebrospinal fluid (CSF) diversionary procedures were performed along with tumor resection in only 12.0%.

4.2. Ideal Candidates for a Neuroendoscopic Approach. Neuroendoscopic resection appears to be most safe and effective [2, 21, 25, 34] when applied in a particular patient population and morphology of tumor. It is often suggested that small tumors, for example, are ideal candidates for neuroendoscopic resection [12, 23, 24, 32, 52]. Soft and/or cystic tumors are also preferred, as they lend themselves to rapid debulking via aspiration and/or other endoscopic techniques [12, 32]. Rigid tumors, in contrast, must be dissected and removed piecemeal with the fairly rudimentary tools available for endoscopic use. This may be too time-consuming of an endeavor to warrant the use of endoscopy in such cases. These principles appear substantiated by our findings that complete or near-complete resection was significantly more common for tumors with a large cystic component and those ≤2 cm in diameter.

Table 1: demonstrating articles included in the study by publication year with corresponding data regarding tumor histology, number of patients (n), presence of preoperative hydrocephalus, use of navigation/stereotactic tools, adjunctive endoscopic procedures, time spent in the operating room (OR time), hospital stay, procedure-related complications, resection success, and recurrence rate for 668 intraventricular tumors in 40 studies that underwent attempted endoscopic resection.

Author	Year	n	Tumor histology (n)	Preoperative Hydro-cephalus (n)	Navigation/ stereotaxy (n)	Adjunctive procedures (n)	Mean OR time (min)	Mean hospital stay (days)	Complications (n)	Complete or near-complete resection (n) (%)	Recurrence (n)
Lewis et al. [11]	1994	7	Colloid cyst (7)	5	0	No	127	1.7	1	7 (100)	1
Abdullah and Caemaert [21]	1995	3	Craniopharyngioma (3)	ND	ND	ND	ND	ND	0	1 (33.4)	2
Abdou and Cohen [3]	1998	13	Colloid cyst (13)	13	0	No	ND	ND	0	10 (76.9)	0
Gaab and Schroeder [12]	1998	19	Colloid cyst (7), Subependymoma (3), low-grade astrocytoma (2), germinoma (1), pineal cyst (1), epidermoid cyst (1), hemangioma (1), cavernoma (1), CPP (1), ependymoma (1)	11	Navigation (4)	ETV (2), septostomy (1), stent (2)	85	ND	3	13 (68.4)	1
King et al. [51]	1999	13	Colloid cyst (13)	12	0	Septostomy (13)	94	2.3	2	10 (83.3)	0
Rodziewicz et al. [36]	2000	12	Colloid cyst (12)	6	0	Septostomy (12)	ND	ND	1	11 (91.7)	1
Decq et al. [55]	2000	22	Colloid cyst (22)	21	0	No	ND	ND	0	14 (63.6)	1
Kehler et al. [8]	2001	10	Colloid cyst (10)	ND	ND	ND	ND	ND	3	9 (90)	1
MacArthur et al. [56]	2002	7	Colloid cyst (3), low-grade astrocytoma (1), ependymoma (1), unknown (2)	ND	ND	ND	ND	ND	ND	4 (57.1)	0
Jho and Alfieri [57]	2002	2	Colloid cyst (2)	ND	0	No	ND	ND	0	2 (100)	0
Sgaramela et al. [58]	2003	1	Colloid cyst (1)	ND	ND	ND	ND	ND	0	1 (100)	0
Hellwig et al. [34]	2003	20	Colloid cyst (20)	19	Stereotaxy (9), Navigation (11)	Intraoperative ventriculogra-phy (11)	250 (stereotactic), 150 (navigated)	7	4	18 (90)	1
Husain et al. [20]	2003	25	Colloid cyst (11), ependymal cyst (2), choroid plexus cyst (2), septum Pellucidum cyst (2), arachnoid cyst (2), neurocysticercosis (2), craniopharyngioma (2), pineoblastoma (1), pineal Cyst (1)	ND	0	No	ND	3	2	20 (80)	ND

Table 1: Continued.

Author	Year	n	Tumor histology (n)	Preoperative Hydro-cephalus (n)	Navigation/ stereotaxy (n)	Adjunctive procedures (n)	Mean OR time (min)	Mean hospital stay (days)	Complications (n)	Complete or near-complete resection (n) (%)	Recurrence (n)
Souweidane [33, 37]	2005	2	Colloid cyst (1), glioneuronal tumor (1)	1	0	No	ND	ND	0	2 (100)	0
Jeon et al. [59]	2005	1	Choroid plexus cyst (1)	1	0	No	ND	37	1	1 (100)	ND
Longatti et al. [43]	2006	61	Colloid cysts (61)	53	0	No	87	6.7	4	38 (62.3)	7
Souweidane and Luther [32]	2006	7	Ependymoma (2), central neurocytoma (2), low-grade glioneuronal tumor (2), subependymoma (1)	7	0	No	117	2.6	2	5 (71.4)	0
Harter et al. [60]	2006	1	Dysembryoplastic neuroepithelial tumor (1)	1	ND	ND	ND	ND	ND	1 (100)	ND
Lekovic et al. [46]	2006	2	Hypothalamic hamartomas (2)	ND	Navigation (2)	No	ND	ND	0	1 (50)	ND
Grondin et al. [2]	2007	25	Colloid cysts (25)	22	0	No	104	3.8	3	24 (96)	1
Horn et al. [48]	2007	28	Colloid cysts (28)	17	Navigation (28)	No	174	5.4	3	10 (52.6), ND × 9	0
Levine et al. [61]	2007	35	Colloid cysts (35)	ND	ND	ND	ND	ND	7	32 (91.4)	7
Greenlee et al. [31]	2008	35	Colloid cysts (35)	ND	Frameless stereotaxy (35)	No	93	3	3	29 (82.8)	1
El-Ghandour [30]	2009	10	Colloid cysts (10)	10	0	ETV (2)	ND	ND	1	8 (80)	0
Stark et al. [38]	2009	1	Papillary ependymoma (1)	1	Navigation (1)	No	ND	ND	1	1 (100)	0
Romano et al. [50]	2009	1	Central neurocytoma (1)	1	0	ETV (1)	ND	ND	0	1 (100)	0
Oertel et al. [19]	2009	11	Unidentified (11)	ND	0	ETV (11)	71	ND	9	4 (36.3)	ND
Mishra et al. [39]	2010	59	Colloid cyst (59)	59	Navigation (59)	No	ND	ND	19	53 (89.8)	0
Najjar et al. [49]	2010	7	Colloid cyst (3), craniopharyngioma (1), low-grade astrocytoma (1), pineal cyst (1), unknown (1)	6	Navigation (2)	ETV (1), Septostomy (2)	ND	ND	0	4 (57.1)	1
Boogaarts et al. [29]	2011	90	Colloid cyst (90)	ND	Stereotaxy (18)	ETV (7)	79	ND	32	46 (57.5), ND × 10	24

Table 1: Continued.

Author	Year	n	Tumor histology (n)	Preoperative Hydro-cephalus (n)	Navigation/stereotaxy (n)	Adjunctive procedures (n)	Mean OR time (min)	Mean hospital stay (days)	Complications (n)	Complete or near-complete resection (n) (%)	Recurrence (n)
Ahmad and Sandberg [16]	2010	1	CPP (1)	1	0	ETV (1)	ND	ND	0	1 (100)	0
Naftel et al. [28]	2011	4	Colloid cyst (2), hypothalamic hamartoma (2)	1	Navigation (2)	No	ND	ND	0	3 (75)	ND
Dlouhy et al. [45]	2011	4	Colloid cyst (3), pineoblastoma (1)	ND	ND	ND	ND	ND	ND	4 (100)	ND
Delitala et al. [27]	2011	7	Colloid cyst (7)	4	Navigation (4)	No	ND	ND	0	6 (85.7)	0
Sood et al. [41]	2011	2	Pineal cyst (1), Pineoblastoma (1)	2	0	No	ND	ND	ND	2 (100)	ND
Wilson et al. [26]	2012	22	Colloid cyst (22)	19	Navigation (19)	No	180	ND	0	21 (95.4)	0
Margetis and Souweidane [25]	2012	67	Colloid cyst (67)	ND	Navigation (67)	No	ND	ND	4	66 (98.5)	3
Mohanty et al. [44]	2012	3	Craniopharyngioma (2), subependymoma (1)	2	0	VP-shunt placement (2)	ND	ND	2	2 (66.7)	0
Selvanathan et al. [42]	2013	1	Ependymoma (1)	1	Navigation	ETV	ND	ND	1	1 (100)	1
Drees et al. [62]	2012	26	Hypothalamic hamartoma (26)	ND	ND	ND	ND	ND	14	0 (0)	ND
Total: 40 studies	Total: 668 patients			Total: 296/352 patients (84.1%)	Total: 262/581 patients (45.1%)	Total: 70/581 patients (12.0%)	Mean: 107.5 minutes	Mean: 4.8 days	Total: 123/592 patients (20.8%)	Total: 487/649 patients (75.0%)	Total: 53/533 patients (9.9%)

CPP: choroid plexus papilloma, ND: no data, ETV: endoscopic third ventriculostomy, VP-shunt: ventriculoperitoneal shunt, and min: minutes.

TABLE 2: displaying the various tumor histologies included in the study with corresponding data regarding the number of studies included, the number of patients, resection success, complication rates, and recurrence rates for each tumor type.

Tumor histology	Studied included (n)	Patients (n)	Complete or near-complete resection (n) (%)	Complications (n)	Recurrence (n)
Colloid Cyst	21	569	441/550 patients (80.2%)	83/556 patients (14.9%)	49/498 patients (9.8%)
Hypothalamic hamartoma	3	30	2/30 patients (6.7%)	14/30 patients (46.7%)	ND
Unidentified	3	14	6/14 patients (42.8%)	9/12 patients (75%)	0/3 patients (0%)
Craniopharyngioma	4	8	4/8 patients (50%)	1/8 patients (12.5%)	2/5 patients (40%)
Ependymoma	5	7	7/7 patients (100%)	4/6 patients (66.6%)	1/7 patients (14.3%)
Subependymoma	3	5	2/5 patients (40%)	2/5 patients (40%)	0/3 patients (0%)
Low-grade astrocytoma	3	4	1/4 patients (25%)	0/3 patients (0%)	0/4 patients (0%)
Pineal cyst	4	4	3/4 patients (75%)	0/3 patients (0%)	0/2 patients (0%)
Pineoblastoma	3	3	3/3 patients (100%)	0/2 patients (0%)	ND
Central neurocytoma	2	3	2/3 patients (33.4%)	0/3 patients (0%)	0/3 patients (0%)
Choroid plexus cyst	2	3	3/3 patients (100%)	1/3 patients (33.4%)	ND
Choroid plexus papilloma	2	2	2/2 patients (100%)	0/2 patients (0%)	0/2 patients (0%)
Septum pellucidum cyst	1	2	2/2 patients (100%)	0/2 patients (0%)	ND
Ependymal cyst	1	2	2/2 patients (100%)	0/2 patients (0%)	ND
Arachnoid Cyst	1	2	0/2 patients (0%)	0/2 patients (0%)	ND
Neurocysticercosis	1	2	1/2 patients (50%)	1/2 patients (50%)	ND
Neuroepithelial tumor	2	2	2/2 patients (100%)	0/1 patient (0%)	0/1 patient (0%)
Glioneuronal tumor	2	2	2/2 patients (100%)	0/2 patients (0%)	0/2 patients (0%)
Cavernoma	1	1	1/1 patient (100%)	1/1 patient (100%)	0/1 patient (0%)
Hemangioma	1	1	1/1 patient (100%)	0/1 patient (0%)	0/1 patient (0%)
Epidermoid cyst	1	1	0/1 patient (0%)	1/1 patient (100%)	1/1 patient (100%)
Germinoma	1	1	1/1 patient (100%)	1/1 patient (100%)	0/1 patient (0%)

ND: no data.

Neuroendoscopic resection is also best suited for relatively avascular tumors [23, 24], as endoscopic methods of acquiring timely hemostasis are lacking, and endoscopic visualization is largely compromised in the setting of active, uncontrolled hemorrhage [12, 32]. In our study, there was insufficient documentation of tumor vascularity within the included studies to draw meaningful conclusions about any relationship between tumor vascularity and variables such as resection success or complication rate.

Ventriculomegaly is another factor which favors a neuroendoscopic approach. Small ventricles are thought to be unfavorable for neuroendoscopy because visibility and maneuverability in this setting are greatly reduced [12, 24, 63, 64], although several series provide evidence that endoscopic therapies are equally feasible in the absence of hydrocephalus [28, 65, 66].

4.3. Weaknesses of Neuroendoscopic Tumor Resection. Several of the limitations of neuroendoscopic tumor resection derive from a fundamental inadequacy of modern neuroendoscopic technology. As previously noted, solid masses greater than 2 cm in diameter, and those with considerable vascularity, are less amenable to neuroendoscopic resection due to the elementary nature of tools currently available for endoscopic dissection and hemostasis.

The large majority of cases included in this study used forceps, suction catheters, and bipolar cautery as the primary tools for dissection, resection, and hemostasis, respectively. Several series, however, report on the use of assistive devices (e.g., CUSA, NICO Myriad aspirator, Micro ENP Ultrasonic Hand Piece, and the Suros device) designed to allow for rapid tumor dissection and removal through an endoscopic approach. Although surgeons who use these devices frequently report their being helpful, objective data regarding their overall benefit is lacking [42, 44, 45]. No significant difference in success of resection, complication rate, or clinical outcome was seen in our study with the use of these assistive devices, although their use was likely too infrequent ($n = 8$) to draw conclusions.

Endoscopic tumor resections are also frequently said to result in inferior rates of gross total resection [25]. The resection rates demonstrated in our study (75.0%) and others (71–100%) [12, 32, 37, 65], however, appear comparable to those reported for microsurgical resection (80.4%–96%), particularly when endoscopic resection attempts are limited to tumors ≤2 cm in diameter (in which case resection rates in our analysis improve to 87.8%) [2, 67].

Some apprehension about the use of endoscopy for tumor resection arises from the perception that tumors resected endoscopically are more likely to recur [12, 21]. There is, in fact, some evidence that the risk of postoperative colloid cyst recurrence is higher with endoscopic resections compared with microsurgery [48]. Other series, however, have shown recurrence rates to be equivalent between the two [2]. The recurrence rate of 9.9% seen in our study is similar to rates reported for microsurgical resections (0.0%–33%) [32, 68–75], although reported recurrence rates vary widely and depend greatly on such variables as tumor type, completeness of initial resection, and the use of adjuvant therapies.

4.4. Stereotactic Tools and Neuronavigation. The use of stereotactic and/or neuronavigational guidance for endoscopic tumor resection is commonly reported in the neurosurgical literature, particularly in cases where ventriculomegaly is absent [12, 33, 65, 66, 76–78]. Some have adopted these adjunctive tools for assistance with burrhole placement, ventricular cannulation, and intraventricular navigation with the expectation that they will simplify the procedure and perhaps improve radiographic and clinical outcomes. Although incorporation of these tools into the procedure may prolong operative time and/or inflate surgical costs, several authors have declared their use to be of substantial benefit [12, 77–79]. Neuronavigation and/or stereotactic techniques were used in 44.1% of the cases in our study, and their use was associated with a significantly higher rate of complete or near-complete tumor resection.

4.5. Complications. The overall complication rate of 20.8% seen in this study is consistent with values reported elsewhere for endoscopic resection (0–25%) [12, 28, 32, 35, 48, 76] and comparable to rates reported for microsurgical interventions (4.3–29.3%) [72, 80–84], although some reports of complications following microsurgical resection approach 70% [5, 11]. The complications seen most commonly in our study were intraventricular hemorrhage (which was frequently minor) and memory disturbance (which was often transient). Many of the complications observed did not translate into increased clinical morbidity, and most of the complication-related clinical morbidity resolved to some degree with time.

4.6. Study Limitations. We present the largest analysis to date of outcomes for endoscopic resection of intraventricular tumors. Limitations of this study include the following: (1) all included publications are retrospective and therefore subject to errors of confounding and bias. A more accurate comparison between surgical and endoscopic resection requires a prospective, randomized trial. (2) Data in our study is collected over an extended period of time. Being that endoscopic techniques have progressed appreciably over the last 25 years, our results may not provide an accurate assessment of the results attainable with modern techniques. A minor percentage of the data included in the study draws from resections utilizing flexible endoscopes, for example. Although some authors are proficient with flexible neuroendoscopes and have reported good outcomes with their use, modern rigid endoscopes offer a vastly improved image quality and are preferred by many neurosurgeons. (3) Available data in the literature draws largely from series of endoscopic colloid cyst resection and thus, represent a slightly skewed picture of endoscopic tumor resection. More data are needed regarding endoscopic resection of other tumor histologies if we hope to gain a truly accurate and complete understanding of the advantages and disadvantages of this technique. (4) Finally, the large majority of cases of endoscopic resection of intraventricular tumors in the literature describe tumors in the region of the third ventricle. The majority of intraventricular tumors, however, are discovered in the body or frontal horn of the lateral ventricle, followed by the atrium, and finally, the foramen of Monro and third ventricle [80, 81, 85]. More data may be needed regarding endoscopic resection of tumors in these more common locations before comments regarding the safety, efficacy, and overall usefulness of endoscopy in the treatment of intraventricular masses can be made.

5. Conclusion

The goal of this study was to better characterize the advantages and disadvantages of the endoscopic approach to intraventricular tumors. Our results indicate that endoscopic tumor resection, when applied in the appropriate setting, is safe and effective.

Further improvements in the outcomes of neuroendoscopic tumor resection rely heavily on the development of endoscopic technology. Dissection tools allowing for the rapid and safe removal of large, solid tumors are lacking, as are effective means of acquiring prompt hemostasis through an endoscopic approach. More data is needed on the outcomes of endoscopic resection of tumors other than colloid cysts. Finally, randomized trials comparing surgical and endoscopic tumor resections would provide a better characterization of the virtues and limitations of each technique.

Microsurgical resection remains the gold standard of intraventricular tumor resection [1–4]. Endoscopic tools and techniques are improving, however, and the applications of endoscopy in the treatment of CNS pathology continue to expand. Though initial results appear promising, the potential of neuroendoscopy and its role in the management of intraventricular tumors are yet to be defined.

References

[1] M. Gazi Yaşargil and S. I. Abdulrauf, "Surgery of intraventricular tumors," *Neurosurgery*, vol. 62, no. 6, pp. SHC1029–SHC1040, 2008.

[2] R. T. Grondin, W. Hader, M. E. MacRae, and M. G. Hamilton, "Endoscopic versus microsurgical resection of third ventricle colloid cysts," *Canadian Journal of Neurological Sciences*, vol. 34, no. 2, pp. 197–207, 2007.

[3] M. S. Abdou and A. R. Cohen, "Endoscopic treatment of colloid cysts of the third ventricle," *Journal of Neurosurgery*, vol. 89, no. 6, pp. 1062–1068, 1998.

[4] A. Goel, "Can the hype of, "Endoscope" become a reality for colloid cyst surgery?" *World Neurosurg*, no. 12, 2012.

[5] B. D. Milligan and F. B. Meyer, "Morbidity of transcallosal and transcortical approaches to lesions in and around the lateral and third ventricles: a single-institution experience," *Neurosurgery*, vol. 67, no. 6, pp. 1483–1496, 2010.

[6] R. L. Jeffree and M. Besser, "Colloid cyst of the third ventricle: a clinical review of 39 cases," *Journal of Clinical Neuroscience*, vol. 8, no. 4, pp. 328–331, 2001.

[7] K. I. Desai, T. D. Nadkarni, D. P. Muzumdar, and A. H. Goel, "Surgical management of colloid cyst of the third ventricle—a study of 105 cases," *Surgical Neurology*, vol. 57, no. 5, pp. 295–302, 2002.

[8] U. Kehler, A. Brunori, J. Gliemroth et al., "Twenty colloid cysts—comparison of endoscopic and microsurgical management," *Minimally Invasive Neurosurgery*, vol. 44, no. 3, pp. 121–127, 2001.

[9] J.-P. Lejeune, D. Le Gars, and E. Haddad, "Tumors of the third ventricle: review of 262 cases," *Neurochirurgie*, vol. 46, no. 3, pp. 211–238, 2000.

[10] T. Mathiesen, P. Grane, L. Lindgren, and C. Lindquist, "Third ventricle colloid cysts: a consecutive 12-year series," *Journal of Neurosurgery*, vol. 86, no. 1, pp. 5–12, 1997.

[11] A. I. Lewis, K. R. Crone, J. Taha, H. R. Van Loveren, H.-S. Yeh, and J. M. Tew Jr., "Surgical resection of third ventricle colloid cysts. Preliminary results comparing transcallosal microsurgery with endoscopy," *Journal of Neurosurgery*, vol. 81, no. 2, pp. 174–178, 1994.

[12] M. R. Gaab and H. W. S. Schroeder, "Neuroendoscopic approach to intraventricular lesions," *Journal of Neurosurgery*, vol. 88, no. 3, pp. 496–505, 1998.

[13] W. Dandy, *Cerebral Ventriculoscopy*, vol. 33, Bull Johns Hopkins Hosp, 1922.

[14] L. Davis, *Neurological Surgery*, Lea & Febiger, Philadelphia, Pa, USA, 1936.

[15] Y. Enchev and S. Oi, "Historical trends of neuroendoscopic surgical techniques in the treatment of hydrocephalus," *Neurosurgical Review*, vol. 31, no. 3, pp. 249–261, 2008.

[16] F. Ahmad and D. I. Sandberg, "Endoscopic management of intraventricular brain tumors in pediatric patients: a review of indications, techniques, and outcomes," *Journal of Child Neurology*, vol. 25, no. 3, pp. 359–367, 2010.

[17] S. Kunwar, "Endoscopic adjuncts to intraventricular surgery," *Neurosurgery Clinics of North America*, vol. 14, no. 4, pp. 547–557, 2003.

[18] F. E. Nulsen and E. B. Spitz, "Treatment of hydrocephalus by direct shunt from ventricle to jugular vain," *Surgical forum*, pp. 399–403, 1951.

[19] J. M. K. Oertel, J. Baldauf, H. W. S. Schroeder, and M. R. Gaab, "Endoscopic options in children: experience with 134 procedures: clinical article," *Journal of Neurosurgery: Pediatrics*, vol. 3, no. 2, pp. 81–89, 2009.

[20] M. Husain, D. Jha, D. K. Vatsal et al., "Neuro-endoscopic surgery—experience and outcome analysis of 102 consecutive procedures in a busy neurosurgical centre of India," *Acta Neurochirurgica*, vol. 145, no. 5, pp. 369–376, 2003.

[21] J. Abdullah and J. Caemaert, "Endoscopic management of craniopharyngiomas: a review of 3 cases," *Minimally Invasive Neurosurgery*, vol. 38, no. 2, pp. 79–84, 1995.

[22] D. Hellwig and B. L. Bauer, "Minimally invasive neurosurgery by means of ultrathin endoscopes," *Acta Neurochirurgica*, vol. 54, pp. 63–68, 1992.

[23] P. Cappabianca, G. Cinalli, M. Gangemi et al., "Application of neuroendoscopy to intraventricular lesions," *Neurosurgery*, vol. 62, no. 2, pp. SHC575–SHC597, 2008.

[24] C. Teo and P. Nakaji, "Neuro-oncologic applications of endoscopy," *Neurosurgery Clinics of North America*, vol. 15, no. 1, pp. 89–103, 2004.

[25] K. Margetis and M. M. Souweidane, *Endoscopic Treatment of Intraventricular Cystic Tumors*, World Neurosurg, 2012.

[26] D. A. Wilson, D. J. Fusco, S. D. Wait, and P. Nakaji, *Endoscopic Resection of Colloid Cysts: Use of A Dual-Instrument Technique and an Anterolateral Approach*, World Neurosurg, 2012.

[27] A. Delitala, A. Brunori, and N. Russo, "Supraorbital endoscopic approach to colloid cysts," *Neurosurgery*, vol. 69, no. 2, pp. 176–182, 2011.

[28] R. P. Naftel, C. N. Shannon, G. T. Reed et al., "Small-ventricle neuroendoscopy for pediatric brain tumor management: clinical article," *Journal of Neurosurgery*, vol. 7, no. 1, pp. 104–110, 2011.

[29] H. D. Boogaarts, P. Decq, J. A. Grotenhuis et al., "Long-term results of the neuroendoscopic management of colloid cysts of the third ventricle: a series of 90 cases," *Neurosurgery*, vol. 68, no. 1, pp. 179–187, 2011.

[30] N. M. F. El-Ghandour, "Endoscopic treatment of third ventricular colloid cysts: a review including ten personal cases," *Neurosurgical Review*, vol. 32, no. 4, pp. 395–402, 2009.

[31] J. D. W. Greenlee, C. Teo, A. Ghahreman, and B. Kwok, "Purely endoscopic resection of colloid cysts," *Neurosurgery*, vol. 62, no. 3, pp. ONS51–ONS55, 2008.

[32] M. M. Souweidane and N. Luther, "Endoscopic resection of solid intraventricular brain tumors," *Journal of Neurosurgery*, vol. 105, no. 2, pp. 271–278, 2006.

[33] M. M. Souweidane, "Endoscopic surgery for intraventricular brain tumors in patients without hydrocephalus," *Neurosurgery*, vol. 57, no. 4, pp. S312–S317, 2005.

[34] D. Hellwig, B. L. Bauer, M. Schulte et al., "Neuroendoscopic treatment for colloid cysts of the third ventricle: the experience of a decade," *Neurosurgery*, vol. 52, no. 3, pp. 525–533, 2003.

[35] H. W. S. Schroeder, M. R. Gaab, and A. R. Cohen, "Endoscopic resection of colloid cysts," *Neurosurgery*, vol. 51, no. 6, pp. 1441–1445, 2002.

[36] G. S. Rodziewicz, M. V. Smith, and C. J. Hodge Jr., "Endoscopic colloid cyst surgery," *Neurosurgery*, vol. 46, no. 3, pp. 655–662, 2000.

[37] M. M. Souweidane, "Endoscopic management of pediatric brain tumors," *Neurosurgical Focus*, vol. 18, no. 6, p. E1, 2005.

[38] A. M. Stark, H. H. Hugo, A. Nabavi, and H. M. Mehdorn, "Papillary ependymoma WHO grade II of the aqueduct treated by endoscopic tumor resection," *Case Reports in Medicine*, vol. 2009, Article ID 434905, 5 pages, 2009.

[39] S. Mishra, S. P. S. Chandra, A. Suri, K. Rajender, B. S. Sharma, and A. K. Mahapatra, "Endoscopic management of third ventricular colloid cysts: eight years' institutional experience and description of a new technique," *Neurology India*, vol. 58, no. 3, pp. 412–417, 2010.

[40] Z. Horváth, F. Vetö, I. Balás, and T. Dóczi, "Complete removal of colloid cyst via CT-guided stereotactic biportal neuroendoscopy," *Acta Neurochirurgica*, vol. 142, no. 5, pp. 539–546, 2000.

[41] S. Sood, M. Hoeprich, and S. D. Ham, "Pure endoscopic removal of pineal region tumors," *Child's Nervous System*, vol. 27, no. 9, pp. 1489–1492, 2011.

[42] S. K. Selvanathan, R. Kumar, J. Goodden, A. Tyagi, and P. Chumas, "Evolving instrumentation for endoscopic tumour removal of CNS tumours," *Acta Neurochirurgica*, vol. 155, no. 1, pp. 135–138, 2013.

[43] P. Longatti, U. Godano, M. Gangemi et al., "Cooperative study by the Italian neuroendoscopy group on the treatment of 61 colloid cysts," *Child's Nervous System*, vol. 22, no. 10, pp. 1263–1267, 2006.

[44] A. Mohanty, B. J. Thompson, and J. Patterson, "Initial experience with endoscopic side cutting aspiration system in pure neuroendoscopic excision of large intraventricular tumors," *World Neurosurgery*, 2012.

[45] B. J. Dlouhy, N. S. Dahdaleh, and J. D. W. Greenlee, "Emerging technology in intracranial neuroendoscopy: application of the NICO Myriad Technical note," *Neurosurgical Focus*, vol. 30, no. 4, article E6, 2011.

[46] G. P. Lekovic, L. F. Gonzalez, I. Feiz-Erfan, and H. L. Rekate, "Endoscopic resection of hypothalamic hamartoma using a novel variable aspiration tissue resector," *Neurosurgery*, vol. 58, no. 1, pp. S166–S168, 2006.

[47] N. Luther and M. M. Souweidane, "Neuroendoscopic resection of posterior third ventricular ependymoma. Case report," *Neurosurgical Focus*, vol. 18, no. 6 A, p. E3, 2005.

[48] E. M. Horn, I. Feiz-Erfan, R. E. Bristol et al., "Treatment options for third ventricular colloid cysts: comparison of open microsurgical versus endoscopic resection," *Neurosurgery*, vol. 60, no. 4, pp. 613–618, 2007.

[49] M. W. Najjar, N. I. Azzam, T. S. Baghdadi, A. H. Turkmani, and G. Skaf, "Endoscopy in the management of intra-ventricular lesions: preliminary experience in the Middle East," *Clinical Neurology and Neurosurgery*, vol. 112, no. 1, pp. 17–22, 2010.

[50] A. Romano, S. Chibbaro, O. Makiese, M. Marsella, P. Mainini, and E. Benericetti, "Endoscopic removal of a central neurocytoma from the posterior third ventricle," *Journal of Clinical Neuroscience*, vol. 16, no. 2, pp. 312–316, 2009.

[51] W. A. King, J. S. Ullman, J. G. Frazee, K. D. Post, and M. Bergsneider, "Endoscopic resection of colloid cysts: surgical considerations using the rigid endoscope," *Neurosurgery*, vol. 44, no. 5, pp. 1103–1111, 1999.

[52] H. W. Schroeder, *Intraventricular Tumors*, World Neurosurg, 2013.

[53] K. Oka, M. Yamamoto, S. Nagasaka, and M. Tomonaga, "Endoneurosurgical treatment for hydrocephalus caused by intraventricular tumors," *Child's Nervous System*, vol. 10, no. 3, pp. 162–166, 1994.

[54] Y. Zhang, C. Wang, P. Liu, and X. Gao, "Clinical application of neuroendoscopic techniques," *Stereotactic and Functional Neurosurgery*, vol. 75, no. 2-3, pp. 133–141, 2000.

[55] P. Decq, C. Le Guerinel, L. Sakka et al., "Endoscopic surgery of third ventricle lesions," *Neurochirurgie*, vol. 46, no. 3, pp. 286–294, 2000.

[56] D. C. Macarthur, N. Buxton, J. Punt, M. Vloeberghs, and I. J. Robertson, "The role of neuroendoscopy in the management of brain tumours," *British Journal of Neurosurgery*, vol. 16, no. 5, pp. 465–470, 2002.

[57] H. D. Jho and A. Alfieri, "Endoscopic removal of third ventricular tumors: a technical note," *Minim Invasive Neurosurg*, vol. 45, no. 2, pp. 114–119, 2002.

[58] E. Sgaramella, S. Sotgiu, and F. M. Crotti, "Neuroendoscopy: one year of experience—personal results, observations and limits," *Minim Invasive Neurosurg*, vol. 46, no. 4, pp. 215–219, 2003.

[59] J. H. Jeon, S. W. Lee, J. K. Ko et al., "Neuroendoscopic removal of large choroid plexus cyst: a case report," *Journal of Korean Medical Science*, vol. 20, no. 2, pp. 335–339, 2005.

[60] D. H. Harter, I. Omeis, S. Forman, and A. Braun, "Endoscopic resection of an intraventricular dysembryoplastic neuroepithelial tumor of the septum pellucidum," *Pediatric Neurosurgery*, vol. 42, no. 2, pp. 105–107, 2006.

[61] N. B. Levine, M. N. Miller, and K. R. Crone, "Endoscopic resection of colloid cysts: indications, technique, and results during a 13-year period," *Minim Invasive Neurosurg*, vol. 50, no. 6, Article ID 993215, pp. 313–317, 2007.

[62] C. Drees, K. Chapman, E. Prenger et al., "Seizure outcome and complications following hypothalamic hamartoma treatment in adults: endoscopic, open, and Gamma Knife procedures," *Journal of Neurosurgery*, vol. 117, no. 2, Article ID 112256, pp. 255–261, 2012.

[63] P. Grunert, N. Hopf, and A. Perneczky, "Frame-based and frameless endoscopic procedures in the third ventricle," *Stereotactic and Functional Neurosurgery*, vol. 68, no. 1-4, pp. 80–89, 1997.

[64] M. J. Torrens, "Endoscopic neurosurgery," *Neurosurgery Quarterly*, vol. 5, no. 1, pp. 18–33, 1995.

[65] M. M. Souweidane, "Endoscopic surgery for intraventricular brain tumors in patients without hydrocephalus," *Neurosurgery*, vol. 62, no. 6, pp. SHC1042–SHC1047, 2008.

[66] M. Yamamoto, K. Oka, S. Takasugi, S. Hachisuka, E. Miyake, and M. Tomonaga, "Flexible neuroendoscopy for percutaneous treatment of intraventricular lesions in the absence of hydrocephalus," *Minimally Invasive Neurosurgery*, vol. 40, no. 4, pp. 139–143, 1997.

[67] T. Hori, T. Kawamata, K. Amano, Y. Aihara, M. Ono, and N. Miki, "Anterior interhemispheric approach for 100 tumors in and around the anterior third ventricle," *Neurosurgery*, vol. 66, no. 3, pp. 65–74, 2010.

[68] G. Kaur, A. J. Kane, M. E. Sughrue et al., "MIB-1 labeling index predicts recurrence in intraventricular central neurocytomas," *Journal of Clinical Neuroscience*, vol. 20, no. 1, pp. 89–93, 2013.

[69] V. V. Nayar, F. DeMonte, D. Yoshor, J. B. Blacklock, and R. Sawaya, "Surgical approaches to meningiomas of the lateral ventricles," *Clinical Neurology and Neurosurgery*, vol. 112, no. 5, pp. 400–405, 2010.

[70] A. Nowak and A. Marchel, "Surgical treatment of intraventricular ependymomas and subependymomas," *Neurologia I Neurochirurgia Polska*, vol. 46, no. 4, pp. 333–343, 2012.

[71] J. Pan, S. Qi, Y. Lu et al., "Intraventricular craniopharyngioma: morphological analysis and outcome evaluation of 17 cases," *Acta Neurochirurgica*, vol. 153, no. 4, pp. 773–784, 2011.

[72] H. Qian, S. Lin, M. Zhang, and Y. Cao, "Surgical management of intraventricular central neurocytoma: 92 cases," *Acta Neurochirurgica*, vol. 154, no. 11, pp. 1951–1960, 2012.

[73] H. I. Seçer, B. Düz, Y. Izci, Ö. Tehli, I. Solmaz, and E. Gönüls, "Tumors of the lateral ventricle: the factors that affected the preference of the surgical approach in 46 patiens," *Turkish Neurosurgery*, vol. 18, no. 4, pp. 345–355, 2008.

[74] K. Stachura, W. Libionka, M. Moskała, M. Krupa, and J. Polak, "Colloid cysts of the third ventricle. Endoscopic and open microsurgical management," *Neurologia I Neurochirurgia Polska*, vol. 43, no. 3, pp. 251–257, 2009.

[75] A. Vasiljevic, P. François, A. Loundou et al., "Prognostic factors in central neurocytomas: a multicenter study of 71 cases," *The American journal of surgical pathology*, vol. 36, no. 2, pp. 220–227, 2012.

[76] H. L. Rekate, I. Feiz-Erfan, Y.-T. Ng, L. F. Gonzalez, and J. F. Kerrigan, "Endoscopic surgery for hypothalamic hamartomas causing medically refractory gelastic epilepsy," *Child's Nervous System*, vol. 22, no. 8, pp. 874–880, 2006.

[77] P. Decq, "Endoscopy or microsurgery: is the never-ending debate concerning the choice of surgical strategy for colloid cysts of the third ventricle still a topical issue or has it been resolved?" *World Neurosurg*, 2012.

[78] H. W. S. Schroeder, W. Wagner, W. Tschiltschke, and M. R. Gaab, "Frameless neuronavigation in intracranial endoscopic neurosurgery," *Journal of Neurosurgery*, vol. 94, no. 1, pp. 72–79, 2001.

[79] V. Rohde, T. Behm, H. Ludwig, and D. Wachter, "The role of neuronavigation in intracranial endoscopic procedures," *Neurosurgical Review*, vol. 35, pp. 351–358, 2012.

[80] H. Z. Gökalp, N. Yüceer, E. Arasil et al., "Tumours of the lateral ventricle. A retrospective review of 112 cases operated upon 1970–1997," *Neurosurgical Review*, vol. 21, no. 2-3, pp. 126–137, 1998.

[81] G. Pendl, E. Ozturk, and K. Haselsberger, "Surgery of tumours of the lateral ventricle," *Acta Neurochirurgica*, vol. 116, no. 2–4, pp. 128–136, 1992.

[82] J. M. Pascual, F. González-Llanos, L. Barrios, and J. M. Roda, "Intraventricular craniopharyngiomas: topographical classification and surgical approach selection based on an extensive overview," *Acta Neurochirurgica*, vol. 146, no. 8, pp. 785–800, 2004.

[83] S. Shapiro, R. Rodgers, M. Shah, D. Fulkerson, and R. L. Campbell, "Interhemispheric transcallosal subchoroidal fornix-sparing craniotomy for total resection of colloid cysts of the third ventricle: clinical article," *Journal of Neurosurgery*, vol. 110, no. 1, pp. 112–115, 2009.

[84] R. Sampath, P. Vannemreddy, and A. Nanda, "Microsurgical excision of colloid cyst with favorable cognitive outcomes and short operative time and hospital stay: operative techniques and analyses of outcomes with review of previous studies," *Neurosurgery*, vol. 66, no. 2, pp. 368–374, 2010.

[85] J. Piepmeier, D. D. Spencer, K. J. Sass, and T. M. George, "Lateral ventricular masses," in *Brain Surgery: Complication Avoidance and Management*, M. Apuzzo, Ed., pp. 581–599, Churchhill Livingstone, New York, NY, USA, 1993.

31

Technical Details of Laparoscopic Sleeve Gastrectomy Leading to Lowered Leak Rate: Discussion of 1070 Consecutive Cases

David L. Warner and Kent C. Sasse

University of Nevada, Reno School of Medicine, 75 Pringle Way, Suite 804, Reno, NV 89502, USA

Correspondence should be addressed to David L. Warner; dwarner@medicine.nevada.edu

Academic Editor: Stephen Kavic

Introduction. Laparoscopic sleeve gastrectomy is a widely utilized and effective surgical procedure for dramatic weight loss in obese patients. Leak at the sleeve staple line is the most serious complication of this procedure, occurring in 1–3% of cases. Techniques to minimize the risk of sleeve gastrectomy leaks have been published although no universally agreed upon set of techniques exists. This report describes a single-surgeon experience with an approach to sleeve leak prevention resulting in a progressive decrease in leak rate over 5 years. *Methods.* 1070 consecutive sleeve gastrectomy cases between 2012 and 2016 were reviewed retrospectively. Patient characteristics, sleeve leaks, and percent body weight loss at 6 months were reported for each year. Conceptual and technical changes aimed towards leak reduction are presented. *Results.* With the implementation of the described techniques of the sleeve gastrectomy, the rate of sleeve leaks fell from 4% in 2012 to 0% in 2015 and 2016 without a significant change in weight loss, as depicted by 6-month change in body weight and percent excess BMI lost. *Conclusion.* In this single-surgeon experience, sleeve gastrectomy leak rate has fallen to 0% since the implementation of specific technical modifications in the procedure.

1. Introduction

Sleeve gastrectomy has become the most widely performed bariatric surgical procedure, with an estimated 75,000 cases performed in 2013 in the United States [1]. Gastric leak remains the most serious complication and occurs in 1 to 3% of all cases and as high as 7% in one case series [2–5]. Gastric staple line leak occurs most commonly at the proximal aspect of the staple line and tends to be subacute in nature [5–9]. Leak is associated with a high degree of morbidity for the patient and cost of care for institutions and payers. Reported techniques to minimize occurrence of leak include changes in calibration tube size, changes in staple cartridge, use of fibrin glues, oversewing of staple line, and use of staple line reinforcement materials [3, 4, 10–12].

2. Methods

All cases of sleeve gastrectomy performed by a single surgeon were reviewed over a 5-year time period, under an IRB-approved protocol. A comprehensive review of the literature of sleeve gastrectomy leak was undertaken. We report 1070 consecutive cases of laparoscopic sleeve gastrectomy and the rate of gastric staple line leak over the time from January 1, 2012, to the end of 2016. The last cases included in the analysis took place in December of 2016 and were monitored for evidence of leaks through March of 2017.

All patients were evaluated with nutritional and psychological evaluations and medical and specialist evaluations in accordance with the nationally accredited center's protocol. Each patient underwent evaluation with either upper GI series or esophagogastroduodenoscopy and responded to clinical questions regarding the presence or absence of GERD symptoms. 18% of patients were diagnosed with hiatal hernia preoperatively and repaired concomitantly with the sleeve, and an additional 9% were diagnosed intraoperatively and repaired. In all cases, the baseline sleeve procedure was performed with laparoscopic technique. After insertion of four trocars, a Nathanson liver retractor was placed to elevate the left lateral segment of the liver. A bougie calibration tube was placed along the lesser curvature, and the greater

Table 1: Sleeve gastrectomy patient characteristics from 2012 to 2016.

	2012	2013	2014	2015	2016
N	158	164	188	240	320
Female (%)	117 (74)	126 (77)	137 (73)	175 (75)	227 (71)
Male (%)	41 (26)	38 (23)	51 (27)	58 (25)	93 (29)
Mean age (years)	37.7	38.2	39.6	38.9	37.4
Mean weight (kg)	125	126	131	128	133
BMI (kg/m^2)	46	47	49	48	47
Revisional	4	4	5	0	0

Table 2: Leak incidence and weight loss results.

Year	Sleeve cases	Leaks	Percent leaks	Initial BMI (kg/m^2)	BMI at 6 mo. (kg/m^2)	Change in BMI (kg/m^2)	6 mo. Wt. loss change in percentage of body weight (% BW)	6 mo. percent excess BMI lost (% EBMIL)
2012	158	6	3.80%	46	36	10	22%	48%
2013	164	6	3.70%	47	36	11	23%	49%
2014	188	2	1.00%	49	36	13	26%	53%
2015	240	0	0%	48	37	11	24%	50%
2016	320	0	0%	47	—	—	—	—

curvature blood supply was divided with radiofrequency sealing, beginning 5 cm from the pylorus. Three Echelon green stapler cartridges were utilized in the antrum, using staple line reinforcement of bovine pericardium (Peristrips). The gastric body and fundus were stapled with varying Echelon stapler cartridges, which became consistent after 2014 with two gold cartridges in the mid body followed by two blue cartridges in the proximal fundus. The left crus was fully exposed. The most proximal stapler was angled 2-3 cm away from the esophagus. The hiatus was repaired with anterior cruroplasty without posterior dissection when a hiatal hernia less than 3 cm was present and with hiatal dissection and anterior and posterior cruroplasty when >3 cm. A methylene blue leak test was performed at the end of the procedure.

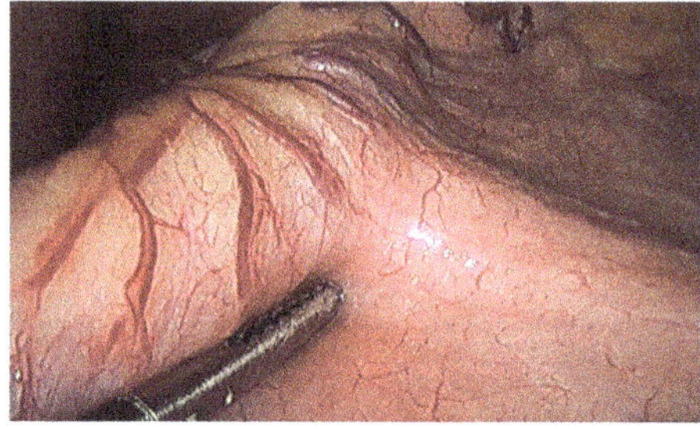

Figure 1: Stomach with 40-French sizing tube within the stomach, positioned along lesser curvature of stomach, in preparation for stapling.

3. Results

Patient characteristics are detailed in Table 1. Over the course of 5 years, 1070 laparoscopic sleeve gastrectomy cases were performed, and a total of 14 leaks occurred (1.3%). During the time studied, the leak rate fell from a rate of 3.8% in 2012, to 3.7% in 2013, to 1% in 2014, and to 0% thereafter (Table 2). All of the leaks (100%) occurred within 3 cm of the gastroesophageal junction, on the proximal sleeve staple line. All of the leaks resolved after treatment with endoscopic stenting, or a combination of endoscopic treatments and surgical reoperation. There was no mortality among any of the 1070 cases, including all of the cases of leak, but one patient did experience a prolonged ICU stay and reoperative surgery with prolonged recovery of approximately 26 weeks.

Weight loss results were compared for cases performed from 2012 to 2015, among the 84% of patients who had weight recorded at 6 months of followup after their sleeve procedure in 2012, 86% in 2013, 81% in 2014, and 88% in 2015. Weight loss results are reported as lost percentage of body weight (% BW) and percentage excess BMI lost (% EBMIL). Mean percent body weight loss at 6 months was 22%, 23%, 26%, and 24%, respectively, not significantly different from year to year ($p = .34$, ANOVA).

The identified technical elements during the change in leak rate from 3.8% to 0% were as follows:

(1) Use of the 40-French sizing calibration tube (Figure 1).

(2) Allowing generous volume around the sizing calibration tube at the curve of the incisura (Figure 2).

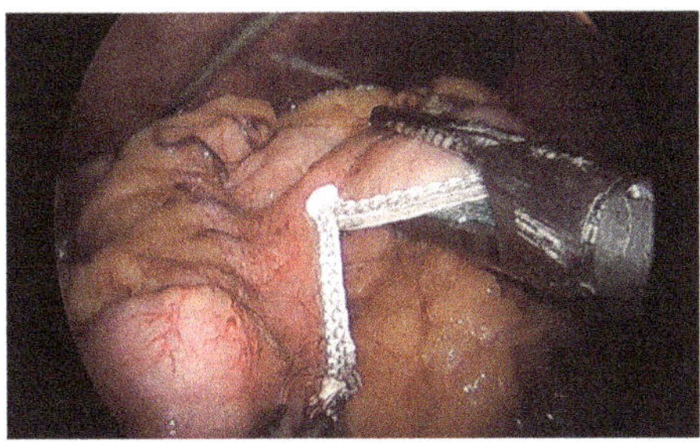

FIGURE 2: Maintaining a wide berth around bougie at incisura region.

(3) Avoidance of the disruption of cardiotuberosity branch arteries serving as the blood supply to the proximal stomach in the cardia region, especially posteriorly (Figure 3).

(4) Angling the linear stapler to the left and more than 15 mm away from the true gastroesophageal junction.

(5) Use of blue or 3.5 mm tissue stapler cartridges in the proximal stomach without staple line reinforcement (Figure 4).

(6) Application of fibrin glue sealant (Tisseel, Baxter Corp.) to the staple line.

(7) Hand-sewn, interrupted sutures to invert the staple line at the proximal 4 cm of the sleeve.

(8) Apposition of omentum to rest in proximity to the completed staple line (Figure 5).

(9) Suturing the omentum back to the mid and lower staple line to prevent a potentially obstructing "wind-sock" deformity.

(10) Avoidance of 1-stage revisional sleeves concomitant with band removal.

A timeline representing the occurrence of leaks and the implementation of the technical changes is displayed in Figure 6.

Each of the 13 revisional cases reported represents concomitant laparoscopic removal of a gastric band and conversion into a sleeve gastrectomy. One leak in each of the years 2013 and 2014 occurred in a revisional case, for a total leak risk of 2/13, or 15%, in revisional cases. The last leak occurred in March of 2014 in a revisional case, after which no further revisional band removals with sleeve were performed. Since March of 2014, over 650 consecutive laparoscopic sleeve procedures have been performed without a leak.

4. Discussion

Gastric leak following sleeve gastrectomy remains the most serious complication of sleeve gastrectomy. Leaks are most commonly subacute in nature and may present with an indolent course, weeks, or even months, after the procedure [5, 13]. Treatment includes establishing adequate drainage and utilizing endoscopic stents, endoluminal suturing, fibrin sealants, and surgical revision [14–21]. Numerous procedures may be required to resolve a sleeve leak, and morbidity and cost to the patient can be considerable.

The etiology of gastric sleeve leaks has been discussed and debated widely. In our center, all of the leaks from all sleeve cases in the past 8 years, whether performed at our center or outside centers and then transferred to our care, occurred in the proximal 4 cm or less of the sleeve. A high percentage of the published cases occur at this location [5–8]. Contributing factors include tissue ischemia, elevated intraluminal pressures, host impaired healing, and suboptimal closure techniques including poor stapler height choice, staple malformation, or hematoma formation. Blood supply has been long held as a key element in determining staple line and anastomotic integrity. The recent elegant cadaveric vascular anatomy study published by Perez demonstrates the fragility of the arterial blood supply to the proximal sleeve, the site of nearly all leaks. Specifically, the disruption of the posterior attachments of the proximal sleeve may be expected to disrupt cardiotuberosity branches of the left gastric artery [6]. It is evident from the anatomical study that the proximal sleeve is vulnerable to compromised blood supply stemming from the division of these small arterioles along the posterior wall of the proximal stomach. During surgery, it is often possible to see small vessels within the posterior attachments as the surgeon marches proximally along the sleeve (Figure 3). Preservation of those attachments and vessels may preserve important blood supply to the proximal sleeve and reduce the risks of leak.

Patient selection is often rightly cited as among the most important factors predictive of leaks and other complications. Tobacco use, steroid and medical immunosuppression, supermorbid obesity, NSAID use, diabetes, malnutrition, Crohn's disease, and revisional procedures have been associated with increased rates of gastric leak [21–23]. While we endeavor to modify risk factors which may be modified and screen out patients with prohibitive risks, we cannot as a practical matter turn away all patients with risk factors. Two of the 8 leak cases in the past 3 years involved a revisional procedure of removing a gastric band and converting into a sleeve. As a result of these cases, and others reported in the literature [22], we changed to a policy of staged conversions with a 6-month interval between band removal and sleeve gastrectomy and have experienced no leaks since.

Intraluminal pressure has been cited as a factor that may lead to increased leaks from the staple line, a logical contention and one that is supported by measurements of higher intraluminal gastric pressure within a sleeve than within a gastric pouch following roux-en-y gastric bypass [24, 25]. Gastric outlet obstruction and subsequent increased intraluminal pressure might be expected to promote staple line leak. Previously described stenosis, twist, or "wind-sock" deformity can each lead to gastric outlet obstruction, and each is prevented or minimized by the technique described [26]. Giving wide berth around the calibration tube or sizing bougie in the antrum and around the incisura minimizes narrowing, and suturing the omentum to the mid and distal staple line pexes the lower stomach to discourage twist or partially obstructing deformity.

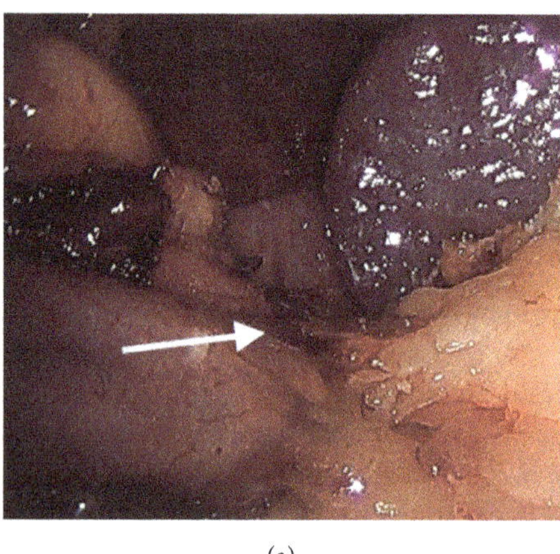
(a)

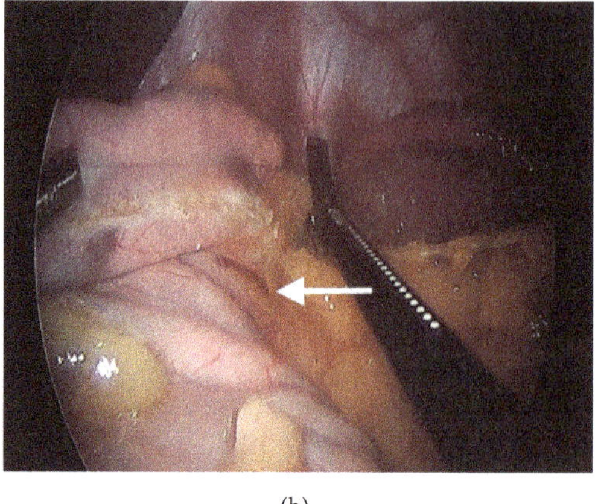
(b)

FIGURE 3: (a) Preserving the proximal posterior attachments and blood supply to the sleeve. (b) Preserving the proximal posterior attachments and blood supply to the sleeve.

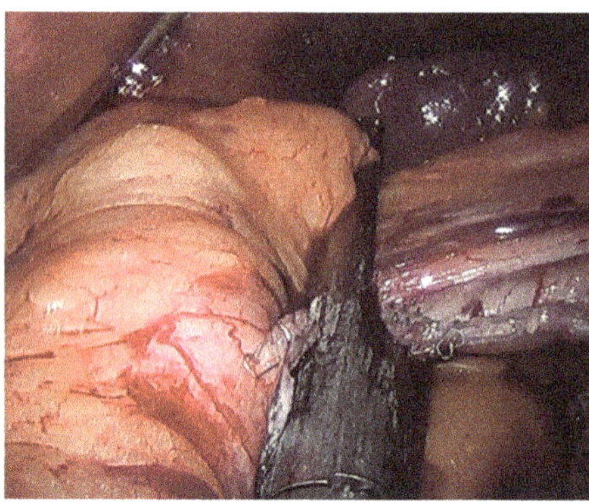

FIGURE 4: Final stapler loads using 3.5 mm staple height (Echelon Blue cartridge) without reinforcement material, angled to the left of the fat pad.

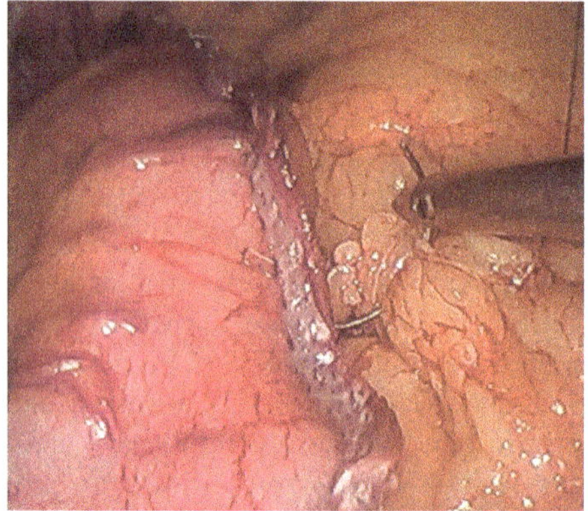

FIGURE 5: Suturing omentum back to sleeve staple line.

Staple height and use of staple line reinforcement material have been widely debated in relation to their association with leak rate. While initial burst pressure is reduced when staple line reinforcement is used [27–29], there is conflicting evidence that reinforcement material reduces leak rates from staple lines in the more delayed time frame most common for gastric sleeve leaks [12]. Greater consensus is present for the finding that staple line bleeding is lessened with staple line reinforcement material, a problem most often encountered in the lower stomach and antrum. What is clear is that the tissue thickness at the proximal stomach is considerably thinner than in the antrum. Prior to 2012, our cases were performed with thick tissue loads (Echelon 4.1 mm, Ethicon Corp.) with staple line reinforcement of the distal stomach using bovine pericardium (Peristrips). Staple height diameter of 3.5 mm for the proximal sleeve has been considered the most appropriate by the sleeve gastrectomy working group [5] and use of this thinner staple height (Echelon 3.5 mm, Ethicon Corp.) without staple line reinforcement at the proximal sleeve has been an element of the technique of 0% leaks.

Calibration tube size remains a debated topic among bariatric surgeons, with the consensus panel recommending a bougie size between 32 Fr and 40 Fr [5]. Some authors have reported greater weight loss success with smaller bougie size, and some authors have noted the association of increased complications of both leak and stenosis with smaller bougie size [3]. Because staple line leaks carry such a high cost in terms of morbidity and health care expense, we have taken the approach that preventing such leaks is of paramount importance. In 2013, the sleeve gastrectomy procedures were performed with 34 Fr bougies; in 2014 a mix of 34 Fr and 40 Fr bougie sizes was utilized, and in 2015 and 2016 all cases were performed with a 40 Fr bougie with 0 leaks.

Fibrin sealants have been promoted for their effectiveness at reducing bleeding from a variety of surgical tissues. Cottam et al. reported the successful use of Tisseel in achieving a 1.6% leak rate in a series of 126 high-BMI individuals undergoing sleeve gastrectomy [30]. There is likely little adverse effect from application of fibrin sealants, and indirect evidence from studies of hepatic and pancreatic tissues, that leaks could potentially be reduced by application of fibrin sealants (Tisseel, Baxter Corp.) [31, 32].

Omental apposition, or omentoplasty, to the staple line may be thought of as a technique which takes a page from

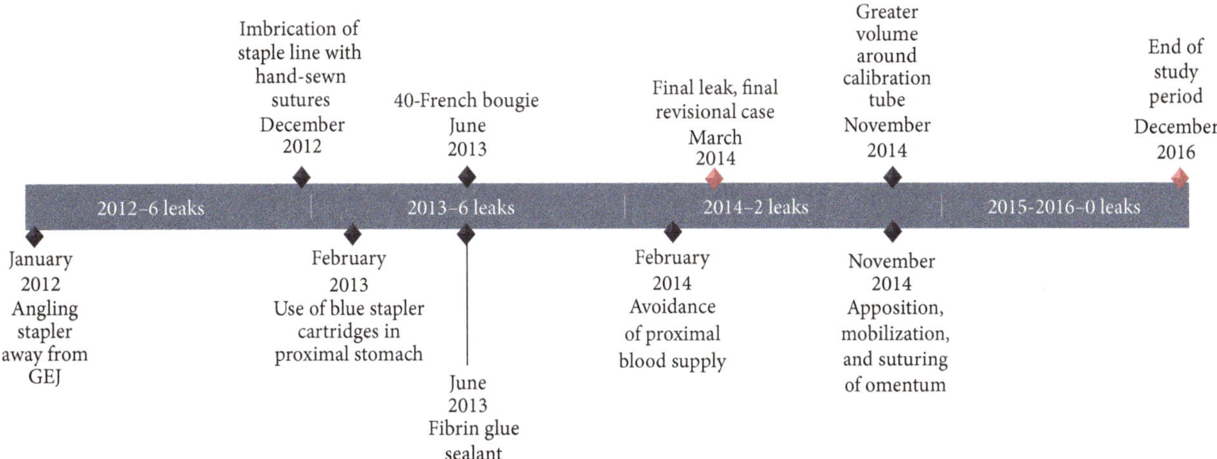

FIGURE 6: Timeline of technique implementation.

historical surgical repairs of perforations of the stomach using an omental patch, a widely successful technique [33]. In some cases, the attachments of the omentum to the spleen or to the abdominal sidewall prevent the omentum from freely migrating to the proximal staple line, and in such cases we believe it makes sense to free the omentum so that it may do so, while maintaining its blood supply.

The role of concomitant hiatal hernia repair, choice of repair technique, and whether or not to reinforce crural repair continue to be defined in the bariatric literature. Increased dissection at the hiatus and angle of His might theoretically exacerbate the already diminished perfusion of the proximal gastric fundus which has been observed among obese individuals [34]. In published studies, there has been no clear relationship between leak rate and performance of concomitant hiatal hernia repair [35, 36] and a recent prospective study in which 96 patients underwent complete GE junction mobilization, exposure, hiatoplasty, and concomitant sleeve resulted in 0 leaks [37]. In this series, repair of hiatal hernia did not appear to influence risk of leak. The optimal role of hiatal hernia repair in sleeve gastrectomy remains to be defined.

"Learning curve" may describe intangible improvements that come from experience and result in reduced complications over time. As has been done with other studies [38], this paper is an attempt to identify granular elements of "learning curve" that may have contributed to reduction in sleeve leaks over time.

Each element may be debated for its contribution to the reduced leak rate, and future studies will undoubtedly shed further light as to which of these elements is simply unnecessary to still achieve a 0% leak rate. It can be argued that, in this series, little undefined learning curve mystery played a role since the surgeon began performing sleeve gastrectomy in 2009 after having performed over 2000 laparoscopic roux-en-y gastric bypass cases. Little change has occurred with assistants and staff over the past 7 years. It remains to be seen if some of these technical elements—namely, the change to a 40 Fr bougie and the reduced tightness around the bougie in the distal stomach and incisura region—will result in compromised weight loss over a longer time period. If this proves to be the case, then we face a complex discussion over the trade-offs of reduced complications versus maximal weight loss results in sleeve gastrectomy. We consider it likely that innovative revisional and medically guided weight loss options including endoscopic revisions, dietary programs, and prescription medication therapy may mitigate differences in weight loss which could potentially occur over a longer time horizon as a result of the technical changes described herein to prevent leak.

Fear of complications remains the most widely cited objection to bariatric surgery referrals among referring doctors, and it remains the most widely cited objection to bariatric surgery among patients who most need it [39]. If we are to bring this life-saving intervention to more individuals, then we must relentlessly reduce complications, the most serious of which is leak in sleeve gastrectomy. The primary weakness of this paper is that these technical elements are offered in an observational manner and each is not rigorously compared in a randomized fashion. It is hoped that identifying these elements in such a granular fashion may help spur more detailed examinations of the optimal methods to reduce complications.

5. Conclusion

In this series over a 5-year period, a sequence of technical changes was made in an effort to prevent the most serious complication of sleeve gastrectomy, namely, staple line leak. Collectively, these technical elements have succeeded in reducing the leak rate from 3.8% in 2012 to 0% in 2015 and 2016 without a change in the 6-month weight loss results. More than 600 consecutive sleeve gastrectomy procedures have now been performed without a leak.

Conflicts of Interest

The authors declare that there are no conflicts of interest regarding the publication of this paper.

Authors' Contributions

Dr. Warner is responsible for data analysis and interpretation of the data for this manuscript. He contributed to drafts and critical revision of the manuscript and approved the final draft. Dr. Warner holds accountability for all aspects of the manuscript. Dr. Sasse is responsible for concept and design of this study, as well as data acquisition and analysis. He drafted and revised the manuscript and approved the final draft. Dr. Sasse holds accountability for all aspects of the manuscript.

References

[1] R. Schroeder, T. D. Harrison, and S. L. McGraw, "Treatment of adult obesity with bariatric surgery," *American Family Physician*, vol. 93, no. 1, pp. 31–37, 2016.

[2] M. Parikh, R. Issa, A. McCrillis, J. K. Saunders, A. Ude-Welcome, and M. Gagner, "Surgical strategies that may decrease leak after laparoscopic sleeve gastrectomy: a systematic review and meta-analysis of 9991 cases," *Annals of Surgery*, vol. 257, no. 2, pp. 231–237, 2013.

[3] R. J. Rosenthal, "International sleeve gastrectomy expert panel consensus statement: best practice guidelines based on experience of >12,000 cases," *Surgery for Obesity and Related Diseases*, vol. 8, no. 1, pp. 8–19, 2012.

[4] R. M. Juza, R. S. Haluck, E. M. Pauli, A. M. Rogers, E. J. Won, and J. R. Lynsue, "Gastric sleeve leak: a single institution's experience with early combined laparoendoscopic management," *Surgery for Obesity and Related Diseases*, vol. 11, no. 1, pp. 60–64, 2015.

[5] M. Gagner, M. Deitel, A. L. Erickson, and R. D. Crosby, "Survey on laparoscopic sleeve gastrectomy (LSG) at the fourth international consensus summit on sleeve gastrectomy," *Obesity Surgery*, vol. 23, no. 12, pp. 2013–2017, 2013.

[6] M. Perez, L. Brunaud, S. Kedaifa et al., "Does Anatomy Explain the Origin of a Leak after Sleeve Gastrectomy?" *Obesity Surgery*, vol. 24, no. 10, pp. 1717–1723, 2014.

[7] G. Donatelli, S. Ferretti, B. M. Vergeau et al., "Endoscopic internal drainage with enteral nutrition (EDEN) for treatment of leaks following sleeve gastrectomy," *Obesity Surgery*, vol. 24, no. 8, pp. 1400–1407, 2014.

[8] T. Oshiro, A. Saiki, J. Suzuki et al., "Percutaneous transesophageal gastro-tubing for management of gastric leakage after sleeve gastrectomy," *Obesity Surgery*, vol. 24, no. 9, pp. 1576–1580, 2014.

[9] A. Csendes, I. Braghetto, P. León, and A. M. Burgos, "Management of Leaks After Laparoscopic Sleeve Gastrectomy in Patients with Obesity," *Journal of Gastrointestinal Surgery*, vol. 14, no. 9, pp. 1343–1348, 2010.

[10] A. Abou Rached, M. Basile, and H. El Masri, "Gastric leaks post sleeve gastrectomy: Review of its prevention and management," *World Journal of Gastroenterology*, vol. 20, no. 38, pp. 13904–13910, 2014.

[11] S. Eubanks, C. A. Edwards, N. M. Fearing et al., "Use of endoscopic stents to treat anastomotic complications after bariatric surgery," *Journal of the American College of Surgeons*, vol. 206, no. 5, pp. 935–938, 2008.

[12] M. Gagner and J. N. Buchwald, "Comparison of laparoscopic sleeve gastrectomy leak rates in four staple-line reinforcement options: A systematic review," *Surgery for Obesity and Related Diseases*, vol. 10, no. 4, pp. 713–724, 2014.

[13] R. C. Moon, N. Shah, A. F. Teixeira, and M. A. Jawad, "Management of staple line leaks following sleeve gastrectomy," *Surgery for Obesity and Related Diseases*, vol. 11, no. 1, pp. 54–59, 2015.

[14] E. El Hassan, A. Mohamed, M. Ibrahim, M. Margarita, M. Al Hadad, and A. A. Nimeri, "Single-stage operative management of laparoscopic sleeve gastrectomy leaks without endoscopic stent placement," *Obesity Surgery*, vol. 23, no. 5, pp. 722–726, 2013.

[15] J. T. Tan, S. Kariyawasam, T. Wijeratne, and H. S. Chandraratna, "Diagnosis and management of gastric leaks after laparoscopic sleeve gastrectomy for morbid obesity," *Obesity Surgery*, vol. 20, no. 4, pp. 403–409, 2010.

[16] M. Corona, C. Zini, M. Allegritti et al., "Minimally invasive treatment of gastric leak after sleeve gastrectomy," *Radiologia Medica*, vol. 118, no. 6, pp. 962–970, 2013.

[17] M. Nedelcu, T. Manos, A. Cotirlet, P. Noel, and M. Gagner, "Outcome of Leaks After Sleeve Gastrectomy Based on a New Algorithm Adressing Leak Size and Gastric Stenosis," *Obesity Surgery*, vol. 25, no. 3, pp. 559–563, 2015.

[18] W. Alazmi, S. Al-Sabah, D. A. Ali, and S. Almazeedi, "Treating sleeve gastrectomy leak with endoscopic stenting: the kuwaiti experience and review of recent literature," *Surgical Endoscopy and Other Interventional Techniques*, vol. 28, no. 12, pp. 3425–3428, 2014.

[19] J. Himpens, G. Dapri, and G. B. Cadiére, *Treatments of Leaks After Sleeve Gastrectomy*, Bariatric Times, 2009.

[20] G. Casella, E. Soricelli, M. Rizzello et al., "Nonsurgical treatment of staple line leaks after laparoscopic sleeve gastrectomy," *Obesity Surgery*, vol. 19, no. 7, pp. 821–826, 2009.

[21] A. R. Aurora, L. Khaitan, and A. A. Saber, "Sleeve gastrectomy and the risk of leak: A systematic analysis of 4,888 patients," *Surgical Endoscopy and Other Interventional Techniques*, vol. 26, no. 6, pp. 1509–1515, 2012.

[22] J. Gagnière, K. Slim, M.-V. Launay-Savary, O. Raspado, R. Flamein, and J. Chipponi, "Previous gastric banding increases morbidity and gastric leaks after laparoscopic sleeve gastrectomy for obesity.," *Journal of visceral surgery*, vol. 148, no. 3, pp. e205–209, 2011.

[23] P. F. Lalor, O. N. Tucker, S. Szomstein, and R. J. Rosenthal, "Complications after laparoscopic sleeve gastrectomy," *Surgery for Obesity and Related Diseases*, vol. 4, no. 1, pp. 33–38, 2008.

[24] R. T. Yehoshua, L. A. Eidelman, M. Stein et al., "Laparoscopic sleeve gastrectomy-volume and pressure assessment," *Obesity Surgery*, vol. 18, no. 9, pp. 1083–1088, 2008.

[25] P. Björklund, H. Lönroth, and L. Fändriks, "Manometry of the upper gut following roux-en-y gastric bypass indicates that the gastric pouch and roux limb act as a common cavity," *Obesity Surgery*, vol. 25, no. 10, pp. 1833–1841, 2015.

[26] E. Brauner, A. Mahajna, and A. Assalia, "Intestinal malrotation presenting as midgut volvulus after massive weight loss following laparoscopic sleeve gastrectomy: Case report and review of the literature," *Surgery for Obesity and Related Diseases*, vol. 8, no. 4, pp. e52–e55, 2012.

[27] W. Arnold and S. A. Shikora, "A comparison of burst pressure between buttressed versus non-buttressed staple-lines in an animal Model," *Obesity Surgery*, vol. 15, no. 2, pp. 164–171, 2005.

[28] D. M. Downey, J. G. Harre, and J. P. Dolan, "Increased burst pressure in gastrointestinal staple-lines using reinforcement with a bioprosthetic material," *Obesity Surgery*, vol. 15, no. 10, pp. 1379–1383, 2005.

[29] K. C. Sasse, D. Warner, S. M. Ward, W. Mandeville, and R. Evans, "Intestinal staple line reinforcement using matristem," *Surgical Science*, vol. 6, no. 1, pp. 65–70, 2015.

[30] D. Cottam, F. G. Qureshi, S. G. Mattar et al., "Laparoscopic sleeve gastrectomy as an initial weight-loss procedure for high-risk patients with morbid obesity," *Surgical Endoscopy and Other Interventional Techniques*, vol. 20, no. 6, pp. 859–863, 2006.

[31] J. A. Sapala, M. H. Wood, and M. P. Schuhknecht, "Anastomotic leak prophylaxis using a vapor-heated fibrin sealant: report on 738 gastric bypass patients," *Obesity Surgery*, vol. 14, no. 1, pp. 35–42, 2004.

[32] K. A. Vakalopoulos, F. Daams, Z. Wu et al., "Tissue adhesives in gastrointestinal anastomosis: a systematic review," *Journal of Surgical Research*, vol. 180, no. 2, pp. 290–300, 2013.

[33] M. Matsuda, M. Nishiyama, T. Hanai, S. Saeki, and T. Watanabe, "Laparoscopic omental patch repair for perforated peptic ulcer," *Annals of Surgery*, vol. 221, no. 3, pp. 236–240, 1995.

[34] A. A. Saber, N. Azar, M. Dekal, and T. N. Abdelbaki, "Computed tomographic scan mapping of gastric wall perfusion and clinical implications," *American Journal of Surgery*, vol. 209, no. 6, pp. 999–1006, 2015.

[35] H. N. Dakour Aridi, H. Tamim, A. Mailhac, and B. Y. Safadi, "Concomitant hiatal hernia repair with laparoscopic sleeve gastrectomy is safe: Analysis of the ACS-NSQIP database," *Surgery for Obesity and Related Diseases*, 2016.

[36] A. Goldenberg-Sandau, W. Good, L. Shaw, and M. Neff, "Laparoscopic sleeve gastrectomy with hiatal hernia repair: a retrospective case series and review of literature," in *Proceedings of the Society of American Gastrointestinal and Endoscopic Surgeons Conference*, San Diego, Calif, USa, 2012.

[37] S. Ruscio, M. Abdelgawad, D. Badiali et al., "Simple versus reinforced cruroplasty in patients submitted to concomitant laparoscopic sleeve gastrectomy: prospective evaluation in a bariatric center of excellence," *Surgical Endoscopy and Other Interventional Techniques*, vol. 30, no. 6, pp. 2374–2381, 2016.

[38] P. Noel, M. Nedelcu, and M. Gagner, "Impact of the Surgical Experience on Leak Rate After Laparoscopic Sleeve Gastrectomy," *Obesity Surgery*, vol. 26, no. 8, pp. 1782–1787, 2016.

[39] E. H. Livingston, "Bariatric surgery in the new millennium," *Archives of Surgery*, vol. 142, no. 10, pp. 919–922, 2007.

32

Prospective Observational Study of Single-Site Multiport Per-umbilical Laparoscopic Endosurgery versus Conventional Multiport Laparoscopic Cholecystectomy: Critical Appraisal of a Unique Umbilical Approach

Priyadarshan Anand Jategaonkar[1] and Sudeep Pradeep Yadav[2]

[1] *Department of General & Laparoscopic Surgery, Mahatma Gandhi Institute of Medical Sciences, Sevagram, Wardha, Maharashtra 442102, India*
[2] *Department of General & Laparoscopic Surgery, Jagjivanram Western Railway Hospital, Mumbai Central, Mumbai, Maharashtra 400008, India*

Correspondence should be addressed to Priyadarshan Anand Jategaonkar; jategaonkarpa@gmail.com

Academic Editor: Stephen Kavic

Purpose. This prospective observational study compares an innovative approach of Single-Site Multi-Port Per-umbilical Laparoscopic Endo-surgery (SSMPPLE) cholecystectomy with the gold standard—Conventional Multi-port Laparoscopic Cholecystectomy (CMLC)—to assess the feasibility and efficacy of the former. *Methods.* In all, 646 patients were studied. SSMPPLE cholecystectomy utilized three ports inserted through three independent mini-incisions at the umbilicus. Only the day-to-day rigid laparoscopic instruments were used in all cases. The SSMPPLE cholecystectomy group had 320 patients and the CMLC group had 326 patients. The outcomes were statistically compared. *Results.* SSMPPLE cholecystectomy had average operative time of 43.8 min and blood loss of 9.4 mL. Their duration of hospitalization was 1.3 days (range, 1–5). Six patients (1.9%) of this group were converted to CMLC. Eleven patients had controlled gallbladder perforations at dissection. The Visual Analogue Scores for pain on postoperative days 0 and 7, the operative time, and the scar grades were significantly better for SSMPPLE than CMLC. However, umbilical sepsis and seroma outcomes were similar. We had no bile-duct injuries or port-site hernias in this study. *Conclusion.* SSMPPLE cholecystectomy approach complies with the principles of laparoscopic triangulation; it seems feasible and safe method of minimally invasive cholecystectomy. Overall, it has a potential to emerge as an economically viable alternative to single-port surgery.

1. Introduction

Conventional *M*ulti-port *L*aparoscopic *C*holecystectomy (CMLC) is the gold-standard for tackling benign gallbladder diseases; it generally requires 4 (sometimes even 5 or more) ports spread across different quadrants of abdomen. Recently, the surgeons' quest for reducing the access-trauma by reducing the number of ports has led to several technical modifications regarding minimally invasive cholecystectomy [1, 2]. And the natural-orifice transluminal endoscopic surgery (NOTES) with its potential to achieve completely scarless abdomen, though the most sought for, seems to have fallen out of favor owing to the technical complexity, the prolonged learning curve, and the questionable safety due to the issues regarding closure of mucosal breach. Logically, the per-umbilical approach, with its potential to produce almost the similar results, has been warmly welcomed by the surgeons and the industry. However, this "third generation" surgery is far from being accepted as the standardized approach due to the lack of ease and uniformity in instrumentation/technique apart from the paucity of convincing data. In this paper, we present an investigational technique—what we called it as the *S*ingle-*S*ite *M*ulti-*P*ort *P*er-umbilical *L*aparoscopic *E*ndo-surgery (SSMPPLE). We further compare it prospectively with CMLC for its critical appraisal. The encouraging results of our first 15 patients (10 straightforward cases and 5 acute cholecystitis cases) prompted us to undertake this comparative analysis. These patients have been excluded from this study. As such, SSMPPLE should be considered distinct methodology from the conventional single-incision technique.

2. Materials and Methods

2.1. Informed Consent. One-to-one discussion sessions were arranged between each of the 646 patients and the surgeon to converse about the technical details of procedure. The investigative nature of the procedure along with its likely advantages and disadvantages/complications at the backdrop of the well-established technique of CMLC were clearly explained to all; subsequently, they were allowed to choose one of the operative techniques. Accordingly, a written informed consent was obtained from everybody.

2.2. Study Population. Following criteria were designed for including or excluding the subjects for this study.

2.3. Inclusion Criteria. The inclusion criteria of this study comprised of: (1) biliary colic, (2) chronic calculus cholecystitis, (3) acute calculus cholecystitis, (4) gallbladder polyps with cholelithiasis, (5) gallbladder mucocele, (6) gallbladder empyema, and (7) biliary pancreatitis.

2.4. Exclusion Criteria. Anticipating the technical difficulty, we offered upfront CMLC or open cholecystectomy to the following patients. Hence, these patients were excluded from the study: (1) patients with choledocholithiasis, (2) perforated gallbladder, (3) remnant calculus cholecystitis, (4) Mirizzi syndrome, (5) suspected carcinoma gallbladder, (6) obese patients with the body mass index (BMI) >35 kg/m^2, and (7) patients unfit for laparoscopy.

2.5. Patient Information

2.5.1. SSMPPLE Group. Three hundred and twenty patients underwent SSMPPLE cholecystectomy from March 2007 to March 2011. Out of them, 221 were females and 99 were males. The mean BMI for the males was 27.7 kg/m^2 (range, 17–31.5) and that for the females was 28.4 kg/m^2 (range, 19–33.7). The mean age of the males was 42.5 years (range, 17–64) and that for the females was 45.3 years (range, 22–68). Eighty patients in this series had some form of medical comorbidity. Indications of surgery included both "simple" as well as "difficult" gallbladder pathologies. We could also successfully apply SSMPPLE technique to patients with abdominal scars of prior surgeries like laparoscopic tubal ligation (n = 22) with umbilical scar, laparoscopic appendectomy (n = 6), and midline laparotomy (n = 6) (Table 1).

2.5.2. CMLC Group. Out of a total of 326 patients operated during the same time frame, 95 were males and 231 were females. The mean BMI for males was 25.3 kg/m^2 (range, 18–30) and that for the females was 27.5 kg/m^2 (range, 18–32.3). Eighty eight patients had some form of medical comorbidity. As with SSMPPLE group, this arm also included similar varieties of straightforward as well as technically difficult cases. Five patients had midline scar of exploratory laparotomy, 25 patients had umbilical scar of laparoscopic tubal ligation, and 4 patients had port scars of laparoscopic appendectomy (Table 1).

2.6. Preoperative Assessment and Preparation. We evaluated all these 646 patients preoperatively by the same biochemical (complete blood count, liver, and renal function tests) and the radiological (abdominal ultrasonography) tests. The decision to offer contrast-enhanced abdominal computed tomography scans or magnetic resonance cholangiography for studying biliary system in detail was taken on case-to-case basis. However, none of the patients from either group needed these special tests. Preanesthesia check was obtained for their fitness to withstand general anesthesia. Preoperative optimization was ensured for all patients from both groups, especially for smokers (by abstinence from smoking) and cardiac patients (by enhancing the exercise tolerance). We do not perform per-operative cholangiography routinely. In an attempt to keep a check on the rate of umbilical sepsis, all patients were subjected to meticulous umbilical cleaning preoperatively (twice the previous evening and once on the day of surgery) with chlorhexidine.

2.7. Instrumentation. Only "day-to-day" autoclavable laparoscopic instruments were used in this study. For SSMPPLE cholecystectomy, we used one 10 mm trocar (for 30° 10 mm laparoscope) and two 5 mm valved threaded plastic trocars (for right and left hand working instruments). Monopolar electrosurgery was used for majority of the cases. Except for the Harmonic scalpel (Ethicon Endosurgery, Cincinnati, OH, USA) engaged selectively for the technically difficult cases (17 from SSMPPLE group and 15 from CMLC group), no other specialized equipment was used. Standard port-closure needle was used for the gallbladder traction when required. Though not used in this series, it would be advisable to use extralong instruments if available.

2.8. Surgical Team. To avoid bias, all the patients of both groups were operated on by the same surgeon and the surgical team.

2.9. Anesthesia and Patient Position. All the patients of both groups were operated under general anesthesia. They were placed in supine position with 30° head-up and 20° right-up position. A nasogastric tube was inserted and single-dose of broad-spectrum antibiotic was administered at induction in all. The monitor was placed at the right shoulder of the patient. The surgeon stood on the left of the patient and the camera assistant stood on the left of the surgeon.

TABLE 1: Patient demographics.

Patient variables	SSMPPLE	CMLC
Number of patients	320	326
Sex (male : female)	99 : 221	95 : 231
Mean age (years)		
Male	42.5 (range, 17–64)	43.8 (range, 15–67)
Female	45.3 (range, 22–68)	44.9 (range, 16–70)
Mean BMI (Kg/m^2)		
Male	27.7 (range, 17–31.5)	25.3 (range, 18–30)
Female	28.4 (range, 19–33.7)	27.5 (range, 18–32.3)
Indications for cholecystectomy		
Biliary colic	161	160
Acute calculus cholecystitis	20	15
Chronic calculus cholecystitis	95	110
Gallbladder polyp with cholelithiasis	7	8
Mucocele of gallbladder	7	15
Empyema of gallbladder	10	4
Biliary pancreatitis	20	14
Medical comorbidities		
HTN	16	15
DM	17	19
HTN + DM	14	15
Heart disease		
Old healed MI	6	5
Left ventricular hypertrophy	5	6
Pulmonary disease		
Old healed tuberculosis	18	21
COPD (controlled)	4	7
Previous abdominal surgery (scar)		
LTL (umbilical)	22	25
LA (umbilical + right iliac fossa + suprapubic)	6	4
Laparotomy (midline)	6	5

HTN: hypertension, DM: diabetes, MI: myocardial infarction, LTL: laparoscopic tubal ligation, OA: open appendectomy, LA: laparoscopic appendectomy, SPC: suprapubic cystostomy, and DL: diagnostic laparoscopy.

2.10. Clinical Parameters Studied. Postoperative outcomes studied for both groups were operative time (defined as the time interval between the first port entry till the last port closure), blood loss, bile duct injury, viscus injury, gallbladder perforation during dissection, conversion to either CMLC or open, postoperative pain, stages of recovery, duration of hospitalization, umbilical seroma/sepsis, cosmetic results, and the rate of port-site hernia. The Visual Analogue Scale (VAS, 0–10) was used for assessing the postoperative pain on days 0, 1, 7, and 30. Considering the suboptimal educational and socioeconomic background of our rural patients, we developed an easy-to-use scar grading scale (I-Thrilled, II-Happy, III-Not bothered, and IV-Unhappy) as per the subjective feeling about the scar they have received. We felt this scale was just the handy method of judging the scar outcomes in our part of the world. Although this system lacked the detailed questionnaire (and hence detailed objective evaluation) regarding the cosmetic outcomes, it assessed the cosmetic results on a gross scale.

2.11. Statistical Analysis. Using SPSS 10.0 software (SPSS Inc., Chicago, IL, USA), Pearson's Chi-square test was applied to assess the statistically significant difference between the variables. This difference was considered significant if the P value was <0.05.

2.12. Surgical Techniques

2.12.1. SSMPPLE Cholecystectomy. The technique of creation of pneumoperitoneum by Veress needle was subject to the shape of umbilicus and the presence of abdominal scar (if any) of previous surgery. In the patient with wide umbilicus (defined as ≥2.5 cm diameter) and without any abdominal scar, a 2 mm stab incision was placed at the 12 O'clock position *on/just inside* the umbilical mound for inserting the Veress needle before creating the pneumoperitoneum. In these patients, we set the intra-abdominal pressure (IAP) at 14 mm Hg. For patients with cardiac and pulmonary comorbidities, we lowered the IAP to 10–12 mm Hg to minimize the

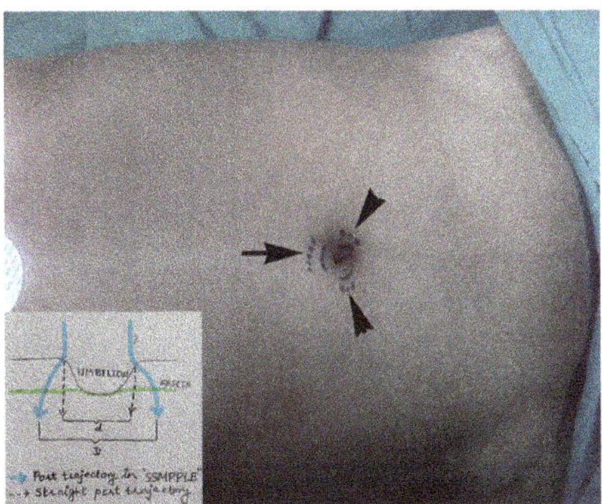

FIGURE 1: Incisions for port placement. Solid lines indicate the skin incisions and dotted lines indicate the fascial trajectories. This resulted in spacing the trocars away. *Inset.* Diagrammatic representation of the ports pathways. Note that the intertrocar distance is more with curved paths (D) than with straight (d).

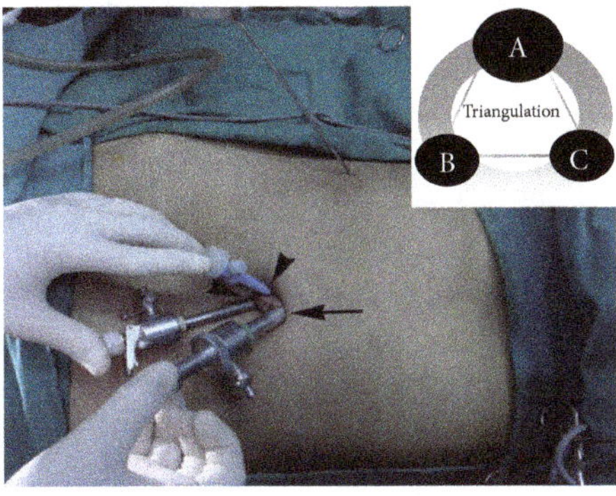

FIGURE 2: Port position. One 10 mm (arrow) and two 5 mm (arrow heads) ports placed *on* the umbilical mound in triangular fashion (*Upper inset*). Note the port-closure needle at the right hypochondrium for gallbladder traction.

detrimental effects of the raised IAP. The pediatric patients were set on 8–10 mm Hg of IAP. The stab incision was then converted into 11 mm curvilinear skin-crease incision (in line with the umbilical mound) through which a 10 mm sharp trocar was introduced. This was used for 10 mm 30° laparoscope. Two 5 mm, one at the 8 O'clock for the left-hand-working instrument and the another at the 4 O'clock position for the right-hand-working instrument were introduced through the similar 5 mm curvilinear skin-crease incisions *on/just inside* the umbilical mound to achieve the triangular trocar ergonomics. The fascial trajectories for all these three trocars were angled centrifugally by 3-4 mm from the respective cutaneous entries (Figures 1 and 2). This modification helped in reducing the intracorporeal "sword-fighting" of the instruments. Moreover, the obliquity of the trocar paths tends to act as a "flap-valve" mechanism in preventing the trocar-site herniation postoperatively.

However, this assembly of 12 O'clock (10 mm)–4 O'clock (5 mm)–8 O'clock (5 mm) can be changed to 6 O'clock (10 mm)–2 O'clock (5 mm)–10 O'clock (5 mm) depending on surgical team's comfort. After this series, we have used the latter in 17 patients with no added advantage.

The pneumoperitoneum helped in stretching the umbilical ring and, thus, purchased some added distance between the trocars and prevented them falling "on-top" of each other (Figure 2, *inset*). Valves of both the 5 mm trocars were kept outwardly placed—one of them was used for CO_2 inflow and other one was used for venting the surgical smoke. Alternatively, the CO_2 cable may be attached to the valve of the 10 mm port. This, along with the light cable, were made to exit from the tops of their respective trocars. Threaded trocars tend to have good grip and prevent gas leak.

Tricks adopted to rectify surgeon-to-camera-assistant collisions and instrument-clashes during the procedure included the following. (1) We adjusted the distant tip of 10 mm cannula to be just inside the peritoneal cavity. This step made it possible to keep the laparoscope withdrawn most of the times, thus, having maximum extracorporeal length of the laparoscope. It could distance the camera-assistant's hand from that of surgeon's. (2) When feasible, extralong laparoscopes were encouraged. (3) Both 5 mm working trocars were inserted 3-4 mm farther into the peritoneal cavity. (4) The camera holding right hand was always laid beneath that of the surgeon's. (5) The surgeon stood on a stool with 0.5 ft height during the whole procedure. This entire surgical assembly gave an adequate "elbow-space" for the operating surgeon as well as the camera-assistant. However, in patients with narrow umbilicus, we preferred to insert all the ports *just outside* umbilical mound to circumvent instrument crowding. Regarding the patients with abdominal scars, anticipating the underlying adhesions in and around the peritoneal side of the umbilicus, we achieved pneumoperitoneum by inserting the Veress needle at the right mid-clavicular line in the right hypochondrium. A miniscope was then inserted through this stab wound and used to visualize the umbilical adhesions if any. Filmy adhesions could be easily swiped with the miniscope itself. In cases of the well-formed adhesions at the umbilicus, instead of using a purely open-laparoscopic technique, a rather safe peritoneal access was achieved by adopting the combination of the "open" laparoscopy (through the curvilinear umbilical incision) counter-monitored by the miniscope via the right hypochondrium.

The problem of the "floppy" fundus/large gallbladder/bulky liver obliterating the view of the cystohepatic triangle in certain patients was tackled by a simple technique. Commercially available catgut loop was introduced through 5 mm right-hand-working trocar and tightened around the fundus before holding and retracting it cephalad with the standard port-closure needle inserted in the right hypochondrium at the anterior axillary line under the laparoscopic vision. Then, the catgut-loop-tail was held and encircled around the jaws of the port-closure needle in such a way that it locks them and prevents it from slipping during the retraction. This reduced the risk of trauma by its sharp tip (nil in our series). Now, it could be easily maneuvered in any direction as per the requirement of the counter traction. Such a dynamic multidirectional retraction provided by the port-closure actually simulated the 4th port traction of CMLC (Figures 2 and 3) and helped us achieving not

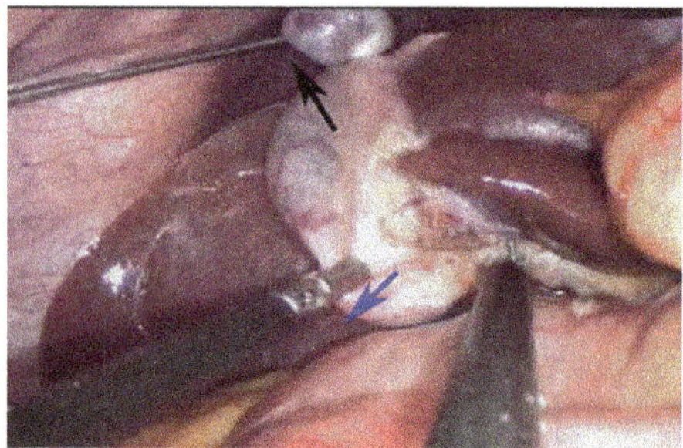

Figure 3: "On road" to the critical view of safety. Note the inferolateral traction (blue arrow) by left-hand grasper and cranial traction (black arrow) by the port closure needle to expose the cystohepatic triangle.

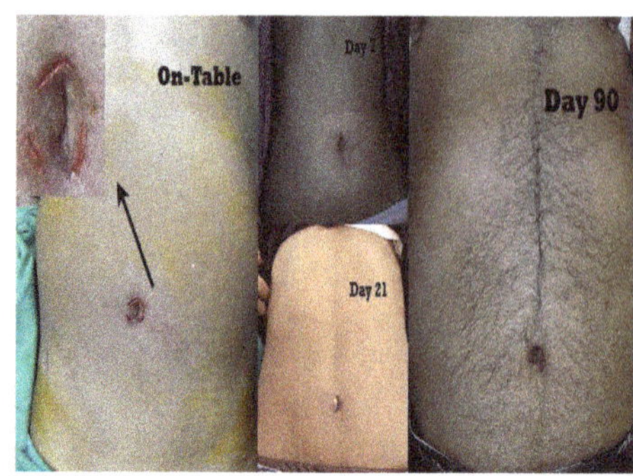

Figure 4: Postoperative scars. Note the undistorted umbilicus with miniscars that are hardly visible. *Inset*. The close-up view of on-table per-umbilical incisions.

only safer but also quicker dissection to accomplish the "critical view of safety" of Strasberg and Soper. Hence, we recommend its liberal use especially for the beginners of the SSMPPLE technique. However, for the thick-walled gallbladders precluding the catgut looping, we performed intracorporeal polypropylene suturing at the fundus before holding and encircling it by the port-closure needle through right hypochondrium in the way described above.

The dissection was commenced by retrograde technique by opening the posterior peritoneal leaf at the cystohepatic triangle first followed by the anterior. While the basic principles of the small controlled moves at one time rather than the haphazard ones and dividing the tissues bit-by-bit rather than the "bulk-division" remained the same, we add the following: instead of inserting and advancing both the instruments simultaneously (like one tends to do in the CMLC), introduce the left-hand retracting instrument till the "target organ" and *then* insert the right-hand dissecting instrument to reach the area of interest (and *vice versa* for the left-hand-dominant surgeon). This has helped us in avoiding the intracorporeal instrument-crossing as well as maintaining an optimum distance (that was necessary for the target-organ manipulation) between the tips of these instruments. Once the "critical view of safety" was convincingly achieved, the cystic duct and the artery were doubly clipped with the medium-sized clips by a 5 mm clip-applier inserted through the right-hand-working port before dividing them in between the clips. If deemed necessary, the medium-large clips were used for the wide cystic ducts by inserting a 10 mm clip applier through the 10 mm port. At this time, we exchanged one of the 5 mm working instruments with a 5 mm laparoscope. We transfixed the cystic ducts (22 biliary colic and 5 acute calculus cholecystitis cases) with 2/0 polyglactic acid by the intracorporeal suturing technique in cases where the clip closure was felt insecure. Once dissected completely from its fossa, the gallbladder was extracted in an endobag via the 10 mm port. None of the patient required merging of these three port incisions. Gallstones >1 cm of size (which were likely to obstruct the safe extraction of specimen) were crushed with the stone-holding forceps before removing them piece-meal. Endobags were used for extracting the gallbladders in all cases. Utmost care was exercised to avoid puncturing these endobag. Hemostasis was checked and saline irrigation was given to the gallbladder fossa and the right subdiaphragmatic region for washing out the acidic milieu in an attempt towards reducing the postoperative shoulder pain. We closed *all* three ports in all cases with 2/0 polyglactic acid suture under direct vision. The skin incisions were infiltrated with the mixture of lignocaine and bupivacaine before closing them by 3/0 monofilament absorbable subcuticular sutures. Thus, it was possible to achieve a good cosmetic outcome without distorting the umbilical anatomy after the closure (Figure 4).

2.12.2. Surgical Technique of CMLC. This was in accordance with the standard steps of 4-port laparoscopic cholecystectomy in "American" patient positioning. None of the patients required any extra port. Similar to SSMPPLE procedure, all the port sites were infiltrated with lignocaine/bupivacaine mixture and closed by 3/0 monofilament absorbable subcuticular sutures.

2.13. Follow-Up Protocol. All the patients from both groups were followed meticulously every 3 months in the first postoperative year and then yearly thereafter. These patients were assessed for port-site hernias by clinical examination and ultrasound if required. However, we lost follow up to 21 patients (SSMPPLE group) and 19 patients (CMLC group).

3. Results

3.1. The SSMPPLE Group. The mean operative time was 43.8 min (range, 20–85). The average blood loss was 9.4 mL (range, 5–55). There was no bile duct injury. However, we had one electrosurgical burn to the second part of the duodenum which was sutured by the intracorporeal technique. Eleven patients (3.4%) had small perforation of gallbladder while dissecting. Spilled bile was sucked and the stones were extracted before giving a thorough peritoneal irrigation with saline. Six patients (1.9%) had to be converted to 4-port CMLC. Five of them had intense pericholecystic adhesions not amenable to this technique and one had ambiguous biliovascular anatomy requiring conversion for better definition of critical structures. Furthermore, we converted five patients to open cholecystectomy; out of these, three

TABLE 2: Results.

Perioperative variables	SSMPPLE	CMLC	P value
Intraoperative			
Camera assistant			
Fellow	216	168	—
Registrar	104	158	—
Mean operative time (min)	43.8 (range, 20–85)	39.5 (range, 28–106)	0.00370
Mean blood loss (mL)	9.4 (range, 5–55)	8.7 (range, 5–40)	<0.0001
Bile duct injury	0	0	—
Major vessel injury	0	0	—
Rate of conversion			
To conventional laparoscopic cholecystectomy	6	Not applicable	—
To open cholecystectomy	5	2	—
Postoperative			
Pain (mean visual analogue score)			
Day 0	3.21 (range, 3–5)	3.89 (range, 3–6)	<0.0001
Day 1	2.09 (range, 1–4)	2.13 (range, 2–4)	NS
Day 7	0	0.04 (range, 0-1)	0.00018
Day 30	0	0	—
Mean postoperative analgesics used (days)	1.7 (range, 0.5–4.8)	3.3 (range, 1–5)	<0.0001
Ambulation (hr)	4.6 (range, 4–8)	4.8 (range, 4–12)	<0.0001
Mean time to solids after surgery (hr)	5.7 (range, 5–12)	6.6 (range, 6–12)	<0.0001
Mean time to discharge after surgery (days)	1.3 (range, 1–5)	1.2 (range, 1–7)	NS
Mean time to normal activity (days)	3.2 (range, 3–7)	3.4 (range, 3–5)	0.00444
Mean time to work (days)	9.6 (range, 7–18)	10.5 (range, 7–15)	<0.0001
Umbilical sepsis	6 (1.9%)	5 (1.5%)	NS
Umbilical seroma	7 (2.2%)	6 (1.8%)	NS
Trocar site hernia	0	0	—
Scar grade	1.28 (range, 1–3)	2.03 (range, 1–3)	<0.0001

were due to uncontrollable cystic artery bleeds and two were due to inadvertent gallbladder fossa bleeds requiring suturing. Eleven patients from this series had low-inserting cystic ducts, 8 had their cystic ducts opening in their right hepatic ducts and 4 had their right hepatic arteries tortuously occupying the cystohepatic triangles—the "caterpillar turns" All the patients were allowed to have solid food by 5.7 h (range, 5–12) after the surgery and were ambulatory by then. Mean VAS applied to all the patients on the days 0, 1, 7, and 30 of the surgery was 3.2 (range, 3–5), 2.1 (range, 1–4), 0, and 0, respectively. Mean postoperative analgesics were used for 1.7 days (range, 0.5–4.8). The postoperative analgesia regimen was standardized for both the groups as follows. All the patient of this study received intravenous aqueous diclofenac sodium at the end of 6th postoperative hour before putting them on oral diclofenac sodium preparation (sustained release) the next day. None of our patients needed opioid analgesics. The patients were discharged after an average of 1.3 days (range, 1–5). The mean time to take up normal activity was 3.2 days (range, 3–7) (Table 2). Except 4, all other patients are under regular follow up. While the first patient of our series has finished 4 years and 9 months of follow up, the last patient has completed 1 year and 10 months of follow up. Two of the four patents lost follow up due to their demise owing to cardiac ailments. Other two have completely lost their follow up due to the reasons unknown. Six patients (1.9%) developed umbilical sepsis which was controlled by antibiotics. Seven patients developed umbilical seroma; they recovered completely by an expectant line of treatment. None of our patients has developed trocar-site hernia till date. Seven patients (4 at the end of 9 months and 4 at the end of 13 months) developed residual bile duct stones which were extracted by endoscopic sphincterotomy. Assessment by the scar grading scale revealed 73.01% patients being thrilled and 25.56% being happy. While nobody was unhappy, 1.42% did not bother about their cosmetic outcome.

3.2. The CMLC Group. In this group, the mean operative time was 39.5 min (range, 28–106) and the blood loss was 8.7 mL (range, 5–40). There were no bile duct or viscus injuries. Nine patients (2.8%) had small gallbladder perforations. Four of them had controlled stone spillages and all the stones could be "berry-picked" into the endobags. The mean VAS applied the patients on the days 0, 1, 7, and 30 of the surgery was 3.9 (range, 3–6), 2.1 (range, 2–4), 0.04 (0-1), and 0, respectively. The mean time to discharge from the hospital was 1.2 days (range, 1–7). Six patients (1.8%) developed umbilical seroma and 5 patients (1.5%) developed umbilical sepsis. All of them recovered with conservative line of management. The

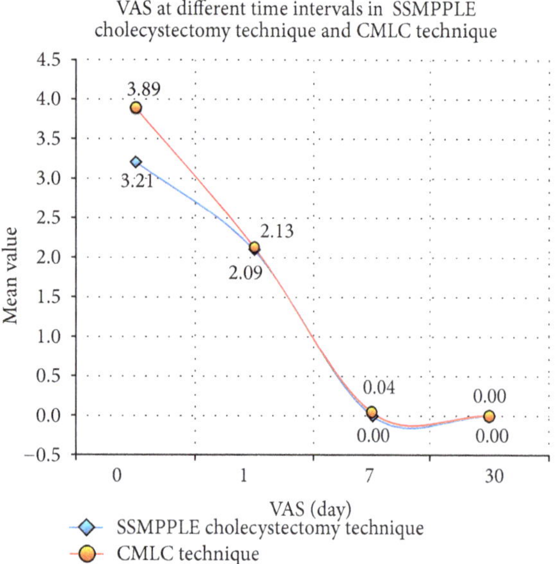

FIGURE 5: Visual Analogue Scale for the SSMPPLE cholecystectomy technique and the CMLC techniques.

blood loss in SSMPPLE (9.4 mL) was significantly more than that in CMLC (8.7 mL). There were statistically significant differences in favor of SSMPPLE over CMLC as far as the operative time, VAS on postoperative days 0 and 7 (Figure 5), time for ambulation and commencing oral intake, resuming normal activities, and scar grading were concerned. We converted two patients to open cholecystectomy for cystic artery bleeds ($n = 1$) and ambiguous biliary anatomy ($n = 1$) (Table 2).

4. Discussion

Owing to the obvious advantages associated with minimally invasive surgery like the less pain and the faster recovery, late 1980s saw the multiport CMLC being quickly accepted as the gold-standard for treating gallstone diseases [2–4]. Once the benefits of minimizing the access trauma, and, at the same time, having a much superior cosmetic outcomes without compromising the safety were further appreciated, the surgeons started attempting different techniques to reduce the number of ports to three or even two for laparoscopic cholecystectomy.

The late 1990s' invention—the natural orifice transluminal endoscopic surgery (NOTES)— could reduce the abdominal access trauma to zero and offered a much sought for outcome—the scarless abdomen [1, 2, 5]. Although better cosmetically, such surgeries, whether pure or hybrid, tend to have a steep learning curve owing to the complex ergonomics, the long flexible instruments with the negligible tactile feedback, and, last but not the least, the high cost factor. Not surprisingly, the transumbilical surgery, considered being the link between the conventional multiport laparoscopic surgery and the NOTES, evolved to be the most user as well as the consumer-friendly alternative. The umbilical cosmetic outcome resembled NOTES. With no risk of visceral transgression, the single-port transumbilical laparoscopic surgery was termed superior to NOTES [6, 7].

Reports discussing the feasibility of single-port transumbilical laparoscopic surgery have peaked only in the last half-a-decade with myriad of modifications [8, 9]. This might be the result of the rising demand of such surgeries producing good cosmetic results (even from the rural population like our center) coupled against the backdrop of the difficulty in learning and affording the NOTES. The single-port transumbilical laparoscopic surgery entails incising the skin and the fascia for up to 3.5 cm at the umbilicus [10, 11]. Raising the skin flap remains the unavoidable step which may contribute to the subcutaneous seroma formation and/or the skin necrosis. This potentially results in poor wound healing and inferior cosmetic results. On the contrary, the SSMPPLE eliminates this step.

We used the standard port-closure needle (coupled with catgut loop) to retract the gallbladder fundus in 46 cases of SSMPPLE. It mirrors the fourth retracting port of conventional laparoscopic cholecystectomy which allows achieving the "critical view of safety" of Strasberg and Soper [12]. Also, it helps to have the perpendicular cystic duct clipping rather than the tangential—an important step to minimize the postoperative bile leak [13]. As the gallbladder wall is not traversed by the needle, it does not violate the basic principles [13]. Further, this site can also be used for the miniscope to visualize umbilical adhesions (if any) before porting. Small drain tube can also be inserted through it, if required. However, its negligent movement can traumatize the diaphragm or the other viscera. Also, for large liver, one should avoid force retraction and opt for an additional 5 mm trocar for safe dissection. We used such an additional 5 mm trocar in the SSMPPLE group for 18 out of 46 patients.

We feel that *all* the three fascial punctures of the ports should be closed under vision. Although the cases discussed here need further long-term followup, none of our patients developed port-site herniation. Port closure under direct vision adds further to the safety.

Umbilical sepsis in the single-port transumbilical laparoscopic surgery is reported in the range of 0 to 14% [14]. We had six patients (1.9%) from the SSMPPLE group that developed umbilical sepsis; three of them were diabetic. All of them recovered completely with antibiotics. As reported earlier, we always use endobags for the gallbladder extraction [15]. This potentially reduces the umbilical contamination. The conversion rates reported in the literature are 0–24% for the single-port transumbilical laparoscopic cholecystectomy [14, 16]. In our series, it was 1.9%. However, we should keep a low threshold for conversion to standard multiport laparoscopy or open surgery [14, 17]. Furthermore, Blinman has elegantly discussed the relationship of tension (and hence pain) at the incision site to the lengths of the incision; the tension is directly proportional to the square of lengths of incisions and not the addition of the lengths [18]. Hence, the projected amount of tension acting at the three ports of SSMPPLE technique (476.1 units) would be lesser by a third than that produced at 25 mm incision of the single-incision surgery (1540.6 units).

A recent meta-analysis of 13 randomized trials (including 923 patients) that studied comparisons between single-incision laparoscopic cholecystectomy and conventional cholecystectomy reported higher failure rate, operative time, and blood loss with the former [19]. The two approaches were found comparable in terms of conversion to open surgery, length of hospital stay, postoperative pain, port-site infections, or hernias. The cosmetic outcomes were better for the former especially when 10 mm ports were used in the latter. However, we feel that, with the technical modifications described in this paper, we could achieve acceptable results. Further, we need to state at this point that the only similarity between SSMPPLE and single-incision laparoscopic cholecystectomy is the very site of access (i.e., the umbilicus). Rest all the elements in this technique (like the number, the placement and the sizes of incisions, the instruments used, the ergonomics, etc.) differ largely. Thus it tends to amalgamate the operative site (umbilicus) of the single-incision laparoscopic cholecystectomy and the instrumentation with operative techniques of the gold-standard—CMLC. Hence it should not be considered a modification of the single-incision laparoscopic cholecystectomy but should rather be taken as a distinct laparoscopic cholecystectomy technique.

A similar technique described in literature [17] used all 5 mm ports and joined the two port sites for the specimen extraction. However, we think that 10 mm laparoscope should always be used right from the commencement of the surgery as it gives much brighter, clearer, and wider vision. Also, it can be used for the 10 mm clip applier and the specimen extraction. For initial few cases of our series, the operative time was longer as our surgical team was under the learning curve of this technique. As the number of cases and the experience increased, the operative time went on decreasing. Another recently reported method uses three ports at periumbilical location to carry out cholecystectomy [20]. Although the reported technique achieved triangulation, the port placement was away from the umbilical fold. Thus, the scars did not recede within the umbilicus. The SSMPPLE helps the scars to recede at the umbilicus to produce better aesthetics.

However, the SSMPPLE has certain limitations. (i) If not precisely and strategically placed, the ports can lie too close to each other leading to extracorporeal clashing. (ii) Although it may be technically easy in wide umbilicus, a narrow or a "slit-like" umbilicus may pose a real challenge. In fact, we should keep a very low threshold for conversion to the CMLC in these cases. (iii) If the cutaneous and the fascial portal punctures lie in vertical line (rather than oblique), one may end up in having the instruments lying parallel to each other leading to difficulty in dissecting. Moreover, notable flaws of this study are (1) limited cohort, (2) nonrandomized study, (3) limited duration of the followup for drawing definitive conclusions about rate of port-site hernia, and (4) the Visual Analogue Scale for incision-related pain and the scar grading scale assessing the respective parameters in a subjective manner rather than the desired objective manner.

Although we have not conducted any cost-analysis comparisons in this study, given that the routine laparoscopic instruments were used with better operative timings without any major complications (Table 2), we feel that the SSMPPLE may become a valuable option of the per-umbilical laparoscopy especially for the patients of the developing nations. However, this technique is a modification of minimally invasive cholecystectomy. We further stress that it is *not* a modification of single incision laparoscopic cholecystectomy in any way because it includes three separate skin incisions/punctures.

5. Conclusion

The presented SSMPPLE cholecystectomy technique does not need any specialized ports or other equipment; it seems safe, efficient, and potentially economically viable alternative to the single-incision laparoscopic cholecystectomy using commercially available specialized port/instruments.

References

[1] T. Kagaya, "Laparoscopic cholecystectomy via two ports, using the "Twin-Port" system," *Journal of Hepato-Biliary-Pancreatic Surgery*, vol. 8, no. 1, pp. 76–80, 2001.

[2] S. Trichak, "Three-port versus standard four-port laparoscopic cholecystectomy: a prospective randomized study," *Surgical Endoscopy and Other Interventional Techniques*, vol. 17, no. 9, pp. 1434–1436, 2003.

[3] M. Gagner and A. Garcia-Ruiz, "Technical aspects of minimally invasive abdominal surgery performed with needlescopic instruments," *Surgical Laparoscopy, Endoscopy and Percutaneous Techniques*, vol. 8, no. 3, pp. 171–179, 1998.

[4] S. Purkayastha, H. S. Tilney, P. Georgiou, T. Athanasiou, P. P. Tekkis, and A. W. Darzi, "Laparoscopic cholecystectomy versus mini-laparotomy cholecystectomy: a meta-analysis of randomised control trials," *Surgical Endoscopy and Other Interventional Techniques*, vol. 21, no. 8, pp. 1294–1300, 2007.

[5] A. N. Kalloo, V. K. Singh, S. B. Jagannath et al., "Flexible transgastric peritoneoscopy: a novel approach to diagnostic and therapeutic interventions in the peritoneal cavity," *Gastrointestinal Endoscopy*, vol. 60, no. 1, pp. 114–117, 2004.

[6] M. T. Gettman and M. L. Blute, "Transvesical peritoneoscopy: initial clinical evaluation of the bladder as a portal for natural orifice translumenal endoscopic surgery," *Mayo Clinic Proceedings*, vol. 82, no. 7, pp. 843–845, 2007.

[7] J. D. Raman, J. A. Cadeddu, P. Rao, and A. Rane, "Single-incision laparoscopic surgery: initial urological experience and comparison with natural-orifice transluminal endoscopic surgery," *BJU International*, vol. 101, no. 12, pp. 1493–1496, 2008.

[8] J. Erbella Jr. and G. M. Bunch, "Single-incision laparoscopic cholecystectomy: the first 100 outpatients," *Surgical Endoscopy and Other Interventional Techniques*, vol. 24, no. 8, pp. 1958–1961, 2010.

[9] B. Bokobza, A. Valverde, E. Magne et al., "Single umbilical incision laparoscopic cholecystectomy: initial experience of the Coelio Club," *Journal of visceral surgery*, vol. 147, no. 4, pp. e253–e257, 2010.

[10] R. Sinha, "Transumbilical single-incision laparoscopic cholecystectomy with conventional instruments and ports: the way forward?" *Journal of Laparoendoscopic and Advanced Surgical Techniques*, vol. 21, no. 6, pp. 497–503, 2011.

[11] T. Adachi, T. Okamoto, S. Ono, T. Kanematsu, and T. Kuroki, "Technical progress in single-incision laparoscopic cholecystectomy in our initial experience," *Minimally Invasive Surgery*, vol. 2011, Article ID 972647, 4 pages, 2011.

[12] P. A. Jategaonkar and S. P. Yadav, "Mirroring dynamic gallbladder retraction of conventional laparoscopic cholecystectomy at the transumbilical approach," *Annals of the Royal College of Surgeons of England*, vol. 96, no. 2, pp. 167–168, 2014.

[13] E. R. Podolsky and P. G. Curcillo II, "Reduced-port surgery: preservation of the critical view in single-port-access cholecystectomy," *Surgical Endoscopy and Other Interventional Techniques*, vol. 24, no. 12, pp. 3038–3043, 2010.

[14] C. Palanivelu, P. A. Jategaonkar, M. Rangarajan, and B. Srikanth, "'Pseudo' cholelithiasis: sequelae of minimally invasive cholecystectomy with maximum surprise: an unusual case," *Endoscopy*, vol. 41, supplement 2, pp. E186–E187, 2009.

[15] P. G. Curcillo II, A. S. Wu, E. R. Podolsky et al., "Single-port-access (SPAŮ) cholecystectomy: a multi-institutional report of the first 297 cases," *Surgical Endoscopy and Other Interventional Techniques*, vol. 24, no. 8, pp. 1854–1860, 2010.

[16] H. Massoumi, N. Kiyici, and H. Hertan, "Bile leak after laparoscopic cholecystectomy," *Journal of Clinical Gastroenterology*, vol. 41, no. 3, pp. 301–305, 2007.

[17] T. A. Azeez and K. M. Mahran, "Transumbilical laparoscopic cholecystectomy: towards a scarless abdominal surgery," *Hepato-Gastroenterology*, vol. 58, no. 106, pp. 298–300, 2011.

[18] T. Blinman, "Incisions do not simply sum," *Surgical Endoscopy and Other Interventional Techniques*, vol. 24, no. 7, pp. 1746–1751, 2010.

[19] S. Trastulli, R. Cirocchi, J. Desiderio et al., "Systematic review and meta-analysis of randomized clinical trials comparing single-incision versus conventional laparoscopic cholecystectomy," *British Journal of Surgery*, vol. 100, pp. 191–208, 2012.

[20] J. Y. Ge, L. Wang, H. Zou, and X. W. Zhang, "Periumbilical laparoscopic surgery through triple channels using common instrumentation," *Experimental and Therapeutic Medicine*, vol. 5, no. 4, pp. 1053–1056, 2013.

33

Robotic-Assisted versus Conventional Laparoscopic Approach for Rectal Cancer Surgery, First Egyptian Academic Center Experience, RCT

Yasser Debakey,[1] **Ashraf Zaghloul**,[2] **Ahmed Farag**,[3] **Ahmed Mahmoud**,[4] **and Inas Elattar**[5]

[1]*Assistant Teacher of Surgical Oncology, National Cancer Institute, Cairo University, Egypt*
[2]*Head of Robotic Surgery Unit, National Cancer Institute, Cairo University, Egypt*
[3]*Head of Colorectal Surgery Unit, Faculty of Medicine, Cairo University, Egypt*
[4]*Associated Professor of Surgical Oncology, National Cancer Institute, Cairo University, Egypt*
[5]*Professor of Biostatistics and Cancer Epidemiology, National Cancer Institute, Cairo University, Egypt*

Correspondence should be addressed to Yasser Debakey; y.eldebakey@cu.edu.eg

Academic Editor: Diego Cuccurullo

Background. Undoubtedly, robotic systems have largely penetrated the surgical field. For any new operative approach to become an accepted alternative to conventional methods, it must be proved safe and result in comparable outcomes. The purpose of this study is to compare the short-term operative as well as oncologic outcomes of robotic-assisted and laparoscopic rectal cancer resections. *Methods.* This is a prospective randomized clinical trial conducted on patients with rectal cancer undergoing either robotic-assisted or laparoscopic surgery from April 2015 till February 2017. Patients' demographics, operative parameters, and short-term clinical and oncological outcomes were analyzed. *Results.* Fifty-seven patients underwent permuted block randomization. Of these patients, 28 were assigned to undergo robotic-assisted rectal surgery and 29 to laparoscopic rectal surgery. After exclusion of 12 patients following randomization, 45 patients were included in the analysis. No significant differences exist between both groups in terms of age, gender, BMI, ASA score, clinical stage, and rate of receiving upfront chemoradiation. Estimated blood loss was evidently lower in the robotic than in the laparoscopic group (median: 200 versus 325 ml, $p = 0.050$). A significantly more distal margin is achieved in the robotic than in the laparoscopic group (median: 2.8 versus 1.8, $p < 0.001$). Although the circumferential radial margin (CRM) was complete in 18 patients (85.7%) in the robotic group in contrast to 15 patients (62.5%) in the laparoscopic group, it did not differ statistically ($p = 0.079$). The overall postoperative complication rates were similar between the two groups. *Conclusion.* To our knowledge, this is the first prospective randomized trial of robotic rectal surgery in the Middle East and Northern Africa region. Our early experience indicates that robotic rectal surgery is a feasible and safe procedure. It is not inferior to standard laparoscopy in terms of oncologic radicality and surgical complications. Organization number is IORG0003381. IRB number is IRB00004025.

1. Background

Over the past two decades, rectal cancer management underwent an immense wave of change from various perspectives. There was a smart shift from open to minimally invasive and robotic techniques, a worldwide application of neoadjuvant multimodal chemoradiation therapy for locally advanced stage disease, as well as optimization of surgical technique with nerve preservation together with the introduction of total mesorectal excision (TME) which were all largely happening in the preceding 10–15 years. The first colorectal laparoscopic procedure was operated upon by Jacobs in 1991 [1]. A decade later, in 2001, the robotic system was introduced to colorectal surgery [2].

To date, laparoscopic surgery has been acknowledged as a safe and effective modality of rectal cancer surgery. However, a randomized controlled multicenter trial has recently suggested that the use of laparoscopic surgery in T3/T4 tumors may result in incomplete resection, affecting the oncological outcome in this group of patients [3]. The challenges of an incomplete TME in laparoscopic surgery are often encountered when faced with anatomical difficulties, for instance, a narrowed male pelvis, bulky tumor, and obese patients. Robotic rectal surgery might be the answer to this quandary.

Why robotics? The company of The da Vinci Surgical System gives many justifications encompassing the high definition 3D image, the wrist-like function, filtration of tremors, microanastomosis, motion scaling, and tele-surgery. Still, we do believe that there are certain perceived advantages during surgery. First is the optimal, stable operative view; the surgeon is no longer assistant-dependent. Second is the high definition 3D image with superior visualization and differentiation between things to be removed from those to be preserved. Moreover, the surgeon's wrist is now incorporated in the technology and he or she would move freely in space deep in the pelvis, a place he could otherwise not get to. Add to that, the countertraction, using the third robotic instrument attached to the fourth robotic arm, with optimal direction and force, may be an operator.

With minimally invasive surgery making headway, we believe that robotic surgery will provide the next major step forward in the treatment of rectal cancer. Like it or not, robotic systems have already revolutionized the surgical field, proving its advantage over laparoscopic techniques in terms of superior visualization, enhanced motion, ergonomics, and comparable clinical outcome.

2. Methods

This is a prospective randomized controlled study that was conducted on all patients of both sexes and definite age group attending the National Cancer Institute and with adenocarcinoma of the rectum located within 15 cm from the anal verge who were eligible to be included in the study. Tumor localization was categorized as the upper rectum (distal border of tumor is from 10 to 15 cm from the anal verge), middle rectum (5 to 10 cm from the anal verge), or lower rectum (less than 5 cm from the anal verge) as measured by colonoscopy and digital rectal examination. Patients were classified into two groups: robotic-assisted rectal surgery "the robotic system that we use is the da Vinci Si (Intuitive Surgical, Inc., Sunnyvale, CA)" and conventional laparoscopic rectal surgery. Baseline demographics (gender, age, ASA, BMI), preoperative data (distance of the tumor from the anal verge, clinical stage, whether preoperative chemoradiation "CRT", presence of residual tumor after CRT), intraoperative data (preparation time, actual operative time, estimated blood loss, and conversion rate to open surgery), postoperative data (pathological stage, number of harvested lymph nodes, macroscopic completeness of resection in the form of proximal margin, distal margin, and circumferential radial margin), and immediate postoperative outcome within one month (days of return of bowel function, days of hospital stay, complications, if any, like anastomotic leakage, ileus, wound problems and others, rate of reoperation, rate of readmission, and 30-day mortality) were analyzed and compared.

The criteria for patients selection were the following: histological diagnosis of adenocarcinoma of rectum, no anesthesiological contraindications to minimally invasive surgery, age ≤ 75 years, ASA ≤ 2, and the procedures performed by the same surgical team. Patients with metastatic disease, malignant bowel obstruction (MBO), and unresectable tumor were excluded from our study.

Preoperative workup (endoscopy with biopsies, radiological imaging including pelvic MRI, liver ultrasound, chest X-ray, and routine abdominal and digital rectal examinations) was routinely carried out. The assignment of patients to either group was done by a permuted block randomization. It was an open-labeled study; i.e., patients, investigators (surgeons, researchers), and data collectors knew which procedure will be done to which patients. The study was approved by the Institutional Review Board (IRB) at NCI, Cairo University. All patients provided written informed consent.

Concerning preoperative preparation; first, mechanical bowel preparation was performed preoperatively with rectal enemas for all patients. A single preoperative dose of antibiotics (oral ciprofloxacin 750 mg and intravenous neomycin 1 gram) was given. Second, from midnight prior to surgery, patients did not receive medications known to cause long-term sedation. Third, for prophylaxis against thromboembolism, subcutaneous enoxaparin 40 mg was given 12 hours before the expected time of the procedure. Fourth, patients received single-dose antibiotic prophylaxis against both anaerobes and aerobes about 1 hour before surgery. Finally, solid diet stopped the day before surgery with no starvation policy as fasting is just for 4 hours for liquids before the procedure.

3. Definitions

Anterior or low anterior resection is defined when the anastomosis is performed above or below the peritoneal reflection, respectively. In ultra-low anterior resection the entire rectum is removed and a coloanal anastomosis is performed. Preparation time is calculated from induction of anesthesia to console and the actual operative time from console to skin closure. Stage migration occurs whenever the final pathological stage differs from the preoperative clinical stage. Operative morbidity is marked by complications in the form of wound infection, ileus. Clinical anastomotic leakage was considered to be present, if any of the following features were observed: presence of peritonitis caused by anastomotic dehiscence, presence of feculent substances coming out through the pelvic drain, or the presence of a pelvic abscess with demonstration of anastomotic leak by rectal examination or contrast study.

4. Work Description [4]

4.1. Operation Room Arrangement. Whichever robotic or laparoscopic is performed, certain principles are adopted: first, patient positioning in a manner precluding pressure or nerve injury so all pressure points were adequately padded; second, patient fixation to the operating table to prevent sliding, so chest strap is placed superior to the xiphoid process and leg strap is also applied over the pneumatic calf; and third, freeing the operative field by positioning IV lines, cardiac monitoring leads, and urinary catheter in a manner that they do not obstruct the surgical team's operative field.

4.2. Patient Positioning. The patient is positioned in a modified lithotomy position with both arms tucked. The patient's abdomen and pelvis are prepared from the xiphoid process to the pubic symphysis and from the right posterior axillary line to the left posterior axillary line. Left docking with an oblique angle (over the hip) is always adopted after the patient is placed in Trendelenburg with the right side tilted downward and the left leg lowered enough to avoid collision during docking, ***Figure 1***.

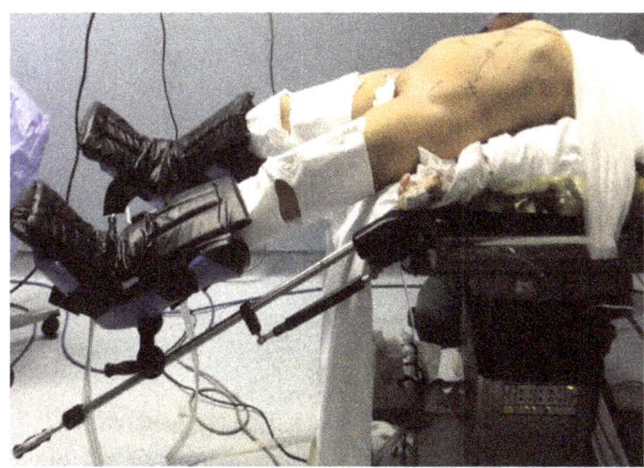

Figure 1: Modified Lloyd-Davis position.

4.3. Mark-Up and Trocar Placement. We adopted a totally robotic approach, so trocars were placed in the right and left lower quadrants (arms 1 and 2, respectively), approximately at the midclavicular lines. Arm 3 is placed in the left lateral abdomen, just superior to anterior iliac spine. An additional 5-mm trocar (assistant port) is placed in right upper quadrant, ***Figure 2***. We avoid placing the trocars too far laterally (particularly in a male patient) because collisions with the lateral pelvic sidewall will make the low pelvic dissection difficult. In the midline just superior and to the right of the umbilicus, we place the camera port which is always a 30-degree camera. Additional trocars are placed once insufflation is achieved to ensure the appropriate 8–10 cm distances between ports.

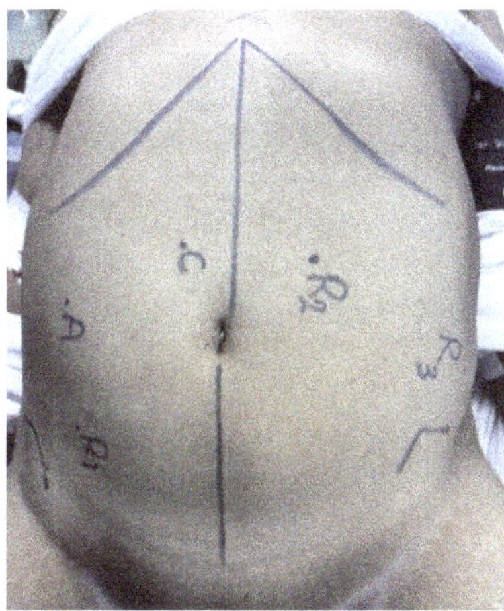

Figure 2: Mark-up.

4.4. Robotic Technique

4.4.1. Abdominal Phase (Part 1). The patient is placed in steep Trendelenburg position with the right side tilted downwards allowing the small bowel and the greater omentum to be reflected toward the right upper quadrant and the liver. We prefer in female patients to put a suture transabdominally straight forwardly through the fundus of the uterus to suspend the uterus in order to get an unhampered see into the pelvis. A monopolar scissors is at first utilized in arm 1, fenestrated bipolar forceps are utilized in arm 2, and a double-fenestrated atraumatic bowel grasper is set in arm 3. Utilizing arm 3, the rectosigmoid junction is gotten a handle on. Instead, a right hand may get a handle on this zone, permitting arm 3 to get a handle on more distally on the rectum to give us extra traction.

Dissection is conveyed upwards along the posterior part of the mesorectum toward the IMA, taking consideration not to break the fascia propria of the rectum and avoiding damage to the superior hypogastric nerves. We dissect specifically underneath the inferior mesenteric artery course and above the retroperitoneal fascial planes, the left ureter and gonadal vessels. The ureter and the gonadal vessels could be distinguished simply over the lateral pelvic wall and the pelvic brim. The IMA is elevated from the retroperitoneum and the ureter and gonadal vessels can be effortlessly swept bluntly posteriorly to keep up their situation inside the retroperitoneum, back and lateral to the IMA. We either control the IMA, IMV with clips, sutures, or sometimes Harmonic. The colonic mesentery would now be able to be lifted off the retroperitoneum proximally and along the side. The extent of dissection is superior to the inferior border of the pancreas and laterally overlying the Gerota's fascia. Now, one can rapidly disengage the lateral peritoneal connections to the left colon and sigmoid by beginning at the pelvic brim and continued proximally toward the splenic flexure.

4.4.2. Abdominal Phase (Part 2). In part 2 of the abdominal phase we deal with freeing the left colonic flexure. A double-fenestrated atraumatic grasper is placed in arm 1; a monopolar curved scissors and a bipolar fenestrated grasper are placed in arms 2 and 3 as required to help mobilizing the splenic flexure in a medial-to-lateral approach keeping the patient in the same position.

4.4.3. Pelvic Phase. We commonly start this dissection along the posterior, right side and proceed caudally, arm 2 pushes the rectum toward the patient's left side, and arm 1 is utilized to perform the dissection which is continued as far to the left pelvic side wall as conceivable to diminish what is needed to be dissected from the patient's left side. The posterior dissection is continued distally just behind the fascia propria of the rectum leaving behind the fascia of the neurovascular corridor intact to protect the hypogastric nerve plexuses. Upon approaching the lateral stalks, they are cut with monopolar cautery. Attention is then turned towards the anterior dissection. The assistant withdraw the rectum down and outside the pelvis. Arm 3 aids tension anterior at the level of the seminal vesicle or posterior vagina by retracting it superiorly and anteriorly. In patients with a tumor involving the posterior rectal wall, our dissection plane is always behind the Denonvilliers' fascia to get it out with the specimen. With anterior-based tumors, our dissection plane is almost always anterior to it.

4.4.4. Anastomotic Technique. If the ECHELON FLEX™ 45 mm stapler can be applied with adequate margin, a double-stapled anastomosis is performed, the rectum was transected with the endoscopic stapler and the specimen was retrieved through a Pfannenstiel or a small incision in the left iliac fossa in most cases. An intracorporeal anastomosis is performed with transanal insertion of a circular stapler. The anastomosis is routinely checked by transanal insufflation of air. When the endoscopic stapler could not be applied with an adequate margin below the tumor, transanal resection and coloanal hand-sewn anastomosis is performed

A diverting loop ileostomy is routinely used in patients with low (below the anterior peritoneal reflection) anastomoses or those patients who received preoperative radiation therapy. Consideration for ileostomy reversal occurs 3 months after the index operation or once any potential adjuvant therapy is completed.

4.4.5. Postoperative Policy. We adopted during this work an enhanced recovery care protocol for patients following either robotic or laparoscopic approach for rectal cancer. Preoperative counseling, adequate fluid and pain management, early feeding, and mobilization following surgery were implemented. The patients were discharged when they fulfilled the discharge criteria which include tolerance to oral diet, adequate pain control with oral analgesics, patient ambulating independently, afebrile patient without tachycardia, nonrising leucocyte count or C-reactive protein (CRP), and adequate home support with ability to take care of the stoma.

5. Statistical Analysis

Data management and analysis were performed using Statistical Package for Social Sciences (SPSS) vs. 23. Numerical data were summarized using medians and ranges. Categorical data were summarized as numbers and percentages. Numerical data were explored for normality using Kolmogorov-Smirnov test and Shapiro-Wilk test. Exploration of data revealed that the collected values were not normally distributed. Comparisons between two groups were done by Mann–Whitney test. Chi-square or Fisher's tests were used to compare between the groups with respect to categorical data, as appropriate. All p-values are two-sided. P-values < 0.05 were considered significant.

6. Results

From April 2015 till February 2017, a total of fifty-seven patients with rectal cancer underwent permuted block randomization, ***Figure 3***. Of these patients, twenty-eight were assigned to undergo robotic-assisted rectal surgery and twenty-nine to undergo laparoscopic rectal surgery. After the exclusion of twelve patients following randomization for different reasons such as consent withdrawal, emergency surgery, or presence of metastasis, forty five patients (twenty-one in the robotic surgery group and twenty-four in the laparoscopic surgery group) were included in the analysis.

Patient demographic data and characteristics are shown in ***Table 1***. There were no significant differences between the groups in terms of age, gender, BMI, ASA score, clinical stage, distance of the tumor from the anal verge, rate of receiving upfront chemoradiation, and rate of no residual lesions after such preoperative therapy. The median age of patients in the robotic surgery group was 53.4 years (range from 32 to 67), while that of those in the conventional laparoscopic surgery group was 50.3 years (range from 36 to 64) ($P = 0.241$). 47.6% of the patients in the robotic group have BMI below 30 kg/m2, while the other 52.4% have BMI above 30. On the other hand, most of the patients in the laparoscopic group (66%) have BMI above 30, while the remaining 33% were below 30 kg/m2 BMI ($P= 0.329$). There was a significant difference in terms of sex, albeit more male patients underwent laparoscopic surgery (42.4% in the robotic group versus 54.2% in the laparoscopic group).

Twelve patients in the robotic group received upfront therapy (57.1%) compared to eleven patients (45.8%) in the laparoscopic group with p value 0.449 and only one patient in each group showed complete clinical and radiological response.

Operative data are compared and recorded in Table 2. In the robotic-assisted surgery group, nine patients underwent anterior resection (42.9%), seven underwent low anterior resection (33.3%), four underwent ultra-low anterior resection (19%), and only one patient (4.8%) underwent abdominoperineal resection (APR). On the other side, the laparoscopic group, thirteen patients underwent anterior resection (54.2%), seven underwent low anterior resection (29.1%), one underwent ultra-low resection (4.2%), and finally four underwent APR (12.5%). The preparation time (time from induction of anesthesia to console) was significantly longer in the robotic group with a median of fifty-five minutes compared to twenty-eight minutes in the laparoscopic group with a p value less than 0.001. Similarity, the actual operative time (time from console to wound closure) was also longer in the robotic group with a median of 201 minutes in contrast to 134.5 minutes in the laparoscopic group with a statistically significant p value of less than 0.001. Although not clinically obvious, the estimated blood loss was statistically significantly lower in the robotic group than

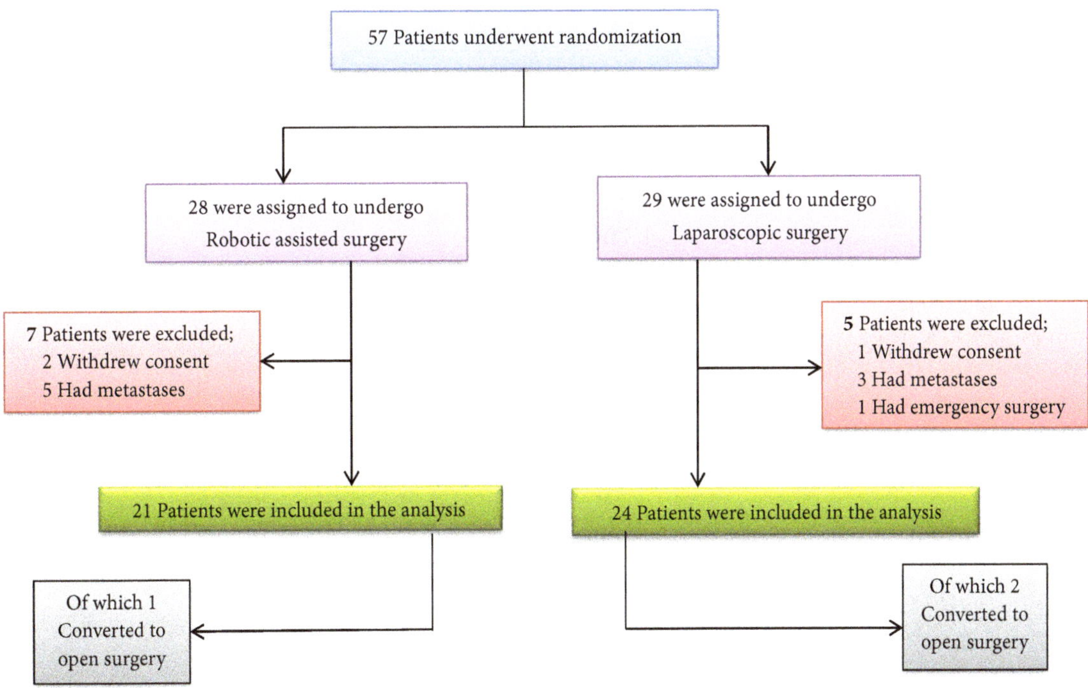

FIGURE 3: Patient enrollment.

TABLE 1: Patients demographic data and characteristics.

	Robotic No. 21	Laparoscopic No. 24	p value
Age	53.4 (32-67)	50.3 (36-64)	0.241
Gender			0.905
Female	10 (47.6%)	11 (45.8%)	
Male	11 (42.4%)	13 (54.2%)	
MBI (kg/m2)			0.329
(i) < 30	10 (47.6%)	08 (33.3%)	
(ii) >/= 30	11 (52.4%)	16 (66.7%)	
ASA score			
(i) Healthy	18 (85.7%)	18 (75%)	
(ii) Mild systemic disease	03 (14.3%)	06 (25%)	
Distance from anal verge			
(i) Upper rectum	9 (42.9%)	13 (54.2%)	
(ii) Middle rectum	10 (47.6%)	8 (33.3%)	
(iii) Lower rectum	2 (9.5%)	3 (12.%)	
Clinical stage			
(i) I	1	4	
(ii) II	15	17	
(iii) III	5	3	
Preoperative chemoradiation	12 (57.1%)	11 (45.8%)	0.449
No residual lesion	01 (4.8%)	01 (4.1%)	

in the laparoscopic group with a median of 200 ml versus 325 ml, respectively, with a p value of 0.050. Despite our initial experience in robotic colorectal surgery only one case required conversion to open surgery compared to two cases in the laparoscopic group. Five cases had stage migration in the robotic group between stages I, II, and III in comparison to eight cases in the laparoscopic group and at the end eleven patients representing 52.4% were in stage II and ten patients (47.6%) were in stage III, in the robotic group. On the other hand, seventeen patients (70.8%) and seven patients

TABLE 2: Operative data.

	Robotic No. 21	Laparoscopic No. 24	p value
Type of operation			
(i) Anterior resection	9 (42.9%)	13 (54.2%)	
(ii) Low anterior resection (LAR)	7 (33.3%)	7 (29.1%)	
(iii) Ultra-LAR	4 (19%)	1 (4.2%)	
(iv) APR	1 (4.8%)	3 (12.5%)	
Median preparation time (min)	55 (39-113)	28 (19-80)	<0.001
Median actual operative time (min)	201 (140-280)	134.5 (110-190)	<0.001
Median estimated blood loss (ml)	200 (50-650)	325 (100-800)	0.050
Convention to open surgery	1 (4.8%)	2 (8.3%)	
Pathological stage			0.203
(i) II	11 (52.4%)	17 (70.8%)	
(ii) III	10 (47.6%)	07 (29.2%)	
Median proximal margin (cm)	13 (10-20)	15 (11-23)	0.270
Median distal margin (cm)	2.8 (1.4-4)	1.8 (1-2.8)	<0.001
CRM quality			0.079
(i) Complete	18 (85.7%)	15 (62.5%)	
(ii) Partly complete	03 (14.3%)	09 (37.5%)	
Median LN retrieved (no.)	14 (8-20)	13 (9-21)	0.498

TABLE 3: Immediate Postoperative Outcomes.

	Robotic No. 21	Laparoscopic No. 24	p value
Flatus (median days)	2 (1-4.3)	1.6 (0.5 -5)	0.017
LOS (median days)	3 (2-14)	2 (2-11)	0.116
Complications			0.965
Anastomotic leakage	1 (4.8%)	1 (4.2%)	
Ileus (median days)	2 (9.5%)	3 (12.5%)	
Wound problems	2 (9.5%)	2 (8.3%)	
Others	1 (DVT)	1(erectile dysfunction)	
Reoperation	0	1 (4.2%)	
Readmission	1 (4.8%)	1 (4.2%)	
Death	0	1 (4.2%)	

(29.2%) in the laparoscopic group were in stages II and III, respectively. The median distal margin was 2.8 cm in the robotic group, while in the laparoscopic group it was 1.8 cm. This was statistically significant with a p value less than 0.001. Although the circumferential radial margin (CRM) was complete in 18 patients (85.7%) in the robotic group in contrast to 15 patients (62.5%) in the laparoscopic group, it did not differ statistically with a p value of 0.079. There was no statistically significant difference in the number of retrieved lymph nodes with a median of fourteen versus thirteen nodes in the robotic and laparoscopic groups, respectively, and a p value of 0.498. In a similar manner, there was no difference between the two groups in the length of the proximal margin.

Postoperatively, ***Table 3***, the median time to passage of first flatus was 2 days in the robotic group and 1.6 days in the laparoscopic group; this was significant statistically with a p value of 0.017. The median length of hospital stay (LOS) was 3 days for patients in the robotic group and only 2 days for patients in the laparoscopic group. This was owing to adoption of a fast track protocol, with no significant statistical difference between the two groups, p value 0.116. The overall postoperative complication rates did not differ between the two groups. Anastomosis leakage occurred once in each group; in the robotic group, the leakage was minimal and was managed successfully conservatively, but unfortunately in the laparoscopic one, the patient was 48-year-old female with mid-rectal cancer who received upfront chemoradiation and known to be diabetic and underwent laparoscopic low anterior resection with covering ileostomy. The leakage was discovered on day 1 with fecal matter coming through the drain with rapid deterioration of the general condition. After adequate resuscitation, a laparoscopic exploration revealed posterior wall disruption with peritoneal soiling. After completion of peritoneal lavage, we thought of two options

TABLE 4: Severity of complications according to Clavien-Dindo classification.

Clavien-Dindo Classification	Robotic No. 21	Laparoscopic No. 24	P Value
No complications	15(71.4%)	18(75%)	0.787
Grade I	4(19.04%) "2 wound infections + 2 ileus"	5(20.83%) "1 erectile dysfunction+ 2 wound infection+2 ileus"	
Grade II	1(4.8%) "DVT"	1(4.2%) "ileus"	
Grade III	1(4.8%) "leakage"	0	
Grade IV	0	0	
Grade V	0	1	

either performing a Hartman's procedure or refashioning the edges and resuturing the two ends, hand sewing and covering the anastomosis with the already present ileostomy and the latter was opted. We thought that adequate lavage, drainage, and the defunctioning ileostomy were sufficient but things do not always go as you wish. The patient was transferred to the ICU, extubated. The next day the general condition continued to deteriorate with tachycardia over 120/min, tachypnea, and metabolic acidosis with rising acute phase reactants. Her duplex study, echocardiography, and cardiac enzymes detected no abnormality. The patient died on day three. In the robotic surgery group, postoperative ileus occurred in two patients compared to three patients in the laparoscopic group and was managed conservatively in both groups. Wound problems in the form of infection or suture disruption (in APR cases) took place in four patients, divided equally between the two groups. One patient had DVT in the robotic group and one in the laparoscopic group complained of erectile dysfunction.

No reoperation or mortality occurred in the robotic surgery group with only one patient readmitted for disrupting perineal wound following abdominoperineal resection. On the other side, one patient was readmitted on postoperative day 3 because of fever and chest infection, also one patient was reoperated upon and unfortunately died.

According to Clavien-Dindo classification of surgical outcomes, complications occurred in six patients in the robotic group and were primarily of grade one, ***Table 4***. One case suffered from deep venous thrombosis and managed with anticoagulants. There was evidence of anastomotic leakage with pelvic collection in another one case of this group dealt with conservatively and with image-guided percutaneous drainage. Comparably, seven cases in the laparoscopic group have complications; five of them in grade one and one case have prolonged paralytic ileus necessitating administration of parenteral nutrition. Grade 5 complications occurred once in this study, Table 4

7. Discussion

Come closer! Do not shake! Stay there! Turn right! Left! This is one of the real practical differences between robotic-assisted and laparoscopic surgery wherein the surgeon is still an assistant-dependent.

Of no doubt, rectal surgery underwent an immense wave of change from various perspectives since the beginning of the twenty-first century. There was a smart shift from open to minimally invasive and robotic techniques, a worldwide application of neoadjuvant multimodal chemoradiation therapy for locally advanced stage disease, as well as optimization of surgical technique with nerve preservation together with the introduction of total mesorectal excision (TME) which was all largely happening in the preceding 10–15 years.

However, laparoscopic rectal cancer resection is a complex procedure with a long learning curve, and conventional laparoscopic surgery in the pelvis is difficult, particularly in cases of a bulky tumor in the deep male pelvis. Thus, the conversion rate to the open approach in the CLASICC trial was over 30% [5] and in the COLOR II trial it was 17% [6].

For any new operative technique to become an accepted alternative to conventional methods, it must be proved safe and must result in comparable outcomes. For instance, studies have emerged since the adoption of laparoscopy for colorectal operations that have shown that it can shorten hospital stay, yielding oncologically adequate resection, with no evident differences in postoperative complications or hospital mortality when compared with a traditional open approach. Because of studies like these, laparoscopy is now considered a reasonable alternative to an open approach in colorectal resection [7, 8]. Moreover, other reviews have already demonstrated robotic rectal surgery to be safe and feasible [9–11], although there are no published studies demonstrating its superiority over the laparoscopic approach mainly due to the lack of randomized control trials.

In our study, there was no significant difference between the robotic and laparoscopic groups in terms of age, gender, BMI, ASA, distance from the anal verge, preoperative clinical stage, and rate of upfront chemoradiation. The operations in the current study were performed by a group of experienced laparoscopic surgeons and honesty considered beginners robotic surgeons. Not surprisingly, we admitted that laparoscopic proctectomy is a challenging particularly with bulky tumors in males with narrow pelvis and required complicated maneuvers to reach the extremes of the pelvis. The sphincter-preserving rate was high in the robotic-assisted group 19% compared to 4.2% in the laparoscopic group and abdominoperineal resection was performed in only one patient (4.8%) in the robotic-assisted group in contrast to nearly triple percentage (12.5%) in the laparoscopic group.

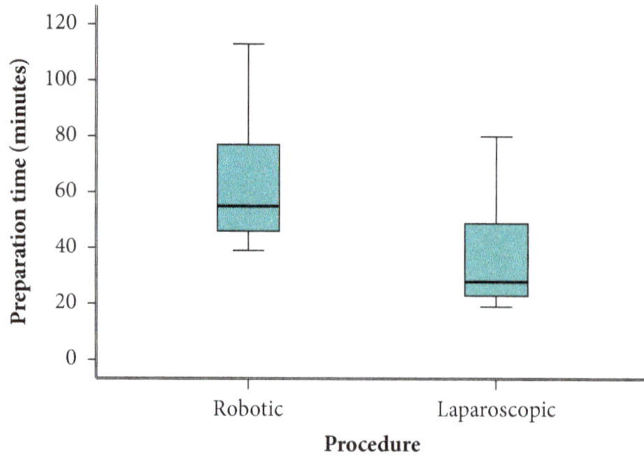

FIGURE 4: Preparation time.

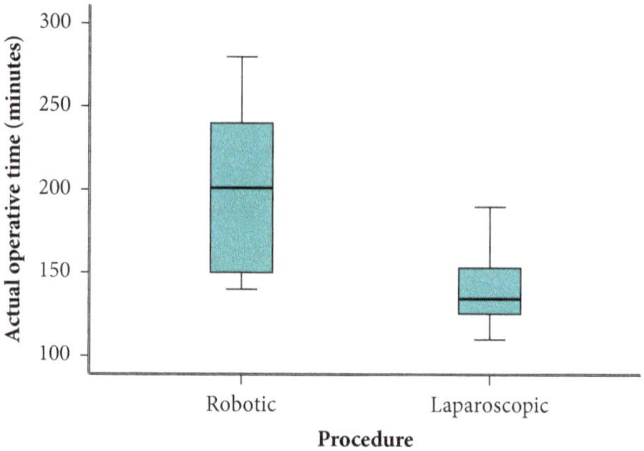

FIGURE 5: Actual operative time.

Such difference may be attributed to the technical characteristics of the robot platform, most importantly, the optimal stable operative pelvic view, the endowrist function, and the countertraction with optimal direction and force using the great third robotic instrument attached to the fourth robotic arm; these are certainly advantageous when compared with the conventional rigid laparoscopic instruments when the pelvis is addressed during surgery.

As regards the conversion rate, only one robotic case was converted to open approach due to bulky mid-rectal tumor in a very narrow male pelvis with no access to reach a comfortable distal margin; it is worth mentioning that it was the second robotic case in the study. On the opposite side, two cases were converted from the laparoscopic approach to the open one. Even though the conversion rate was almost doubled in the laparoscopic approach, this could not be evident statistically due to the small number of cases but resembles the results of Ielpo and associates [12] who suggested that the robotic approach has lower conversion rates when the tumor location requests a low anterior resection and as a consequence, the operation is technically more challenging. In converted cases being associated with greater morbidity and tumor recurrence [13], robotic surgery could provide better oncologic long-term results as well as decreased perioperative morbidity.

An obvious finding of this trial is the longer preparation time ***(Figure 4)*** (median time 55 versus 28 minutes) and actual operative time ***(Figure 5)*** (201 versus 134.5 minutes) of robotic surgery and laparoscopic surgery, respectively, with a very significant p value in both times of less than 0.001. These results are justified by the time used to dock and undock the robotic system, even in presence of an experienced surgical team. It happens not infrequently that patients on the surgical table require different positions, so the robotic cart needs to be undocked and redocked several times during the same procedure. This extends the operative time. Undoubtedly, the standardization of step by step surgical procedures together with the continuous training of the whole surgical team (surgeons, nurses, anesthesiologists, and operation room staff) can improve the quality of the operations and lead to a progressive reduction of the operative time. Classically speaking, longer operative time is related to increased morbidity, most likely related to the difficulty of the operation [11]; however, prolonged times in robotic surgery are not associated with increased complications as declared by this study and previously published review and meta-analysis of Luca and associates [14].

This randomized trial reported a significantly lower estimated blood loss after robotic rectal surgery (p value =0.050). A recent case-controlled analysis comparing TME between robotic and laparoscopic methods did not show any significant difference in the amount of blood loss [15]. A separate meta-analysis review reaffirmed these findings [16]. The number of harvested lymph nodes is indispensable in the postoperative tumor staging and hence the right treatment for more patients. Of course, its accuracy increases with the number of nodes retrieved within the surgical specimen and should be at least 12, as settled by the last AJCC [17]. In this work, this target was always respected by the high ligation policy of the IMA, both in the laparoscopic and in the robotic group. The difference between the harvested lymph nodes in the robotic (median: 14, range: 8 to 20) and laparoscopic (median: 13, range 9 to 21) groups was not substantial in our study; p value was 0.498. Comparably, previous studies comparing robotic and laparoscopic rectal cancer surgery have shown no significant differences in the number of lymph nodes harvested [18–22]. Eight cases in our study have less than 12 lymph nodes retrieved in their final surgical specimens of which there are 5 in the robotic group and 3 cases in the other arm. Remarkably, 7 cases have received neoadjuvant chemotherapy and two of which have shown complete radiological response with no residual tumor or induration but only one of these two cases showed complete pathological response.

Tumor response assessment of the other 5 cases after upfront chemoradiation by MRI showed partial regression. Coincidence of good tumor response and the low number of harvested lymph nodes raises the probability of better locoregional disease control rather than poor diligence of the surgical or pathological teams. Unfortunately, the small number of cases stands as an obstacle to draw a definitive commentary.

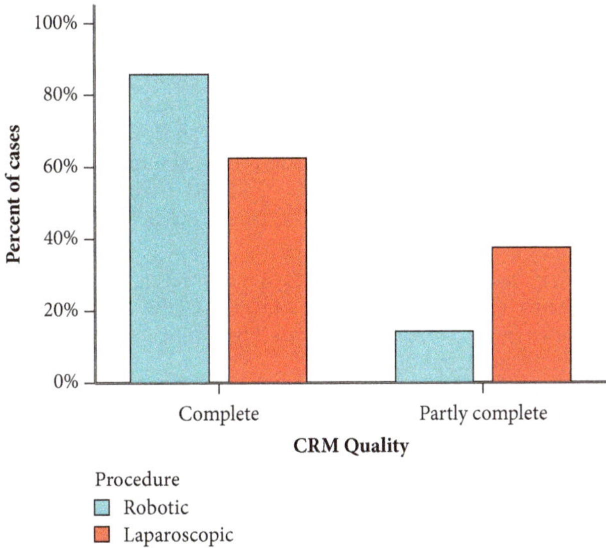

FIGURE 6: CRM quality.

The quality of the circumferential radial margin together with the distal margin is considered leading parameters in evaluating the treatment of rectal cancer. Findings from the present work seem to determinate the superiority of robotic surgery over the laparoscopic approach, ***Figure 6,*** with ability to dissect adequately beyond the lower limit of the tumor in the robotic group (median: 2.8, range: 1.4-4 cm) when compared to the laparoscopic group (median: 1.8, range: 1-2.8). This was evident statistically with a p value of less than 0.001. Even though not statistically significant, achievement of a complete circumferential radial margin, i.e., completeness of the fascia propria of the rectum, occurred in more than 85% of case in the robotic group compared to 62.5% in the laparoscopic group (p value: 0.079). In a similar fashion, a significant wider CRM in their robotic series when compared to the laparoscopic ones was reported by Barnajian [23] and D'Annibale [24].

One of the main benefits of minimally invasive surgery is the early recovery. During this trial we adopted an enhanced recovery protocol wherein sips of water were started on postoperative day (POD) 0, liquid diet on POD 1, and soft diet on POD 2. Patients were nursed in an environment that encouraged independence and mobilization. Patients were strongly encouraged to be out of bed longer than 2 hours beginning on the day after operation. Our discharge criteria included afebrile patient without tachycardia, tolerance of oral feeding, adequate control of pain with oral analgesia, patient ambulating independently, nonrising leucocyte count or CRP, and adequate support at home. Despite being indistinct clinically, there was a significant difference in the day of first flatus in favor of the laparoscopic group 1.6 days compared to 2 days in the robotic group, p value: 0.017.

This study did not show a significant difference between both groups in terms of hospitalization (LOS), complication rate, reoperation, or readmission. Anastomotic leak is the most severe surgical complication in colorectal surgery. Endorsed risk factors for anastomotic leak are cancers located below the peritoneal reflection, irradiated pelvis, obesity, and intraoperative blood transfusions [25, 26]. A covering ileostomy was adopted in presence of any of these hazardous criteria. In this study, the overall anastomotic leakage rates in the robotic and laparoscopic series were similar (4.8% versus 4.2%).

The discern advantage of the robotic high definition 3D image allows better identification of autonomic nerves. Potential sites of nerve damage are the superior hypogastric plexus, leading to ejaculatory dysfunction in males and impaired lubrication in females, and the pelvic splanchnic nerves deep in the lateral pelvic wall leading to erectile dysfunction in men which occurred in one patient in the laparoscopic group representing 4.2% compared to 0% in the robotic group in sight of this study. We adopt a short questionnaire to assess the sexual function including failure of ejaculation or erection and whether failure of the latter is complete or partial i.e., difficulty in penetration or in maintaining erection. We have only one case who complained of partial erectile dysfunction. According to results of the CLASSIC trial [27], autonomic injury risk with sexual dysfunction in males is significantly higher in laparoscopic surgery when compared to the open approach. In the same context, two studies suggested that robotic-assisted rectal surgery is better than conventional laparoscopic surgery in preventing sexual or urinary dysfunction [26, 28].

It is worth mentioning than the most important point of strength in this work is being randomized by permuted block randomization trying to minimize the selection bias.

We have also to mention about the weakness of this study. First, the small sample size prevents us from drawing proper conclusions, especially for each type of procedure. Moreover, this study did not focus properly in the functional outcome aside from a short follow-up period of one month. Finally, the different stand points of experience between robotic and laparoscopic rectal surgery among surgeons may fail to signify the great technical characteristics of the robotic platform.

8. Conclusion

To our knowledge, this is the first prospective randomized trial of robotic rectal surgery in the Middle East and Northern Africa region.

Our early experience indicates that robotic rectal surgery is a feasible and safe procedure. It is not inferior to standard laparoscopy in terms of oncologic radicality and surgical complications.

This randomized control trial on 45 patients has demonstrated that the distal margin and the quality of the CRM with the robotic system are better than conventional laparoscopy but with an obvious weak spot of longer operative time. Of course more randomized trials with larger sample size are needed to stabilize the robotic approach in rectal cancer surgery. Furthermore, the current commercial robotic platform is best suited for a single quadrant confined dissection. As such, it has some limitations in rectal surgery where more than one quadrant is involved. On the contrary, the perfect stable operative view, the wrist-like function, and the optimal direction and force created by the third robotic instrument might improve the diffusion of this minimally invasive technology in the treatment of rectal cancer.

Finally, it is just a beginning, as we believe; it is very difficult to imagine a surgeon in the further future working without interface.

Abbreviations

RCT: Randomized controlled trial
BMI: Body mass index
ASA: American Society of Anesthesiologists
CRM: Circumferential radial margin
TME: Total mesorectal excision
CRT: Chemoradiation therapy
MBO: Malignant bowel obstruction
IRB: Institutional Review Board
NCI: National Cancer Institute
LOS: Length of stay
IMA: Inferior mesenteric artery
CRP: C-reactive protein
SPSS: Statistical package for social sciences
LAR: Low anterior resection
APR: Abdominoperineal resection
DVT: Deep venous thrombosis
POD: Postoperative day.

Consent

All of the patients provided written informed consent before the surgical procedures.

Authors' Contributions

All authors participated in writing the different sections of the current study and have read and approved the final manuscript.

Acknowledgments

This study was supported by Professor Dr. Sherif Maamoun, Head of Surgical Oncology Department at NCI, Cairo University, Egypt, and Professor Dr. Omar Zakaria, President Elect of Breast Cancer International (BSI). This study was all funded by the National Cancer Institute, Cairo University, Egypt.

References

[1] M. Jacobs, J. C. Verdeja, and H. S. Goldstein, "Minimally invasive colon resection (laparoscopic colectomy)," in *Surgical Laparoscopy Endoscopy*, vol. 1, pp. 144–150, 1991.

[2] G. B. Makin, D. J. Breen, and J. R. T. Monson, "The impact of new technology on surgery for colorectal cancer," *World Journal of Gastroenterology*, vol. 7, no. 5, pp. 612–621, 2001.

[3] H. J. Bonjer, C. L. Deijen, G. A. Abis et al., "A randomized trial of laparoscopic versus open surgery for rectal cancer," *The New England Journal of Medicine*, vol. 372, no. 14, pp. 1324–1332, 2015.

[4] A. Adkins, M. Albert, D. Alsaleh et al., "Low Anterior Resection/Proctectomy," in *Robotic Approaches to Colorectal Surgery*, H. Ross et al., Ed., pp. 157–164, Springer International Publishing, Switzerland.

[5] P. J. Guillou, P. Quirke, H. Thorpe et al., "Short-term endpoints of conventional versus laparoscopic-assisted surgery in patients with colorectal cancer (MRC CLASICC trial): multicentre, randomised controlled trial," *The Lancet*, vol. 365, no. 9472, pp. 1718–1726, 2005.

[6] M. H. van der Pas, E. Haglind, M. A. Cuesta et al., "Laparoscopic versus open surgery for rectal cancer (COLOR II): short-term outcomes of a randomised, phase 3 trial," *The Lancet Oncology*, vol. 14, no. 3, pp. 210–218, 2013.

[7] A. Biondi, G. Grosso, A. Mistretta et al., "Laparoscopic-assisted versusopen for colorectal cancer: short- and long-term outcomes comparison," *Journal of Laparoendoscopic & Advanced Surgical Techniques*, vol. 23, pp. 1–7, 2013.

[8] D. L. Vendramini, M. M. D. Albuquerque, E. M. Schmidt, E. E. Rossi-Junior, W. D. A. Gerent, and V. J. L. D. Cunha, "Laparoscopic and open colorectal resections for colorectal cancer.," *Arquivos brasileiros de cirurgia digestiva : ABCD = Brazilian archives of digestive surgery*, vol. 25, no. 2, pp. 81–87, 2012.

[9] A. Mirnezami, R. Mirnezami, A. K. Venkatasubramaniam, K. Chandrakumaran, T. Cecil, and B. Moran, "Robotic colorectal surgery: hype or new hope? A systematic review of robotics in colorectal surgery," *Colorectal Disease*, 2010.

[10] R. Scarpinata and E. H. Aly, "Does robotic rectal cancer surgery offer improved early postoperative outcomes?" *Diseases of the Colon & Rectum*, vol. 56, no. 2, pp. 253–262, 2013.

[11] T. W. Mak, J. F. Lee, K. Futaba, S. S. Hon, D. K. Ngo, and S. S. Ng, "Robotic surgery for rectal cancer: A systematic review of current practice," *World Journal of Gastrointestinal Oncology*, vol. 6, no. 6, p. 184, 2014.

[12] B. Ielpo, R. Caruso, Y. Quijano et al., "Robotic versus laparoscopic rectal resection: Is there any real difference? A comparative single center study," *The International Journal of Medical Robotics and Computer Assisted Surgery*, vol. 10, no. 3, pp. 300–305, 2014.

[13] J. Hance, T. Rockall, and A. Darzi, "Robotics in Colorectal Surgery," *Digestive Surgery*, vol. 21, no. 5-6, pp. 339–343, 2005.

[14] F. Luca, M. Valvo, T. L. Ghezzi et al., "Impact of robotic surgery on sexual and urinary functions after fully robotic nerve-sparing total mesorectal excision for rectal cancer," *Annals of Surgery*, vol. 257, no. 4, pp. 672–678, 2013.

[15] P. Allemann, C. Duvoisin, L. Di Mare, M. Hübner, N. Demartines, and D. Hahnloser, "Robotic-Assisted Surgery Improves the Quality of Total Mesorectal Excision for Rectal Cancer Compared to Laparoscopy: Results of a Case-Controlled Analysis," *World Journal of Surgery*, vol. 40, no. 4, pp. 1010–1016, 2016.

[16] S. H. Lee, S. Lim, J. H. Kim, and K. Y. Lee, "Robotic versus conventional laparoscopic surgery for rectal cancer: Systematic review and meta-analysis," *Annals of Surgical Treatment and Research*, vol. 89, no. 4, pp. 190–201, 2015.

[17] SB. Edge, DR. Byrd, CC. Compton, AG. Fritz, FL. Greene, and A. Trotti, *AJCC Cancer Staging Handbook*, Springer-Verlag, NewYork, NY, 7th edition, 2010.

[18] P. P. Bianchi, C. Ceriani, A. Locatelli et al., "Robotic versus laparoscopic total mesorectal excision for rectal cancer: A comparative analysis of oncological safety and short-term outcomes," *Surgical Endoscopy*, vol. 24, no. 11, pp. 2888–2894, 2010.

[19] J.-H. Baek, C. Pastor, and A. Pigazzi, "Robotic and laparoscopic total mesorectal excision for rectal cancer: A case-matched study," *Surgical Endoscopy*, vol. 25, no. 2, pp. 521–525, 2011.

[20] S. H. Baik, H. Y. Kwon, J. S. Kim et al., "Robotic versus laparoscopic low anterior resection of rectal cancer: Short-term outcome of a prospective comparative study," *Annals of Surgical Oncology*, vol. 16, no. 6, pp. 1480–1487, 2009.

[21] J. M. Kwak, S. H. Kim, J. Kim, D. N. Son, S. J. Baek, and J. S. Cho, "Robotic vs laparoscopic resection of rectal cancer: Short-term outcomes of a case-control study," *Diseases of the Colon & Rectum*, vol. 54, no. 2, pp. 151–156, 2011.

[22] J. S. Park, G.-S. Choi, K. H. Lim, Y. S. Jang, and S. H. Jun, "Robotic-assisted versus laparoscopic surgery for low rectal cancer: Case-matched analysis of short-term outcomes," *Annals of Surgical Oncology*, vol. 17, no. 12, pp. 3195–3202, 2010.

[23] M. Barnajian, D. Pettet, E. Kazi, C. Foppa, and R. Bergamaschi, "Quality of total mesorectal excision and depth of circumferential resection margin in rectal cancer: A matched comparison of the first 20 robotic cases," *Colorectal Disease*, vol. 16, no. 8, pp. 603–609, 2014.

[24] A. D'Annibale, G. Pernazza, I. Monsellato et al., "Total mesorectal excision: A comparison of oncological and functional outcomes between robotic and laparoscopic surgery for rectal cancer," *Surgical Endoscopy*, vol. 27, no. 6, pp. 1887–1895, 2013.

[25] Y. Liu, X. Wan, G. Wang et al., "A scoring system to predict the risk of anastomotic leakage after anterior resection for rectal cancer," *Journal of Surgical Oncology*, vol. 109, no. 2, pp. 122–125, 2014.

[26] N. C. Buchs, P. Gervaz, M. Secic, P. Bucher, B. Mugnier-Konrad, and P. Morel, "Incidence, consequences, and risk factors for anastomotic dehiscence after colorectal surgery: a prospective monocentric study," *International Journal of Colorectal Disease*, vol. 23, no. 3, pp. 265–270, 2008.

[27] M. Broholm, H.-C. Pommergaard, and I. Gögenür, "Possible benefits of robot-assisted rectal cancer surgery regarding urological and sexual dysfunction: A systematic review and meta-analysis," *Colorectal Disease*, vol. 17, no. 5, pp. 375–381, 2015.

[28] I. D. Nagtegaal, C. J. H. van de Velde, E. van der Worp, E. Kapiteijn, P. Quirke, and J. H. J. M. van Krieken, "Macroscopic evaluation of rectal cancer resection specimen: clinical significance of the pathologist in quality control," *Journal of Clinical Oncology*, vol. 20, no. 7, pp. 1729–1734, 2002.

34

Laparoscopic Cystectomy In-a-Bag of an Intact Cyst: Is It Feasible and Spillage-Free After All?

Stelios Detorakis, Dimitrios Vlachos, Stavros Athanasiou, Themistoklis Grigoriadis, Aikaterini Domali, Ioannis Chatzipapas, Emmanuel Stamatakis, Athanasios Mousiolis, Apostolos Patrikios, Aris Antsaklis, Dimitrios Loutradis, and Athanasios Protopapas

1st Department of Obstetrics and Gynecology of the University of Athens, Alexandra Hospital, 80 Queen Sophie Avenue and Lourou Street, 11528 Athens, Greece

Correspondence should be addressed to Athanasios Protopapas; prototha@otenet.gr

Academic Editor: Peng Hui Wang

This prospective study was conducted to assess the feasibility of laparoscopic cystectomy of an intact adnexal cyst performed inside a water proof endoscopic bag, aiming to avoid intraperitoneal spillage in case of cyst rupture. 102 patients were recruited. Two of them were pregnant. In 8 of the patients the lesions were bilateral, adding up to a total of 110 cysts involved in our study. The endoscopic sac did not rupture in any case. Mean diameter of the cysts was 5.7 cm (range: 2.3–10.5 cm). In 75/110 (68.2%) cases, cystectomy was completed without rupture, whereas in the remaining 35/110 (31.8%) cases the cyst ruptured. Minimal small spillage occurred despite every effort only in 8/110 (7.2%) cases with large (>8 cm) cystic teratomas. There were no intraoperative or postoperative complications. We concluded that laparoscopic cystectomy in-a-bag of an intact cyst is feasible and oncologically safe for cystic tumors with a diameter < 8 cm. Manipulation of larger tumors with the adnexa into the sac may be more difficult, and in such cases previous puncture and evacuation of the cyst contents should be considered.

1. Introduction

Advances in laparoscopic surgery over the past 3 decades have made the removal of most benign ovarian masses that previously required laparotomy technically possible. Laparoscopic surgery is less invasive, requires shorter hospitalization and recovery times, and is usually favored by young patients due to its better aesthetic results [1, 2]. However its role in the management of adnexal masses has become controversial, in terms of the oncological safety of such a procedure. The main concern is that iatrogenic rupture and spillage of contents of a malignant adnexal mass would upgrade the disease stage, resulting in a need for adjuvant chemotherapy and possibly compromising the overall survival of the patient [3, 4]. These concerns have led to several guidelines and restrictions concerning laparoscopic management of adnexal masses throughout the years, which are not generally adopted and change quite often [5, 6].

Laparoscopic cystectomy in-a-bag is a technique proposed for the management of suspicious adnexal cystic masses and has been described in the early '90s [7, 8]. Nevertheless, its real value in preventing spillage of contents in case of intraoperative rupture of a cyst has not been properly assessed in a prospective manner. Furthermore, under the preoperative term "suspicious adnexal masses" a variety of pathologies will be included with the majority representing benign ovarian swellings [9, 10].

Our study was designed to investigate prospectively the true value of a large waterproof and handle-free endoscopic sac in preventing spillage of contents after rupture of laparoscopically managed cystic adnexal masses. We also attempted to determine the probabilities of rupture for each of the several histologically different cystic masses encountered in a group of young patients, in whom an effort to excise the lesion intact was made. Our purpose was to recognize preoperative and intraoperative risk factors for rupture, and spillage after rupture, and set the limits for attempting excision of an intact cyst versus performing puncture and evacuation of its contents.

2. Materials and Methods

Patients with cystic adnexal masses referred for laparoscopic management to the Gynecological Endoscopy Unit of the 1st Department of Obstetrics & Gynecology of the University of Athens, "Alexandra" Hospital, Athens, Greece, from January 2009 to September 2013, were recruited for this prospective cohort study. The study was approved by our institution's scientific committee, and a detailed informed consent was obtained from all patients.

The standard preoperative triage included a complete clinical and gynecological examination and tumor markers (CEA, CA-125, CA19-9, a-fetoprotein, and β-hCG), plus a detailed pelvic transvaginal (TVS) and/or transabdominal (TAS) ultrasound scan. During ultrasonographic examination the following characteristics of the adnexal mass were looked for and recorded: size, appearance of fluid content, presence of a solid component, septations, papillary projections into the cyst or surface excrescences, the thickness of the cyst wall, presence of neovascularization, and the cyst's uni- or bilateral localization. An abdominal CT scan or MRI was occasionally performed to assist in the differential diagnosis. Women > 45 years old, those with a preoperative diagnosis of an endometrioma, and those with probable invasive ovarian cancer were excluded from this study. Cases with possible functional cysts were reexamined after 3-4 months and were scheduled for laparoscopy were the lesion persisted.

Ovarian masses included in our sample were allocated into four groups regarding their sonographic characteristics: fluid filled structures, anechoic or of low echogenicity, possible teratomas, paraovarian cysts, and masses that could not be classified as benign or malignant based on their sonographic appearance. Fluid filled ovarian lesions were subgrouped into unilocular and multilocular. Ovarian lesions presenting with mixed echogenicity, consisting of longitudinal white lines or a Rokitansky nodule, and showing acoustic shadows were categorized as teratomas. Unilocular, anechoic cystic masses observed nearby the ovary were allocated in a separate group. Finally, ovarian cystic lesions that could not be preoperatively reported as definitely benign were characterized as suspicious. Presence of papillary projections, meaning inner irregularities of cystic wall > 3 mm, and presence of a solid component were taken into account. Solid parts, in particular, were differentiated from Rokitansky nodules based on the presence or not of acoustic shadows. Because of the expected high prevalence of benign masses in our group of patients, size per se was not considered a single criterion to characterize the mass as suspicious or not, despite the fact that lesion size may affect preoperative diagnosis [11–13].

Laparoscopic surgery was performed using the technique of 4 trocars: one primary trocar was placed through a vertical intraumbilical incision, allowing the use of a 10 mm, 0-degree laparoscope. Another two accessory trocars (5 mm) were inserted in the lower abdomen lateral to the inferior

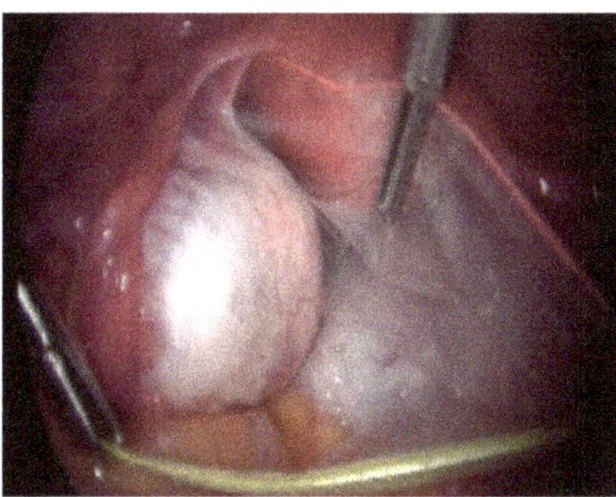

FIGURE 1: Cyst-harboring adnexa inside handle-free endoscopic sac.

epigastric vessels and a fourth accessory trocar (5 mm) was inserted above the pubic hairline.

After insertion of the laparoscope, a careful and thorough inspection of the pelvis and abdomen was performed and peritoneal washings or free peritoneal fluid was taken for cytological examination. The waterproof endoscopic bag (Unimax, Medical Technology Promedt, Consulting GmBH, $5'' \times 7''$) was inserted blindly into the peritoneal cavity wrapped tightly into its plastic applicator through the umbilical trocar and opened by unrolling it with atraumatic forceps, after replacing the laparoscope. The lesion-harboring adnexa was placed and kept inside the bag throughout its dissection (Figure 1). The endoscopic bag used in our study was not attached to an external manipulator; instead it was supplied with a lasso at its rim made of a memory wire aimed to be tightened in the end of the procedure to allow for safe specimen extraction. Laparoscopic cystectomy was performed without previous evacuation of the cyst, making an effort to keep the adnexa inside the sac throughout the procedure and excise the cyst intact. In case of inadvertent rupture even minimal leakage was recorded. In cases with bilateral cysts the side harboring the smaller cyst was treated first.

The ovarian capsule was incised with scissors and the cleavage plane between cyst and ovary was identified. The cyst was enucleated from the surrounding ovarian tissue mainly by means of blunt dissection and/or aqua dissection. Dense adhesions between the cyst and ovarian stroma were divided sharply with scissors after bipolar coagulation, closer to the surface of the cyst. In cases with suspicious masses the technique was slightly modified and the adhesions were divided closer to the ovary than the cyst to allow for a safety margin. In case of rupture during cyst dissection the instrument tips were washed with normal saline, while inside the bag, before removing them from the peritoneal cavity.

After excision of the cyst, the left 5 mm accessory trocar was replaced by a 10 mm trocar. The end of the wire was pulled outside the peritoneal cavity through this trocar which was removed, and the closed mouth of the bag was retrieved through the skin incision and opened extracorporeally. The cyst was deflated inside the bag using a needle or another cutting instrument and a suction pump, in order to reduce its volume and make the extraction of the bag and the remaining cyst possible without contamination of the abdominal wall.

TABLE 1: Distribution of our cases according to the final histological diagnosis.

Final histology	Rupture		Spillage		MCD		Total
	No N (%)	Yes N (%)	No N (%)	Yes N (%)	Mean cm	Range cm	N
Serous cystadenoma	10 (62.5)	6 (37.5)	14 (87.5)	2 (12.5)	6.98	4.8–9.5	16
Mucinous cystadenoma	3 (18.8)	13 (81.3)	11 (68.8)	5 (31.3)	7.61	4.3–10.5	16
Serous cystadenofibroma	5 (83.3)	1 (16.7)	6 (100.0)	0 (0.0)	6.43	5.0–10.0	6
Simple serous cyst	11 (91.7)	1 (8.3)	12 (100.0)	0 (0.0)	4.47	3.2–6.1	12
Benign cystic teratoma	33 (73.3)	12 (26.7)	44 (97.8)	1 (2.2)	5.17	2.3–8.2	45
Borderline ovarian tumor	2 (50.0)	2 (50.0)	0 (0.0)	0 (0.0)	7.40	5.2–8.6	4
Paraovarian cyst	11 (100.0)	0 (0.0)	11 (100.0)	0 (0.0)	6.25	4.0–9.0	11
Total	75 (68.2)	35 (31.8)	102 (92.7)	8 (7.3)	5.70	2.3–10.5	110

Whenever a solid component was prominent the incision was enlarged to allow for easier and safer extraction.

Based on final histology the following histological groups emerged and are used for analysis: serous cystadenoma, mucinous cystadenoma, benign cystadenofibroma, simple serous cyst, benign mature cystic teratoma, paraovarian cyst, and borderline ovarian tumor.

3. Statistics

Statistical analysis was performed with the Statistics Package for Social Sciences (SPSS) version 15. An independent samples t-test and the nonparametric Mann-Whitney U test were used to compare MCDs between cases with and without rupture, and between cases with and without spillage. The Chi-square and Fisher's exact tests were used to determine the statistical significance during comparisons of categorical data.

The logistic regression model provided the estimated probability of rupture and spillage for any particular case. In this model the MCD was used as an independent variable. A p value of less than 0.05 was considered as statistically significant.

4. Results

All 102 cases included in this study were operated on by a single senior surgeon (AP) to ensure consistency in the operative technique. In 8 cases the lesions were bilateral, which made a total of 110 cysts available for analysis. Two patients were pregnant and their procedure was performed during the second trimester of pregnancy. Another 6 cases, 4 with endometriomas and 2 with functional cysts with an erroneous preoperative diagnosis discovered during surgery, were excluded from this study.

Patients and maximum cyst diameters per group of final histology are summarized in Table 1. Mean patient age was 28.9 years (range: 12–44). Mean maximum diameter of the cysts (MCD) was 5.7 cm (range: 2.3–10.5 cm). The endoscopic sac did not rupture in any case. In 75/110 (68.2%) cases, cystectomy was completed without rupture, whereas in the remaining 35/110 (31.8%) cases the cyst ruptured. Spillage occurred despite every effort in 8/110 (7.2%) cases, all with large (>8 cm) cystic teratomas. Rupture occurred in 32.1% (17/53) of the cysts with sonolucent fluid content, whereas, in 26.4% (14/53) of those with mixed solid and sonolucent contents and in 100% (4/4) of those with internal echos, the cyst ruptured.

The mean MCD of the cysts that ruptured independent of spillage was 6.75 cm and the mean MCD of those without rupture was 5.60 cm. This difference was statistically significant ($p < 0.001$). In the group of patients with rupture but no spillage the MCD was 6.10 cm and did not differ significantly compared with that of the no-rupture group. When attempting to determine a cutoff point of the MCD above which the probability of rupture (with or without spillage) increases significantly, this was set at 7.3 cm. Among ovarian cysts with a MCD $\geq$ 7.3 cm 57.7% (15/26) ruptured, compared with 23.8% (20/84) of those with a MCD < 7.3 cm ($p = 0.003$). The relative risk (RR) of rupture was 4.36 times greater for cysts with MCD $\geq$ 7.3 cm than for those with MCD < 7.3 cm (Figure 2).

Combining the final histological diagnosis and the MCD of the cyst with the probability of rupture, we found that ovarian cysts with a MCD $\geq$ 7.3 cm had an almost threefold (×2.94) higher RR of rupture than those with a MCD < 7.3 cm for a given histological type ($p = 0.040$). Mucinous cystadenomas in particular were more likely to rupture during their excision compared with other histological types of the same diameter; 81.3% (13/16) of the mucinous cystadenomas ruptured, whereas only 23.4% of the other histological types (22/94) did so during their excision ($p < 0.0001$). The RR of rupture for mucinous cystadenomas was 10.7 times higher compared with other histological types, for the same MCD (Figures 3 and 4).

In our study 31.8% of the ovarian cysts (35/110) ruptured during their excision with the previously described technique. In 22.9% (8/35) of these, spillage of their contents into the peritoneal cavity was recorded, and therefore the percentage of rupture and spillage in our study was 7.2% (8/110). The mean MCD of the ovarian cysts with spillage of their contents was 8.94 cm, which was significantly higher than the mean MCD of 5.74 cm of those without spillage (independent of rupture), and the mean MCD of 6.10 cm

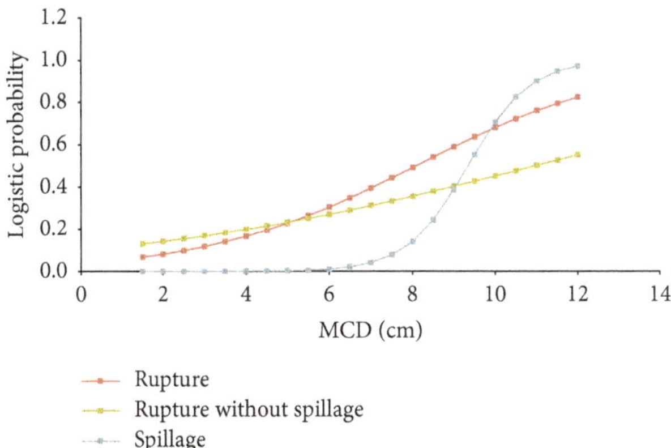

FIGURE 2: Probabilities of rupture with and without spillage in relation to MCD (cm).

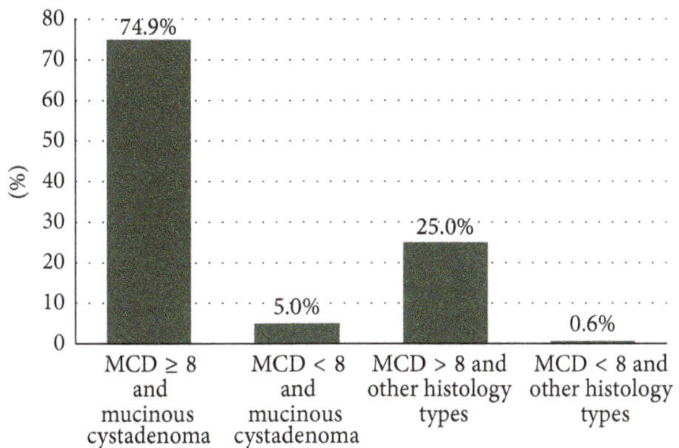

FIGURE 3: Probabilities of rupture in relation to MCD (cm) and cyst histology.

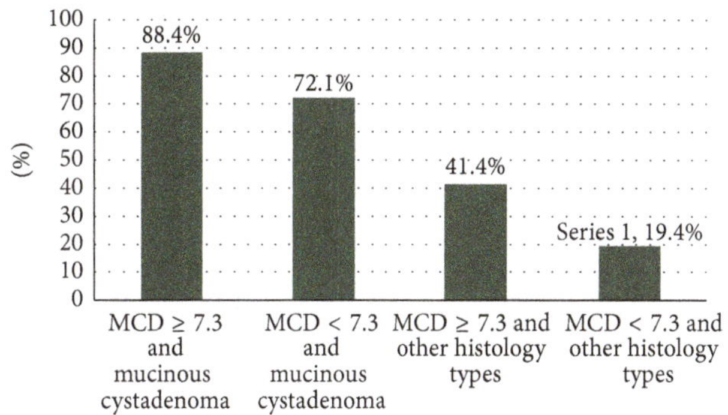

FIGURE 4: Probabilities of spillage in relation to MCD (cm) and cyst histology.

of those with rupture but no spillage ($p < 0.0001$, each comparison). In the group with rupture and spillage 5 of the 8 (62.5%) cases had mucinous cystadenomas. Moreover, 31.3% (5/16) of mucinous cystadenomas sustained spillage of their content. The percentage of spillage in all other histological types grouped together was significantly lower ($p = 0.002$).

We also tried to determine a cutoff point of statistical significance (according to what we did for cyst rupture) above which the probability of spillage of contents of a ruptured ovarian cyst into the peritoneal cavity increases significantly. This cutoff point was set at 8 cm. Among ovarian cysts with MCD ≥ 8 cm, 43.8% (7/16) sustained spillage, compared with only 1.1% (1/94) of those with MCD < 8 cm ($p < 0.0001$). In other words, the RR of spillage was 72 times higher for cysts ≥ 8 cm than for those < 8 cm. In the group of 35 cysts that ruptured during their excision and in relation to the cutoff point of 8 cm, in only 3.6% (1/28) of those with a MCD < 8 cm their contents were spilled after rupture, compared with 100% (7/7) of those with MCD ≥ 8 cm ($p < 0.001$).

Regarding the relation between the histological diagnosis of the cyst and the probability of spillage, we found that cysts with MCD ≥ 8 cm had a RR for spillage 56 times higher than those with MCD < 8 cm, among cysts with the same final histology (FH) ($p = 0.001$). Mucinous cystadenomas in particular, for the same MCD, had a RR for spillage 8.9 times higher than other histological types ($p = 0.033$). Borderline tumors, in particular, ruptured in 2/4 (50%) cases, including a pregnant patient, but without any spillage, whereas in none of the 11 paraovarian cysts ruptured.

Another interesting aspect in our study was to investigate how the increase of the MCD affects the probability of rupture and spillage. In order to determine that aspect, we developed three statistical models using as an independent variable the MCD and as a dependent variable the event of rupture with or without spillage (model 1), rupture without spillage (model 2), and finally rupture with spillage (model 3). For every 1 cm increase of the MCD, there is an average increase of the RR of rupture by 1.48 times ($p = 0.02$). For every 1 cm increase of the MCD, there is an average increase of the RR of rupture with spillage by 3.8 times ($p = 0.001$) (Figure 2).

5. Discussion

This prospective study was conducted to determine safety criteria for attempting the laparoscopic excision of an intact adnexal cyst using a handle-free endoscopic sac as protection from spillage. Our study population consisted exclusively of young patients desiring preservation of their full reproductive capacity. We believe that avoidance of spillage during cystectomy is of great importance not only for malignant cysts (because of disease upstaging), but also for benign ones, because of the possibility that the spilled content might cause chemical peritonitis and result in future periadnexal and intraperitoneal adhesions, even in the absence of symptoms [14, 15].

The operative management of adnexal cystic swellings (ACS) represents one of the commonest indications for laparoscopic gynecological surgery. Such a preoperative diagnosis may include several pathological entities: ovarian and nonovarian lesions, nonneoplastic and neoplastic masses, and, among these, benign, borderline, and even invasive neoplasms. Accurate preoperative and/or intraoperative diagnosis may be feasible on many occasions and impossible in others, for the reason that different pathologies may share a variety of similar morphological features [16–18].

"Suspicious adnexal mass" is a term used to describe a lesion that does not appear to be overt cancer but possesses several sonographic or morphologic characteristics that increase its likelihood of proving malignant at final histology [7, 19]. Despite the fact that even today many authorities consider laparoscopy an inappropriate tool to treat invasive ovarian cancer, the laparoscopic approach has been established over the years as the first-line operative modality to evaluate suspicious adnexal masses [19–21].

The prevalence of invasive ovarian cancer is highly variable in groups of patients with ovarian cystic swellings treated with laparoscopy. It depends on the studied population and is lowest in young patients < 40 years old [19, 22]. In this reproductive age group, laparoscopic cystectomy with ovarian preservation represents the treatment of choice for all benign lesions. After careful patient selection, even suspicious cystic masses may be treated conservatively, providing that all measures are taken to avoid intraoperative spillage in case of rupture. Obviously, removal from the peritoneal cavity of an intact cyst with extraperitoneal evacuation inside a waterproof endoscopic sac has the lowest risk of intraperitoneal spillage and contamination.

The main parameter that should be considered when choosing the right method to excise a cyst (with or without previous evacuation of its contents) is its maximal diameter. Rupture of a cyst does not necessarily lead to spillage of its contents into the peritoneal cavity, providing that it is always being excised in a waterproof laparoscopic sac, whereas rupture is obviously a prerequisite for spillage. Our study showed that the RR for rupture increases by 48% for every 1 cm rise in cyst diameter, whereas the RR for spillage quadruples, respectively. From a clinical perspective, the main concern is not so much to avoid rupture of a cyst but to avoid spillage. Therefore the cutoff point in cyst diameter with a major clinical significance was set at 8 cm. Based on our results, showing that 43.8% of the cysts with MCD ≥ 8 cm sustained spillage of their contents, compared with only 1.1% of those < 8 cm (in other words the RR of spillage was 72 times higher for cysts ≥ 8 cm), we can conclude that the technique of excision of an intact cyst, without previous evacuation of its contents, is effective and oncologically safe for lesions ≤ 8 cm. For larger ovarian cystic masses it is recommended to puncture and evacuate the cyst inside the sac and then remove its residual wall from the ovary.

Mucinous cystadenomas (the majority of which were multilocular) were associated with an almost 10-fold higher RR for rupture compared with other histological types (for the same MCD). It can be safely concluded that for cysts that give us morphologically the impression of a mucinous cystadenoma, it is safer to previously evacuate their content (always in a laparoscopic bag in order to avoid microspillage) and then excise the remaining cystic wall. This may require more than a single puncture.

An interesting finding of our study was the low rate of rupture for those cystic masses that were characterized as suspicious. Overall, only 3/14 (21.4%) cysts in this group (4 borderlines, 5 cystadenofibromas, 2 serous cystadenomas, and 3 teratomas) ruptured, with 0% spillage. For this group of patients the cystectomy technique, as it was mentioned above, was slightly different. With the modified technique, even in the group of patients with borderline ovarian tumors ($N = 4$), the rupture rate was 50% (one in a pregnant patient) with 0% spillage. This indicates (a) that laparoscopic cystectomy may be performed safely in a BOT without spillage and (b) that oophorectomy should not be the obligatory treatment of choice for suspicious cystic masses.

In conclusion, taking into account two major parameters in an adnexal cyst to be treated with laparoscopic cystectomy (maximum diameter and morphological profile) we were able to come up with a guideline concerning choice of the proper technique for its safe excision without spillage of its contents into the peritoneal cavity. Similarly, with proper patient selection, rupture could be avoided in a significant percentage of cases. In any case the adnexa harboring the lesion should be placed inside a waterproof laparoscopic sac and particular attention must be paid to keep it inside the sac throughout the procedure. In the unfortunate event that spillage occurs, cyst contents must be immediately removed by repeated washing and aspiration. Vigorous irrigation of the peritoneal cavity with saline solution, combined with positioning of the patient in the anti-Trendelenburg position by the end of the surgery, minimizes the risk of chemical peritonitis and possibly implantation of malignant cells.

Competing Interests

Drs. Stelios Detorakis, Dimitrios Vlachos, Stavros Athanasiou, Themistoklis Grigoriadis, Aikaterini Domali, Ioannis Chatzipapas, Emmanuel Stamatakis, Athanasios Mousiolis, Apostolos Patrikios, Aris Antsaklis, Dimitrios Loutradis, and Athanasios Protopapas have no competing interests or financial ties to disclose.

References

[1] L. Mettler, K. Semm, and K. Shive, "Endoscopic management of adnexal masses," *Journal of the Society of Laparoendoscopic Surgeons*, vol. 1, no. 2, pp. 103–112, 1997.

[2] M. Canis, B. Rabischong, C. Houlle et al., "Laparoscopic management of adnexal masses: a gold standard?" *Current Opinion in Obstetrics and Gynecology*, vol. 14, no. 4, pp. 423–428, 2002.

[3] A. J. Dembo, M. Davy, A. E. Stenwig, E. J. Berle, R. S. Bush, and K. Kjorstad, "Prognostic factors in patients with stage I epithelial ovarian cancer," *Obstetrics and Gynecology*, vol. 75, no. 2, pp. 263–273, 1990.

[4] I. Vergote, J. De Brabanter, A. Fyles et al., "Prognostic importance of degree of differentiation and cyst rupture in stage I invasive epithelial ovarian carcinoma," *The Lancet*, vol. 357, no. 9251, pp. 176–182, 2001.

[5] American College of Obstetricians and Gynecologists, "ACOG Practice Bulletin (2007) Management of adnexal masses," *Obstetrics & Gynecology*, vol. 110, no. 1, pp. 201–214, 2007.

[6] French College of Gynecologists and Obstetricians, "Recommendations for clinical practice: presumed benign ovarian tumors," *Journal de Gynécologie Obstétrique et Biologie de la Reproduction*, vol. 42, no. 8, pp. 856–866, 2013.

[7] A. Shushan, A. Protopapas, and A. L. Magos, "Laparoscopic "oophorectomy-in-a bag"-an alternative to laparotomy for the evaluation of suspicious ovarian masses," *Journal of Obstetrics and Gynaecology*, vol. 21, no. 4, pp. 399–401, 2001.

[8] A. Zanatta, M. M. S. Rosin, and L. Gibran, "Laparoscopy as the most effective tool for management of postmenopausal complex adnexal masses when expectancy is not advisable," *Journal of Minimally Invasive Gynecology*, vol. 19, no. 5, pp. 554–561, 2012.

[9] T. Slangen, P. Beretta, G. Catalano, R. Marana, and B. van Herendael, "Bag surgery as part of a protocol to treat ovarian masses by laparoscopy," *The Journal of the American Association of Gynecologic Laparoscopists*, vol. 1, no. 4, part 2, article S34, 1994.

[10] P. M. Yuen and M. S. Rogers, "Laparoscopic removal of ovarian cysts using a zipper storage bag," *Acta Obstetricia et Gynecologica Scandinavica*, vol. 73, no. 10, pp. 829–831, 1994.

[11] D. Timmerman, L. Valentin, T. H. Bourne, W. P. Collins, H. Verrelst, and I. Vergote, "Terms, definitions and measurements to describe the sonographic features of adnexal tumors: a consensus opinion from the International Ovarian Tumor Analysis (IOTA) group," *Ultrasound in Obstetrics and Gynecology*, vol. 16, no. 5, pp. 500–505, 2000.

[12] L. Savelli, A. C. Testa, D. Timmerman, D. Paladini, O. Ljungberg, and L. Valentin, "Imaging of gynecological disease (4): clinical and ultrasound characteristics of struma ovarii," *Ultrasound in Obstetrics and Gynecology*, vol. 32, no. 2, pp. 210–219, 2008.

[13] A. Di Legge, A. C. Testa, L. Ameye et al., "Lesion size affects diagnostic performance of IOTA logistic regression models, IOTA simple rules and risk of malignancy index in discriminating between benign and malignant adnexal masses," *Ultrasound in Obstetrics and Gynecology*, vol. 40, no. 3, pp. 345–354, 2012.

[14] S. Milingos, A. Protopapas, P. Drakakis et al., "Laparoscopic treatment of ovarian dermoid cysts: eleven years' experience," *Journal of the American Association of Gynecologic Laparoscopists*, vol. 11, no. 4, pp. 478–485, 2004.

[15] W. Kondo, N. Bourdel, B. Cotte et al., "Does prevention of intraperitoneal spillage when removing a dermoid cyst prevent granulomatous peritonitis?" *BJOG—An International Journal of Obstetrics and Gynaecology*, vol. 117, no. 8, pp. 1027–1030, 2010.

[16] S. Takemoto, K. Ushijima, R. Kawano et al., "Validity of intraoperative diagnosis at laparoscopic surgery for ovarian tumors," *Journal of Minimally Invasive Gynecology*, vol. 21, no. 4, pp. 576–579, 2014.

[17] A. L. Covens, J. E. Dodge, C. Lacchetti et al., "Surgical management of a suspicious adnexal mass: a systematic review," *Gynecologic Oncology*, vol. 126, no. 1, pp. 149–156, 2012.

[18] M. Canis, R. Mashiach, A. Wattiez et al., "Frozen section in laparoscopic management of macroscopically suspicious ovarian masses," *Journal of the American Association of Gynecologic Laparoscopists*, vol. 11, no. 3, pp. 365–369, 2004.

[19] M. Canis, G. Mage, J. L. Pouly, A. Wattiez, H. Manhes, and M. A. Bruhat, "Laparoscopic diagnosis of adnexal cystic masses: a 12-year experience with long-term follow-up," *Obstetrics and Gynecology*, vol. 83, no. 5, pp. 707–712, 1994.

[20] R. H. Demir and G. J. Marchand, "Adnexal masses suspected to be benign treated with laparoscopy," *Journal of the Society of Laparoendoscopic Surgeons*, vol. 16, no. 1, pp. 71–84, 2012.

[21] D. J. Quinlan, D. E. Townsend, and G. H. Johnson, "Safe and cost effective laparoscopic removal of adnexal masses," *Journal of the American Association of Gynecologic Laparoscopists*, vol. 4, no. 2, pp. 215–218, 1997.

[22] A. Mahdavi, B. Berker, C. Nezhat, F. Nezhat, and C. Nezhat, "Laparoscopic management of ovarian cysts," *Obstetrics and Gynecology Clinics of North America*, vol. 31, no. 3, pp. 581–592, 2004.

35

Elective "True Day Case" Laparoscopic Inguinal Hernia Repair in a District General Hospital: Lessons Learned from 1000 Consecutive Cases

A. Solodkyy, M. Feretis, A. Fedotovs, F. Di Franco, S. Gergely, and A. M. Harris

Department of Upper Gastrointestinal Surgery, Hinchingbrooke Hospital, Hinchingbrooke Park, Huntingdon, Cambridgeshire PE29 6NT, UK

Correspondence should be addressed to A. Solodkyy; sladkiy61@hotmail.com

Academic Editor: Peng Hui Wang

Introduction. Laparoscopic inguinal hernia repair (LIHR) is ideal for day case surgery. It is recommended that at least 70% should be day cases as a measure of cost-effectiveness. The aims of this study were to (i) assess the rate of true day case (TDC) surgery and (ii) identify predictors associated with unexpected overnight stay (UOS). *Methods*. Data was collected prospectively on 1000 consecutive elective LIHR performed in a District General Hospital (DGH) over a 7-year period. Data was collected on baseline patient demographics, ASA grade, and intraoperative details. A multivariate analysis was performed in order to identify predictors of UOS. *Results*. 1000 patients (927 males) underwent elective LIHR. Mean age was 57.3±15.2 years. 915 patients were planned as day case procedures. 822/915 day cases (89.8%) were discharged on the same day and 93 (10.2%) stayed overnight unexpectedly. Patient age, duration of procedure, and patient slot in the operating list were found to be independent predictors ($p<0.05$) of UOS. *Conclusion*. Our results demonstrate that LIHR is a "true" day case procedure in a DGH. Although some factors associated with UOS cannot be altered, careful patient selection and operating list planning are of paramount importance in order to minimise the burden on healthcare resources.

1. Introduction

In 2009, the European Hernia Society (EHS) published guidelines with indications for laparoscopic and open inguinal hernia repair. They recommend a laparoscopic approach to be considered for bilateral hernias and recurrent hernias after previous anterior repair and for all females. A Lichtenstein repair is recommended for large scrotal hernias, after previous abdominal surgery, and when general anaesthesia is not advised. Primary unilateral hernias can be repaired using a Lichtenstein or laparoscopic approach depending on surgeon expertise [1]. In the United Kingdom (UK) the National Institute for Clinical Excellence (NICE) has revised their guidance on the surgical management of inguinal hernias to recommend that laparoscopic repair be considered for first-line management of unilateral primary hernias [2]. The change in the recommendation resulted from the findings of a meta-analysis which highlighted the lower rate of wound-related complications, lower postoperative pain symptoms experienced by patients, and earlier return to daily activities [3]. Laparoscopic hernia repair has the advantage by reducing the time and effort that a patient's family or other carers devote to care, following discharge from hospital [4]. Stylopoulos et al. concluded the laparoscopic hernia repair is cost effective approach and associated with higher quality-of-life benefits at lower cost in their huge study population [5].

Despite the potential role LIHR has to play in the management of patients with symptomatic inguinal hernias, the procedure has not gained universal acceptance amongst surgeons. In the United States (US) only 14–19% of inguinal hernia operations were reported to be repaired using the laparoscopic approach [6, 7]. One population-based analysis in Florida revealed that even the majority of recurrent hernias was being repaired using an open approach [6]. In the UK the trend regarding the repair of choice for inguinal hernias appears to be similar to the US with only 4.9% of all hernia repairs being performed using the laparoscopic approach in Scotland [8]. We were unable to find published data on the

UK-wide proportion of laparoscopic hernia repair (versus open) but anecdotally it is thought to be around 20-25%. The low uptake has been thought to be due to the fact that LIHR is a challenging procedure with a steep learning curve and the benefits for patients are still being debated. One concern surgeons have when considering a switch to routine laparoscopic repair of primary inguinal hernias is the increased operating time indicated in some of the trials. A meta-analysis of eight randomised controlled trials reported in the NICE guidelines quotes a mean increase in operating time of 7.9 minutes for TEP repair, when compared to standard open mesh repair [2]. Although this increase in operating time is not great, when the large number of repairs performed annually is considered (10 hernia repairs per 10,000 population per year in the UK), even a small increase could have a significant impact on health care resources, efficiency, and waiting lists in Day Surgery Units. It is however recognised that with experience the duration of the laparoscopic technique can reduce to parity with open surgery (personal data). Within the National Health Service (NHS), there is a drive to consider day surgery as first-line, rather than inpatient surgery, with the Department of Health recommendation that 75% of all elective surgeries be performed as day case procedures [9].

The aims of this report were (i) to assess the "true" rate of LIHR performed as "day cases", (ii) to identify the immediate postoperative complications experienced by patients, and (iii) to identify predictors of unexpected patient overnight stay in a DGH.

2. Methods

Data was prospectively collected on 1000 consecutive patients who underwent LIHR using the trans-abdominal preperitoneal (TAPP) approach in our institution's Day Case Unit (DCU) over a 7-year period (2010-2017). Data was collected on baseline patient demographics, preoperative body mass index (BMI), American Society of Anaesthetists (ASA) patient grade, level of experience of operating surgeon, duration of procedure, laterality of the hernia, and immediate postoperative complications. Day case surgery was defined as '*admission and discharge on the same day as surgery, with day case surgery as the intended management*', as recently described by Anderson et al. [10].

Continuous variables are reported as "mean" values and Standard Deviation (SD). Categorical variables are reported as absolute frequencies/percentages (%). Continuous variables were compared (univariate analysis) using the Mann–Whitney or independent samples t-test, depending on the distribution of the data. The chi-square or Fisher's exact test was used for comparison purposes between categorical variables. A binary, logistic regression model was developed in order to identify independent predictors of unexpected patient overnight stay. A p-value <0.05 was considered to be statistically significant. The Statistical Package for the Social Science (SPSS, version 24.0 Armonk, NY) was used for analysis purposes.

TABLE 1: Baseline characteristics of the study's population.

	Total (N=1000)
Age∗ (years)	57.3±15.2
Gender† (Male: Female)	927:73
Single side hernia†	761(76.1%)
Bilateral hernia†	239(23.9%)
BMI∗ (Kg/m^2)	26.3±3.5
ASA grade†	
(i) 1	454(45.4%)
(ii) 2	487(48.7%)
(iii) 3	59 (5.9%)

∗ → values as mean/SD and † → values as frequencies/ percentages.

Surgical Technique

3-Port Placement. 1 x 10mm supraumbilical, 2 x 5mm left and right lateral. Patient placed in slight head-down position.

Peritoneum. Transverse peritoneal incision was extended medially to lateral umbilical ligament, 3-4cm above hernia deficit, using diathermy scissors; preperitoneal space was developed with blunt dissection. Hernia sac reduced using blunt dissection; vas and testicular vessels were clearly seen and preserved.

Mesh. 15 x 10cm Premilene™ mesh [*B. Braun: Melsungen, Germany*] was placed in preperitoneal space and fixed with Securestrap™ [*Ethicon: New Jersey, USA*] tacks placed at lower medial, upper medial, and upper lateral corners, avoiding lower lateral corner (so-called 'triangle of sorrow'). Peritoneum was closed with tacks avoiding inferior epigastric artery.

Closure. 'J' PDS to deep fascia, 3/0 prolene to skin.

3. Results

During the study period, 1000 patients (927 males) underwent elective LIHR in our institution's day case surgery unit. Mean age of the patients at the time of surgery was 57.3±15.2 years. Within this group 761 (76.1%) cases were unilateral and 239 (23.9%) cases were bilateral hernia repairs. The median body mass index (BMI) (kg/m^2), as recorded on patients' visit to our institution's preassessment clinic prior to surgery, was 26.3 ±3.5. The patients' American Society of Anaesthetists (ASA) patient grade was as follows: ASA 1 n= 454 (45.4%); ASA 2 n= 487 (48.7%); and ASA 3 = 59 (5.9%), respectively. Mean operating time for performing the LIHR was 60.9 ± 21.3 minutes. This includes unilateral and bilateral cases. Only 5 out of 1000 (0. 5%) laparoscopic procedures were converted to open surgery due to technical difficulty (e.g., irreducibility of incarcerated hernia). Patient baseline and operative characteristics are summarised in Table 1.

Nine hundred and fifteen patients (91.5%) were scheduled to undergo LIHR as "day case admissions", whereas 85 patients (8.5%) were prebooked for overnight hospital stay case by case taking into consideration multiple factors

TABLE 2: Reasons for unexpected overnight hospital stay (n=93).

Reason	Number of Patients (%)
Retention of urine	44 (47.3%)
Complications related to general anaesthesia/ slow recovery	23 (24.7%)
Post-operative pain	16 (17.2%)
Bleeding post operatively	5 (5.4%)
Other	5 (5.4%)

(patient premorbid status/social reasons). These patients were excluded from further analysis.

With regard to those patients (n=915) who were scheduled to be discharged on the day of their procedure, 822 out of 915 (89.8%) achieved the TDC target, whereas 93 out of 915 patients (10.2%) required UOS due to a variety of reasons, summarised in Table 2. Forty-four patients (47.3%) experienced urinary retention in the immediate postoperative period and a urethral catheter was inserted. One patient was catheterised for urinary retention but was discharged home on the same day with catheter. Anaesthetic issues such as prolonged postoperative nausea and vomiting, hypotension, and desaturation were documented in 23 patients (24.7%). The other common reasons for UOS were postoperative pain in 16 patients; 5 patients experienced immediate post-operative bleeding causing haematoma and were admitted for observation; 5 patients stayed due to unexpected other reasons.

3.1. TDC Versus UOS (Univariate Analysis). Patients who required an unexpected overnight hospital stay were older (63.22±13.83 years) compared to the TDC group (55.5±14.8 years, p<0.0001). Furthermore, the mean operating time was significantly longer in the UOS group (66.8±24.2) compared to the TDC patient group (60.3±21.0 min, p=0.0091). The LIHR took more than 90 minutes in 15/93(16.1%) of patients in the UOS group, whereas only 78/822(9.4%) in the TDC group had procedure which was longer than this time. The difference, however, did not reach statistical significance (p=0.068).

The majority of patients [68/93(73.1%)] in the UOS group were operated in the second half of the operating list when compared to the TDC group 447/822 (54.4%, p=0.0009). This also explains why significant proportion of UOS patients left recovery after 18:30 hrs and did not have adequate time to recover prior to the same day discharge, when compared to those who were discharged on the same day [23/93 (24.7%) versus. 50/822(6%), p<0.0001].

There was no difference in the intraoperative complications experienced by patients of the two groups; however, immediate postoperative complications such as urinary retention were significantly higher in the UOS group (47.3% versus. 0.0%; p<0.0001). The primary surgeon was of training grade in 84 out of 822 cases (10.2%) in the TDC group versus 6 out of 93 procedures (6.5%) in the UOS group (p>0.05). The proportion of patients who underwent bilateral LIHR in the UOS group (28/93, 30%) was comparable to that of the TDC group [178/822, 21.6% (p=0.067)]. Finally, there was no significant difference between the two groups in terms of patient gender, BMI values, and ASA grade (p>0.05).

3.2. Independent Predictors of Unexpected Overnight Stay. We created a logistic regression model in order to identify independent predictors of unscheduled overnight patient stay following LIHR. The following variables were entered into the model: patient age, ASA grade, BMI, duration of procedure, hernia laterality (i.e., bilateral versus. unilateral), grade of operating surgeon, and patient slot in the operating list (i.e., a.m. versus p.m.). The following 3 variables were independent predictors of unexpected overnight patient stay: patient age, duration of procedure, and patient slot in the operating list. The univariate and multivariate analysis is shown in Table 3.

4. Discussion

In this report, we present data from 1000 consecutive patients undergoing elective LIHR in a DGH. In our experience, LIHR can be safely offered as a day case procedure thereby minimising the financial burden on healthcare resources. Furthermore, we identified three factors (patient age, duration of surgery, and patient slot in the operating list) as predictors of UOS. The authors suggest that taking these factors into account early in the preoperative stage could lead to maximal utilisation of operating list and would also lead to further reduction of healthcare expenses.

Groin hernia repairs are amongst the most commonly performed general surgical operations with over 71,000 inguinal and femoral hernias repairs carried out in England in 2014/15. Previous economic analyses have estimated that, in England alone, surgical repair of inguinal hernias utilised over 100,000 NHS bed-days of hospital resources. The British Association of Day Surgery has suggested that 80% of inguinal hernia repairs should be carried out as day case procedures, regardless of the technique used. In 2014/15, 77.8% of primary inguinal hernia repairs (unilateral) were carried out as a day case, and rates varied from 67% to 88% across institutions. Furthermore, surgeons have a variety of approaches and materials in their armamentarium [2, 11]. It has long been established that LIHR can be performed safely and effectively as a day case procedure. However, the uptake of the technique has not been endorsed by many surgeons for a variety of reasons. A recent survey amongst members of the American Hernia Society revealed that just over 50% of surgeons utilise the laparoscopic approach for repair of inguinal hernias, with lack of training, increased operating time, and costs being the commonest reasons to opt for the open approach [12]. In our unit, the laparoscopic approach has been the method of choice for repairing symptomatic unilateral or bilateral inguinal hernias for the past 15 years. A typical straightforward unilateral hernia repair will take around 30-45 mins and bilateral 45-60 mins. As our results demonstrate, operation time achieves equivalence (to open surgery) with experience; conversion rates to open surgery have been extremely low and morbidity associated with the procedure has been minimal.

TABLE 3: Comparison (univariate and multivariate analysis) of baseline demographic and operative characteristics of "true day cases" (TCD) and patients who required an unexpected overnight stay (UOS).

Parameter	TDC (N=822)	UOS (n=93)	Univariate Analysis	Multivariate Analysis
Age years ∗(Mean ± SD)	55.5±14.8	63.2±13.83	p<0.0001	**P=0.0001**
Age ∗ ≥60	377(45.9%)	63(67.8%)	p<0.0001	
Male gender †	769(93.5%)	84 (90.3%)	p=0.2723	
BMI∗ (Kg/m2)	26.4±3.5	25.8±3.5	p>0.05	P=0.110
BMI∗ ≥ 35 Kg/m^2	18(2.2%)	2 (2.1%)	p=0.3457	
ASA1/2 vs ASA3	798/23	87/6	p=0.1126	P=0.582
Mean operation time (mins)∗	60.3±21.0	66.8±24.2	p=0.0091	**p=0.021**
Length of procedure (>90 minutes†)	78 (9.4%)	15 (16.1%)	p=0.068	
Time leaving recovery (after 18:30 hr) †	50(6%)	23 (24.7%)	p<0.0001	
Recovery time (min) ∗	68.7±31.4	80.3±46.9	p=0.0226	
Timing of procedure (PM list) †	447(54.4%)	68 (73.1%)	p=0.0009	**p=0. 001**
Immediate post-operative complications (urine retention, bleeding) †	1 (0.00%)	49(52.7%)	p<0.0001	
Operations by trainee(SAS/Registrar) †	84 (10.2%)	6(6.5%)	p>0.05	P=0.375
Bilateral/unilateral	178/644	28/65	p=0.067	p=0.267

∗ → values as mean/SD and † →values as frequencies/ percentages.

The criteria for selecting patients suitable for day case surgery have changed over the past 15 years as a result of the pressure on healthcare resources, lack of hospital capacity, and the obesity pandemic. However, the current practice for many units in the United Kingdom (UK) is to routinely book patients with high BMI (>30kg/m^2), diabetic patients, and all those classified ASA 3 for an overnight hospital stay. NHS Modernisation in 2002 raised the BMI limit for day surgery procedures, from 30kg/m^2 in 1992 (Royal College of Surgeons recommendation) to 35 kg/m^2; however, other professional bodies (Association of Anaesthetists of Great Britain and Irelands) recommend that the patients are not excluded from day surgery on BMI alone [10]. Our experience over a seven-year period was that BMI alone should not be a limiting factor for the surgeon to perform LIHR as day case procedure. Nevertheless, our standard practice as a unit is to encourage obese patients to lose weight prior to elective surgery.

According to British Hernia Society (BHS), the strict patient selection criteria are becoming less common and, in principle, an inguinal hernia repair as day surgery could be potentially offered for virtually every patient who has satisfactory care at home [13]. As our results demonstrate, ASA grade should not be a limiting factor for offering patients LHR as day case, provided that patients attend a preassessment clinic. In a large American cohort study, the costs of an inguinal hernia repair in a clinical setting were found to be 56% higher than those for day surgery [14]. Also, in Germany, day case surgery has been reported to generate lower costs [15]. It is therefore evident, in an era where healthcare resources are not unlimited, that accurate preoperative assessment is essential in order to keep expenses as low as possible.

Similar to others, our departmental policy is to repair bilateral inguinal hernias laparoscopically from a cost-utility and patient perspective [16–20]. Our analysis did not reveal hernia laterality (i.e., bilateral versus unilateral repair) to be an independent predictor of UOS. However, the regression model identified duration of procedure as an independent predictor of UOS. Changes in patient physiological parameters whilst under anaesthesia along with difficult dissection at the level inguinal region could be potential explanations for this finding. Furthermore, given that laparoscopic hernia repair has a relatively slow learning curve, as previous reports have demonstrated, one might expect a difference in the rates of UOS between qualified surgeons and surgeons in training. Comparison of the figures did not show a statistically significant difference. This can be explained by that fact that as a laparoscopic training unit the consultants are present for all training hernia cases and will step in if difficulties are encountered, which helps to control operation time and minimises morbidity/complications. A few trainees become very proficient at this procedure requiring less intervention (as would be expected) and as such their cases will not unduly affect the UOS rate.

In our day case surgery unit we apply only one absolute exclusion criterion which is the absence of a responsible adult to stay with the patient for the first 24 hours following discharge. We suggest that criteria other than social should be considered relative and selection should be done on a case by case basis. However, patients older than 60 years or/and have other significant comorbidities (e.g., diabetes) should be listed for morning rather than afternoon procedure to allow for longer recovery time before discharge. Both these variables were independent predictors of UOS in our patient cohort and highlight the necessity of preoperative patient planning in order to minimise costs and the impact on bed availability.

5. Conclusion

Our results demonstrate that LIHR can be offered as a "true" day case procedure with high same day discharge rate of around 90% in a DGH. Although some factors associated with UOS cannot be altered, careful patient selection and operating list prioritisation are of paramount importance in order to minimise number of unexpected overnight stay. We recommend that patients who are older and have multiple comorbidities should be booked on a morning list to allow adequate recovery time and thus increase the chance of same day discharge. Patients with BMI $\geq$ 35 or ASA 3 who are routinely scheduled for overnight stay in many units are in our experience often suitable for day case surgery with careful planning, good preoperative advice, and established communication channels, should they require advice or support after discharge. These measures may increase the overall rate of true day case surgery for LIHR and have a significant cost benefit by reducing the added bed pressures and financial costs of overnight or further hospital stay.

Authors' Contributions

A. Solodkyy, M. Feretis, and A. M. Harris conceptualised and designed the study. A. Solodkyy and A. Fedotovs collected the data. A. Solodkyy and M. Feretis performed the statistical analysis and wrote the manuscript and prepared the final draft. F. Di Franco, S. Gergely, and A. M. Harris reviewed the manuscript and made the necessary corrections. A. M. Harris made the final corrections to the manuscript.

Disclosure

Manuscript was orally presented in" 26th International Congress of the European Association for Endoscopic Surgery (EAES), London, United Kingdom, 30 May–1 June 2018.

References

[1] M. P. Simons, T. Aufenacker, M. Bay-Nielsen et al., "European Hernia Society guidelines on the treatment of inguinal hernia in adult patients," *Hernia*, vol. 13, no. 4, pp. 343–403, 2009.

[2] National Institute for Clinical Excellence (NICE), "Laparoscopic surgery for inguinal hernia repair," 2018, https://www.nice.org.uk/guidance/ta83/documents/final-appraisal-determination-laparoscopic-surgery-for-inguinal-hernia-repair2.

[3] M. A. Memon, N. J. Cooper, B. Memon, M. I. Memon, and K. R. Abrams, "Meta-analysis of randomized clinical trials comparing open and laparoscopic inguinal hernia repair," *British Journal of Surgery*, vol. 90, no. 12, pp. 1479–1492, 2003.

[4] K. McCormack, B. Wake, J. Perez et al., "Laparoscopic surgery for inguinal hernia repair: Systematic review of effectiveness and economic evaluation," *Health Technology Assessment*, vol. 9, no. 14, 2005.

[5] N. Stylopoulos, G. S. Gazelle, and D. W. Rattner, "A cost-utility analysis of treatment options for inguinal hernia in 1,513,008 adult patients," *Surgical Endoscopy*, vol. 17, no. 2, pp. 180–189, 2003.

[6] D. S. Smink, I. M. Paquette, and S. R. G. Finlayson, "Utilization of laparoscopic and open inguinal hernia repair: A population-based analysis," *Journal of Laparoendoscopic & Advanced Surgical Techniques*, vol. 19, no. 6, pp. 745–748, 2009.

[7] I. M. Rutkow, "Demographic and socioeconomic aspects of hernia repair in the United States in 2003," *Surgical Clinics of North America*, vol. 83, no. 5, pp. 1045–1051, 2003.

[8] M. Duff, R. Mofidi, and S. J. Nixon, "Routine laparoscopic repair of primary unilateral inguinal hernias - A viable alternative in the Day Surgery Unit?" *The Surgeon*, vol. 5, no. 4, pp. 209–212, 2007.

[9] DOH, *Day Surgery: Operational Guide*, Department of Health, 2002.

[10] T. Anderson, M. Walls, and R. Canelo, "Day cases surgery guidelines," *Surgery-Oxford International Edition*, vol. 35, no. 2, pp. 85–91, 2016.

[11] Royal College of Surgeons, "Commissioning Guide Groin Hernia," 2016, https://www.rcseng.ac.uk/-/.../groin-hernia-commissioning-guide_published-2016.pdf.

[12] M. Trevisonno, P. Kaneva, and Y. Watanabe, "A survey of general surgeons regarding laparoscopic inguinal hernia repair: practice patterns, barriers, and educational needs," *Hernia*, 2014.

[13] *Groin Hernia Guidelines*, British Hernia Society, 2013, http://www.britishherniasociety.org/wp-content/uploads/2015/07/iipp_-_groin_hernia_guidelines_as_gone_to_press_-4.pdf.

[14] J. B. Mitchell and B. Harrow, "Costs and outcomes of inpatient versus outpatient hernia repair," *Health Policy*, vol. 28, no. 2, pp. 143–152, 1994.

[15] D. Weyhe, C. Winnemoller, A. Hellwig et al., "(Section sign) 115 b SGB V threatens outpatient treatment for inguinal hernia. Analysis of outcome and economics," *Chirurg*, vol. 77, pp. 844–855, 2006.

[16] P. Caudill, J. Nyland, C. Smith, J. Yerasimides, and J. Lach, "Sports hernias: A systematic literature review," *British Journal of Sports Medicine*, vol. 42, no. 12, pp. 954–964, 2008.

[17] R. Bittner, M. E. Arregui, T. Bisgaard et al., "Guidelines for laparoscopic (TAPP) and endoscopic (TEP) treatment of inguinal hernia [International Endohernia Society (IEHS)]," *Surgical Endoscopy*, vol. 25, no. 9, pp. 2773–2843, 2011.

[18] K. McCormack, N. W. Scott, P. M. Go, S. Ross, and A. M. Grant, "Laparoscopic techniques versus open techniques for inguinal hernia repair.," *Cochrane Database of Systematic Reviews (Online)*, no. 1, p. CD001785, 2003.

[19] C. G. Schmedt, S. Sauerland, and R. Bittner, "Comparison of endoscopic procedures vs Lichtenstein and other open mesh techniques for inguinal hernia repair: a meta-analysis of randomized controlled trials," *Surgical Endoscopy*, vol. 19, no. 2, pp. 188–199, 2005.

[20] A. Karthikesalingam, S. R. Markar, P. J. E. Holt, and R. K. Praseedom, "Meta-analysis of randomized controlled trials comparing laparoscopic with open mesh repair of recurrent inguinal hernia," *British Journal of Surgery*, vol. 97, no. 1, pp. 4–11, 2010.

36

Complications, Not Minimally Invasive Surgical Technique, Are Associated with Increased Cost after Esophagectomy

Sue J. Fu,[1] Vanessa P. Ho,[2] Jennifer Ginsberg,[1] Yaron Perry,[1] Conor P. Delaney,[3] Philip A. Linden,[1] and Christopher W. Towe[1]

[1]*Division of Thoracic and Esophageal Surgery, University Hospitals Cleveland Medical Center and Case Western Reserve School of Medicine, Cleveland, OH, USA*
[2]*Department of Surgery, University Hospitals Cleveland Medical Center and Case Western Reserve School of Medicine, Cleveland, OH, USA*
[3]*Digestive Disease Institute, The Cleveland Clinic and Cleveland Clinic Lerner School of Medicine, Cleveland, OH, USA*

Correspondence should be addressed to Christopher W. Towe; christopher.towe@uhhospitals.org

Academic Editor: Stephen Kavic

Background. Minimally invasive esophagectomy (MIE) techniques offer similar oncological and surgical outcomes to open methods. The effects of MIE on hospital costs are not well documented. *Methods.* We reviewed the electronic records of patients who underwent esophagectomy at a single academic institution between January 2012 and December 2014. Esophagectomy techniques were grouped into open, hybrid, MIE, and transhiatal (THE) esophagectomy. Univariate and multivariate analyses were performed to assess the impact of surgery on total hospital cost after esophagectomy. *Results.* 80 patients were identified: 11 THE, 11 open, 41 hybrid, and 17 MIE. Median total cost of the hospitalization was $31,375 and was similar between surgical technique groups. MIE was associated with higher intraoperative costs, but not total hospital cost. Multivariable analysis revealed that the presence of a complication, increased age, American Society of Anesthesiologists class IV (ASA4), and preoperative coronary artery disease (CAD) were associated with significantly increased cost. *Conclusions.* Despite the association of MIE with higher operation costs, the total hospital cost was not different between surgical technique groups. Postoperative complications and severe preoperative comorbidities are significant drivers of hospital cost associated with esophagectomy. Surgeons should choose technique based on clinical factors, rather than cost implications.

1. Introduction

Minimally invasive techniques are a popular alternative to traditional open methods in nearly all surgical disciplines. An early concern with these techniques was potential increased operative cost relative to open surgery [1]. Studies of cost in abdominal surgical procedures, including cholecystectomy, appendectomy, reflux surgery, gastric bypass, ventral hernia repair, and colectomy, have refuted this concern and shown that minimally invasive techniques are associated with reduced ICU admissions, fewer complications, shorter length of stay, and decreased postdischarge resource utilization, all of which contribute to overall hospital costs [2–4]. As health care budgets come under scrutiny, the cost of surgical procedures should be assessed to ensure optimal use of health care resources relative to their clinical benefit. This is especially true for patients undergoing esophagectomy which is associated with high rates of complications and long term morbidity [5].

Advances in surgical techniques and perioperative standards have significantly decreased morbidity and mortality associated with esophagectomy [6]. A large body of research focused on clinical outcomes of minimally invasive esophagectomy (MIE) has demonstrated improved surgical and clinical outcomes, such as decreased blood loss, reduced length of stay, and fewer pulmonary complications [7–9]. Hybrid approaches, utilizing a combination of endoscopic and traditional approaches, have also been studied and show evidence of clinical benefit compared to traditional techniques [10, 11]. However, there is little data on economic outcomes of MIE and hybrid procedures compared to traditional approaches. The scant published data suggest MIE may result in decreased or similar costs [12]. A 2009 European study of MIE and open Ivor Lewis esophagectomy reported similar costs and safety, but this report was not adjusted for cost confounders in their analysis [13].

We aimed to analyze the costs associated with esophagectomy to assess whether a cost difference exists between minimally invasive, hybrid, and open approaches and, if so, which areas of the patient encounter contain cost differences. We hypothesized that there would be cost differences between minimally invasive and open techniques and that individual components, such as intraoperative cost or ICU cost, would account for the majority of the differences.

2. Methods

All patients undergoing esophagectomy at an academic medical center were identified via a prospectively maintained database between January 2012 and December 2014. Clinical data were extracted from the institution's database and were matched with institutional cost data pulled from UH-Socrates platform (Socrates Analytics, Cleveland, OH). This study was approved by the institution's Institutional Review Board. All data were analyzed using STATA/SE, version 13.0 (Stata Corp., College Station, TX).

Variables extracted from the clinical database included demographics, preoperative comorbidities, procedure characteristics, and postoperative complications. Preoperative characteristics extracted included age, body mass index (BMI), hypertension, coronary artery disease (CAD), prior chemotherapy or radiation, chronic obstructive pulmonary disease (COPD), diabetes, congestive heart failure (CHF), Zubrod class, and American Society of Anesthesiologists (ASA) class. Preoperative chemotherapy and/or radiotherapy was used as a proxy for tumor characteristics. Surgery type was classified as transhiatal (neck and abdominal incisions), open (open thoracotomy and open laparotomy), hybrid (either video assisted thoracic surgery (VATS) or laparoscopy for one part of the procedure), or purely minimally invasive (both VATS and laparoscopy). Both Ivor Lewis and tri-incisional esophagectomy could be performed using hybrid and MIE techniques. Full explanations of these procedures are available elsewhere [7]. The decision to use a specific technique was at the discretion of the attending surgeon. Reoperation and/or preoperative chemotherapy or radiation therapy were not contraindications to performing a minimally invasive approach. Complications were extracted from the database and were verified with chart review. Complications recorded included return to the operating room, postoperative infections, arrhythmias, respiratory issues (including reintubation and pneumonia), postoperative transfusions, and unexpected admission to the intensive care unit and were categorized as defined by the Society of Thoracic Surgeons [14]. Patients who had any recorded complication, regardless of complication severity, were categorized as having a complication.

The primary outcome of interest was total cost of the hospitalization. Actual hospital cost data were extracted from the institution's financial database. Patients with incomplete cost data were excluded. Costs were grouped into the following cost center categories: anesthesia, intensive care unit (ICU), laboratory, operating room, telemetry floor, and all other costs, which included cardiac, pharmacy, radiology, and physical therapy costs. The total cost for each patient was calculated by summation of the costs for all the cost center categories.

Descriptive analysis was performed to determine distribution of preoperative characteristics and complications. Due to nonnormal distribution of cost data due to several high outliers, nonparametric tests were utilized for cost analysis. Data are presented as median and interquartile range. Chi-square or Fisher's Exact test, as appropriate, was utilized to determine differences between groups for categorical variables. Kruskal-Wallis one-way analysis of variance was performed to determine whether there were cost differences between groups; pairwise comparisons between groups were then performed when differences were identified. p value less than 0.05 was considered significant.

Multivariable regression was utilized to examine the effect of preoperative and operative variables on cost, including pertinent preoperative variables as well as surgery type. Preoperative clinical variables, such as age, preoperative chemotherapy, and radiation, were included in the model as potential confounders. Complications were found to be a significant cost driver in the initial multivariate regression analysis and therefore we further stratified our multivariate regression analysis based on the occurrence of postoperative complications. Model 1 includes all patients. In order to differentiate the effect of complications on cost, we created two additional multivariable models. Model 2 includes only patients without complications and Model 3 includes only patients with complications.

3. Results

During the study period, 86 esophagectomies were performed by 4 surgeons. Eighty patients had complete medical records and cost data available and were included in the analysis (Table 1). Patient ages ranged from 32 to 85 years, with median age of 65 years. The most common preoperative comorbidity was hypertension ($n = 44$, 55%) followed by diabetes ($n = 16$, 20%). There were no differences in the preoperative characteristics between operative technique groups. The majority of the patients received preoperative chemotherapy ($n = 52$, 65%) and radiation therapy ($n = 51$, 63.8%), and the rate of preoperative chemotherapy and radiation was similar between operative groups. The hybrid approach was most common ($n = 41$, 51.25%) and was most commonly performed with a laparotomy and VATS ($n = 38$, 47.5%). The median length of stay (LOS) after esophagectomy was 8 (IQR 7–9) days. There was no difference in LOS between surgery types ($p = 0.48$). There were no deaths in the 30-day period following esophagectomy in this cohort. Complications occurred in 42 patients (52.5%). The most common complications were atrial fibrillation ($n = 12$, 15%), anastomotic leak ($n = 11$, 13.75%), and pneumonia ($n = 11$, 13.75%). Sixteen patients (20%) required return

TABLE 1: Overview of study population.

	Median (IQR) or N frequency (%)					p value
	All	THE	Open	Hybrid	MIE	
Patient variables						
N (%)	80 (100)	11 (13.75)	11 (13.75)	41 (51.25)	17 (21.25)	
Age	65.2 (59.6–75.3)	67.4 (60.4–76.2)	65.1 (59.7–75.6)	64.7 (56.8–75.4)	63.4 (59.5–73.8)	0.891
Gender						0.241
Male	59 (73.8)	10 (90.9)	6 (54.6)	29 (70.7)	14 (82.4)	
Female	21 (26.2)	1 (9.1)	5 (45.5)	12 (29.3)	3 (17.7)	
Preoperative comorbidities or treatments						
Hypertension	44 (55.0)	4 (36.4)	6 (54.6)	25 (61.0)	9 (52.9)	0.550
CAD	15 (18.8)	4 (36.4)	1 (9.1)	7 (17.1)	3 (17.7)	0.502
Prior CTS	11 (13.8)	1 (9.1)	2 (18.2)	6 (14.6)	2 (11.8)	1.000
Preop XRT	51 (63.8)	7 (63.6)	5 (45.5)	29 (70.7)	10 (58.8)	0.455
Preop Chemo	52 (65.0)	7 (63.6)	6 (54.6)	29 (70.7)	10 (58.8)	0.729
COPD	10 (12.5)	1 (9.1)	2 (18.2)	5 (12.2)	2 (11.8)	0.955
CHF	5 (6.3)	2 (18.2)	1 (9.1)	2 (4.9)	0 (0.0)	0.189
Diabetes	16 (20.0)	2 (18.2)	1 (9.1)	9 (22.0)	4 (23.5)	0.904
Zubrod class						0.851
Normal Activity	33 (41.3)	5 (45.5)	4 (36.4)	15 (36.6)	9 (52.9)	
Symptomatic	47 (58.8)	6 (54.6)	7 (63.6)	26 (63.4)	8 (47.1)	
ASA class						0.573
II	7 (8.8)	2 (18.2)	0 (0.0)	4 (9.8)	1 (5.9)	
III	69 (86.3)	9 (81.8)	11 (100.0)	33 (80.5)	16 (94.1)	
IV	4 (5.0)	0 (0.0)	0 (0.0)	4 (9.8)	0 (0.0)	
Operative outcomes						
OR time (min)	441 (399–511)	330 (307–348)	449 (397–486)	437 (410–480)	527 (461–581)	<0.001
LOS (days)	8 (7–9)	7 (7–12)	8 (7–13)	8 (7–9)	7 (6–9)	0.476
Postoperative complications	42 (52.5)	5 (45.5)	5 (45.5)	23 (56.1)	9 (52.9)	0.912

Data presented as n (%) for categorical variables or median (interquartile range) for continuous variables.
p values indicate Fisher's Exact test for categorical variables and Kruskal-Wallis one-way test analysis of variance for continuous variables.
IQR: interquartile range. THE: transhiatal esophagectomy. MIE: minimally invasive esophagectomy. Preop: preoperative. CAD: coronary artery disease. CTS: cardiothoracic surgery. XRT: radiotherapy. COPD = chronic obstructive pulmonary disease. CHF: congestive heart failure. ASA: American Society of Anesthesiologist. LOS: length of stay.

to the OR, which included patients that required endoscopy or bronchoscopy (even if no intervention was performed). A table which lists the frequency of all complications and reasons for return to OR is available in the online supplement (Table S1, in Supplementary Material available online at http://dx.doi.org/10.1155/2016/7690632). There was no difference in complication rate for the different procedure types ($p = 0.88$).

The median total cost of the procedure and the associated hospitalization was $31,375 (IQR $26,487–$48,906). Figure 1 depicts the range of total cost for each surgical technique. Operating room cost was the largest subtype of cost and accounted for $10,449 (IQR $9,108–$14,599) or approximately 33% of the total cost associated with the procedure. Median total cost and cost subgroups associated with each surgical technique are listed in Table 2. The total hospital costs for each procedure type were similar ($p = 0.14$). Anesthesia, OR, and non-ICU room and board floor costs, however, were different among the groups ($p < 0.05$). Specifically, MIE was associated with increased OR costs relative to each of the 3 other surgery types, increased anesthesia costs relative to transhiatal and hybrid esophagectomy, and increased non-ICU room and board costs relative to THE. There was a trend towards lower ICU costs in MIE patients ($p = 0.08$). The median operation time was 441 minutes for all surgeries. Operation time for MIE was significantly longer compared to the other surgeries ($p < 0.01$, Table 1). Operative time was related to OR cost (Figure S1), and this accounts for of the majority of the higher variable OR costs associated with MIE.

We also noted that, for all procedures performed, the occurrence of complications significantly increased total hospital cost. The unadjusted total cost increase for an associated postoperative complication was $17,804 ($p = 0.0006$, 95% CI $7,840–$27,758). The complication associated with largest cost increase was reintubation and was associated with a cost increase of $20,777. Anastomotic leak was associated with an average additional cost of $14,025.

By multivariable regression, ASA class IV, increasing age, preoperative coronary artery disease, and the presence of complications were associated with increased total hospital

TABLE 2: Median cost (% of total cost) [IQR] by cost center.

Cost center	Median (%) [IQR] All patients (n = 80)	THE (n = 11)	Open (n = 11)	Hybrid (n = 41)	MIE (n = 17)	p value
OR	$10,449 (33%) [$9,108–14,599]	$7,703 (28%) [$7,274–10,060]	$10,903 (31%) [$9,992–16,816]	$10,099 (35%) [$9,081–11,300]	$15,732 (44%) [$11,721–25,218]	<0.001
Non-ICU room and board	$8,294 (26%) [$6,791–10,995]	$5,556 (20%) [$5,261–6,945]	$8,334 (24%) [$6,660–10,933]	$8,294 (29%) [$6,945–9,675]	$10,845 (31%) [$8,294–13,556]	0.005
ICU	$4,414 (14%) [$3,111–8,632]	$8,117 (29%) [$4,139–16,207]	$8,277 (24%) [$4,541–12,948]	$4,316 (15%) [$2,270–6,811]	$4,139 (12%) [$2,270–8,277]	0.085
Anesthesia	$2,204 (7%) [$1,918–2,713]	$1,644 (6%) [$1,413–2,146]	$2,374 (7%) [$2,016–3,443]	$2,148 (7%) [$1,920–2,525]	$2,946 (8%) [$2,382–4,237]	<0.001
Lab	$1,807 (6%) [$1,274–3,027]	$1,610 (6%) [$1,294–5,872]	$2,238 (6%) [$1,782–4,054]	$1,692 (6%) [$1,167–2,499]	$1,817 (12%) [$1,570–3,118]	0.271
Other*	$3,706 (12%) [$749–5,744]	$3,411 (12%) [$1,311–5,937]	$6,067 (17%) [$1,544–10,509]	$3,518 (12%) [$0–4,907]	$4,151 (12%) [$2,241–5,550]	0.659
Total	$31,375 [$26,487–48,484]	$27,835 [$23,626–45,267]	$35,002 [$24,589–62,223]	$28,710 [$26,469–34,186]	$35,508 [30,101–61,623]	0.135

*Other costs comprise pharmacy, radiology, cardiac, and physical therapy costs.
p values indicate Kruskal-Wallis one-way test analysis of variance for continuous variables.
IQR: interquartile range. ICU: intensive care unit. OR: operating room. THE: transhiatal esophagectomy. MIE: minimally invasive esophagectomy.

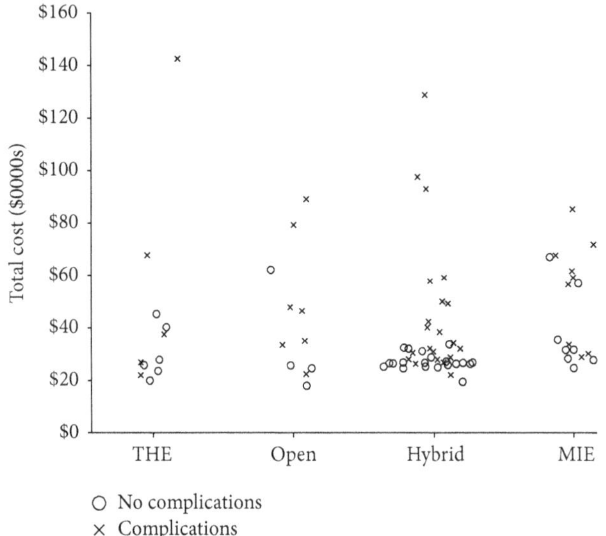

FIGURE 1: Range of cost for each procedure and by presence of postoperative complications. THE: transhiatal esophagectomy. MIE: minimally invasive esophagectomy.

cost (Table 3). The total costs associated with each surgery type were statistically comparable. A preoperative diagnosis of hypertension appeared to be cost "saving" by $21,226. Among patients without complications, there was no single factor associated with increased (or decreased) total cost. Among patients with complications, age, preoperative coronary artery disease, and ASA class IV were associated with higher hospital cost, and hypertension was also cost "saving" in this group.

4. Discussion and Conclusions

In this study, we report that complications and preoperative characteristics, not surgical technique, affect inpatient hospital cost after esophagectomy. We found no difference in index hospitalization cost between the various surgical procedures performed. In the only other study that has assessed costs of minimally invasive and open esophagectomy, Parameswaran et al. found higher operative costs and lower inpatient care costs for MIE versus open transthoracic surgeries, but similar costs overall [13]. Notably, their cost analysis utilized calculated costs, whereas the current study was able to extract actual hospital costs. To our knowledge, the current study is the first to analyze the effect of esophagectomy surgery technique on hospital costs using actual patient costs. Our study corroborates the findings from Parameswaran and expands upon them using risk-adjusted analysis.

In breakdown of cost, we found that MIE was associated with increased OR, anesthesia, and telemetry floor costs among all patients and especially among patients who did not experience complications. The increased telemetry floor costs findings for MIE reflect increased non-ICU based room and board cost due to decreased proportion of time in the ICU. Despite not reaching statistical significance, we believe that MIE achieves cost parity with the other procedures by offsetting higher intraoperative cost with lower cost of postoperative care, largely by reducing cost related to ICU utilization. This is similar to results proposed in other fields of surgery since 2003 [3].

Our data supports a growing body of literature that minimally invasive procedures may be associated with increased OR cost but are potentially overall cost saving when other variables are considered [4, 15, 16]. This study corroborates those findings in that we also found that MIE was associated

TABLE 3: Multivariate regression analysis.

Variable	All cases		Cases without complications		Cases with complications	
	Coefficient	*p* value	Coefficient	*p* value	Coefficient	*p* value
Complications	$17,385	<0.001				
Age (y)	$695	0.001	$240	0.196	$804	0.025
HTN	−$21,226	0.000	−$1,438	0.770	−$33,324	0.001
CAD	$16,189	0.006	−$5,831	0.502	$22,838	0.008
Preop ChemoXRT	−$5,173	0.252	$6,317	0.186	−$10,660	0.119
COPD	−$7,118	0.341	$5,156	0.555	−$17,171	0.152
CHF	$2,995	0.770	−$4,522	0.745	$6,547	0.680
Diabetes	−$630	0.910	$9,901	0.142	−$216	0.980
Zubrod symptomatic	$90	0.984	$4,887	0.270	$2,197	0.777
ASA class						
II	1		1		1	
III	$13,691	0.076	$7,406	0.246	$28,676	0.053
IV	$47,180	<0.001	n/a		$60,294	0.003
Procedure						
THE	1		1		1	
Open	$8,332	0.308	$2,304	0.746	$13,865	0.319
Hybrid	−$2,581	0.698	−$6,988	0.259	$13,858	0.907
MIE	$9,127	0.216	$6,457	0.353	$1,375	0.909
Constant	−$17,170	0.275	$2,845	0.838	−$11,753	0.655
Observations	80		38		42	
R-squared	.5546		.4349		.6713	

THE: transhiatal esophagectomy. MIE: minimally invasive esophagectomy. HTN: hypertension. CAD: coronary artery disease. CTS: cardiothoracic surgery. XRT: radiotherapy. COPD: chronic obstructive pulmonary disease. CHF: congestive heart failure. ASA: American Society of Anesthesiologist.

with longer and more expensive operations but was not associated with increased total hospital cost. Although the majority of the cost increase in MIE was related to longer operative time, other causes of higher MIE operating costs may be related to use of specialized and/or disposable instruments.

Because operative time is such a significant factor in cost, we believe that continued implementation of minimally invasive techniques may lead to cost saving over time as surgeons become more facile with these approaches and operative time decreases accordingly. Nguyen et al. reported a reduction of 108 minutes in MIE operating times in a series of 104 minimally invasive cases, eventually leading to shorter operating times in comparison to open esophagectomy [17].

While surgery type was not associated with significant cost differences, postoperative complications were revealed to be a significant cost driver in our analysis. When corrected for preoperative comorbidities and surgical technique, a hospital stay associated with a postoperative complication (or complications) was associated with an overall cost increase of $17,835. This supports previous data that postoperative events are associated with increased costs [18]. However, it should be noted that, for the purposes of this study, we did not differentiate severity of complications. Complication severity grade has been found to significantly increase hospital costs [19]. The relationship of postoperative complications on hospital costs may be related to different types of complications or their severity. In our cohort, for example, postoperative atrial fibrillation did not alter cost, while pneumonia and anastomotic leak led to increased cost. These subgroups also differed in that pneumonia was associated with increased ICU and radiology related cost, while anastomotic leak increased cost related to non-ICU room and board (and not ICU or radiology).

Two unexpected findings from this study were the independent effects of hypertension and coronary artery disease on hospital costs, as revealed by multivariate analysis. A preoperative diagnosis of hypertension was associated with cost *savings* of $21,226 among all patients and savings of $33,324 among patients that experienced a postoperative complication. Coronary artery disease was associated with additional costs of $16,189 overall, and again this effect was even more pronounced in patients with complications at $22,838, even when correcting for the occurrence of postoperative cardiac complications. Our data does not explain how hypertension could be cost saving, but we hypothesize that a diagnosis of hypertension may be a surrogate for improved preoperative medical management. Perioperative treatment of patients with diagnosis of hypertension with beta-blockers or aspirin, for example, may affect perioperative outcomes (or their severity) and therefore cost [20, 21]. Further research into this association is required.

Our study design has several limitations. Surgical technique was at the surgeon's discretion, creating bias in how patients were selected for the procedures. We have attempted to mitigate this bias in our analysis, by adjusting available confounders, but the potential for the effect remains given the retrospective nature of this study. Furthermore, the analysis was not adjusted to cancer stage, which may be a confounder in cost related to surgery. We have attempted to minimize the effect of clinical stage as a confounder by including preoperative chemotherapy and radiation, which we believe is a surrogate for advanced stage disease, in our multivariable analysis. Another limitation is that these cost data may not be generalizable to other institutions. Our use of postoperative pathways to decrease length of stay and avoid unnecessary radiographic studies may not be representative of a broader population. Additionally, the size of our cohort, while being larger than those of other studies on cost analysis of minimally invasive surgical techniques, is relatively small. Further subdivision into 4 groups may make the groups too small to identify differences even if they exist (type II error). The last weakness is that the data presented examines only inpatient hospital cost from the index hospital admission and does not reflect the true economic impact on the health care "system," including costs associated with readmission. We believe that our data is nonetheless important in examining this "narrow" segment of cost because this cost remains the largest cost associated with esophagectomy and should include cost associated with most complications.

As the cost of health care is increasingly scrutinized, we believe that surgeons should take an active role in cost containment. Emerging technology has the potential to increase cost without leading to significant clinical benefit. This study demonstrates that minimally invasive techniques are no more costly than open procedures at our institution. Given that there were no differences in cost amongst these groups, we advocate that surgeons should choose technique based on clinical factors, not cost. We also show that patients with certain preoperative characteristics and postoperative complications can have significantly increased hospital costs. We would not advocate in any way that this data be used to "ration" care to patients that might cost less. Instead, we believe that this data supports using evidence based guidelines to reduce complications; reduction of cost would be a welcome secondary effect of having fewer complications. Future research is warranted to determine whether care pathways in esophagectomy can reduce associated hospital cost at a multi-institution level. In light of the escalating cost of healthcare, we believe that protocols that consider cost optimization (in addition to other clinical factors) should be implemented and studied.

Abbreviations

ASA: American Society of Anesthesiologists
BMI: Body mass index
CAD: Coronary artery disease
CHF: Congestive heart failure
COPD: Chronic obstructive pulmonary disease
ICU: Intensive care unit
IQR: Interquartile range
LOS: Length of stay
MIE: Minimally invasive esophagectomy
OR: Operating room
VATS: Video assisted thoracic surgery.

Competing Interests

The authors have no competing interests regarding the publication of this paper.

References

[1] R. M. Newman and L. W. Traverso, "Cost-effective minimally invasive surgery: what procedures make sense?" *World Journal of Surgery*, vol. 23, no. 4, pp. 415–421, 1999.

[2] M. M. Tiwari, J. F. Reynoso, R. High, A. W. Tsang, and D. Oleynikov, "Safety, efficacy, and cost-effectiveness of common laparoscopic procedures," *Surgical Endoscopy*, vol. 25, no. 4, pp. 1127–1135, 2011.

[3] C. P. Delaney, R. P. Kiran, A. J. Senagore, K. Brady, and V. W. Fazio, "Case-matched comparison of clinical and financial outcome after laparoscopic or open colorectal surgery," *Annals of Surgery*, vol. 238, no. 1, pp. 67–72, 2003.

[4] C. P. Delaney, E. Chang, A. J. Senagore, and M. Broder, "Clinical outcomes and resource utilization associated with laparoscopic and open colectomy using a large national database," *Annals of Surgery*, vol. 247, no. 5, pp. 819–824, 2008.

[5] M. Scarpa, S. Valente, R. Alfieri et al., "Systematic review of health-related quality of life after esophagectomy for esophageal cancer," *World Journal of Gastroenterology*, vol. 17, no. 42, pp. 4660–4674, 2011.

[6] S. Paul and N. Altorki, "Outcomes in the management of esophageal cancer," *Journal of Surgical Oncology*, vol. 110, no. 5, pp. 599–610, 2014.

[7] M. C. J. Anderegg, S. S. Gisbertz, and M. I. van Berge Henegouwen, "Minimally invasive surgery for oesophageal cancer," *Best Practice & Research: Clinical Gastroenterology*, vol. 28, no. 1, pp. 41–52, 2014.

[8] S. Sihag, C. D. Wright, J. C. Wain et al., "Comparison of perioperative outcomes following open versus minimally invasive Ivor Lewis oesophagectomy at a single, high-volume centre," *European Journal of Cardio-thoracic Surgery*, vol. 42, no. 3, pp. 430–437, 2012.

[9] S. S. A. Y. Biere, M. I. van Berge Henegouwen, K. W. Maas et al., "Minimally invasive versus open oesophagectomy for patients with oesophageal cancer: a multicentre, open-label, randomised controlled trial," *The Lancet*, vol. 379, no. 9829, pp. 1887–1892, 2012.

[10] N. Briez, G. Piessen, F. Torres, G. Lebuffe, J.-P. Triboulet, and C. Mariette, "Effects of hybrid minimally invasive oesophagectomy on major postoperative pulmonary complications," *British Journal of Surgery*, vol. 99, no. 11, pp. 1547–1553, 2012.

[11] L. Bailey, O. Khan, E. Willows, S. Somers, S. Mercer, and S. Toh, "Open and laparoscopically assisted oesophagectomy: a prospective comparative study," *European Journal of Cardio-Thoracic Surgery*, vol. 43, no. 2, pp. 268–273, 2013.

[12] L. Lee, M. Sudarshan, C. Li et al., "Cost-effectiveness of minimally invasive versus open esophagectomy for esophageal

cancer," *Annals of Surgical Oncology*, vol. 20, no. 12, pp. 3732–3739, 2013.

[13] R. Parameswaran, D. Veeramootoo, R. Krishnadas, M. Cooper, R. Berrisford, and S. Wajed, "Comparative experience of open and minimally invasive esophagogastric resection," *World Journal of Surgery*, vol. 33, no. 9, pp. 1868–1875, 2009.

[14] Society of Thoracic Surgeons, Data Collection, http://www.sts.org/sites/default/files/documents/AnnotatedDataCollectionFormV2_81%20April.2015.pdf.

[15] K. C. Harth, J. Rose, C. P. Delaney, J. A. Blatnik, I. Halaweish, and M. J. Rosen, "Open versus endoscopic component separation: a cost comparison," *Surgical Endoscopy and Other Interventional Techniques*, vol. 25, no. 9, pp. 2865–2870, 2011.

[16] B. P. Crawshaw, H.-L. Chien, K. M. Augestad, and C. P. Delaney, "Effect of laparoscopic surgery on health care utilization and costs in patients who undergo colectomy," *JAMA Surgery*, vol. 150, no. 5, pp. 410–415, 2015.

[17] N. T. Nguyen, M. W. Hinojosa, B. R. Smith, K. J. Chang, J. Gray, and D. Hoyt, "Minimally invasive esophagectomy lessons learned from 104 operations," *Annals of Surgery*, vol. 248, no. 6, pp. 1081–1091, 2008.

[18] M. N. Short, T. A. Aloia, and V. Ho, "The influence of complications on the costs of complex cancer surgery," *Cancer*, vol. 120, no. 7, pp. 1035–1041, 2014.

[19] P. W. Carrott, S. R. Markar, M. K. Kuppusamy, L. W. Traverso, and D. E. Low, "Accordion severity grading system: assessment of relationship between costs, length of hospital stay, and survival in patients with complications after esophagectomy for cancer," *Journal of the American College of Surgeons*, vol. 215, no. 3, pp. 331–336, 2012.

[20] T. Stern and A. S. Cifu, "Perioperative β-blocker therapy," *JAMA: Journal of the American Medical Association*, vol. 313, no. 24, pp. 2486–2487, 2015.

[21] N. S. Gerstein, M. C. Carey, J. E. Cigarroa, and P. M. Schulman, "Perioperative aspirin management after POISE-2: some answers, but questions remain," *Anesthesia and Analgesia*, vol. 120, no. 3, pp. 570–575, 2015.

Residency Training in Robotic General Surgery: A Survey of Program Directors

Lea C. George, Rebecca O'Neill, and Aziz M. Merchant

Department of Surgery, Rutgers New Jersey Medical School, Newark, NJ 07103, USA

Correspondence should be addressed to Aziz M. Merchant; aziz.merchant@rutgers.edu

Academic Editor: Peng Hui Wang

Objective. Robotic surgery continues to expand in minimally invasive surgery; however, the literature is insufficient to understand the current training process for general surgery residents. Therefore, the objectives of this study were to identify the current approach to and perspectives on robotic surgery training. *Methods.* An electronic survey was distributed to general surgery program directors identified by the Accreditation Council for Graduate Medical Education website. Multiple choice and open-ended questions regarding current practices and opinions on robotic surgery training in general surgery residency programs were used. *Results.* 20 program directors were surveyed, a majority being from medium-sized programs (4–7 graduating residents per year). Most respondents (73.68%) had a formal robotic surgery curriculum at their institution, with 63.16% incorporating simulation training. Approximately half of the respondents believe that more time should be dedicated to robotic surgery training (52.63%), with simulation training prior to console use (84.21%). About two-thirds of the respondents (63.16%) believe that a formal robotic surgery curriculum should be established as a part of general surgery residency, with more than half believing that exposure should occur in postgraduate year one (55%). *Conclusion.* A formal robotics curriculum with simulation training and early surgical exposure for general surgery residents should be given consideration in surgical residency training.

1. Introduction

Since its emergence, robotic surgery technology has seen rapid global adoption across many surgical disciplines including urology, gynecology, and general surgery and, now, robotic surgery is a mainstay of minimally invasive surgery in the United States [1–4]. The growth of robotics into general surgery is partially due to its continuous advancements, such as enhanced visual control and quality, improved manipulation of instruments, and elimination of tremor [1, 5–7]. However, despite the growing field of robotic surgery, there have been only minor changes in the general surgery residency curriculum to incorporate robotic surgery education [8].

In the first few years following robotic surgery FDA approval, several studies explored methods of implementing robotic surgery into general surgery residency training. In 2002, Donias et al. found that only 23% of responding general surgery program directors wished to incorporate robotic training into their residency programs [9]. A year later, Patel et al. discovered that 57% of residents had a strong interest in robotic surgery, yet 80% of them did not have an established robotics training program at their institution [10]. More recently, based on a survey study from 2013, Farivar et al. uncovered that while 96% of US residents have a surgical robot system at their institution, only 63% of residents have participated in a robotic case. Furthermore, 60% of those residents did not receive any robotics training prior to participation [5].

Since these studies, the use of the surgical robot in general surgery has expanded significantly, along with an increased exposure to surgical residents. Very few studies since then have surveyed the current status of robotics training in general surgery residency which is evolving rapidly, with the last survey of general surgery program directors dating back to 2002. Further investigations are needed to determine how different residency programs have adapted to incorporate robotic surgery, especially since the usage of robotics in surgery has increased. In addition, even with the incorporation of robotic surgery training, it is unclear how this training is evaluated, since each institution may have developed different methods to assess proficiency.

With robotic technology continuing to grow, minimally invasive surgery may be applicable to a more extensive array of procedures in the future. The objectives of this study were to (1) understand how much exposure general surgery residents currently have to robotic-assisted operations, (2) whether they have received any formal or informal training to robotic surgery, and (3) the effect of this platform on general surgical training.

2. Methods

2.1. Study Population. With Rutgers New Jersey Medical School Institutional Review Board approval, all study members were recruited from accredited general surgery training programs in the United States. The Accreditation Council for Graduate Medical Education website was used to identify 281 general surgery residency programs in October of 2017. Of those listed, 236 programs had email contact information for residency program directors.

2.2. Questionnaire. An online, Rutgers-associated survey tool, Qualtrics, was used to develop a 33-question survey, of which 5 were follow-up questions based on a skip pattern, in which the questions appeared based on the response to the certain questions (Appendix A). The purpose of this survey was to evaluate different perspectives of program directors on robotic surgery education. Specifically, participants were asked about their area of interest in general surgery, years of experience as a surgeon, and amount of experience with robotic surgery. Furthermore, the survey inquired about general aspects of their own surgical residency program, the volume of robotic surgery performed at their institution, and robotic surgery training in their residency program. Lastly, participants were requested to provide their view toward robotic surgery training for residents and achieving proficiency. Some survey questions were modified from previous studies that assessed the prevalence and application of robotic surgery education in residency programs and were therefore found to be still relevant [5, 9, 10].

An initial email was sent to the study population requesting their participation in December of 2017. The email contained an informed consent letter stating the objectives of the study and rights as a participant, an electronic link to the online questionnaire, and contact information of the principal investigator. An electronic reminder was sent to all participants three weeks later to maximize the response rate. The survey did not include any names or identifying information, ensuring privacy and confidentiality. The responses were password protected by the authors.

2.3. Statistical Analysis. The responses were automatically compiled descriptively as percentages for statistical analysis by the Qualtrics program. Basic statistics and table creation were performed with Microsoft Excel 2016.

3. Results

3.1. Demographics. The study sample included 20 total respondents; 18 respondents fully completed the survey, 1 respondent completed all 33 questions except the last 5 questions, and 1 respondent only completed the last 12 questions. The overall survey response rate was 8% (20 of 236 potential respondents). Of the participants who elected to answer, 10 were directors of a university residency program (52.63%), 2 of a university-affiliated residency program (10.53%), and 7 of a community/independent residency program (36.84%), as represented in Table 1. The majority of responding program directors were from medium-sized programs, defined in this study as 4–7 graduating residents per year. Specifically, these responses included 3 program directors of programs with 1–3 graduating residents per year (15.79%), 15 program directors of programs with 4–7 graduating residents per year (78.95%), and 1 program director of a program with 8+ graduating residents per year (5.26%). Next, there was a range of responses for number of attending general surgeons performing robotic surgery at each of the responding program directors' institution with 4 participants having 0–2 robotic surgeons (21.05%), 5 with 3–5 robotic surgeons (26.32%), 5 with 6–8 robotic surgeons (26.32%), and 5 with 8+ robotic surgeons (26.32%), as stated in Table 1. However, there was more variation between the number of cases performed each year for each respondent's institution: 6 reported their institutions performed less than 50 cases per year (33.33%), 4 reported their institutions performed 51–100 cases per year (22.22%), 3 reported their institutions performed 101–200 cases per year (16.67%), and 5 reported their institutions performed over 200 cases per year (27.78%).

The program directors' experiences and interests were also investigated (Table 2). When asked of their primary surgical interest, most program directors responded that they were interested in general surgery (6 of 19, 31.58%). There were 3 participants who responded in each of the specialties: surgical oncology, trauma surgery, and vascular surgery (15.79% each). Additionally, 2 participants specialized in colorectal surgery (10.53%) and another 2 were interested in minimally invasive surgery/laparoscopic surgery (10.53%). No program directors responded that they would be interested in any other field, including bariatric surgery, cardiothoracic surgery, dermatological surgery, endocrine surgery, neurosurgery, ophthalmology, oral and maxillofacial surgery, orthopedic surgery, otorhinolaryngology, pediatric surgery, plastic surgery, thoracic surgery, and urology. Additionally, most responding program directors did not currently use robotic surgery in their practice (73.68%). Of those who do, 3 participants have 0–3 years of experience in robotic surgery (60%) and 2 have for 4–6 years of experience (40%). Of the 5 who perform robotic surgery, 4 included the number of robotic cases they perform each month, varying from 1 to 6 cases (Table 2). Additionally, of the 14 respondents who do not currently use robotic surgery in their practice, only 2 have ever used robotic surgery in their practice (14.29%).

3.2. Current Robotic Surgery Training in General Surgery Residency. To understand the general trends in robotic surgery education and any differences between training, residency directors were questioned about their current training programs (Tables 3 and 4). The majority of responding program directors indicated that their institutions did have a formal

Table 1: Institution demographics.

Question	Response
Residency program type ($N = 19$)	University (52.63%) University affiliated (10.53%) Community/independent (36.84%)
Number of graduating residents per year ($N = 19$)	1–3 residents (15.79%) 4–7 residents (78.95%) 8+ residents (5.26%)
Number of attending surgeons performing robotic surgery ($N = 19$)	0–2 surgeons (21.05%) 3–5 surgeons (26.32%) 6–8 surgeons (26.32%) 9+ surgeons (26.32%)
Number of general surgery robotic cases each year ($N = 18$)	Less than 50 cases (33.33%) 51–100 cases (22.22%) 101–200 cases (16.67%) Over 200 cases (27.78%)

Table 2: Program director demographics.

Question	Response
Area of specialty interest or expertise within general surgery ($N = 19$)	Colorectal surgery (10.53%) General surgery (31.58%) Surgical oncology (15.79%) Trauma surgery (15.79%) Vascular surgery (15.79%) Other (10.53%, MIS/GI surgery/abdominal wall reconstruction, laparoscopic surgery) All others* (0%)
Number of years as a practicing surgery ($N = 19$)	0–4 years (0%) 5–9 years (26.32%) 10–14 years (15.79%) 15–19 years (21.05%) 20+ years (36.84%)
Use of robotic surgery in current practice ($N = 19$)	Yes (26.32%) No (73.68%)
If yes, amount of years using robotic surgery in practice ($N = 5$)	0–3 years (60%) 4–6 years (40%) 7–9 years (0%) 10+ (0%)
If yes, number of cases performed each month ($N = 4$)	1 case 2 cases 1–3 cases 6 cases
If no, any experience in robotic surgery in practice ($N = 14$)	Yes (14.29%) Never used robotic surgery (85.71%)

*Other options included: Bariatric Surgery, Cardiothoracic Surgery, Dermatologic Surgery, Endocrine Surgery, Neurosurgery, Ophthalmology, Oral and Maxillofacial Surgery, Orthopedic Surgery, Otorhinolaryngology, Pediatric Surgery, Plastic Surgery, Thoracic Surgery, Urology.

TABLE 3: Comparison of current robotic surgery training to program director beliefs.

Question	Current practice	PG opinion
Is there/should there be a formal clinical curriculum for robotic surgery training of general surgery residents at your institution? (N = 19)	Yes (73.68%) No (26.32%)	Yes (63.16%) No (36.84%)
At which postgraduate year (PGY) level, do/should your residents first have exposure to robotic surgery? (N = 19, 20, resp.)	PGY1 (42.11%) PGY2 (10.53%) PGY3 (31.58%) PGY4 (10.53%) PGY5 (5.26%)	PGY1 (55%) PGY2 (15%) PGY3 (30%) PGY4 (0%) PGY5 (0%)
What is your program's current/the best method to deliver robotic surgery training during residency? (N = 19, 20, resp.)	Conference/didactic session (0%) Teaching labs/simulation (10.53%) Operating room experience (5.26%) Combination of the above (84.21%)	Conference/didactic session (0%) Teaching labs/simulation (30%) Operating room experience (0%) Combination of the above (70%)*
Does/should your program collaborate with industry to provide robotic surgery training to residents? (N = 20, 19, resp.)	Yes (80%) No (20%)	Yes (63.16%) No (36.84%)
Do/should all graduating chief residents in your program achieve competency in this operation prior to graduation? (N = 20)	Yes (30%) No (70%)	Yes (35%) No (65%)
If not currently a competency, is resident achievement of competency based on resident's interest in robotic surgery? (N = 14)	Yes (78.57%) No (21.43%)	

*By selecting "combination of the above," respondents were requested to further elaborate. The responses included (N = 12) all 3 listed above (75%), computer based training, followed by simulation, followed by beside assist, finally console (8.33%), and simulation modulates then OR (16.67%).

clinical curriculum for robotic surgery training for their general surgery residents (73.68%, Table 3). Additionally, most have a formal simulation curriculum established for robotic surgery training (63.16%, Table 4). Regarding those without a formal simulation curriculum, most respondents perceived funding/cost (20.83%), faculty availability (20.83%), and access to simulators and facilities (20.83%) as the top barriers to including robotic simulation into their program (Table 4). Dedicated time for simulation (16.67%) and lack of facilities (16.67%) were also selected as barriers preventing the incorporation of a formal simulation curriculum. Only one participant found lacking national standards for robotic simulation as a barrier.

Most responding program directors stated that their residency programs incorporate residents' first exposure to robotic surgery in either postgraduate year 1 or 3 (41.11% and 31.58%, resp., Table 3). The postgraduate year (PGY) level at which residents begin to assist at the bedside of a robotic case varied, with a third of the programs beginning in PGY2 (33.33%, Table 4). As to when residents begin to perform as a console surgeon in a robotic case, many respondents reported that their programs allowed their residents to do so once they were a PGY4 (44.48%).

Currently, a majority of the participants with programs that included robotic surgery into their residency training, reported the use of a combination of teaching labs/simulation and operating room experience (84.21%, Table 3). Furthermore, most programs had a specific simulation training for residents in docking, instrument exchange, and console skills (73.68%, 82.35%, and 84.21%, resp.), but most did not have specific simulation training for specific robotic procedures such as cholecystectomy and hernia repair (57.89%, Table 4). To provide robotic surgery training to general surgery residents, most respondents indicated collaborating with industry (80%, Table 3).

Prior to allowing residents to assist in or perform a robotic surgery case, most respondents required residents to achieve proficiency on a robotic simulator (70%, Table 4). However, the majority did not require all graduating chief residents at their program to achieve competency in basic robotic operation prior to graduating (70%, Table 3). In these programs that did not require competency, most residents who do achieve competency in robotic surgery do so because of their interest in robotic surgery (78.57%). Unfortunately, for those graduating residents interested in further developing their robotic surgery skills, most program directors surveyed did not offer a minimally invasive and robotic surgery fellowship at their institution (89.47%).

3.3. Views on Robotic Surgery Education in General Surgery Residency. To understand future directions of robotic surgery training for general surgery residents, the current opinions on robotic surgery education were investigated (Tables 3 and 5). About two-thirds of the surveyed program directors believe that a formal robotics surgery curriculum should be incorporated in general surgery residency training (63.16%, Table 3). All respondents believe that residents should be first exposed to robotic surgery training within

TABLE 4: Current robotic surgery education method.

Question	Response		
Is there a formal simulation curriculum for robotic surgery training of general surgery residents at your institution? (N = 19)	Yes (63.16%) No (36.84%)		
What do you perceive as a barrier(s) to including robotic simulation in your program? (N = 24)	Funding/cost (20.83%) Faculty availability (20.83%) Dedicated time for simulation (16.67%) Lack of facilities (16.67%) Access to simulators and facilities (20.83%) Lack of scientific evidence (0%) Lack of national standards in robotic simulation (4.17%) Other (0%)		
At which postgraduate year (PGY) level do most residents in your program begin to assist at the bedside of a robotic case? (N = 18)	PGY1 (22.22%) PGY2 (33.33%) PGY3 (27.78%) PGY4 (11.11%) PGY5 (5.56%)		
At which postgraduate year (PGY) level do most residents in your program begin to perform as a console surgeon in a robotic case? (N = 18)	PGY1 (5.56%) PGY2 (0%) PGY3 (27.78%) PGY4 (44.44%) PGY5 (22.22%)		
Does your program have specific simulation training for residents in any of the following tasks:	Docking (N = 19)	Yes (73.68%)	No (26.32%)
	Instrument exchange (N = 17)	Yes (82.35%)	No (17.65%)
	Console skills (N = 19)	Yes (84.21%)	No (15.79%)
	Specific robotic procedures [cholecystectomy, hernia repair, etc.] (N = 19)	Yes (42.11%)	No (57.89%)
Does your program require residents to achieve proficiency on a robotic simulator prior to assisting in, or performing, a robotic surgery case? (N = 20)	Yes (70%) No (20%)		
Does your institution offer a minimally invasive and robotic surgery fellowship? (N = 19)	Yes (10.53%) No (89.47%)		

TABLE 5: Views on robotic surgery education method.

Question	Response
Should more time be dedicated to robotic surgery training during general surgery residency? (N = 19)	Yes (52.63%) No (47.37%)
Should more time be dedicated to robotic simulation training prior to resident console use in the operating room? (N = 19)	Yes (84.21%) No (15.79%)
How should proficiency/mastery of robotic surgery be determined? (N = 20)	Number of cases completed (20%%) Level of involvement on RS cases (40%) Other (40%)**
Do you believe a fellowship in robotic surgery should be required to safely perform robotic surgery cases? (N = 19)	Yes (15.79%) No (84.21%)

**By selecting "other," respondents were requested to further elaborate. The responses included (N = 6) measured performance of surgeons with excellent robotic surgery outcomes, validated metrics, a combination of standardized evaluation, competency evaluations, and procedures, PD evaluation, and EPA's such as -- can the resident dock/can the resident dissect/can the resident maneuver the camera/change. Instruments/can the resident sew simple versus complex cases, and OSATs.

their first 3 years, with a majority thinking this should occur at the PGY1 level (55%). Interestingly, more than half of the participating program directors believe that more time should be dedicated to robotic surgery training during general surgery residency (52.63%, Table 5). More specifically, that more training time should be dedicated to robotic simulation training prior to console use in the operating room (84.21%).

As to the best method to deliver robotic training to general surgery residents, more than two-thirds (70%, Table 3) found it best to use a combination. The most common combination included using conference/didactic session, teaching labs/simulators, and the operating room. One participant suggested computer-based training, followed by simulation, then by bedside assisting, and finally console use. Others found that teaching labs/simulators are the best method to deliver robotic training (30%), as reported in Table 3. Consistent with current practice, many respondents still believe industry should play a role in this robotic training and simulation (63.16%).

With all the training and proficiencies required of graduating residents, most program directors do not find that proficiency in robotic surgery should be a required competency (Table 3). However, if proficiency/mastery needed to be determined, most participants would base it off of either a resident's level of involvement on a robotic surgery case or some sort of evaluation method of their robotic skills (40% for each method, Table 5), with one participant responding "Can the resident dock? Can the resident dissect? Can the resident maneuver the camera/change instruments? Can the resident sew simple versus complex cases?" as ways to assess robotic skills. Very few thought that the number of cases completed would be enough to determine proficiency of robotic surgery (20%). Lastly, a majority of program directors did not believe that a fellowship in robotic surgery should be required to safely perform robotic surgery cases (84.21%).

4. Discussion

This survey provided a unique opportunity to understand the perspectives of program directors on the implementation, usage, and assessment of robotic surgery training in general surgery residency programs. We found that the majority of responding program directors do not currently use robotic surgery in their practice, but their general surgery residency programs did have a formal robotic surgery curriculum as well as simulation training. For those that did not have simulation, the most common perceived barriers were cost, faculty availability, and access to simulators. With cost and access as two major barriers, industry may be able to play an important role in robotic surgery training. In fact, most respondents are of programs that currently collaborate with industry to provide robotic surgery training to residents and most responding program directors believe that they should continue to play a role in the future. This suggests that respondents acknowledge the importance of robotic surgery training, but its implementation may be impeded by financial or technical constraints. This is supported by the fact that a majority of the responding program directors believe a formal robotic surgery curriculum should be incorporated and that more time should be spent on robotic surgery training, especially with simulation prior to operating room experiences.

Responding program directors not only support increased emphasis on robotic surgery training but also advocate for early exposure. Program directors responded that, in both current practice and their perspective, residents have early exposure to robotic surgery, commonly in the first year. Program directors responded that the robotic surgery training commonly occurs as follows: introduction to robotic surgery during PGY1, achievement of proficiency via simulation prior to bedside assisting during PGY2, and then practicing and advancing until they can control the console, which usually occurs during PGY4. Despite this stepwise training, we found that chief residents are not required to attain competency in robotic surgery prior to graduation. Similarly, responding program directors did not feel this competency requirement should be implemented. Interestingly, a majority of the responding program directors believe that a fellowship is not necessary to safely perform robotic surgery cases. Essentially, general surgery residents are educated in robotic surgery throughout their residency, though it is not a required competency for graduation. Despite the lack of competency requirement, responding program directors feel the robotic surgery training during residency is sufficient for graduates to safely perform robotic surgery.

These results were supported by current literature. This survey revealed that most respondents' programs now provide exposure to robotics surgery during residency, which is supported by a more recent study surveying general surgery residents in 2013 [5]. Comparable to previous studies about robotics education, this study finds that there needs to be greater emphasis on robotics surgery education during residency [5, 10]. Furthermore, results from robotics education studies in other surgical specialties also support the results of this survey that there is a need to develop a structured curriculum in robotic surgery [11–14].

Similar to results of this study, recent studies also found that a majority of programs offer their residents early robotic training, with most beginning at the PGY1 levels [5, 10]. According to older studies, most programs used experiences assisting in the operating room as the main teaching method for residents, with minimal augmentation from teaching labs and conference/didactic session [5, 9, 10]. The results of this study do not support this result and, along with more recent studies, found that many programs have now switched to using a combination of teaching methods to educate residents in robotics [14, 15]. This difference may be due to the fact that robotics technology is rapidly developing, with more developed and accessible simulation training tools. By standardizing robotics education, general surgery residency programs can incorporate protected time toward developing this surgical method, which would ultimately improve surgical outcomes and better our patients.

This study had several limitations typical of survey-based studies. First, the response rate was low resulting in not enough responses to perform robust statistical analysis; therefore, only descriptive analysis was used. This low response rate makes it difficult to apply the conclusions of this paper to all general surgery residency programs and their program directors. Another limitation was that participation was voluntary, meaning it is possible that people who had strong opinions regarding robotic surgery were more likely to complete the survey, resulting in selection bias. Perhaps another method of distribution besides email would have increased the response rate, thereby reducing these limitations and enabling the application of these conclusions on a greater scale.

Overall, despite several limitations, this study has provided useful insights into the realities and program director perspectives of robotic surgery training. This information may contribute to the further incorporation of robotic training into the general surgery residency programs.

5. Conclusion

In conclusion, this study found that the majority of responding general surgery residency programs have robotic surgery training with the use of simulation. Respondents support this training, even though few perform robotic surgery themselves and in fact advocate for increased time and emphasis on robotic surgery training as well as early exposure for residents. This study has obtained valuable results regarding robotic surgery training and the perspectives of general surgery residency program directors which will contribute towards the continued progress of robotic surgery education in general surgery residency programs.

Disclosure

This research did not receive any specific grant from funding agencies in the public, commercial, or not-for-profit sectors.

Supplementary Materials

Appendix A contains our 33-question survey. Both multiple choice and open-ended questions were used. Five questions were follow-up questions based on a skip pattern, in which the questions appeared based on the response to certain questions. *(Supplementary Materials)*

References

[1] J. H. Palep, "Robotic assisted minimally invasive surgery," *Journal of Minimal Access Surgery*, vol. 5, no. 1, pp. 1–7, 2009.

[2] L. B. Conrad, P. T. Ramirez, W. Burke et al., "Role of minimally invasive surgery in gynecologic oncology," *International Journal of Gynecological Cancer*, vol. 25, no. 6, pp. 1121–1127, 2015.

[3] S. D. Herrell, "Robotic surgery: past, present, and future," *Atlas of Robotic Urologic Surgery*, pp. 459–472, 2017.

[4] R. Sudan and S. S. Desai, "Emergency and weekend robotic surgery are feasible," *Journal of Robotic Surgery*, vol. 6, no. 3, pp. 263–266, 2011.

[5] B. S. Farivar, M. Flannagan, and I. M. Leitman, "General surgery residents' perception of robot-assisted procedures during surgical training," *Journal of Surgical Education*, vol. 72, no. 2, article no. 990, pp. 235–242, 2015.

[6] J. Y. Lee, P. Mucksavage, C. P. Sundaram, and E. M. Mcdougall, "Best practices for robotic surgery training and credentialing," *The Journal of Urology*, vol. 185, no. 4, pp. 1191–1197, 2011.

[7] T. L. Ghezzi and O. C. Corleta, "30 Years of Robotic Surgery," *World Journal of Surgery*, vol. 40, no. 10, pp. 2550–2557, 2016.

[8] B. Morris, "Robotic surgery: Applications, limitations, and impact on surgical education," *The Medscape Journal of Medicine*, vol. 7, no. 3, article no. 72, 2005.

[9] H. W. Donias, R. L. Karamanoukian, P. L. Glick, J. Bergsland, and H. L. Karamanoukian, "Survey of resident training in robotic surgery," *The American Surgeon*, vol. 68, no. 2, pp. 177–181, 2002.

[10] Y. R. Patel, H. W. Donias, and D. W. Boyd, "Are you ready to become a robo-surgeon?" *The American Surgeon*, vol. 69, pp. 599–603, 2003.

[11] M. H. Vetter, M. Palettas, E. Hade, J. Fowler, and R. Salani, "Time to consider integration of a formal robotic-assisted surgical training program into obstetrics/gynecology residency curricula," *Journal of Robotic Surgery*, pp. 1–5, 2017.

[12] J. M. Gobern, C. M. Novak, and E. G. Lockrow, "Survey of robotic surgery training in obstetrics and gynecology residency," *Journal of Minimally Invasive Gynecology*, vol. 18, no. 6, pp. 755–760, 2011.

[13] G. Dulan, D. Hogg, K. Gilbert-Fischer et al., "Developing a proficiency-based training program for robotic surgery," *Journal of Surgical Research*, vol. 165, no. 2, p. 334, 2011.

[14] S. M. Sperry, B. W. O'Malley Jr., and G. S. Weinstein, "The University of pennsylvania curriculum for training otorhinolaryngology residents in transoral robotic surgery," *ORL*, vol. 76, no. 6, pp. 342–352, 2014.

[15] J. S. Winder, R. M. Juza, J. Sasaki et al., "Implementing a robotics curriculum at an academic general surgery training program: our initial experience," *Journal of Robotic Surgery*, vol. 10, no. 3, pp. 209–213, 2016.

38

Robot-Assisted Hybrid Esophagectomy Is Associated with a Shorter Length of Stay Compared to Conventional Transthoracic Esophagectomy: A Retrospective Study

Hans C. Rolff, Rikard B. Ambrus, Mohammed Belmouhand, Michael P. Achiam, Marianne Wegmann, Mette Siemsen, Steen C. Kofoed, and Lars B. Svendsen

Department of Surgical Gastroenterology, Rigshospitalet, University of Copenhagen, Blegdamsvej 9, 2100 Copenhagen, Denmark

Correspondence should be addressed to Hans C. Rolff; hc.rolff@gmail.com

Academic Editor: Casey M. Calkins

Aim. To compare the peri- and postoperative data between a hybrid minimally invasive esophagectomy (HMIE) and the conventional Ivor Lewis esophagectomy. *Methods.* Retrospective comparison of perioperative characteristics, postoperative complications, and survival between HMIE and Ivor Lewis esophagectomy. *Results.* 216 patients were included, with 160 procedures performed with the conventional and 56 with the HMIE approach. Lower perioperative blood loss was found in the HMIE group (600 ml versus 200 ml, $p < 0.001$). Also, a higher median number of lymph nodes were harvested in the HMIE group (median 28) than in the conventional group (median 23) ($p = 0.002$). The median length of stay was longer in the conventional group compared to the HMIE group (11.5 days versus 10.0 days, $p = 0.03$). Patients in the HMIE group experienced fewer grade 2 or higher complications than the conventional group (39% versus 57%, $p = 0.03$). The rate of all pulmonary (51% versus 43%, $p = 0.32$) and severe pulmonary complications (38% versus 18%, $p = 0.23$) was not statistically different between the groups. *Conclusions.* The HMIE was associated with lower intraoperative blood loss, a higher lymph node harvest, and a shorter hospital stay. However, the inborn limitations with the retrospective design stress a need for prospective randomized studies. Registration number is DRKS00013023.

1. Introduction

Surgery is the treatment of choice for resectable tumors in the distal esophagus and at the gastroesophageal junction. However, the surgical procedure is associated with a high incidence of postoperative morbidity and mortality with the latter ranging from 2 to 10% [1, 2]. In order to minimize postoperative morbidity and mortality, minimally invasive esophagectomy has been implemented. Minimally invasive surgery diminishes the surgical trauma [3], reduces blood loss and overall hospital stay [4–6], and has comparable oncological results to open surgery [7, 8]. Nevertheless, the conventional minimally invasive surgical methods are challenged by technical aspects, such as two-dimensional view with lack of depth perceptions, long and rigid instruments, and uncomfortable positions for the surgeon [9]. These limitations are less prominent with the implementation of robot-assisted esophagectomy, which allows three-dimensional view and improved articulation of instruments with seven degrees of freedom [10]. Still, data on the clinical effects of robot-assisted esophagectomy are scarce with only few studies published [11, 12].

At our department, a hybrid minimally invasive Ivor Lewis esophagectomy (HMIE), with robot-assisted laparoscopic access to the abdominal cavity and conventional thoracotomy, was implemented during spring 2013. Accordingly, both the HMIE and the conventional Ivor Lewis esophagectomy have been standard procedures since the implementation of the robot-assisted procedure. The aim of this study was to compare the intra- and postoperative data between the two surgical approaches.

2. Materials and Methods

2.1. Patients. Data from all patients operated for adenocarcinoma in the distal esophagus, at a tertiary referral center in the period from January 1, 2013, to June 1, 2015, were included in the analysis. The patients were retrospectively identified by using the operation codes of The Nordic Medico-Statistical Committee related to resection of distal EC [13]. The presented results from the HMIE group included the learning curve. Initially the operating Robot (daVinci® Si System, Intuitive Surgical Inc., Sunnyvale, CA, USA) was available for 1 day a week; however, resections for distal EC were performed 3 days weekly; thus patients were allocated randomly according to the operation day. However patients that were initially allocated to the HMIE procedure were disqualified if obese (BMI ≥ 35), had a history of previous open abdominal surgery, or were suspected for having a T4-tumor. After two months, the restriction regarding obesity was revised due to good experience with borderline obese cases.

2.2. Preoperative Management. All patients followed a standard program after referral to our center. Accordingly, the patients underwent a confirmatory esophagogastroduodenoscopy followed by a contrast enhanced thoracoabdominal computed tomography (CT) scan (or positron emission tomography- (PET-) CT scan if indicated). These examinations were supplemented by an ultrasound examination of the neck and a pulmonary function test, prior to a multidisciplinary conference with the presence of specialists within the fields of surgery, oncology, radiology, pathology, and nuclear medicine. If a patient was considered eligible for surgery, a diagnostic laparoscopy was performed to evaluate the resectability. Prior to definitive surgery, patients with adenocarcinoma were referred for perioperative oncological adjuvant chemotherapy according to the MAGIC-regimen [14].

2.3. Surgical Procedures. The conventional transthoracic esophagectomy started with upper laparotomy. Hereafter resectability was again evaluated by ruling out any signs of distant or nonresectable spread. The gastroesophageal junction and the hiatus is hereafter exposed by division of the gastrohepatic and the phrenoesophageal ligaments. The stomach is mobilized at the greater curvature by division of the short gastric vessels and the gastrocolic ligament under the consideration of the right gastroepiploic artery. The stomach is lifted up and the left gastric vessels are identified and divided. The stomach is then mobilized from the lesser curvature to the right gastric artery. This step is followed by Kocher Maneuver. The stomach conduit was then prepared and a pyloromyotomy was performed.

In contrast, the robot-assisted laparoscopy started with insufflation (12 mmHg) with the patient in a supine position, followed by mobilization of the stomach, lymphadenectomy, and division of arteries with the patient in a 13-degree head-up tilt position, as described for the open procedure. After the closure of abdomen (conventional procedure) and desufflation (robot-assisted laparoscopy), the thoracic surgical procedure was identical in both groups; a right thoracotomy at the sixth intercostal space to remove the tumor en bloc along with mediastinal, subcarinal, and paraesophageal lymph nodes (D1+ lymphadenectomy). After resection of the tumor, gastric continuity was reestablished between the esophagus and the remnant corpus part of the stomach, and the surgery was concluded with the placement of a nasogastric tube and a chest tube.

2.4. Postoperative Management. All patients followed a standardized postoperative care regimen and were mobilized from day one. Pain was managed using epidural analgesia until the postoperative day three, and patients were individually supplemented with paracetamol, tramadol, or morphine if indicated. During the first week after surgery, patients followed a strict nil-by-mouth regimen and were instead supplied with intravenous nutrition. At the 7th postoperative day, an X-ray with orally administered contrast swallow was performed to evaluate the integrity of the anastomosis, with reintroduction of liquid oral intake if no sign of anastomotic leakage was detected.

2.5. Study Design. The present study was a retrospective, nonrandomized, single center evaluation, comparing the conventional with the HMIE. In cases where the HMIE were converted into a conventional open procedure, the results were presented as a conventional procedure.

As this was a retrospective study assessing the treatment quality no ethical approval was required. All patient sensitive data were treated anonymously and were not directly transferable to the individual patient.

2.6. Patient Data Registration. All preoperative data regarding demography, comorbidities, height, and weight were retrieved from the electronic patient records. Also, data regarding postoperative morbidity and mortality were registered according to the Clavien-Dindo classification [15] (Table 1), followed by the calculation of the comprehensive complication index (CCI) score [16] using the online tool available at http://www.assessurgery.com/about_cci-calculator/. All events were recorded individually by two investigators and disagreements were settled by discussion within the group. Anastomotic insufficiency was confirmed by either contrast enhanced CT scan/X-ray or by endoscopy and was graded according to Svendsen et al. [17].

2.7. Statistics. Descriptive statistics for continuous variables are presented as median (min., max.) and dichotomous variables are presented by the absolute number and the percentage of positives. Continuous variables were compared using Mann-Whitney U test, while χ^2-test was used for categorical variables.

The statistical analyses were performed using the SPSS-software (IBM SPSS statistics for Windows, Version 22.0. Armonk, NY). p values < 0.05 were considered significant. The comparison of long-term survival between groups was conducted through a Log-Rank test.

TABLE 1: Clavien-Dindo classification of postoperative complications.

Grade I	Any deviation from the normal postoperative course without the need for pharmacological treatment or surgical, endoscopic, and radiological interventions. Allowed therapeutic regimens are drugs as antiemetics, antipyretics, analgetics, diuretics, electrolytes, and physiotherapy. This grade also includes wound infections opened at the bedside.
Grade II	Requiring pharmacological treatment with drugs other than such allowed for grade I complications. Blood transfusions and total parenteral nutrition are also included.
Grade III	Requiring surgical, endoscopic, or radiological intervention.
(i) IIIa	Intervention not under general anesthesia.
(ii) IIIb	Intervention under general anesthesia
Grade IV	Life-threatening complications (including CNS complications) requiring IC/ICU management.
(i) IVa	Single organ dysfunction (including dialysis).
(ii) IVb	Multiorgan dysfunction.
Grade V	Death of the patient.

3. Results

During the period of January 1, 2013, to June 1, 2015, a total of 216 patients were included in the statistical analysis, with 160 procedures performed with the conventional approach and 56 with the HMIE approach. Two cases were converted due to obesity and severe adhesions.

There were no differences regarding age and gender distribution, body mass index (BMI), or ASA-scores between the two groups (Table 2).

A significantly lower total blood loss was found in the HMIE group compared to the conventional group (600 ml versus 200 ml, $p < 0.001$). Also, the median number of harvested lymph nodes was significantly higher in the HMIE group (median 28) than in the conventional group (median 23) ($p = 0.002$). In contrast, neither the time of general anaesthesia, operating time, nor the total procedure time was statistically different between the groups.

The median length of hospital stay was significantly longer in the conventional group compared to the HMIE group (11.5 days versus 10.0 days, $p = 0.03$). There were no differences in postoperative complications between the conventional and the HMIE group regarding the proportion of patients experiencing one or more complications of grade I or higher (76% versus 65%, $p = 0.12$), just as no difference in CCI score (12.2 versus 20.9, ($p = 0.12$)) was found. The proportion of patients in the HMIE group which experienced one or more complications of grade II or higher was significantly lower than in the conventional group (39% versus 57%, $p = 0.03$). The rate of anastomotic insufficiency was identical (7%) ($p = 1.00$), and there were no significant differences regarding the 30- and 90-day mortality between the groups.

The rate of all pulmonary complications is shown in Table 3 and shows no statistical differences between the two groups, both regarding the sum of pulmonary complications and when looking isolated at the severe pulmonary complications. However there was a trend towards fewer severe complications in the HMIE groups, but this finding was not statistically significant.

There was no statistically significant difference between the two groups regarding the long-term survival ($p = 0.7$).

4. Discussion

In the present study, we found that patients operated with the HMIE approach had a lesser surgical blood loss, had more lymph nodes harvested, and had a shorter hospital stay compared to patients undergoing conventional Ivor Lewis esophagectomy. Furthermore, the HMIE group experienced fewer grade ≥II complications than the conventional group.

The abovementioned perioperative benefits regarding blood loss and lymph node harvest related to the HMIE approach could reflect that the robot assistance offers a more precise and refined dissection phase compared to the conventional approach. This has benefits, as it has been proposed that blood transfusions are associated to a poorer long-term outcome in cancer patients [18] and are thus important to avoid. The impact of the extent of lymph node resection on long-term survival is much debated. Some papers advocate that the number of removed lymph nodes is an independent prognostic marker [19]. Other reports state that increasing the number of harvested lymph nodes does not per se offer any improvement in the survival [20]. However, the number of metastatic nodes removed and increasing positive-to-negative node ratio were strongly negatively associated to survival [20]. Thus an increased lymph node harvest leads to a better staging. In the present series the increased number of harvested lymph nodes in the HMIE group did not translate into an improved survival, indicating that there is little or no impact on survival. The presented number of harvested lymph nodes in this series is the total amount, and the lymph nodes therefore originate from both the thorax and abdomen. As the thoracic approach was identical it is plausible that the difference in lymph node harvest was due to the different abdominal approaches.

The findings, regarding the postoperative complications, were not entirely clear. No difference in the CCI score between the groups was found; however, a significantly lower proportion of the patients in the HMIE group experienced

Table 2: Comparison of pre-, peri-, and postoperative data between cohorts.

	Conventional (n = 160)	HMIE (n = 56)	p value
Age*	65 (28–88)	66 (39–86)	0.65
Gender			
(i) Male	125 (78%)	50 (88%)	
(ii) Female	35 (22%)	6 (12%)	0.12
BMI*	26.6 (15.6–43.7)	25.8 (18.8–31.2)	0.19
ASA-score			
(i) ASA 1 (%)	41 (26%)	17 (30%)	0.73
(ii) ASA 2 (%)	80 (50%)	28 (50%)	1
(iii) ASA 3 (%)	39 (24%)	12 (21%)	0.72
(iv) ASA 4 (%)	0 (0%)	1 (2%)	
Operating time* (minutes)	248 (100–420)	232 (174–800)	0.2
Blood loss* (ml)	600 (100–4400)	200 (50–1970)	<0.001
Harvested lymph nodes*	23 (11–60)	28 (15–61)	0.002
Length of stay* (days)	11.5 (8–101)	10 (8–69)	0.03
CCI-score	20.9 (0–100)	12.2 (0–100)	0.22
Complications**			
(i) ≥Grade I complications (%)	122 (76%)	37 (65%)	0.12
(ii) ≥Grade II complications (%)	91 (57%)	22 (39%)	0.02
(iii) ≥Grade III complications (%)	51 (32%)	14 (25%)	0.32
Anastomotic insufficiency	11 (7%)	4 (7%)	1
30-day mortality (%)	3 (2%)	0 (0%)	0.57
90-day mortality (%)	5 (3%)	3 (5%)	0.43

HMIE: hybrid minimally invasive esophagectomy; CCI: comprehensive complication index. These scores are generated from http://www.assessurgery.com/about_cci-calculator/; *continuous covariates are presented with median and minimum and maximum values; **complications are graded according to the Clavien-Dindo score. The numbers represents the proportion of patients experiencing one or more complications of at least the grade indicated in the table.

Table 3: Pulmonary complications.

	Conventional (n = 160)	HMIE (n = 56)	p value
All pulmonary complications	51% (81/160)	43% (24/56)	0.32
Severe pulmonary complications*	38% (41/160)	18% (10/56)	0.24

*Severe respiratory complications are defined as grade III or higher on the Clavien-Dindo score.

one or more grade II complications, compared to the conventional group in the current study. These findings are in accordance with the available literature, where the majority of studies report no major differences between the minimally invasive and conventional approaches [21]. Accordingly, some studies report fewer complications with a minimally invasive approach [22, 23], but reports have also indicated that the minimally invasive approach was associated with a higher frequency of acute reoperation [24]. In this study, there was no difference in the pattern of grade II complications between the groups, and thus no apparent explanation for this difference. There was no difference between groups regarding the more severe grade ≥III complications.

In general, the quantification of postoperative complications is semiquantitative by nature, making direct comparison between studies difficult. The Clavien-Dindo grading system does offer some standardization, but different interpretations of the grading system, especially in the low-grade complication range, are likely to occur. Due to these difficulties in getting an objective measure, surrogate markers for the quantification of the complexity of the postoperative course could be used. One such parameter is the total length of hospital stay, which in this study was shorter in the HMIE group compared to the conventional group. This fact may have important economic implications, as a shortening of the admission time may level out the higher costs associated with the robot-assisted procedure. This benefit has been reported for gynecological and urological cancers [25, 26]. More interestingly, it is conceivable that the length of stay and rate of postoperative complications may be further reduced by introducing MIS in the thoracic part of the procedure.

Currently, no consensus regarding the role of MIS in the surgical treatment of upper gastrointestinal cancers exists. A consensus is difficult to define, since the surgical strategies for treating upper gastrointestinal cancers cover a very heterogeneous group of procedures, both regarding the type of access, that is, laparoscopy and robot-assisted laparoscopy, and whether or not these modalities should be applied in the abdomen and/or the thorax. Furthermore, the study designs in previous studies investigating the role of MIS have been suboptimal, with the vast majority being retrospective with small patient volume and with great variation of the surgical techniques among the studies. This aspect is also a limitation in the present study, as this was conducted retrospectively at a single center. This only highlights the need for large prospective randomized trials. Such trials have been registered [7, 27, 28]. Trials comparing the HMIE with the conventional Ivor Lewis esophagectomy especially are relevant due to the similar surgical techniques between the studies [27, 29]. Messager et al. showed significantly reduced perioperative mortality when comparing the HMIE with the conventional procedure [29]. This feat was achieved without a higher rate of reoperation, which had been a concern in previous reports. However, the rate and type of postoperative complications were not reported in the study [29]. Data from the MIRO-trial [27] do show that the rate of pulmonary complications was significantly decreased in the hybrid group. We were unable to reproduce these results; however, there was a trend towards fewer severe pulmonary complications in the HMIE group. Most significantly we found that the length of stay was reduced for the HMIE group. The findings from our study in combination with randomized HMIE studies indicate that HMIE could offer important advantages and may be the future standard surgical strategy for patients with malignant tumors in the distal esophagus.

5. Conclusion

This study shows that HMIE was associated with a significantly reduced intraoperative blood loss, a higher number of harvested lymph nodes, and a shorter hospital stay. Whether this is solely due to the less invasiveness of the HMIE compared to conventional Ivor Lewis esophagectomy needs to be investigated further and the possible advantages must be confirmed in a prospective randomized setting.

References

[1] T. Kim, S. N. Hochwald, G. A. Sarosi, A. M. Caban, G. Rossidis, and K. Ben-David, "Review of minimally invasive esophagectomy and current controversies," *Gastroenterology Research and Practice*, vol. 2012, Article ID 683213, 7 pages, 2012.

[2] C. Mariette, G. Piessen, and J.-P. Triboulet, "Therapeutic strategies in oesophageal carcinoma: role of surgery and other modalities," *The Lancet Oncology*, vol. 8, no. 6, pp. 545–553, 2007.

[3] C. Okholm, J. P. Goetze, L. B. Svendsen, and M. P. Achiam, "Inflammatory response in laparoscopic vs. open surgery for gastric cancer," *Scandinavian Journal of Gastroenterology*, vol. 49, no. 9, pp. 1027–1034, 2014.

[4] P. Nafteux, J. Moons, W. Coosemans et al., "Minimally invasive oesophagectomy: A valuable alternative to open oesophagectomy for the treatment of early oesophageal and gastro-oesophageal junction carcinoma," *European Journal of Cardio-Thoracic Surgery*, vol. 40, no. 6, pp. 1455–1464, 2011.

[5] S. Law, "Is minimally invasive preferable to open oesophagectomy?" *The Lancet*, vol. 379, no. 9829, pp. 1856–1858, 2012.

[6] J. D. Luketich, P. R. Schauer, N. A. Christie et al., "Minimally invasive esophagectomy," *The Annals of Thoracic Surgery*, vol. 70, no. 3, pp. 906–912, 2000.

[7] P. C. van der Sluis, J. P. Ruurda, S. van der Horst et al., "Robot-assisted minimally invasive thoraco-laparoscopic esophagectomy versus open transthoracic esophagectomy for resectable esophageal cancer, a randomized controlled trial (ROBOT trial)," *Trials*, vol. 13, article 230, 2012.

[8] R. J. J. Verhage, E. J. Hazebroek, J. Boone, and R. Van Hillegersberg, "Minimally invasive surgery compared to open procedures in esophagectomy for cancer: A systematic review of the literature," *Minerva Chirurgica*, vol. 64, no. 2, pp. 135–146, 2009.

[9] V. Falk, D. Mintz, J. Grunenfelder, J. I. Fann, and T. A. Burdon, "Influence of three-dimensional vision on surgical telemanipulator performance," *Surgical Endoscopy*, vol. 15, no. 11, pp. 1282–1288, 2001.

[10] K. H. Kernstine, "The first series of completely robotic esophagectomies with three-field lymphadenectomy: Initial experience," *Surgical Endoscopy*, vol. 22, no. 9, article 2102, 2008.

[11] N. T. Nguyen, D. M. Follette, B. M. Wolfe, P. D. Schneider, P. Roberts, and J. Goodnight J.E., "Comparison of minimally invasive esophagectomy with transthoracic and transhiatal esophagectomy," *JAMA Surgery*, vol. 135, no. 8, pp. 920–925, 2000.

[12] V. Bresadola, G. Terrosu, A. Cojutti, E. Benzoni, E. Baracchini, and F. Bresadola, "Laparoscopic versus open gastroplasty in esophagectomy for esophageal cancer: a comparative study," *Surgical Laparoscopy Endoscopy & Percutaneous Techniques*, vol. 16, no. 2, pp. 63–67, 2006.

[13] NOMESCO NM-SC. NOMESCO Classification of Surgical Procedures. 2009.

[14] D. Cunningham, W. H. Allum, S. P. Stenning et al., "Perioperative chemotherapy versus surgery alone for resectable gastroesophageal cancer," *The New England Journal of Medicine*, vol. 355, no. 1, pp. 11–20, 2006.

[15] D. Dindo, N. Demartines, and P. Clavien, "Classification of surgical complications: a new proposal with evaluation in a cohort of 6336 patients and results of a survey," *Annals of Surgery*, vol. 240, no. 2, pp. 205–213, 2004.

[16] K. Slankamenac, R. Graf, J. Barkun, M. A. Puhan, and P.-A. Clavien, "The comprehensive complication index: A novel continuous scale to measure surgical morbidity," *Annals of Surgery*, vol. 258, no. 1, pp. 1–7, 2013.

[17] L. B. Svendsen, L. S. Jensen, J. Holm et al., "Differences in the pattern of anastomotic leakage after oesophagectomy in two high-volume centres," *Danish Medical Journal*, vol. 60, no. 12, Article ID A4733, 2013.

[18] J. P. Cata, J. Lasala, G. Pratt, L. Feng, and J. B. Shah, "Association between perioperative blood transfusions and clinical outcomes in patients undergoing bladder cancer surgery: a systematic review and meta-analysis study," *Journal of Blood Transfusion*, vol. 2016, Article ID 9876394, 8 pages, 2016.

[19] S.-G. Wu, Z.-Q. Zhang, W.-M. Liu et al., "Impact of the number of resected lymph nodes on survival after preoperative

radiotherapy for esophageal cancer," *Oncotarget* , vol. 7, no. 16, pp. 22497–22507, 2016.

[20] M. van der Schaaf, A. Johar, B. Wijnhoven, P. Lagergren, and J. Lagergren, "Extent of lymph node removal during esophageal cancer surgery and survival," *Journal of the National Cancer Institute*, vol. 107, no. 5, 2015.

[21] S. Sihag, A. S. Kosinski, H. A. Gaissert, C. D. Wright, and P. H. Schipper, "Minimally Invasive Versus Open Esophagectomy for Esophageal Cancer: A Comparison of Early Surgical Outcomes from the Society of Thoracic Surgeons National Database," *The Annals of Thoracic Surgery*, vol. 101, no. 4, pp. 1281–1288, 2016.

[22] S. S. A. Y. Biere, M. A. Cuesta, and D. L. Van Der Peet, "Minimally invasive versus open esophagectomy for cancer: A systematic review and meta-analysis," *Minerva Chirurgica*, vol. 64, no. 2, pp. 121–133, 2009.

[23] S. S. A. Y. Biere, M. I. van Berge Henegouwen, K. W. Maas et al., "Minimally invasive versus open oesophagectomy for patients with oesophageal cancer: a multicentre, open-label, randomised controlled trial," *The Lancet*, vol. 379, no. 9829, pp. 1887–1892, 2012.

[24] R. Mamidanna, A. Bottle, P. Aylin, O. Faiz, and G. B. Hanna, "Short-term outcomes following open versus minimally invasive esophagectomy for cancer in England: A population-based national study," *Annals of Surgery*, vol. 255, no. 2, pp. 197–203, 2012.

[25] S. F. Herling, C. Palle, A. M. Møller, T. Thomsen, and J. Sørensen, "Cost-analysis of robotic-assisted laparoscopic hysterectomy versus total abdominal hysterectomy for women with endometrial cancer and atypical complex hyperplasia," *Acta Obstetricia et Gynecologica Scandinavica*, vol. 95, no. 3, pp. 299–308, 2016.

[26] S. Buse, C. E. Hach, P. Klumpen et al., "Cost-effectiveness of robot-assisted partial nephrectomy for the prevention of perioperative complications," *World Journal of Urology*, vol. 34, no. 8, pp. 1131–1137, 2016.

[27] N. Briez, G. Piessen, F. Bonnetain et al., "Open versus laparoscopically-assisted oesophagectomy for cancer: a multicentre randomised controlled phase III trial - the MIRO trial," *BMC Cancer*, vol. 11, article 310, 2011.

[28] N. Briez, G. Piessen, F. Torres, G. Lebuffe, J.-P. Triboulet, and C. Mariette, "Effects of hybrid minimally invasive oesophagectomy on major postoperative pulmonary complications," *British Journal of Surgery*, vol. 99, no. 11, pp. 1547–1553, 2012.

[29] M. Messager, A. Pasquer, A. Duhamel, G. Caranhac, G. Piessen, and C. Mariette, "Laparoscopic gastric mobilization reduces postoperative mortality after esophageal cancer surgery: A French nationwide study," *Annals of Surgery*, vol. 262, no. 5, pp. 817–823, 2015.

39

Laparoscopic Repair of Congenital Diaphragmatic Hernia in Adults

Sanjay Kumar Saroj,[1] Satendra Kumar,[2] Yusuf Afaque,[3] Abhishek Kumar Bhartia,[4] and Vishnu Kumar Bhartia[4]

[1]*Minimal Access Surgery, Institute of Medical Sciences, BHU, Varanasi, India*
[2]*General Surgery, Institute of Medical Sciences, BHU, Varanasi, India*
[3]*AIIMS, New Delhi, India*
[4]*CMRI, Kolkata, India*

Correspondence should be addressed to Sanjay Kumar Saroj; drsahilsaroj@gmail.com

Academic Editor: Diego Cuccurullo

Background, Aims, and Objectives. Congenital diaphragmatic hernia typically presents in childhood but in adults is extremely rare entity. Surgery is indicated for symptomatic and asymptomatic patients who are fit for surgery. It can be done by laparotomy, thoracotomy, thoracoscopy, or laparoscopy. With the advent of minimal access techniques, the open surgical repair for this hernia has decreased and results are comparable with early recovery and less hospital stay. The aim of this study is to establish that laparoscopic repair of congenital diaphragmatic hernia is a safe and effective modality of surgical treatment. *Materials and Methods.* A retrospective study of laparoscopic diaphragmatic hernia repair done during May 2011 to Oct 2014. Total $n = 13$ (M/F: 11/2) cases of confirmed diaphragmatic hernia on CT scan, 4 cases Bochdalek hernia (BH), 8 cases of left eventration of the diaphragm (ED), and one case of right-sided eventration of the diaphragm (ED) were included in the study. Largest defect found on the left side was 15×6 cm and on the right side it was 15×8 cm. Stomach, small intestine, transverse colon, and omentum were contents in the hernial sac. The contents were reduced with harmonic scalpel and thin sacs were usually excised. The eventration was plicated and hernial orifices were repaired with interrupted horizontal mattress sutures buttressed by Teflon pieces. A composite mesh was fixed with nonabsorbable tackers. All patients had good postoperative recovery and went home early with normal follow-up and were followed up for 2 years. *Conclusion.* The laparoscopic repair is a safe and effective modality of surgical treatment for congenital diaphragmatic hernia in experienced hands.

1. Introduction

Congenital diaphragmatic hernia typically presents in childhood. However, its clinical manifestation and diagnosis in adults are extremely rare. They occur due to failure of the development of muscular diaphragm, which leads to displacement of the abdominal component into thorax. The diagnosis of congenital diaphragmatic hernia is based on clinical investigation and is confirmed by plain X-ray film barium study and computed tomography scans.

There are four types of congenital diaphragmatic hernia: posterolateral hernia of Bochdalek, parasternal hernia of Morgagni-Larrey, eventration of diaphragm, and peritoneal-pericardial hernia. Bochdalek hernia is the most common type of congenital diaphragmatic hernia, which was first described by Bochdalek in 1848 [1]. It develops due to the failure of closure of the posterolateral aspect of pleuroperitoneal canal, which takes place between 8 and 10 weeks of gestation. As the left canal closes later than the right, it occurs on the left side in 85% of cases [2].

Eventration of the diaphragm is a congenital anomaly consisting of failure of muscular development of part or all of one or both hemidiaphragms [3]. Clinically, eventration of diaphragm refers to an abnormal elevation of one leaf of an intact diaphragm as a result of paralysis, aplasia, or atrophy of varying degrees of muscle fibers [4]. In some cases, it may be difficult or impossible to distinguish from diaphragmatic paralysis. Complete eventration almost invariably occurs on

TABLE 1: Demographic profile of patients.

Number of patients $N = 13$	
Average age (yrs)	36 yrs
Range of age	28 yrs to 54 yrs
Sex	M : F = 11 : 2
Left sided	12
Right sided	1
Associated factors	
Trauma	7
Congenital	5
Pregnancy	1
Other associated anomalies	Nil

TABLE 2: Clinical manifestation.

Clinical features	Number of patients	Percentage (%)
Abdominal pain	10	76.9
Respiratory distress	3	23%
Cough	2	15.3%
Vomiting	2	15.3%
Intestinal obstruction	1	7.69%
Strangulation	0	—
Asymptomatic	1	7.69%
GERD	7	53.8%
Dysphagia	4	30.77%

TABLE 3: Hernial description.

Pathology		
Type of defect	Bochdalek hernia = 4 Eventration of left side diaphragm = 8 Eventration of right side = 1	
Size of defect	Largest = 15 × 8 cm	Smallest 8 × 8
Content of defect	Right side = liver Left side = stomach = 4 Colon = 3 Stomach with spleen = 1 Omentum = 2	

the left side [5] and is rare on the right [6]. There are very few cases of the right-sided diaphragmatic hernia reported in adults in the literature.

It may be associated with other congenital anomalies. The prevalence of Bochdalek hernia is one in 2,200 births [7] and only 5–10% of them remain undetected in childhood, which presents in adults [8].

Surgery is indicated for symptomatic [6] as well as asymptomatic patients who are fit for surgery [4, 7, 9]. It can be done by laparotomy, thoracotomy, thoracoscopy, or laparoscopy [10, 11]. With the advent of minimal access techniques, the open surgical repair for this hernia has decreased. The results of thoracoscopy and laparoscopy in such cases have been found to be comparable. Laparoscopic repair helps in delineating clear anatomy, working space, early recovery, and return to home and work. Campos and Sipes [12] did the first laparoscopic repair of diaphragmatic hernia in 1991. Kuster et al. followed it in 1992 [13]. Till now only small case series and case report are available in the literature. The aim of this study is to establish that laparoscopic repair of congenital diaphragmatic hernia is a safe and effective modality of surgical treatment in experienced hands.

2. Material and Methods

We present a retrospective study of diaphragmatic hernia repair done laparoscopically during period of May 2011 to Oct 2014. Total $n = 13$ (M/F: 11/2) cases of diaphragmatic hernia were treated (Table 1). Average age of presentation was 36 years (28–54 years). One patient was having right-sided eventration of the diaphragm, while another 12 were presented with left-sided eventration. Bochdalek hernia (BH) was found in 4 patients while the remaining 9 patients were having eventration of the diaphragm. Most patients were having a complex of clinical features.

Abdominal pain (Table 2) and discomfort were the most common presenting complaints in 10 (76.9%) patients followed by dysphagia and GERD in 7 (23%) patients and respiratory distress and cough in 3 (23%) patients. One patient presented with features of small bowel obstruction while one patient was clinically asymptomatic. On clinical examination there was decreased breath sound on left lower chest and also on the right side in a right-sided eventration of the diaphragm. Routine blood investigations were normal. X-ray of the chest showed an elevated left hemidiaphragm and pleural effusion in the left sided diaphragmatic hernia while the elevation of the right hemidiaphragm appeared in the right sided. CT thorax and abdomen were used as a diagnostic modality showing the splenic flexure of the colon and small intestine in the left chest causing mediastinal shift to right. Stomach, 1st, and 2nd part of the duodenum were grossly distended in an obstructed diaphragmatic hernia (Figure 5). In right-sided diaphragmatic hernia there was a large protuberance of liver pushing the right lung (Figure 3).

With a preoperative diagnosis of diaphragmatic hernia, the laparoscopic repair was planned. The patient was placed in 30° reverse trendelenburg position with a sand bag under left lower chest. After insufflations of abdomen, five ports were placed. Presence of diaphragmatic hernia (Table 3) was confirmed, and 4 cases of Bochdalek hernia (BH), 8 cases of left eventration of diaphragm, and one case of right-sided eventration of the diaphragm were included in this study. Largest defect found on the left side was 15 × 6 cm (Figure 1) and on the right side it was 15 × 8 cm. Stomach, small intestine, transverse colon, and omentum were found to be in the hernial sac on left side.

The contents were reduced with the help of harmonic scalpel dissection and however thin sacs were excised. After reduction of contents, hernial orifice was repaired with Polypropylene—1/0 (Ethibond/Prolene). Interrupted horizontal mattress sutures were placed buttressed by Teflon pieces. A 20 × 15 cm (Figure 2) composite mesh (Parietex)

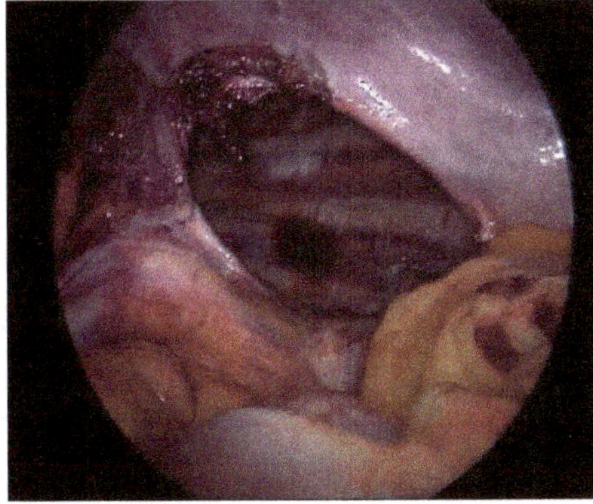

Figure 1: Large Bochdalek hernia on left side.

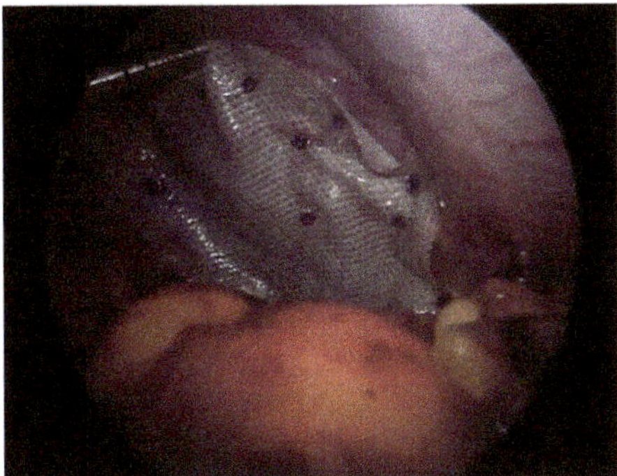

Figure 2: Composite mesh fixed with tackers.

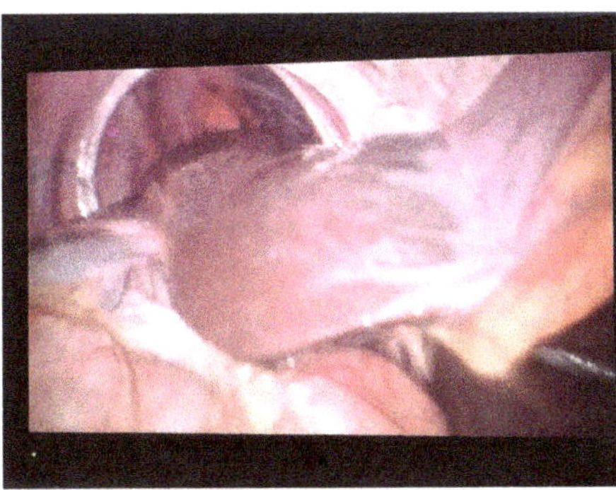

Figure 3: Right-sided eventration of diaphragm content as liver protuberance.

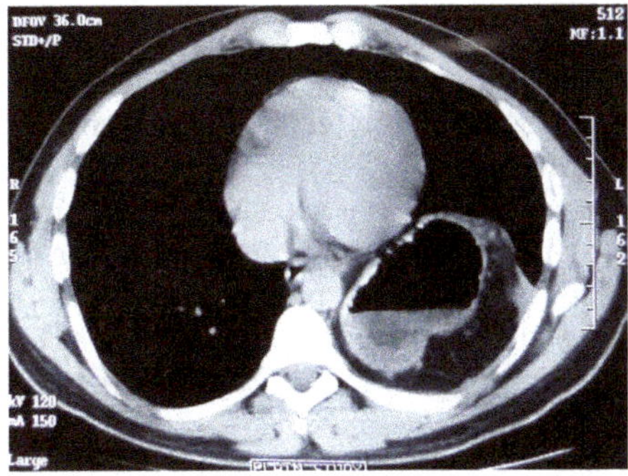

Figure 4: CT scan showing stomach herniation in left Bochdalek hernia.

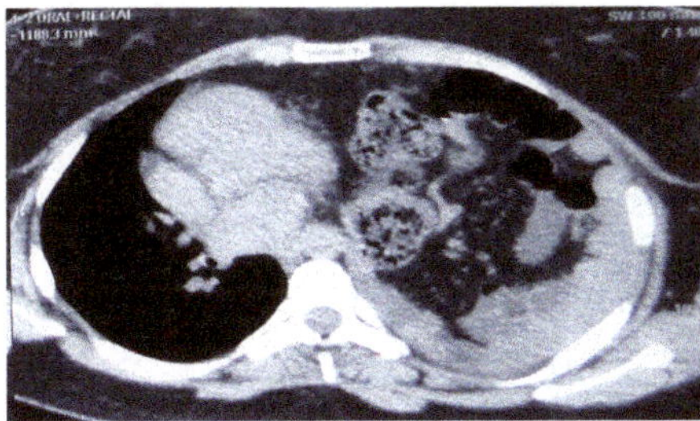

Figure 5: CT scan showing small intestine herniation in left Bochdalek hernia.

was placed over the defect fixed with nonabsorbable tackers. Diaphragmatic plication with (Ethibond) mesh placement was a procedure done in all 9 cases of eventration of the diaphragm.

On the right-sided diaphragmatic hernia the content was liver protuberance, which was reduced with limited conversion procedure compared to the plication of diaphragm with mesh placement being done. Average operating time was 145 mins (110–180 mins). Patients were ambulated and next day liquid diet was given. A postoperative chest X-ray was done on postoperative day one. The average hospital stay was 4 days (2–6 days) and patients were discharged on PPI and analgesic. All patients were followed up for 2 years and one patient was lost in follow-up after one year. All of them were having improvement in clinical symptoms while there was persistent dull aching pain in 3 patients; dyspepsia and fullness in 4 patients were having respiratory distress.

3. Discussion

Congenital diaphragmatic hernia presents in different ways in adults and pediatric age group. Cyanosis and respiratory distress are predominant features in neonates and infancy, while in adults it presents with chest pain, difficulty in breathing, abdominal pain, and sometimes intestinal obstruction [14]. Some cases may remain asymptomatic and it may be due to the occlusion of diaphragmatic defect by the intra-abdominal viscous [15]. Two-thirds of asymptomatic cases have been found to be on the right side and it is mainly because of the liver which prevents herniation of other organs [16].

In congenital diaphragmatic hernia various intra-abdominal organs can herniate into the thorax. Organs that commonly herniate are stomach (Figure 4), ileum, colon, and spleen and on the right side liver and right kidney may also herniate along with the bowel loops. A left side Bochdalek hernia may be associated with lung hypoplasia, extralobar sequestration, malrotation of midgut, and cardiac defects and on the right side, it is often associated with hypoplasia of the right lobe of liver [17].

Bochdalek hernia is a rare hernia in adults, so misdiagnosis is common. Inappropriate intervention, such as chest tube placement, can occur in the cases of misdiagnosis [18–21]. The delay in diagnosis may also result in strangulation and

TABLE 4: Treatment option and complications.

Treatment	
Laparoscopic	10
Open repair	1
Plication with mesh repair	10
Mesh repair	3
Postoperative complication	
Persistence of pain	3
Dyspepsia	4
Respiratory distress	2

death [22]. CT scan is the most accurate imaging modality for the diagnosis and evaluation of the contents of this hernia, especially when it is small [23, 24]. About 38% of these adults are misdiagnosed as pleural effusion, empyema, lung cyst, and pneumothorax when CT scan is not done [25]. One of our patients was also diagnosed as a case of pleural effusion before CT scan was done. The other advantage of the CT scan was here to detect the presence of spleen as one of the contents and helped in cautious handling of this friable organ to prevent the catastrophe [26]. MRI is an alternative diagnostic modality.

In the laparoscopic repair of Bochdalek hernia visualisation and working space is excellent (Table 4) [27]. One difficulty faced is that the contents tend to go back in the thorax because of the positive intra-abdominal pressure due to pneumoperitoneum and it is overcome by holding it back in the abdomen with a grasper. In incarcerated cases the part of diaphragm forming the neck of the hernia may need to be opened to reduce the contents. The hernial sac in Bochdalek hernia is present in only 10–15% of patients and it can be excised or left as such. The dissection of the sac may also lead to pleural injury [28]. A study was performed in which a CT scan was done on postoperative day 30 to see what happens to the left over hernial sac, and it was seen that the sac had disappeared [29].

The closure of the defect can be done by different methods. When the defect is small it can be simply sutured closed, but when it is large (>10 cm square) it will need a prosthetic reinforcement [9, 30]. Sufficient evidence favoring any particular type of mesh is lacking [31]. In our practice, we close the defect with horizontal mattress over the Teflon sheets with the nonabsorbable sutures. And then we put a large piece of composite mesh to cover the whole hemidiaphragm. The advantage of Teflon sheet is that it prevents the cutting of the diaphragmatic edges when the tension is high during approximation in large defects. Mesh repair was used to strengthen the weak diaphragm.

4. Conclusion

CDH in adults is an uncommon form of diaphragmatic hernia. The laparoscopic repair is a safe and effective modality of surgical treatment in experienced hands.

Competing Interests

The authors declare that they have no competing interests.

References

[1] V. A. Bochdalek, "Einige betrechtugen uber die entsehung des angerborenen zwerchfellbruches zur pathologischen anatomien des hernien," *Vrlijschr Prakti Heilk*, vol. 19, article 89, 1848.

[2] L. A. Christiansen, M. Blichert-Toft, and S. Bertelsen, "Strangulated diaphragmatic hernia. A clinical study," *The American Journal of Surgery*, vol. 129, no. 5, pp. 574–578, 1975.

[3] R. Prasad, J. Nath, and P. K. Mukerji, "Eventration of diaphragm," *Journal of the Indian Medical Association*, vol. 84, no. 6, pp. 187–189, 1986.

[4] B. K. P. Goh, M. C. C. Teo, S.-P. Chng, and K.-C. Soo, "Right-sided Bochdalek's hernia in an adult," *American Journal of Surgery*, vol. 194, no. 3, pp. 390–391, 2007.

[5] T. V. Thomas, "Congenital eventration of the diaphragm," *The Annals of Thoracic Surgery*, vol. 10, no. 2, pp. 180–192, 1970.

[6] M. Al-Emadi, H. Ismail, M. A. Nada, and H. Al-Jaber, "Laparoscopic repair of bochdalek hernia in an adult," *Surgical Laparoscopy and Endoscopy*, vol. 9, no. 6, pp. 423–425, 1999.

[7] J. M. Swain, A. Klaus, S. R. Achem, and R. A. Hinder, "Congenital diaphragmatic hernia in adults," *Seminars in Laparoscopic Surgery*, vol. 8, no. 4, pp. 246–255, 2001.

[8] D. S. Thoman, T. Hui, and E. H. Phillips, "Laparoscopic diaphragmatic hernia repair," *Surgical Endoscopy and Other Interventional Techniques*, vol. 16, no. 9, pp. 1345–1349, 2002.

[9] G. D. Rice, C. J. O'Boyle, D. I. Watson, and P. G. Devitt, "Laparoscopic repair of Bochdalek hernia in an adult," *ANZ Journal of Surgery*, vol. 71, no. 7, pp. 443–445, 2001.

[10] D. Weissberg and Y. Refaely, "Symptomatic diaphragmatic hernia: surgical treatment," *Scandinavian Cardiovascular Journal*, vol. 29, no. 4, pp. 201–206, 1995.

[11] N. T. Liem and L. A. Dung, "Thoracoscopic repair for congenital diaphragmatic hernia: lessons from 45 cases," *Journal of Pediatric Surgery*, vol. 41, no. 10, pp. 1713–1715, 2006.

[12] L. I. Campos and E. K. Sipes, "Laparoscopic repair of diaphragmatic hernia," *Journal of Laparoendoscopic Surgery*, vol. 1, no. 6, pp. 369–373, 1991.

[13] G. G. R. Kuster, L. E. Kline, and G. Garzo, "Diaphragmatic hernia through the foramen of Morgagni: laparoscopic repair case report," *Journal of Laparoendoscopic Surgery*, vol. 2, no. 2, pp. 93–100, 1992.

[14] A. Alam and B. N. Chander, "Adult Bochdalek hernia," *Medical Journal Armed Forces India*, vol. 61, no. 3, pp. 284–286, 2005.

[15] S. Nitecki and J. A. Bar-Maor, "Late presentation of Bochdalek hernia: our experience and review of the literature," *Israel Journal of Medical Sciences*, vol. 28, no. 8-9, pp. 711–714, 1992.

[16] M. E. Mullins, J. Stein, S. S. Saini, and P. R. Mueller, "Prevalence of incidental Bochdalek's hernia in a large adult population," *American Journal of Roentgenology*, vol. 177, no. 2, pp. 363–366, 2001.

[17] R. Marleta, "Diaphragmatic anomalies," in *Swenson's Textbook of Paediatric Surgery*, J. G. Raffensperger, Ed., pp. 721–735, Appleton and Lange, New York, NY, USA, 5th edition, 1990.

[18] Y. Chai, G. Zhang, and G. Shen, "Adult Bochdalek hernia complicated with a perforated colon," *Journal of Thoracic and Cardiovascular Surgery*, vol. 130, no. 6, pp. 1729–1730, 2005.

[19] R. E. Berkowitz, "Foramen of Bochdalek hernia in an adult: case report," *Military Medicine*, vol. 146, no. 5, pp. 356–357, 1981.

[20] C. O. McDonnell, P. Naughton, A. Aziz, and T. N. Walsh, "Laparoscopic repair of a strangulated Bochdalek hernia," *Irish Journal of Medical Science*, vol. 172, no. 3, pp. 145–146, 2003.

[21] A. M. Dalton, R. S. Hodgson, and C. Crossley, "Bochdalek hernia masquerading as a tension pneumothorax," *Emergency Medicine Journal*, vol. 21, no. 3, pp. 393–394, 2004.

[22] E. S. Dhaka, M. I. Hasan, K. K. Mutatkar, and M. L. Sapra, "Strangulated diaphragmatic hernia simulating hydropneumothorax (case report)," *The Journal of the Association of Physicians of India*, vol. 27, no. 8, pp. 777–779, 1979.

[23] M. S. Shin, S. A. Mulligan, W. A. Baxley, and K.-J. Ho, "Bochdalek hernia of diaphragm in the adult: diagnosis by computed tomography," *Chest*, vol. 92, no. 6, pp. 1098–1101, 1987.

[24] A. C. Wilbur, A. Gorodetsky, and J. F. Hibbeln, "Imaging findings of adult bochdalek hernias," *Clinical Imaging*, vol. 18, no. 3, pp. 224–229, 1994.

[25] S. Thomas and B. Kapur, "Adult Bochdalek hernia—clinical features, management and results of treatment," *The Japanese Journal of Surgery*, vol. 21, no. 1, pp. 114–119, 1991.

[26] G. Harinath, P. S. Senapati, M. J. K. Pollitt, and B. J. Ammori, "Laparoscopic reduction of an acute gastric volvulus and repair of a hernia of Bochdalek," *Surgical Laparoscopy, Endoscopy and Percutaneous Techniques*, vol. 12, no. 3, pp. 180–183, 2002.

[27] M. Taskin, K. Zengin, E. Unal, D. Eren, and U. Korman, "Laparoscopic repair of congenital diaphragmatic hernias," *Surgical Endoscopy*, vol. 16, no. 5, p. 869, 2002.

[28] N. T. Liem, "Thoracoscopic surgery for congenital diaphragmatic hernia: a report of nine cases," *Asian Journal of Surgery*, vol. 26, no. 4, pp. 210–212, 2003.

[29] M. E. Mullins and S. Saini, "Imaging of incidental Bochdalek hernia," *Seminars in Ultrasound, CT and MRI*, vol. 26, no. 1, pp. 28–36, 2005.

[30] Y. Kitano, K. P. Lally, and P. A. Lally, "Congenital diaphragmatic hernia study group: late-presenting congenital diaphragmatic hernia," *Journal of Pediatric Surgery*, vol. 40, no. 12, pp. 1839–1843, 2005.

[31] C. Palanivelu, M. Rangarajan, S. Rajapandian, V. Amar, and R. Parthasarathi, "Laparoscopic repair of adult diaphragmatic hernias and eventration with primary sutured closure and prosthetic reinforcement: a retrospective study," *Surgical Endoscopy*, vol. 23, no. 5, pp. 978–985, 2009.

40

Laparoscopic Choledochotomy in a Solitary Common Duct Stone: A Prospective Study

K. B. Deo, S. Adhikary, S. Khaniya, V. C. Shakya, and C. S. Agrawal

Department of Surgery, B. P. Koirala Institute of Health Sciences, Dharan, Nepal

Correspondence should be addressed to K. B. Deo; kunalbikramdeo@gmail.com

Academic Editor: Diego Cuccurullo

Background. Laparoscopic common bile duct exploration has all the advantages of minimal access and is also the most cost effective compared to the other options. *Objective.* To study a profile on laparoscopic common bile duct exploration for a single common duct stone. *Methods.* A total of 30 consecutive patients with solitary common bile duct stone attending our hospital over a period of one year were enrolled in the study. Laparoscopic common bile duct exploration was done by transductal route in all the patients. *Results.* There were 18 females and 12 males with age ranging from 28 to 75 years. Jaundice was present in 12 (40%) patients. Twenty-four (80%) patients had raised alkaline phosphatase. The mean size of CBD on ultrasound was 11.55 mm. The mean size of calculus was 11.06 mm and was located in the distal CBD in 26 (86.7%) patients. The mean operative time was 158.4 ± 57.89 min. There were 8 (26.6%) conversions to open procedure. T-tube was used in 26 (86.7%) patients. The postoperative complications were hospital acquired chest infection in 3 (10%), surgical site infection in 3 (10%), acute coronary syndrome in one (3.3%), and bile leak after T-tube removal in one (3.3%) patient. *Conclusions.* Laparoscopic common bile duct exploration is an effective, safe management of common bile duct stone.

1. Introduction

Approximately 10% of patients who undergo laparoscopic cholecystectomy harbor common bile duct stones [1, 2]. With continual improvement in the technology and expertise in laparoscopic techniques, laparoscopic common bile duct exploration is becoming more popular and may be the next paradigm in the management of choledocholithiasis [3]. Clearance rates of more than 90% are accepted as the standard of care [4].

During the early days of laparoscopic cholecystectomy, the use of intraoperative laparoscopic common bile duct exploration (LCBDE) was limited. Surgeons relied on methods like ERCP ± sphincterotomy with morbidity (15%) and mortality (1%), which increased the hospital stay and cost with additional risk of acute pancreatitis [5]. This has led to resurgence of LCBDE in common duct stones [5]. We conducted this study to find out the safety of LCBDE in our patients.

2. Materials and Methods

It is a prospective study in patients with solitary duct stones with or without jaundice. Multiple duct stones, CBD diameter < 6 mm, cholangitis or pancreatitis, previous history of cholecystectomy, dense and ugly abdominal scars, and those unwilling to undergo surgery and unfit for surgery were excluded.

A good history and clinical examination followed by routine work-up and ultrasonography was done to see the gall stones, number, size, and location of common duct stones, and diameter of common duct. The diagnosis of single choledocholithiasis was made only after sonologist confirmed visualizing entire common duct in one or more than one setting.

Laparoscopic CBD exploration was done with 10 mm umbilical and epigastric ports followed by two small accessory subcostal ports. The first 5 mm trocar was placed along the right anterior axillary line and second 5 mm port at the right subcostal region. An additional right epigastric

5 mm port was useful for inserting a rigid ureteroscope. The choledochotomy was closed with 3-0 polyglactin acid over the T-tube. The T tubes were made up of polyvinyl chloride. A subhepatic closed suction drainage (14 F) was then inserted. Visual analogue scale scoring was done in the postoperative period for assessment of pain. T-tube cholangiogram was done on 10th day to look for any retained stones or abnormal findings. T-tube was removed only after confirmation of normal findings in cholangiogram. All the data were entered in Microsoft excel and converted to SPSS version 11.5.

3. Results

Thirty subjects of LCBDE included 14 (46.7%) cases in the age group between 40 and 60 years. The mean age was 49.2 ± 12.89 years with a male to female ratio of 1.5 : 1 (Table 1).

All cases had abdomen pain and duration varied from 15 days to 9 months with a mean of 94.7 days. Jaundice was seen in 12 (40%) patients with mean duration of 16.25 days. Eight patients had comorbid conditions, namely, hypertension (4), chronic obstructive pulmonary disease (2), and type II diabetes mellitus and hypertension (2), and two cases had abdominal hysterectomy in the past. On physical examination, icterus was present in 12 (40.0%) patients, pallor in two (6.6%) patients, and hepatomegaly in two (6.6%) patients. Twenty-four (80%) patients had deranged liver function test. Total bilirubin was raised in 12 (40.0%) and alkaline phosphatase was raised in 24 (80.0%) patients. The prothrombin time and international normalized ratio (INR) were raised in 11 (36.7%) patients.

Abdominal ultrasonography was the main tool for diagnosis as our institution does not have magnetic resonance cholangiography (MRC) facility. All had associated gallstones. The most common location of stone was at the distal common duct 26 (86.7%) and in four (6.6%) cases it was in the mid part of duct. The mean diameter was 11.55 ± 2.43 mm (range 8 to 17 mm); the mean size of the stone was 11.06 ± 4.42 mm (range 5.7 to 25.0 mm).

The mean operative time for laparoscopic surgery was 158.40 ± 57.89 minutes (range 75 to 360 mins) (Table 1). In those who had to be converted, one patient had a prolonged operative interval (360 mins) because we performed Roux en Y hepaticojejunostomy for choledochal cyst.

Laparoscopic exploration was done successfully (Figures 1 and 2) in 22 (73.3%) cases and 8 (26.6%) had to be converted (Table 1). The reasons for conversion were: multiple stones (1), impacted calculus in the distal end of duct which was difficult to extract (2), frozen anatomy of Calot's triangle (1), nonretrieval of a stone (1), and requirement of choledochoduodenostomy (2). One patient had to undergo a Roux en y hepaticojejunostomy after excision of choledochal cyst (accidental discovery, not picked up by imaging). There were no intraoperative complications except bleeding from one branch of common hepatic artery to CBD (around 50 ml) which was controlled by application of pressure followed by electrocoagulation.

The postoperative period was fairly stable. The mean duration of analgesics administered was 5.9 ± 1.51 days (range 4 to 11 days). The visual analogue scale was used to assess the pain on days 1 and 2. The mean VAS score on the first postoperative day was 6.6 ± 1 (range 5 to 8 days). Similarly, the mean VAS score on the second day was 3.33 ± 0.76 (range 2 to 5 days).

Table 1

Parameters	Numbers (n = 30)
Age group in years	
<40	9
40–60	14
≥60	7
Gender	
Male	12
Female	18
Symptoms	
Abdomen pain	30
Jaundice	12
Fever	5
Mean operative time	158.40 ± 57.89 (75–360) min
Total conversions	8 (26.7%)
Reasons for conversion	
Impaction	2
Frozen anatomy	1
Multiple stones	1
Nonretrieval of stone	1
Choledochoduodenostomy	2
Hepaticojejunostomy (choledochal cyst)	1
Complications	
Morbidity	7 (23.3%)
Chest infection	3
Surgical site infection	3
Acute coronary syndrome	1
Mortality	0

Majority, 26 (86.7%), of patients recovered from ileus on the first day. Feeding was started on the second day for 24 (80%) patients. The mean complete ambulation time was 4.33 ± 1.49 days (range 3 to 10 days). Two patients had delayed ambulation due to cardiac (1) and chest complications (1). The mean hospital stay was 6.76 ± 1.33 days (range 5 to 11 days).

T-tube was used in 26 (86.7%) patients. One patient underwent primary closure after choledochotomy and the remaining two underwent choledochoduodenostomy as CBD diameter was more than 15 mm. Remaining one had Roux en Y hepaticojejunostomy after excision of choledochal cyst. Twenty-four had normal findings with free flow of contrast to the duodenum. Two patients had filling defect which was seen in the common bile duct. The T-tube removal was done before 21 days in 19 patients but all after 15 days. T-tube was removed after 21 days in 7 patients.

Three (10%) patients had developed hospital acquired chest infection. Surgical site infection (SSI) was present in

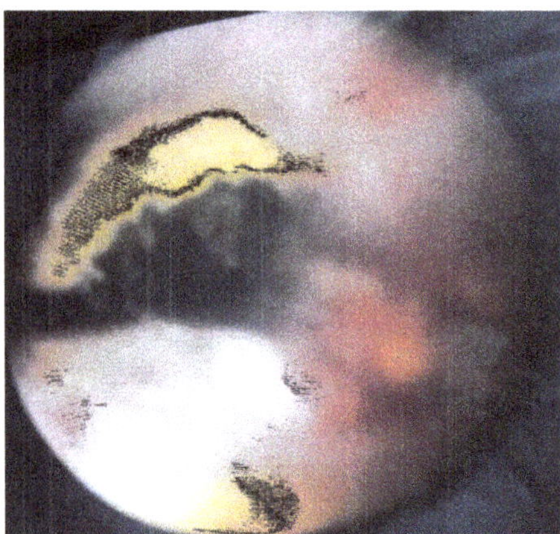

Figure 1

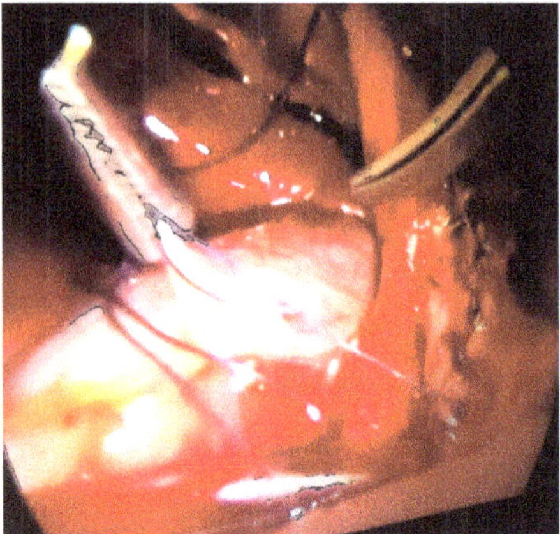

Figure 2

three (10%) patients (two in conversion and one had port site infection following laparoscopic drainage of pyoperitoneum following bile leak after T-tube removal). SSI were managed with dressings and antibiotics. One patient developed acute coronary syndrome on the first day and he recovered with no further complication and was successfully discharged. Two patients with filling defect underwent endoscopic retrograde cholangiography and stone extraction for residual stones. One case had bile leak followed by pyoperitoneum following T-tube removal (at the end of 3rd week) and was subsequently managed with laparoscopic peritoneal lavage and drainage after readmission. She recovered gradually and had an incisional hernia in the umbilical port following a port site infection. The hernia was later managed with overlay mesh.

4. Discussion

Common bile duct stones are commonly managed by ERCP ± sphincterotomy, followed by laparoscopic cholecystectomy. The risks associated with ERCP and the morbidity associated with open surgery have paved the way for considering Laparoscopic common bile duct exploration [5]. Recently a single stage Laparoscopic common bile duct exploration has been increasingly reported as a safe and effective treatment option [6].

It is a prospective study of 30 consecutive patients of solitary common bile duct stone showing a higher prevalence in females (60.0%) comparable to other studies [7–10], which could be due to female gender, hormones, and increased fat consumption with less physical work. The mean age was 49.2 ± 12.89 years with majority between 40 and 60 years of age similar to other studies [11–13]; their mean age varied from 42.25 to 47 years; but in some other studies [8, 9, 14] they had presented in older age (mean age 63 to 66.1 years). In our study the mean age of presentation was 56.0 years in males and 44.66 years in females. This shows that common bile duct stone occurs early in females. The importance of age, as it affects a postoperative outcome, was shown in the study by Noble et al. [15] where patients beyond 60 years were more likely to suffer from respiratory and urinary complications.

The pain was present in all patients and it varied from 15 days to 9 months. Jaundice was present in 12 (40.0%) patients with a mean of 16.25 days and fever in 5 (16.7%) patients. Riciardi et al. [7] and Shelat et al. [10] also showed that abdomen pain was the major complaint which was present in 93% and 80% of the total cases, respectively. The presence of jaundice was similar in a study by Shelat et al. [10] but less (27%) in study by Riciardi et al. [7] possibly due to increased concerns shown by patients once jaundice appeared and also a small sample size of our study, and so on. Similarly fever was present in 14.7% and 15% in the study done by Riciardi et al. [7] and Rogers et al. [12], respectively, which was similar to our study. The late presentation seen in our few patients was because of difficult access to hospital.

Alkaline phosphatase was raised in 24 (80.0%) patients with a median of 253 U/L, higher than that in the study by Ricardi et al. [7] where alkaline phosphatase was raised only in 56% of the patients with a mean value of 216 ± 10 U/L. Similar findings were noticed by Rogers et al. [12] and Wani et al. [13].

Ultrasonogram of the abdomen was the main tool to diagnose common bile duct stone as magnetic resonance cholangiopancreaticography (MRCP) was not available at our institute and many of our patients cannot afford the cost of MRCP outside. The decision to operate was made only after sonologist had confirmed having visualized entire common duct and single stone in one or more setting. The most common location of the stone was distal CBD with as many as 26 (86.7%) patients with a mean diameter of 11.5 ± 2.43 mm (range 8 to 17 mm) comparable to a study by Chander et al. [11] where the average diameter was 11.7 mm and majority (63%) of patients had the diameter between 8 mm and 15.4 mm and Topal et al. [9] where the average diameter was 11.5 mm. However, Wani et al. [13] and Khan et al. [16] studies showed the mean common bile duct of 15 mm diameter. We chose to have solitary calculus as inclusion criteria as we were in the beginning of learning curve.

We used rigid ureteroscope for the visualization of common bile duct stone. Khan et al. [16] had also reported a successful use of a rigid nephroscope for laparoscopic common bile duct explorations. LCBDE was successfully done in 22 (73.3%) patients. The conversion was needed in

8 (26.6%) patients for impacted stones, frozen anatomy due to dense adhesions, multiple stones and associated technical difficulties, and nonretrieval of a stone. The finding of multiple stones in one case was in intraoperative period which was missed in imaging. Conversion rate was high in our study than other studies [7–10, 17–21] where it varied between no conversions in Bandyopadhaya et al. [18] study to 4% in others [10, 20]. The reasons for conversion in their studies were learning curve, dense adhesions, bleeding, technical difficulties, impacted stones, and so on. These reasons were similar to our study. Similar to our study choledochal cyst was one of the causes for conversion in study by Petelin [17] and Paganini and Lezoche [19] where two cases had bile duct cyst. The high conversion in our study could be due to a steep learning curve, being in early part of the study (initial thirty cases), the operative findings, technical difficulties, and so on. Due to the initial part of our learning curve we chose to convert two cases requiring choledochoduodenostomy due to hugely dilated CBD of almost two centimeters (we usually perform choledochoduodenostomy in case of CBD dilatation > 1.5 cm). The decision to perform choledochotomy was purely due to preoperative and intraoperative findings as we do not have facilities like laparoscopic ultrasound or intraoperative cholangiogram. However none of the patients had negative choledochotomy.

In our study the mean operative time was 158.4 ± 57.89 minutes (range 75 to 360 minutes). Our operative time was comparable with some studies [7, 11, 19] where mean operative time varied from 126 minutes to 139 minutes. Shorter operative time was seen in other studies [16, 18, 21] (range 71 mins to 83 mins). Some studies [10, 22] had a longer operative time (185 to 191 mins).

We started feeding on 2nd day and ambulation on the third day. However in study by Bandyopadhyay et al. [18] patients were started orally on the day of surgery and were ambulatory next day. The mean hospital stay was 6.76 ± 1.33 days ranging from 5 to 11 days. The hospital stay in our study was longer than other studies [7, 10, 11, 16, 18, 21, 23] where mean hospital stay varied from 1.95 days to 4.6 days. The mean hospital stay was longer in study by Tang et al. [14] and Huang et al. [22] (range 9 and 10.4 days). Longer hospital stay in our study was because of complications like chest infections, surgical site infections, and acute coronary syndrome.

The choledochotomy was closed over T-tube in majority (86.7%) of our patients. The decision of primary closure in one case was as per decision of operating surgeon. T-tube was used in all laparoscopic common bile duct explorations by Huang et al. [22]. However in some studies [7, 8, 13, 14, 16, 18] T-tube had been used in limited number of patients. They did primary closure of choledochotomy or used antegrade biliary stents. Wani et al. [13] had shown successful use of endonasobiliary drainage. Shimizu et al. [24] have described the use of the C tube through the cystic duct with a better outcome in terms of technical feasibility, lesser complication, early removal, and decreased hospital stay as compared to the use of T-tube. In our study average removal time was 20.92 ± 8.0 days (range 15 to 42 days). This was quite long as compared to a study by Chander et al. [11] where the average removal time was 13.1 ± 5 days. The reason for variation in the removal of T-tube in our study was the removal on an outpatient basis as some patients presented late, as well as presence of filling defects in CBD in two (6.6%) patients where we had to continue with the tube till a definitive treatment was done. Similarly other studies also had retention of stones (2 to 8%) in their patients [7, 11, 14, 19, 22].

The postoperative complications were similar to other studies [7, 8, 11, 14, 16, 19, 21] which include bile leak, chest and port site infection, and myocardial infarction. Bile leak leading to pyoperitoneum was present in one of our patients following T-tube removal at the end of 3rd week. It was unusual compared to our past experience with PVC T-tube. Though formation of fibrous tract is slow as compared to latex tube, 3 weeks used to be a sufficient time. Though this study did not have mortality, it was present (1 to 3%) in other studies [14, 19, 21]. It could be due to selection bias, a small sample size, and less patients with comorbid condition. The technique has been reported to be associated with morbidity and mortality rates that range as high as 5% to 7% and 1% to 2%, respectively [25].

5. Limitations of Our Study

This is a prospective study with a small sample size. Moreover, it was our initial experience that there could have been a little selection bias. We look to conduct future studies with a much bigger sample size and conduct a prospective randomized controlled trial comparing it with other options available. We had to deviate from established methods of investigations like MRCP and few intraoperative steps (like choosing only transductal approach over transcystic approach, using intraoperative cholangiogram or laparoscopic ultrasound) due to unavailability and cost factor in our patients.

6. Conclusion

In the era of minimal access surgeries, laparoscopic common bile duct exploration is an effective, safe management of common bile duct stone. Besides advantages of laparoscopic surgery, it offers a single stage management of common bile duct stone reducing the hospital stay and financial load to the patients.

Consent

Patients and their relatives were informed in their native language regarding their disease, options, choice of procedure, advantages, and disadvantages of both open and laparoscopic common bile duct exploration. Informed consent was taken and signed.

References

[1] S. A. Ahewndt, "The biliary system," in *Sabistons Textbook of Surgery*, W. E. Saunders, Ed., pp. 1597–1639, Elseveir, Philadelphia, 17th edition, 2004.

[2] L. W. Way, W. H. Admirand, and J. E. Dunphy, "Management of choledocholithiasis.," *Annals of Surgery*, vol. 176, no. 3, pp. 347–359, 1972.

[3] G. Berci and L. Morgenstern, "Laparoscopic management of common bile duct stones. A multi-institutional SAGES study. Society of American Gastrointestinal Endoscopic Surgeons," *Surgical Endoscopy*, vol. 8, no. 10, pp. 1168–1174, 1994.

[4] J. Escat, G. Fourtanier, C. Maigne, C. Vaislic, D. Fournier, and F. Prevost, "Choledochoscopy in common bile duct surgery for choledocholithiasis: A must. Eight years experience in 441 consecutive patients," *The American Surgeon*, vol. 51, no. 3, pp. 166-167, 1985.

[5] A. S. Fink, "To ERCP or not to ERCP? That is the question," *Surgical Endoscopy*, vol. 7, no. 5, pp. 375-376, 1993.

[6] K. K. Tan and K. H. Liau, "Laparoscopic Common Bile Duct Exploration: Our First 50 Cases," *Ann Acad Med Singapore*, vol. 39, pp. 136–142, 2010.

[7] R. Riciardi, S. Islam, J. J. Canete, P. L. Arcand, and M. E. Stoker, "Effectiveness and long-term results of laparoscopic common bile duct exploration," *Surgical Endoscopy*, vol. 17, no. 1, pp. 19–22, 2003.

[8] C. J. Taylor, J. Kong, M. Ghusn, S. White, N. Crampton, and L. Layani, "Laparoscopic bile duct exploration: Results of 160 consecutive cases with 2-year follow up," *ANZ Journal of Surgery*, vol. 77, no. 6, pp. 440–445, 2007.

[9] B. Topal, R. Aerts, and F. Penninckx, "Laparoscopic common bile duct stone clearance with flexible choledochoscopy," *Surgical Endoscopy*, vol. 21, no. 12, pp. 2317–2321, 2007.

[10] V. G. Shelat, C. Y. Chan, K. H. Liau, and C. K. Ho, "Laparoscopic exploration can salvage failed endoscopic bile duct stone extraction," *Singapore Medical Journal*, vol. 53, no. 5, pp. 313–317, 2012.

[11] J. Chander, A. Vindal, P. Lal, N. Gupta, and V. K. Ramteke, "Laparoscopic management of CBD stones: An Indian experience," *Surgical Endoscopy*, vol. 25, no. 1, pp. 172–181, 2011.

[12] S. J. Rogers, J. P. Cello, J. K. Horn et al., "Prospective randomized trial of LC+LCBDE vs ERCP/S+LC for common bile duct stone disease," *JAMA Surgery*, vol. 145, no. 1, pp. 28–33, 2010.

[13] M. A. Wani, N. A. Chowdri, S. H. Naqash, F. Q. Parray, R. A. Wani, and N. A. Wani, "Closure of the Common Duct - Endonasobiliary Drainage Tubes vs. T Tube: A Comparative Study," *Indian Journal of Surgery*, vol. 72, no. 5, pp. 367–372, 2010.

[14] C. N. Tang, K. K. Tsui, J. P. Ha, W. T. Siu, and M. K. Li, "Laparoscopic exploration of the common bile duct: 10-year experience of 174 patients from a single centre," *Hong Kong Med J*, vol. 12, no. 3, pp. 191–196, 2006.

[15] H. Noble, E. Whitley, S. Norton, and M. Thompson, "A study of preoperative factors associated with a poor outcome following laparoscopic bile duct exploration," *Surgical Endoscopy*, vol. 25, no. 1, pp. 130–139, 2011.

[16] M. Khan, S. J. F. Qadri, and S. S. Nazir, "Use of rigid nephroscope for laparoscopic common bile duct exploration - A Single-center experience," *World Journal of Surgery*, vol. 34, no. 4, pp. 784–790, 2010.

[17] J. B. Petelin, "Laparoscopic common bile duct exploration," *Surgical Endoscopy*, vol. 17, no. 11, pp. 1705–1715, 2003.

[18] S. K. Bandyopadhyay, S. Khanna, B. Sen, and O. Tantia, "Antegrade common bile duct (CBD) stenting after laparoscopic CBD exploration," *Journal of Minimal Access Surgery*, vol. 3, no. 1, pp. 19–25, 2007.

[19] A. M. Paganini and E. Lezoche, "Follow-up of 161 unselected consecutive patients treated laparoscopically for common bile duct stones," *Surgical Endoscopy*, vol. 12, no. 1, pp. 23–29, 1998.

[20] H. Tokumura, A. Umezawa, H. Cao et al., "Laparoscopic management of common bile duct stones: Transcystic approach and choledochotomy," *Journal of Hepato-Biliary-Pancreatic Sciences*, vol. 9, no. 2, pp. 206–212, 2002.

[21] R. Tinoco, A. Tinoco, L. El-Kadre, L. Peres, and D. Sueth, "Laparoscopic common bile duct exploration," *Annals of Surgery*, vol. 247, no. 4, pp. 674–679, 2008.

[22] S.-M. Huang, C.-W. Wu, G.-Y. Chau, S.-C. Jwo, W.-Y. Lui, and F.-K. P'eng, "An alternative approach of choledocholithotomy via laparoscopic choledochotomy," *JAMA Surgery*, vol. 131, no. 4, pp. 407–411, 1996.

[23] C. M. Ferguson, "Laparoscopic common bile duct exploration: Practical application," *JAMA Surgery*, vol. 133, no. 4, pp. 448–451, 1998.

[24] S. Shimizu, K. Yokohata, K. Mizumoto, K. Yamaguchi, K. Chijiiwa, and M. Tanaka, "Laparoscopic choledochotomy for bile duct stones," *Journal of Hepato-Biliary-Pancreatic Sciences*, vol. 9, no. 2, pp. 201–205, 2002.

[25] M. E. Franklin, "Laparoscopic choledochotomy," in *Operative Strategies in Laparoscopic Surgery*, E. H. Phillips and R. J. Rosenthal, Eds., p. 59, Springer-Verlag, New York, NY, USA, 1995.

Permissions

All chapters in this book were first published in MIS, by Hindawi Publishing Corporation; hereby published with permission under the Creative Commons Attribution License or equivalent. Every chapter published in this book has been scrutinized by our experts. Their significance has been extensively debated. The topics covered herein carry significant findings which will fuel the growth of the discipline. They may even be implemented as practical applications or may be referred to as a beginning point for another development.

The contributors of this book come from diverse backgrounds, making this book a truly international effort. This book will bring forth new frontiers with its revolutionizing research information and detailed analysis of the nascent developments around the world.

We would like to thank all the contributing authors for lending their expertise to make the book truly unique. They have played a crucial role in the development of this book. Without their invaluable contributions this book wouldn't have been possible. They have made vital efforts to compile up to date information on the varied aspects of this subject to make this book a valuable addition to the collection of many professionals and students.

This book was conceptualized with the vision of imparting up-to-date information and advanced data in this field. To ensure the same, a matchless editorial board was set up. Every individual on the board went through rigorous rounds of assessment to prove their worth. After which they invested a large part of their time researching and compiling the most relevant data for our readers.

The editorial board has been involved in producing this book since its inception. They have spent rigorous hours researching and exploring the diverse topics which have resulted in the successful publishing of this book. They have passed on their knowledge of decades through this book. To expedite this challenging task, the publisher supported the team at every step. A small team of assistant editors was also appointed to further simplify the editing procedure and attain best results for the readers.

Apart from the editorial board, the designing team has also invested a significant amount of their time in understanding the subject and creating the most relevant covers. They scrutinized every image to scout for the most suitable representation of the subject and create an appropriate cover for the book.

The publishing team has been an ardent support to the editorial, designing and production team. Their endless efforts to recruit the best for this project, has resulted in the accomplishment of this book. They are a veteran in the field of academics and their pool of knowledge is as vast as their experience in printing. Their expertise and guidance has proved useful at every step. Their uncompromising quality standards have made this book an exceptional effort. Their encouragement from time to time has been an inspiration for everyone.

The publisher and the editorial board hope that this book will prove to be a valuable piece of knowledge for researchers, students, practitioners and scholars across the globe.

List of Contributors

Arjan J. F. P. Verhaegh, Ryan E. Accord, Leen van Garsse and Jos G. Maessen
Department of Cardiothoracic Surgery, Maastricht University Medical Center, P. Debyelaan 25, 6202 AZ Maastricht, The Netherlands

Sarah E. Franjoine and James H. Liu
Division of Reproductive Endocrinology and Infertility, Department of Obstetrics and Gynecology, University Hospitals Case Medical Center, MacDonaldWomen's Hospital, Cleveland, OH 44106, USA

Mohamed A. Bedaiwy
Division of Reproductive Endocrinology and Infertility, Department of Obstetrics and Gynecology, University Hospitals Case Medical Center, MacDonaldWomen's Hospital, Cleveland, OH 44106, USA
Division of Reproductive Endocrinology and Infertility, Department of Obstetrics and Gynaecology, The University of British Columbia, D415A, 4500 Oak Street, Vancouver, BC, Canada V6H 3N1
Women's Health University Center, Department of Obstetrics and Gynecology, Faculty of Medicine, Assiut University, Assiut 71515, Egypt

Faten F. Abdel Hafez
Women's Health University Center, Department of Obstetrics and Gynecology, Faculty of Medicine, Assiut University, Assiut 71515, Egypt

Cuiyu Geng
Department of Biostatistics and Epidemiology, CaseWestern Reserve University School of Medicine, Cleveland, OH 44106, USA

Chee Wei Tay, Shridhar Ganpathi Iyer, Krishnakumar Madhavan and Stephen Kin Yong Chang
Department of Surgery, Division of Hepatobiliary and Pancreatic Surgery, National University Health System, Singapore 119228

Mikael Hartman
Department of Surgery, Division of Hepatobiliary and Pancreatic Surgery, National University Health System, Singapore 119228
Department of Medical Epidemiology and Biostatistics, Karolinska Institute, 17177 Stockholm, Sweden
Saw Swee Hock School of Public Health, NationalUniversity of Singapore, Singapore

Liang Shen
Division of Biostatistics, Yong Loo Lin School of Medicine, National University of Singapore, Singapore 119228

Melissa A. Christino
Division of Sports Medicine, Boston Children's Hospital, Boston, MA 02215, USA

Bryan G. Vopat
Department ofOrthopaedic Surgery, Massachusetts General Hospital, Boston, MA 02114, USA

Alexander Mayer and Robert M. Shalvoy
Department of Orthopaedic Surgery, Rhode Island Hospital, Brown University, Providence, RI 02903, USA

Andrew P. Matson
Department of Orthopaedic Surgery, Duke University Medical Center, Durham, NC 27710, USA

Steven E. Reinert
Department of Information Services, Rhode Island Hospital, Lifespan, Providence, RI 02903, USA

Sakol Manusook and Charintip Somprasit
Department of Obstetrics and Gynaecology, Faculty of Medicine, Thammasat University, Pathum Thani 12120, Thailand

Chamnan Tanprasertkul
Department of Obstetrics and Gynaecology, Faculty of Medicine, Thammasat University, Pathum Thani 12120, Thailand
Center of Excellence in Applied Epidemiology, Thammasat University, PathumThani 12120, Thailand

Sophapun Ekarattanawong
Division of Physiology, Department of Preclinical Science, Faculty ofMedicine, Thammasat University, PathumThani 12120, Thailand

Opas Sreshthaputra and Teraporn Vutyavanich
Department of Obstetrics and Gynecology, Faculty of Medicine, Chiang Mai University, Chiang Mai 50000, Thailand

D. Ryan Ormond and Costas G. Hadjipanayis
Department of Neurosurgery, Emory University School of Medicine, Atlanta, GA 30322, USA

Guy David
Associate Professor of Health Care Management, The Wharton School, University of Pennsylvania, 202 Colonial Penn Center, 3641 Locust Walk, Philadelphia, PA 19104, USA

Candace L. Gunnarsson
S2 Statistical Solutions, Inc., 11176 Main Street, Cincinnati, OH 45241, USA

Matt Moore
Healthcare Policy and Economics, Ethicon Endo-Surgery, 4545 Creek Road, Cincinnati, OH 45252, USA

John Howington
Division of Thoracic Surgery and Surgical Quality, NorthShore UniversityHealth System, 2650 Ridge Avenue, 3507Walgreen Buliding, Evanston, IL 60201, USA

Daniel L. Miller
Division of Thoracic Surgery, Emory University Healthcare, 1365 Clifton Rd NE, Atlanta, GA 30322, USA

Michael A. Maddaus
Division of Thoracic Surgery, University of Minnesota, 420 Delaware Street SE, Mayo Mail Code 195, Minneapolis, MN 55455, USA

Robert Joseph McKenna Jr.
Division of Thoracic Surgery, Cedars Sinai Medical Center, 8635 West Third, Suite 675, Los Angeles, CA 90048, USA

Bryan F. Meyers
Division of Cardiothoracic Surgery, Barnes-Jewish Hospital Plaza, Washington University in St. Louis, Queeny Tower, Suite 3108, St. Louis, MO 63110-1013, USA

Scott J. Swanson
Division of Minimally Invasive Thoracic Surgey, Brigham and Women's Hospital, Dana-Farber Cancer Institute, Harvard Medical School, 75 Francis Street, Boston, MA 02115, USA

Nirali Shah and Sandhya Iyer
Department of General Surgery, Lokmanya TilakMunicpalMedical College and GeneralHospital, Sion, Mumbai 400022, India

Medhat M. Ibrahim
Pediatric Surgery Unit, Faculty of Medicine, Al-Azhar University, Nasr City, Cairo 11884, Egypt

Mustafa Hasbahceci
Department of General Surgery, Faculty of Medicine, Bezmialem Vakif University, Vatan Street, Fatih, 34093 Istanbul, Turkey

Fatih Basak
Department of General Surgery, Umraniye Education and Research Hospital, Umraniye, 34766 Istanbul, Turkey

Aylin Acar
Department of General Surgery, Lutfi Kirdar Kartal Education and Research Hospital, Kartal, 34890 Istanbul, Turkey

Orhan Alimoglu
Department of General Surgery, Faculty of Medicine, Istanbul Medeniyet University, Kadikoy, 34722 Istanbul, Turkey

Sergio B. Sesia and Frank-Martin Haecker
Department of Pediatric Surgery, University Children's Hospital Basel, Spitalstrasse 33, 4056 Basel, Switzerland

Eric M. Haas, Rodrigo Pedraza, Madhu Ragupathi, Ali Mahmood and T. Bartley Pickron
Division of Minimally Invasive Colon and Rectal Surgery, Department of Surgery, e University of Texas Medical School at Houston, Houston, TX 77030, USA
Colorectal Surgical Associates, LLP, Ltd., Houston, TX, USA

Abdulkadir Bedirli, Bulent Salman and Osman Yuksel
Department of General Surgery, Gazi University Medical Faculty, Besevler, 06510 Ankara, Turkey

Sedat Dalbayrak, Kadir Öztürk, Mesut YJlmaz, Mahmut GökdaL and Murat Ayten
Neurospinal Academy, Neurosurgery, 34940 Istanbul, Turkey

Onur Yaman
Tepecik Education and Training Hospital, Clinic of Neurosurgery, 35120 Izmir, Turkey

Siripong Sirikurnpiboon and Paiboon Jivapaisarnpong
Colorectal Division, General Surgery Department, Rajavithi Hospital, Rangsit University, Bangkok 10400, Thailand

Apollon Zygomalas
Life Science Informatics-Medical Informatics, Department of Surgery, University of Patras, Rio, 26500 Patras, Greece

Konstantinos Giokas and Dimitrios Koutsouris
Biomedical Engineering Laboratory, School of Electrical and Computer Engineering, National Technical University of Athens, 15780 Zografou, Athens, Greece

Polat Dursun, Hulusi B. Zeyneloglu, Irem Alyazıcı, Ali Haberal and Ali Ayhan
Department of Obstetrics and Gynecology, Baskent University, School of Medicine, Ankara, Turkey

Tugan Tezcaner
Department of Surgery, Baskent University, School of Medicine, Ankara, Turkey

Megan R. Hsu
Department of Orthopedic Surgery, Beaumont Hospital Research Institute, 3811West 13 Mile Road, Suite #404, Royal Oak, MI 48073, USA

Meraaj S. Haleem and Wellington Hsu
Department of Orthopedic Surgery, Northwestern University Feinberg School of Medicine, 676 Saint Clair St. Suite #1350, Chicago, IL 60611, USA

Dariusz Dziedzic and Tadeusz Orlowski
Department ofThoracic Surgery, National Research Institute of Chest Diseases, Warsaw, Poland

Gopala Krishna Alaparthi
Department of Physiotherapy, Kasturba Medical College, Manipal University, Bejai, Mangalore 575004, India

Alfred Joseph Augustine
Department of Surgery, Kasturba Medical College, Manipal University, Mangalore 575004, India

R. Anand
Department of Pulmonary Medicine, Kasturba Medical College, Manipal University, Mangalore 575004, India

Ajith Mahale
Department of Radiodiagnosis, Kasturba Medical College, Manipal University, Mangalore 575004, India

Michael B. Cloney, Angela M. Bohnen, Zachary A. Smith, Tyler Koski and Nader Dahdaleh
Department of Neurological Surgery, Feinberg School of Medicine, Chicago, IL, USA

Jack A. Goergen
Feinberg School of Medicine, Chicago, IL, USA

AliM. El Saman, Faten F. AbdelHafez, KamalM. Zahran, Hazem Saad, Mohamed Khalaf and Mostafa Hussein
Women's Health Center, Department of Obstetrics and Gynecology, Faculty of Medicine, Assiut University, Assiut, Egypt

Ibrahim M. A. Hassanin
Department of Obstetrics and Gynecology, Faculty of Medicine, Sohag University, Sohag, Egypt

Saba M. Shugaa Al Deen
Department of Obstetrics and Gynecology, University Hospital of Sana'a, Yemen

Entidhar Al Sawah, Anthony N. Imudia and Emad Mikhail
Department of Obstetrics and Gynecology, University of South Florida Morsani College of Medicine, Tampa, FL, USA

Jason L. Salemi
Department of Family and Community Medicine, Baylor College of Medicine, Houston, TX, USA

Mitchel Hoffman
Division of Gynecologic Oncology, Moffitt Cancer Center, University of South Florida, Tampa, FL, USA

Manuneethimaran Thiyagarajan and Chandru Ravindrakumar
General Surgery Department, Sri Ramachandra MedicalUniversity, Chennai, India

Stephan Klessinger
Department of Neurosurgery, Nova Clinic Biberach, Eichendorffweg 5, 88400 Biberach, Germany
Department of Neurosurgery, University of Ulm, Albert-Einstein-Allee 23, 89081 Ulm, Germany

Roop Singh, Paritosh Gogna and Parmod Kumar Karwasra
Department of Orthopaedic Surgery, Paraplegia and Rehabilitation, Pt. B.D. Sharma PGIMS, 52 / 9-J, Medical Enclave, Rohtak, Haryana 124001, India

Sanjeev Parshad and Rajender Kumar Karwasra
Department of Surgery, Pt. B.D. Sharma PGIMS, Rohtak, Haryana 124001, India

Kiranpreet Kaur
Department of Anaesthesia and Critical Care, Pt. B.D. Sharma PGIMS, Rohtak, Haryana 124001, India

David Breuskin, Jana DiVincenzo, Steffi Urbschat and Joachim Oertel
Department of Neurosurgery, Saarland University, 66421 Homburg, Germany

Yoo-Jin Kim
Department of Pathology, Saarland University, 66421 Homburg, Germany

Natalie De Cure
Centenary Hospital for Women and Children, Woden, ACT 2606, Australia

Stephen J. Robson
Department of Obstetrics and Gynaecology, Australian National University Medical School, Garran, ACT 2605, Australia

Nikolaos A. Chatzizacharias, Khaled Dajani and Asif Jah
Department of HPB and Transplant Surgery, Addenbrooke's Hospital, Cambridge University Hospitals NHS Foundation Trust, Cambridge, UK

Jun Kit Koong
Department of HPB and Transplant Surgery, Addenbrooke's Hospital, Cambridge University Hospitals NHS Foundation Trust, Cambridge, UK
Department of Surgery, Faculty of Medicine, University of Malaya, Kuala Lumpur, Malaysia

Sean M. Barber, Leonardo Rangel-Castilla and David Baskin
Houston Methodist Neurological Institute, Department of Neurological Surgery, Suite 944, 6560 Fannin Street, Houston, TX 77030, USA

David L. Warner and Kent C. Sasse
University of Nevada, Reno School of Medicine, 75 PringleWay, Suite 804, Reno, NV 89502, USA

Priyadarshan Anand Jategaonkar
Department of General and Laparoscopic Surgery, Mahatma Gandhi Institute of Medical Sciences, Sevagram, Wardha, Maharashtra 442102, India

Sudeep Pradeep Yadav
Department of General and Laparoscopic Surgery, JagjivanramWestern Railway Hospital, Mumbai Central, Mumbai, Maharashtra 400008, India

Yasser Debakey
Assistant Teacher of Surgical Oncology, National Cancer Institute, Cairo University, Egypt

Ashraf Zaghloul
Head of Robotic Surgery Unit, National Cancer Institute, Cairo University, Egypt

Ahmed Farag
Head of Colorectal Surgery Unit, Faculty of Medicine, Cairo University, Egypt

Ahmed Mahmoud
Associated Professor of Surgical Oncology, National Cancer Institute, Cairo University, Egypt

Inas Elattar
Professor of Biostatistics and Cancer Epidemiology, National Cancer Institute, Cairo University, Egypt

Stelios Detorakis, Dimitrios Vlachos, Stavros Athanasiou, Themistoklis Grigoriadis, Aikaterini Domali, Ioannis Chatzipapas, Emmanuel Stamatakis, AthanasiosMousiolis, Apostolos Patrikios, Aris Antsaklis, Dimitrios Loutradis, and Athanasios Protopapas
1st Department of Obstetrics and Gynecology of the University of Athens, Alexandra Hospital, 80 Queen Sophie Avenue and Lourou Street, 11528 Athens, Greece

A. Solodkyy, M. Feretis, A. Fedotovs, F. Di Franco, S. Gergely and A.M. Harris
Department of Upper Gastrointestinal Surgery, Hinchingbrooke Hospital, Hinchingbrooke Park, Huntingdon, Cambridgeshire PE29 6NT, UK

Sue J. Fu, Jennifer Ginsberg, Yaron Perry, Philip A. Linden and Christopher W. Towe
Division ofThoracic and Esophageal Surgery, University Hospitals Cleveland Medical Center and CaseWestern Reserve School of Medicine, Cleveland, OH, USA

Vanessa P. Ho
Department of Surgery, University Hospitals Cleveland Medical Center and CaseWestern Reserve School of Medicine, Cleveland, OH, USA

Conor P. Delaney
Digestive Disease Institute, The Cleveland Clinic and Cleveland Clinic Lerner School of Medicine, Cleveland, OH, USA

Lea C. George, Rebecca O'Neill and Aziz M. Merchant
Department of Surgery, Rutgers New Jersey Medical School, Newark, NJ 07103, USA

Hans C. Rolff, Rikard B. Ambrus, Mohammed Belmouhand, Michael P. Achiam, Marianne Wegmann, Mette Siemsen, Steen C. Kofoed and Lars B. Svendsen
Department of Surgical Gastroenterology, Rigshospitalet, University of Copenhagen, Blegdamsvej 9, 2100 Copenhagen, Denmark

Sanjay Kumar Saroj
Minimal Access Surgery, Institute of Medical Sciences, BHU, Varanasi, India

Satendra Kumar
General Surgery, Institute of Medical Sciences, BHU, Varanasi, India

Yusuf Afaque
AIIMS, New Delhi, India

Abhishek Kumar Bhartia and Vishnu Kumar Bhartia
CMRI, Kolkata, India

K. B. Deo, S. Adhikary, S. Khaniya, V. C. Shakya and C. S. Agrawal
Department of Surgery, B. P. Koirala Institute of Health Sciences, Dharan, Nepal

Index

www.ingramcontent.com/pod-product-compliance
Lightning Source LLC
Chambersburg PA
CBHW061329190326
41458CB00011B/3947
9781632428097